# CONTEMPORARY ISSUES IN HEALTH SERVICES

Health Services Administration Series
by Delmar Publishers, Inc.

# CONTEMPORARY ISSUES IN HEALTH SERVICES

*Edited by:*

**Stephen J. Williams, Sc.D.**

Professor of Public Health and
Head, Division of Health Services Administration
Graduate School of Public Health
San Diego State University

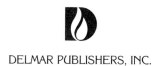

DELMAR PUBLISHERS, INC.

# NOTICE TO THE READER

Delmar staff:
Senior Administrative Editor: Bill Burgower
Associate Editor: Elisabeth F. Williams
Editorial Assistant: Debra Flis
Project Editor: Mary Beth Ray
Senior Production Supervisor: Larry Main
Art/Design Manager: Russell Schneck
Electronic Publishing Supervisor: Lisa Santy

For information, address Delmar Publishers Inc.
3 Columbia Circle, Box 15–015,
Albany, NY 12212–5015

Printed in the United States of America
Published simultaneously in Canada
by Nelson Canada,
a divison of The Thomson Corporation

1 2 3 4 5 6 7 8 9 10 XXX 99 98 97 96 95 94 93

Library of Congress Cataloging-in-Publication Data

Contemporary issues in health services/edited by Stephen J. Williams.
    p. cm. — (Delmar series in health services administration)
    Consists of articles reprinted from various sources.
    Includes bibliographical references.
    ISBN 0-8273-5575-0 (textbook)
    1. Medical care—United States.  2. Medical policy—United States.
3. Medical economics—United States.  I. Williams, Stephen J.
Stephen Joseph, 1948–    .  II. Series.
    [DNLM: 1. Health Services—United States—collected works.  W 84
AA1 C741]
RA395.A3C73 1992
362.1'0973—dc20
DNLM/DLC
for Library of Congress                           92–49604
                                                     CIP

# Introduction to the Series

This Series in Health Services is now in its second decade of providing top quality teaching materials to the health administration/public health field. Each year has witnessed further strengthening of the market position of each of the principal books in the Series, also reflecting the continued excellence of the products. Each author, book editor, and contributor to the Series has helped build what is widely recognized as the top textbook and issues collection of books available in this field today.

But we have achieved only a beginning. Everyone involved in the Series is committed to further expansion of the scope, technical excellence, and usability of the Series. Our goal is to do more for you, the reader. We will add new books in important areas, seek out more excellent authors, and increase the physical attributes of the book to make them easier for you to use.

We thank everyone, the authors and users in particular, who have made this Series so successful and so widely used. And we promise that this second decade will be dedicated to further expansion of the Series, and to enhancement of the books it contains to provide still greater value to you, our constituency.

*Stephen J. Williams*
*Series Editor*

# Delmar Series in Health Services Administration
Stephen J. Williams, Sc.D., Series Editor

*Introduction to Health Services,* fourth edition
   Stephen J. Williams and Paul R. Torrens, Editors

*Health Care Economics,* fourth edition
   Paul J. Feldstein

*Health Care Management: A Text in Organization Theory and Behavior,* second edition
   Stephen M. Shortell and Arnold D. Kaluzny, Editors

*Ambulatory Care, Management,* second edition
   Austin Ross, Stephen J. Williams, and Eldon L. Schafer, Editors

*Health Politics and Policy,* second edition
   Theodor J. Litman and Leonard S. Robins, Editors

*Strategic Management of Human Resources in Health Services Organizations*
   Myron D. Fottler, S. Robert Hernandez, and Charles L. Joiner, Editors

SUPPLEMENTAL READER:
*Contemporary Issues in Health Services*
   Stephen J. Williams

# Including Contributions By

Geoffrey M. Anderson, M.D., Ph.D.
University of British Columbia,
Vancouver, British Columbia, Canada

DeWitt C. Baldwin, Jr., M.D.
American Medical Association
Chicago, IL

Morris L. Barer, M.B.A, Ph.D.
University of British Columbia,
Vancouver, British Columbia, Canada

Edmund R. Becker, Ph.D.
Harvard University
Boston, MA

Thomas E. Bittker, M.D.
CIGNA Healthplan of Arizona
Glendale, AZ

Peter Braun, M.D.
Harvard University
Boston, MA

Robert H. Brook, M.D., Sc.D.
The Rand Corporation
Santa Monica, CA

Mark B. Chassin, M.D., M.P.P
The Rand Corporation
Santa Monica, CA

Cathy A. Cowan
Office of National Health Statistics
Baltimore, MD

Karen Davis, Ph.D.
Johns Hopkins University
Baltimore, MD

Steven DiCarlo
Health Insurance Association of America
Washington, DC

Avedis Donabedian, M.D., M.P.H
University of Michigan
Ann Arbor, MI

Robert A. Dorwart, M.D., M.P.H
Harvard University
Cambridge, MA

Alain C. Enthoven, Ph.D.
Stanford University
Stanford, CA

Arnold M. Epstein, M.D., M.A.
Harvard School of Public Health
Boston, MA

Robert G. Evans, Ph.D.
University of British Columbia
Vancouver, British Columbia, Canada

David Feeny, Ph.D.
McMaster University
Hamilton, Ontario, Canada

Arlene Fink, Ph.D.
The Rand Corporation
Santa Monica, CA

Catherine Fooks, M.A.
McMaster University
Hamilton, Ontario, Canada

Jon Gabel
Health Insurance Association of America
Washington, DC

Amiram Gafni, Ph.D.
McMaster University
Hamilton, Ontario, Canada

Howard H. Goldman, M.D., Ph.D.
University of Maryland School of Medicine
Baltimore, MD

Gerald W. Grumet, M.D.
Rochester General Hospital
Rochester, NY

David C. Hadorn, M.D., M.A.
The Rand Corporation
Santa Monica, CA

David U. Himmelstein, M.D.
Cambridge Hospital and Harvard Medical School
Cambridge, MA

William C. Hsiao, Ph.D.
Harvard University
Boston, MA

Katherine Kahn, M.D.
The Rand Corporation
Santa Monica, CA

Arnold D. Kaluzny, Ph.D.
University of North Carolina
Chapel Hill, NC

Joan Keesey
The Rand Corporation
Santa Monica, CA

Peter Kemper, Ph.D.
Center for Intramural Research
Agency for Health Care Policy Research
Rockville, MD

Phillip R. Kletke, Ph.D.
American Medical Association Center for Health
   Policy Research
Chicago, IL

Jacqueline Kosecoff, Ph.D.
The Rand Corporation
Santa Monica, CA

Chris Koyanagi
National Mental Health Association
Alexandria, VA

Richard Kronick, Ph.D.
University of California
San Diego, CA

Roberta J. Labelle, M.A.
McMaster University
Hamilton, Ontario, Canada

H. Richard Lamb, M.D.
University of Southern California School of Medicine
Los Angeles, CA

Helen C. Lazenby
Office of National Health Statistics,
Baltimore, MD

Jeffrey A. Lemieux
United States Department of Health and Human Services
Baltimore, MD

Suzanne W. Letsch
Office of National Health Statistics
Baltimore, MD

Katharine R. Levit
Office of National Health Statistics,
Baltimore, MD

Jonathan Lomas, M.A.
McMaster University
Hamilton, Ontario, Canada

Neil Love, M.D.
University of Miami
Miami, FL

Carrie Lynn Manning, B.A.
Rutgers University
New Brunswick, NJ

William D. Marder, A.M.
Abt Associates, Inc.
Cambridge, MA

Mary B. McGuire, M.P.H.
American Medical Association
Chicago, IL

David R. McKusick
United States Department of Health and Human Services
Baltimore, MD

Curtis P. McLaughlin, D.B.A.
University of North Carolina
Chapel Hill, NC

Daniel N. Mendelson, M.P.P.
Tufts University School of Medicine
Boston, MA

Nancy Merrick, M.D.
The Rand Corporation
Santa Monica, CA

Charlotte Muller, Ph.D.
City University of New York
New York, NY

Christopher M. Murtaugh, Ph.D.
Center for Intramural Research
Agency for Health Care Policy Research
Rockville, MD

R.E. Park, Ph.D.
The Rand Corporation
Santa Monica, CA

Uwe E. Reinhardt, Ph.D.
Princeton University
Princeton, NJ

Peter Ries
National Center for Health Statistics
Hyattsville, MD

Beverley Davies Rowley, Ph.D.
American Medical Association
Chicago, IL

Louise B. Russell, Ph.D.
Rutgers University
New Brunswick, NJ

**William B. Schwartz, M.D.**
Tufts University School of Medicine
Boston, MA

**Anne B. Silberger, A.M.**
American Medical Association Center for Health
  Policy Research
Chicago, IL

**David H. Solomon, M.D.**
The Rand Corporation
Santa Monica, CA

**Sally T. Sonnefeld**
United States Department of Health and Human Services
Baltimore, MD

**Gregory L. Stoddart, Ph.D.**
McMaster University
Hamilton, Ontario, Canada

**William G. Tholl**
Health and Welfare Canada and the Canadian
Health Economics Research Association

**George W. Torrance, Ph.D.**
McMaster University
Hamilton, Ontario, Canada

**Daniel R. Waldo**
United States Department of Health and Human Services
Baltimore, MD

**John E. Wennberg, M.D.**
Dartmouth Medical School
Hanover, NH

**Mark B. Wenneker, M.D.**
Harvard Medical School
Boston, MA

**Steffie Woolhandler, M.D., M.P.H.**
Harvard Medical School
Boston, MA

**Douwe Yntema, Ph.D.**
Harvard University
Boston, MA

# Contents

# Preface

A huge and dramatically diffuse body of literature has now accumulated in the areas of health services research and medical care organization over the last twenty-five years. This literature reflects thoughtful analysis of the many aspects and problems involved in the provision of health care to the American population.

The published literature in health services and related areas provides a wealth of resources for both students and practitioners to understand better the challenges facing the health care system and its managers. The increasing complexity of the health care system, and of the underlying forces that affect health and health care outcomes, and the rapid diffusion and proliferation of health care resources themselves, suggest the need for a better understanding of the results of this research and analysis. Finally, a careful study of this body of literature can help in each individual's analysis of policy alternatives facing the nation and in the selection of the best course for the future for us all.

## SELECTION OF ARTICLES

This book pulls together from this body of literature selected published articles that provide provocative, thoughtful, and insightful information regarding various aspects of the health care system. Selecting articles for inclusion here from the wealth of material available was a challenging task. Priority was given to review articles and to those articles which reflect more completely the underlying challenges and paradoxes of providing health care services to our nation. In addition, selected descriptive articles that help lay the framework for understanding the existing structure of the system were also included.

## WHO CAN USE THIS BOOK

This collection of readings is designed to facilitate a comprehensive understanding of the health care system. As such, this book is useful for both students and practitioners. Students in fields related to health services, such as health services administration, medicine, nursing, and other clinical areas, public policy administration, business administration, and related fields will benefit from reading the material contained in this book. Practitioners and policy makers seeking a better understanding of the system within which they work, and for which they make critical decisions, will also benefit from these readings.

## ORGANIZATION OF THE BOOK

The structure of *Contemporary Issues in Health Services* is designed to parallel the structure of *Introduction to Health Services, Fourth Edition,* coedited by Stephen J. Williams and Paul R. Torrens. The individual sections of this book parallel the sections of *Introduction to Health Services* so that, where appropriate, this collection of readings can be used to supplement the content of *Introduction to Health Services.* However, the articles selected for inclusion here have great value in and of themselves and bear witness to the evolution of our thought processes regarding the nation's health care system.

This book is organized into seven sections. Each section is prefaced with its own brief introduction. The first part of the book contains articles addressing issues of disease and illness and their definitions. Part Two addresses issues related to utilization of health services. Part Three examines institutions providing services, including the hospital, mental health organizations, and long-term care providers. Part Four discusses nonfinancial resources, specifically technology and health care personnel. Part Five addresses the critically important issue of financial resources, including national health expenditures and health insurance mechanisms. Part Six examines issues related to the assessment and regulation of health care system performance including evaluating the quality of care provided. Finally, Part Seven examines issues of national health policy and directions for the future of our nation's health care system.

## IN CONCLUSION

Regardless of each individual's political and ideological orientation, everyone can agree that the health care system is immensely complex and requires thoughtful analysis and evaluation. The published material presented here is a source of valuable information for everyone involved in the operation of our nation's health care system.

As our nation struggles to address the complex problems involved in the provision of health services, those involved in the system must also better understand the complexities, politics, financial limitations, and other constraints under which they operate. These articles go a long way toward helping each of us achieve that task.

Stephen J. Williams
San Diego, California

# PART ONE
## Disease and Illness

This section of the book addresses the underlying causes and characteristics of disease and illness in the United States. Two selections are included in this section. The first, by John E. Wennberg, critically addresses the relationship, or lack thereof, between illness rates and the use of health services, suggesting that appropriate use of our nation's health care system is difficult to achieve and that a better understanding of the underlying causes of disease and illness, and the subsequent need for health care services, requires further investigation.

The second selection, by Neil Love, describes patient care-seeking behavior in response to potential cancer-related symptoms. This article reflects nicely many of the complex emotional, psychological, and behavioral aspects of disease and illness, using cancer as an example. Providers in the nation's health care system can be modified and channeled in ways that improve the nation's health status and reduce health care costs.

# Chapter 1
# Population Illness Rates Do Not Explain Population Hospitalization Rates

## A Comment on Mark Blumberg's Thesis That Morbidity Adjusters Are Needed to Interpret Small Area Variations

John E. Wennberg, M.D.

Under pressure from escalating health care costs, government, business, and insurers are striving to decrease health care utilization. At the same time, many Americans lack adequate access to health care services. In this charged atmosphere, Mark Blumberg's concern about the appropriate application of epidemiologic research to health policy[1] is both legitimate and important. I share with Dr. Blumberg the fundamental goal of bringing the scientific method to bear on available data to better inform public and private decisions in health care.

Dr. Blumberg is correct in his assertion that there are differences in morbidity between regions and cities in the United States and that these differences are not (fully) explained by differences in the population's age structure. Small area studies consistently confirm this point. Small area studies are also compatible with the notion that illness is the major factor in the individual patient's decision to consult a physician. On these issues we are not in conflict. However, his conclusion that small area studies cannot be interpreted without adjusting for regional differences in both age and morbidity must be addressed.

Small area studies conclusively demonstrate the following: 1) Population characteristics such as age and morbidity cannot explain the degree of variation found in health care utilization among small areas. Indeed, variations in population, age, and morbidity among small areas are hardly correlated with variations in hospitalization rates for most diagnoses or operations. 2) The pattern of variations of the population-based rate of hospitalization for specific diagnoses or surgical conditions is best explained by differences in clinical judgment on the appropriateness of treatment. The differences arise from professional disagreements and lack of consensus on the value and outcomes of alternative ways of solving clinical problems. 3) Because utilization is not closely limited by scientific consensus, non-health factors such as the supply of resources can influence clinical decisions. Small area studies support the findings of other research showing that the supply of such resources as the numbers of beds and physicians clearly influence utilization.

Let me review the evidence for each of these contentions before turning to the important public policy implications of small area analyses.

## MORBIDITY, ILLNESS, AND THE PATTERN OF VARIATION IN HOSPITALIZATION RATES

Small area studies show statistically (and clinically) significant differences in the incidence of hospitalization rates for treatment of hip fractures, heart attacks, and

Reprinted with permission from J.B. Lippincott Company. *Medical Care,* April 1987, Vol. 25, No. 4.

strokes between communities and regions. Since virtually all patients with symptoms of these conditions will seek care and since the standards of practice throughout the United States call for the hospitalization of patients with these conditions, most of the variation in the age-adjusted rate of hospitalization must reflect underlying differences between communities in the incidence of illness. For these conditions, non–health-related factors play little role either in the decision to hospitalize or in variation in utilization rates.

As it turns out, however, these conditions are unique in that their pattern of variation is extremely low compared with most other causes of hospitalization. Orthopedic injuries provide a typical example. It can be asserted with some confidence that in the United States virtually all patients with fractures of the hip, ankle, or forearm seek and receive care. But is hospitalization necessary? For hip fractures, there is no question; all physicians agree on the need to hospitalize. It is of interest that the range of variation in the incidence of hip fracture hospitalization is similar to that of another measure of morbidity, the bed disability day indicator used by Blumberg (column 1 of his Table 4). In contrast to hip fracture, the hospitalization rates for ankle fractures show substantially greater variation. Ankle fractures are less severe than hip fractures: some cases can be and often are treated in the outpatient department. The increased variation in the hospitalization rates for this condition suggests that this decision is made differently from place to place—i.e., in some communities, the standard of care is such that a greater proportion of ankle fractures are treated on an outpatient basis than in other communities. While it is theoretically possible that the incidence of ankle fractures is much more variable than hip fracture from community to community, there is no good epidemiologic reason why this should be so. Hospitalization for fracture of the forearm is considerably more variable than ankle fractures, showing an eightfold range in variation, from a low in one market area that is only 30% of the state average to more than twice the state rate in another. Hospitalization rates for knee injuries, and low back injuries are even more variable, showing a 12–fold to 15–fold variation.

The inference I make from my analyses of the pattern of variation is that the amount and type of prescribed hospital-based care often vary from physician to physician in a fashion that is substantially unrelated to the underlying severity or incidence of the relevant illness. It is possible to estimate the percentage of the variation in the incidence of hospitalization for the injuries in Figure 1 that might reasonably be attributed to differences in morbidity between communities. Klim McPherson and Peter Clifford developed a statistic for estimating the magnitude of variation that improves upon traditional measures by removing the component of variation at-

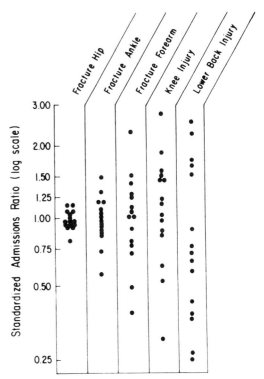

**Figure 1.** The incidence of hospitalization for common injuries among Maine hospital market areas, 1980–1982. Each dot represents the rate for a hospital market. The rates are age-adjusted and expressed as a ratio to the state average.

tributable to sample size.[2] Using their systematic component of variation (SCV), the magnitude of variation in the incidence of hospitalization can be compared directly without confounding owing to differences in the size of the numerators for the rates. Under the assumption that the magnitude of variation in the hospitalization (incidence) of hip fractures provides a reasonable estimate for the magnitude of variation in incidence for other injuries, the SCV for hip fractures can be used to estimate the proportion of total variation in hospitalization rates attributable to differences in the incidence of the injury. Table 1 shows that variation in the incidence of injuries appears to play a very minor role in the overall variation in hospitalization rates.

Most causes of medical and surgical admissions show wide variations in hospitalization rates. Hysterectomy is

Table 1. Systematic Component of Variation (SCV) and SCV for Hip Fracture as Percent of SCV for Selected Orthopedic Injuries

| Type of Injury | SCV | SCV Hip SCV × |
|---|---|---|
| Hip Fracture | 7.0 | 100.0% |
| Fracture of the ankle | 47.2 | 14.8 |
| Fracture of the forearm | 138.0 | 5.1 |
| Knee Injury | 161.1 | 4.8 |
| Back Injury | 295.7 | 2.0 |

recognized as a surgical procedure where professional discretion plays an important role. Typically, 90% of the medical and surgical admissions are for DRGs that show greater intrinsic variation than hysterectomy.[3,4]

## CORRELATIONS BETWEEN POPULATION MORBIDITY AND HOSPITALIZATION RATES

The theory that the amount and type of care prescribed for many conditions is substantially unrelated to the underlying incidence of the relevant illness is also supported by studies using morbidity measures obtained from personal interviews. When Alan Gittelsohn and I first described the small area variation phenomenon in Vermont,[5] the conventional wisdom of the day held that demand in medical markets was controlled by a central consensus among practicing physician on the appropriateness of medical care. Out findings (for example, that the per capita cost for hospitalization in Burlington, Vermont, was twice that of Middlebury, Vermont, or that the chance of having a tonsillectomy by age 15 was 60% in Stowe, Vermont, but only 12% in neighboring Waterbury) evoked a long and sometimes quite imaginative list of possible population- or patient-based reasons for variation.

Unease about the theoretical as well as the practical implications of the Vermont variations led Jack Fowler and me to undertake a formal test of the hypothesis that differences in the distribution of patient or population characteristics could account for the variations we found.[6,7] We set out to see if the variables that Ronald Andersen and his colleagues[8] had found useful in predicting individual patient demand for care were distributed differently among Vermont communities with up to a twofold

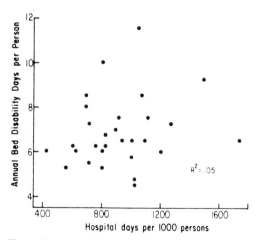

**Figure 2.** Association between a population morbidity measure and hospital patient day rate. The bed-disability data are from column A and the patient day rate from column four of Blumberg's Table 4. Even though about 15% of bed-disability days occur in the hospital,[1] only 5% of the variation in total patient days is explained by bed-disability days.

Table 2. Hospital Statistics in Two Iowa Communities (1980)

|  | Iowa City | Des Moines | IC/DM |
|---|---|---|---|
| Beds per 1,000 | 3.8 | 5.4 | 1.42 |
| Occupancy rate | 60.5% | 72.6% | 1.20 |
| Expend./capita | $200 | $323 | 1.47 |
| Part A Reim./enrollee | $734 | $1320 | 1.80 |
| Admissions/10,000 for: | | | |
| Low-variation conditions | 44 | 45 | 1.02 |
| High-variation conditions | 77 | 108 | 1.40 |
| Very high-variation conditions | 109 | 217 | 2.00 |

variation in costs and hospitalization rates. The members of some 300 households in each of six different hospital market areas were interviewed. In summary, we could find no difference in socioeconomic characteristics or morbidity rates (including the bed disability indicator). Indeed, the populations of the six communities were remarkably similar in their actual behavior in contacting their physicians for an episode of illness or for preventive services. The survey supported the conclusion that the differences in utilization we were measuring resulted from decisions physicians made after their patients contacted them—that is, as a result of differences in the way the agency role was exercised by Vermont physicians.

It is of interest that the data Dr. Blumberg presents in his Table 4 also support the theory that the amount of hospital care populations receive is substantially unrelated to morbidity. Figure 2 shows the relationship between bed disability days and hospitalization rates. There is virtually no relationship, even though more than 15% of bed disability days occur in the hospital.[1] The same is true for age structure. The $R^2$ statistic for the explained variation between the expected hospitalization rate based on age (column D) and the observed (column F) is 0.06 ($P = 0.192$). This is similar to my experience with small area studies where age structure and crude admission or patient day rates show very weak and sometimes paradoxic correlations. In view of the importance Dr. Blumberg places on knowing the morbidity level of the population before interpreting small area variations, some may find it ironic that both age and Dr. Blumberg's own morbidity measures are statistically unrelated to the total hospitalization rate. This is not surprising, however, since such a small proportion of the variation in specific causes of admission (e.g., Table 2) is related to variation in population need.

## CORRELATION BETWEEN SUPPLY FACTORS AND UTILIZATION

Supply factors, however do have a strong statistical association with utilization, particularly the association

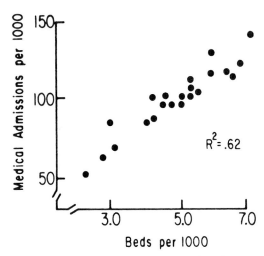

**Figure 3.** Association between medical admission rates and the numbers of hospital market areas, 1980. Each dot represents the rate for a hospital market area. The beds per 1,000 are corrected for boundary crossing.[10]

between available beds per capita and the admission rate for medical admissions (Fig. 3). A strong relationship between allocated beds per capita and medical admissions is consistent among small area studies. I agree with Dr. Blumberg that correlation does not mean causation. However, the theory that more beds are built in communities where populations are sicker is discredited by the observation that morbidity measures are uncorrelated with hospital utilization. Moreover, a review of the dynamics of growth that led to the construction of new beds points out the important role numerous non–health-related factors play in the decision to build hospital beds.[9,10] It is of great interest that when communities have relatively more beds, their physicians tend to admit proportionately more highly variable *medical conditions*—those conditions for which hospitalization rates are substantially uncorrelated with morbidity.

The situation vis-a-vis available beds per capita, occupancy rate, costs, patient days, and admission rates for medical conditions is illustrated in Table 2 for Des Moines and Iowa City. The incidence of hospitalization for strokes and heart attacks—low-variation conditions—are virtually identical, suggesting similar incidence rates for coronary artery disease in the two communities. However, the incidence of hospitalization for high-variation medical conditions is substantially greater in Des Moines. The high-variation conditions include many other manifestations of coronary artery disease such as heart failure, atherosclerosis, chest pain, angina, and cardiac arrhythmia.

The lower rate of use of services among residents of Iowa City does not seem to imply local rationing of care owing to insufficient resources. The occupancy rates of the two hospitals in the area indicate that additional resources are available if needed. Indeed, there is little

correlation between occupancy rates of local hospitals and utilization among small areas,[11,12] suggesting that clinicians in low-utilization communities tend to hold as many resources in reserve as their counterparts in high-rate areas. They could hospitalize more patients with high-variation conditions, if they thought it clinically indicated. For some reason, they prefer not to. I interpret this to mean that if there is marginal medical utility to individual patients associated with higher rates of hospitalization, this utility is not recognized by clinicians practicing in low-utilization communities.

## WHICH RATE IS RIGHT?

The fundamental reason why non–health-related factors can influence utilization rates can be traced to the lack of professional consensus on appropriate standards for the management of the majority of medical and surgical conditions. The extent of this uncertainty poses serious challenges to public policy for health. Traditional notions about efficiency and equity depend largely on an implicit belief in the value of medical care. I share Blumberg's concern that the misinterpretation of small area data could lead policy makers to deny care to those in need by assuming that the lowest rate of utilization is the correct rate. This is a nonsense assumption that could lead to serious limitations on resources for necessary services. However, the contrasting assumption that high rates of care necessarily reflect rational clinical decisions on the marginal return of medical care is equally uninformed. Although it is indisputably true that hospitalization is needed for many people who are sick, it is also very likely that for many other people the discomfort and cost associated with hospitalization and the risks of iatrogenesis combine to produce a negative outcome.

The challenge of small area analysis is answering this question: Which rate is right[13] Some health care services are overutilized. Others are certainly underutilized, especially by the increasing numbers of uninsured in America. Although the savings achieved by decreasing overutilization might be used to ease the plight of those with limited access and avoid unnecessary rationing of valuable care for all Americans, this opportunity is not now seriously pursued. In the absence of outcome-based standards of care and protocols to assure that patient values guide the clinical decision process, unwanted variations are inevitable. The most important policy conclusion of small area analysis is the need to study the outcomes of medical and surgical care.

## References

1. Blumberg MS. Inter-area variations in age-adjusted health status. *Med Care* 1987;25:340–353.

2. McPherson K, Wennberg JE, Hovind OB, et al. Small-area variations in the use of common surgical procedures: An international comparison of New England, England, and Norway. *N Engl J Med* 1982;307:1310–1314.

3. Wennberg JE, McPherson K, Caper P. Will payment based on diagnostic-related groups control hospital costs? *N Engl J Med* 1984;311:295–300.

4. Wennberg JE. Small area variations in hospitalized dose mix for DRGs in Maine, Massachusetts, Iowa. Final report of project supported by the National Center for Health Services Research, Grant No. HS-04932, 1984.

5. Wennberg J, Gittelsohn A. Small area variations in health care delivery. *Science* 1973;182:1102–1108.

6. Wennberg J, Fowler FJ. A test of consumer contributions to small area variations in health care delivery. *J Maine Med Assoc* 1977;68:275–279.

7. Wennberg JE. On patient need, equity, supplier-induced demand, and the need to assess the outcome of common medical practices. *Med Care* 1985;23:512–520.

8. Andersen R, Newman J. Societal and individual determinants of medical care utilization. *Milbank Mem Fund Q* 1973(Winter);51:95–124.

9. Altman D, Greene RJ, Sapolsky HM. Health Planning and Regulation: The Decision-Making Process. Ann Arbor, MI: AUPHA Press, 1981:74–97.

10. Wennberg JE, Gittelsohn AM. A Small Area Approach to the Analysis of Health Systems Performance. Washington, DC: Government Printing Office (DHHS publication no. [HRA]80–14012), 1980:137–176.

11. Wennberg J, Gittelsohn A. Health care delivery in Maine III: Evaluating the performance of hospitals. *J Maine Med Assoc* 1975;66:298–306.

12. McCracken S, Latessa P, Wennberg J. A Study of Hospital Utilization in Iowa in 1980. Des Moines, IA: Servi-Share of Iowa, 1982.

13. Wennberg JE. Which rate is right? *N Engl J Med* 1986;314:310–311.

# Chapter 2

# Why Patients Delay Seeking Care for Cancer Symptoms

## What You Can Do About It

Neil Love, M.D.

## PREVIEW

Why do many patients hesitate to seek care for cancer symptoms? Can primary care physicians help prevent tragic delays? Dr. Love proposes that by being aware of the factors involved, including fear and denial, physicians can educate their patients about warning signals and the importance of early diagnosis. The article emphasizes the benefits of patient education, particularly regarding breast cancer and malignant melanoma.

*It was my doleful observation, repeated again and again, that the metaphoric trappings that deform the experience of having cancer have very real consequences: they inhibit people from seeking treatment early enough, or making a greater effort to get competent treatment. The metaphors and myths, I was convinced, kill.*[1]
　　　　　　　　—Susan Sontag, author and cancer patient

One of the most established of oncologic dicta, "the earlier the diagnosis, the better the prognosis," is the foundation for cancer screening programs. Unfortunately, most cases of cancer are not diagnosed until patients recognize the symptoms themselves. In contemporary practice, a surprisingly high percentage of patients with newly diagnosed cancer report a prolonged delay in seeking care.

Nothing is more frustrating to either patient or physician than the realization that potentially avoidable delay may have adversely influenced the prognosis. Why do patients hesitate? Does fear of the disease block our logic? Is the public ignorant of the warning signs of cancer? Do economic barriers cause hesitation in seeking medical care? The answer is, All of the above.

The next question then is, Can primary care physicians help prevent these tragic delays? The medical literature provides some intriguing answers.

## KEY FACTORS

Knowledge of and attitudes toward cancer are so varied that, given the same symptoms, people often resort to different actions. Common factors in patient delay include fear and denial, lack of information, and financial considerations.

### Fear and Denial

Rational and irrational fears are important elements in the decision to seek care for warning signals. In "normal" adults, denial is a common adaptive response to threat and loss that allows one to buy time in assimilating a painful realization without being overwhelmed.[2]

A survey at Massachusetts General Hospital[3] showed that patients with newly diagnosed cancer who had

Reprinted with permission from Postgraduate Medicine, March 1991, Vol. 89, No. 4.

delayed seeking medical care generally did so as "a conscious and deliberate act rather than a failure to perceive the neoplasm or to comprehend its consequences." The study found that 39% of patients waited more than 4 months to seek medical care and that one in six patients waited more than a year. The role of fear and denial in this process was suggested by the fact that patients who labeled their condition as a "tumor" waited significantly longer than those who called it "cancer." Duration of delay was not related to age or sex; however, patients with lower income and less education delayed longer.

The decision to seek care requires a cognitive grasp of the medical implications of symptoms and a belief in the benefits of diagnosis and treatment. Unfortunately, negativism about cancer therapy is widespread. For example, a 1986 survey[4] revealed that two thirds of the respondents agreed with the statement that "treatments for cancer are worse than the disease." Almost half believed that "there is no point to having cancer tests, because it is only looking for trouble." People with this attitude may be expected not to seek care unless symptoms are exerting a significantly adverse effect on their lifestyle.

Cancer's image as a relentless and devastating disease that is treated with toxic and disfiguring methods undoubtedly promotes unconscious denial mechanisms. This concept can be combated in daily office practice, where up to 20% of visits are the result of "fear or thoughts of cancer" and half of all patients admit to a general fear of the disease.[5] In *Early Diagnosis of Cancer in General Practice,*[6] Holtedahl notes that primary care physicians diagnose cancer only about once a month, but they rule out the disease every day.

In an evaluation of psychosocial factors that predict patient delay, Samet and associates[7] found that cancer patients who had regular checkups with primary care physicians had the shortest delays in diagnosis. This study and other reports have shown that patients who have a positive, trusting relationship with their physician delay seeking care for cancer symptoms for a significantly shorter period.

## Lack of Information

To minimize diagnostic delay, public awareness programs such as the American Cancer Society's Seven

Table 1. The seven warning signals of cancer

1. Change in bowel or bladder habits
2. A sore that does not heal
3. Unusual bleeding or discharge
4. Thickening or lump in breast or elsewhere
5. Indigestion or difficulty swallowing
6. Obvious change in wart or mole
7. Nagging cough or hoarseness

*American Cancer Society.*

Table 2. Prevalence of cancer symptoms in a "healthy" population

| | Prevalence(%) | |
| SYMPTOM | MEN | WOMEN |
| --- | --- | --- |
| Frequent urination | 13.2 | 14.8 |
| Change in bowel habits | 9.6 | 9.7 |
| Bloody or black stools | 6.4 | 3.2 |
| Hoarseness, change in voice | 7.5 | 9.1 |
| Cough for more than a month | 8.5 | 9.1 |
| Breast mass | NA | 4.4 |
| Testicular mass | 2.3 | NA |
| Change in mole | 4.2 | 5.9 |

*Adapted from Balshem et al.[9]*

Warning Signals of Cancer have been developed (table 1).[8] However, a major problem with this approach is the high prevalence and nonspecific nature of many of the warning signals in apparently healthy adults. One population-based survey[9] found that about half of those interviewed had at least one current symptom (table 2). Furthermore, warning signs were more common in respondents aged 25 to 44 years than in persons older than 65. This finding contrasts with the much greater incidence of cancer in the elderly.[10]

Another study[11] found that more than 5% of patients who visited a primary care physician were experiencing a warning signal. Follow-up revealed that only 25% of patients with subsequent cancer had previously reported a warning signal. These data suggest that nontargeted patient education efforts about cancer symptoms may be relatively unproductive and that a more individualized approach is needed.

## Financial Considerations

Greenwald[12] found that cancer patients with copaid fee-for-service healthcare coverage waited longer to seek care than patients with coverage from a health maintenance organization. This finding suggests that financial factors may contribute to patient delay.

A particular concern is the lack of efficient access to care for indigent people. For example, the majority of medical care for indigent people in Dade County, Florida, is provided by Jackson Memorial Hospital, the main teaching center for the University of Miami School of Medicine. At the hospital, we have found that the stage of cancer at initial diagnosis in "staff" patients is far more advanced than that in private patients. This phenomenon may be partially explained by educational and cultural factors. However, overcrowded clinics for the indigent and lack of inpatient resources also have important roles.

Indigent patients with cancer symptoms often wait many months for an initial clinic appointment, and definitive diagnosis and treatment may result in a delay within the healthcare system of up to a year. The apparent result can be seen in cases of breast cancer, where 22% of staff patients at Jackson Memorial Hospital initially present with metastases, compared with 6% of private patients. Average tumor size and degree of axillary node involvement are also much more advanced in indigent patients. As a result, although patients matched for stage have similar survival rates, the overall 5-year mortality rate of staff patients is 52% compared with 30% in private patients.

The lack of access to care for uninsured patients not only has direct effects on the patients involved but also sends the message to the indigent community at large that "if it doesn't bother you, don't bother it." This thinking reinforces the psychological denial normally experienced when cancer symptoms occur.

## PRIORITIES IN PATIENT EDUCATION

It is generally agreed that cancer is a heterogeneous group of diseases with a plethora of biomedical and psychosocial characteristics. Although physicians can generally encourage patients to seek care for medical symptoms, patient education can also be directed to specific types of cancer. This strategy should be based on several key questions.

- *What is the patient's cancer risk?* Patient education efforts targeting rare diseases are not cost-effective. For example, occult presentations of hypoglycemia from pancreatic insulinomas often result in diagnostic delays of a year or more.[13] However, this tumor is too unusual to include in routine office education efforts.

  In some situations, education can be directed at those patients who are at high risk for particular cancers. For example, patients with a history of tobacco and alcohol use can be instructed regarding the early signs of oral cancer. The mouth is easily accessible, and there is a direct correlation between stage of disease at diagnosis and prognosis. Unfortunately, early lesions are often overlooked by both patients and physicians.[14]

- *Is the patient capable of identifying a cancer warning signal?* Unfortunately, the presenting symptoms of many common cancers are nonspecific and difficult to separate from those of benign conditions. For example, colorectal cancer is the second most common cause of cancer mortality,[1] and the average diagnostic delay with this disease exceeds 5 months.[15] However, the initial symptoms of colorectal cancer are extremely common in apparently healthy adults. One study[16] found that one in six persons had experienced rectal bleeding in the previous 6 months, and one third described a significant alteration in bowel habits, including straining, incomplete emptying, and uncomfortable fullness of the abdomen.

  Should all patients with these symptoms be counseled to seek attention, or should more specific symptoms be targeted as warning signals? Physician efforts in colorectal cancer control probably would be more productive if focused on prevention (counseling for low-fat, high-fiber diets) and screening (rectal examination, flexible sigmoidoscopy, and fecal testing for occult blood).

  The dilemma of warning signals can also be seen with ovarian cancer, where nonspecific symptoms such as fatigue

and urinary frequency are common initial signs. Unfortunately, more distinctive symptoms, such as abdominal pain and swelling, often accompany advanced tumors.[17] Many experts believe that the key to early diagnosis of visceral cancers will be the development of accurate screening tests to detect disease at an asymptomatic stage.

- *Does earlier diagnosis of cancer improve prognosis?* With the growing concern for more cost-effective medical care, physicians rely on documented research findings to guide clinical practice. Not all studies have demonstrated a significant relationship between patient delay and disease stage and survival. For example, studies of patients with testicular cancer have consistently shown a median patient delay of at least 2 months.[18] Although larger tumors are more common in men who delay longer, there has been little evidence that delay is a major factor in the stage at diagnosis or the prognosis. Inherent tumor biology and growth characteristics may be more important factors in determining stage of disease at presentation. Also, the evolution of increasingly successful treatment for all stages of testicular cancer has improved 5-year relapse-free survival rates from 62% in 1960 to higher than 90% currently.[8] Perhaps the effectiveness of treatment regardless of stage supersedes the effect of delay, although earlier diagnosis may permit therapy with fewer adverse effects.

These data should not necessarily discourage physicians from teaching self-examination of the testicles and using other means of promoting earlier diagnosis of highly curable tumors. However, time constraints of office practice require prioritization of efforts. From this perspective, two specific cancers, breast cancer and malignant melanoma, deserve particular attention.

### Breast Cancer

Although mammographic screening is capable of detecting clinically occult tumors, most patients present with masses noticed on self-palpation.[19] Breast cancer may be the most important target of public education to prevent diagnostic delay. In a study of the effect of delay on stage at diagnosis for cancers at a number of sites,[20] the most significant correlation was noted with breast cancer. Stage of disease is important not only because of the direct relationship to survival but also because smaller tumors are more likely to be treatable with limited breast surgery such as lumpectomy.

Wilkinson and associates[21] found that one in seven patients with breast cancer waited more than 7 months after noticing a mass, and about one fourth of patients who delayed had metastases. Although breast cancer is no longer considered an emergent condition requiring immediate surgery, this study showed that delays of longer than 2 months correlated with disease stage and survival.

Although a painless breast mass is the most common initial symptom of breast cancer, the disease has many other presentations, including focal pain, nipple discharge, and dimpling. Patients with these less characteristic findings delay treatment more than twice as long as patients who palpate lumps.[19]

The importance of the patient in detection of breast cancer is supported by a meta-analysis encompassing 12 studies of more than 8,000 patients.[22] This analysis concluded that women who regularly examined themselves had significantly smaller tumors and a 36% lower incidence of positive axillary lymph nodes. Both of these staging factors are highly predictive of prognosis.

Despite controversy over the precise impact of self-examination, the accessibility of the breasts to palpation and the extensive data showing that women often delay seeking evaluation of breast masses suggest that breast cancer education should be a routine part of office care. When teaching self-examination,* the physician also has the opportunity to assure patients that most breast lumps are benign and that an office visit to evaluate a breast mass may avoid needless worry. Patients can also be taught that when breast cancer does occur, lumpectomy is an option for most patients and that important treatment advances have improved the outlook for this disease.

### Malignant Melanoma

Timely diagnosis of this skin tumor is important. Surgery is highly effective for early lesions, but treatment of metastases is generally ineffective. The incidence of melanoma is increasing by about 4% a year; it was estimated that 6,000 people would die of the disease in 1990.[8] The average time between first noticing a lesion and becoming suspicious is about 6 months, and patients generally wait an additional 3 months before seeking medical care.[23] Delay in this situation is significantly longer in women.[23] Patients with melanomas in less accessible areas, such as the upper and lower back, delay longer.[24]

Radial tumor growth seen in superficial spreading melanomas generally provokes quicker patient action than the elevation that occurs with nodular melanomas.[24] Patient delay correlates with stage and prognosis with both types of lesions, but more so with nodular melanoma, because more advanced lesions are often seen with the latter.[24]

Patients with melanoma respond most quickly to symptoms that elicit anxiety, such as bleeding, ulceration, itching, and tenderness.[25] Unfortunately, these findings usually accompany more advanced lesions. Earlier signs of the disease (eg, changes in the size, color, or elevation of a nevus) are often less stress-producing and do not elicit a behavioral response; thus, they are associated with greater delay. Previous public education efforts have emphasized changes in moles. However, tu-

mors often grow very slowly and may not be noticed by the patient. As a result, more emphasis needs to be placed on the inherent characteristics of melanoma, such as irregular shape and color.

The question remains whether the public can be successfully trained to identify these tumors at an earlier stage. During an educational campaign on pigmented lesions in Scotland, posters and leaflets were distributed to libraries and clinics, and patients who recognized early lesions were encouraged to seek attention.[26] A massive media blitz was also organized. Patient referrals after this campaign increased dramatically, and the percentage of melanomas diagnosed at an early stage increased from 38% to 62%.[26] Similar educational programs have been launched in the United States.

Examination of the patient's skin during a routine office visit provides the physician with an excellent opportunity to give instruction regarding the characteristic changes of melanoma. Educational pamphlets that assist in these efforts are available through a variety of organizations.**

## ROLE OF THE PRIMARY CARE PHYSICIAN

Primary care physicians see their patients an estimated 2.5 to 4 times a year.[27] With the average American immediate family containing 3.5 members, this provides physicians the opportunity to have frequent contact with the family unit. When a patient makes an office visit for a benign, self-limited problem, the physician has an excellent opportunity for preventive health education. Cancer control should be one of the primary targets for these efforts and can include discussion of prevention (emphasizing smoking cessation and dietary intervention), screening (particularly for breast and cervical cancer), and prompt diagnosis. Patient education about melanoma, breast cancer, and other neoplastic conditions may be an important factor in decreasing the length of delay before diagnosis and in improving treatment outcome.

In addition to providing information, physicians can also attempt to change attitudes and address specific fears. Many observers believe that the most important and central patient concern related to cancer is loss of control. Patients may be more likely to seek care if they believe that their physician will ensure that no intervention will be forced on them and that their autonomy will be respected. This trust may take years to develop, particularly for patients who have already had adverse experiences with cancer in family members.

Another important primary care aspect of patient delay has received little attention: the feelings of a cancer patient who has delayed seeking care. What goes through

*For a patient handout on self-examination, see the October 1989 issue of *Cancer Evaluation,* page 167.

**American Academy of Dermatology, 1567 Maple Ave, Evanston, IL 60201; Skin Cancer Foundation, Box 561, New York, NY 10156.

the mind of a patient with melanoma who first noticed the lesion a year ago or a patient with breast cancer who has palpated a mass for 6 months? Many of these patients are sick with guilt and self-reproach for not having sought attention earlier.

Primary care physicians are on the front line of cancer diagnosis and have the opportunity to assess these issues and attempt to comfort and reassure patients. An extensive data base demonstrates that patient delay is extremely common and that many people do not know when to seek care or are afraid to do so. Patients with newly diagnosed cancer must attempt to shed negative concerns and prepare for treatment and rehabilitation.

## SUMMARY

Patient delay in seeking care for cancer symptoms is common and well documented by research studies. Fear and denial, lack of information about cancer, and financial considerations all contribute to this delay. Patient education may be an important factor in decreasing the length of delay and thereby improving treatment outcome. By making good use of opportunities for patient education, primary care physicians may positively influence the prognosis of several types of cancer, particularly breast cancer and malignant melanoma of the skin.

## References

1. Sontag S. Illness as metaphor and AIDS and its metaphor. New York: Doubleday, 1990:102
2. Wool MS. Understanding denial in cancer patients:. In: Goldberg RJ, ed. Psychiatric aspects of cancer. Advances in psychosomatic medicine. Vol 18. Basel: Karger, 1988:37–53
3. Hackett TP, Cassem NH, Raker JW. Patient delay in cancer. N Engl J Med 1973;289(1):14–20
4. Aging and wellness. (Videotape) Tampa, FL: American Cancer Society, 1986
5. Nylenna M. Fear of cancer among patients in general practice. Scand J Prim Health Care 1984; 2(1):24–6
6. Holtedahl K. Early diagnosis of cancer in general practice: a manual. New York: Springer-Verlag, 1990
7. Samet JM, Hunt WC, Lerchen ML, et al. Delay in seeking care for cancer symptoms: a population-based study of elderly New Mexicans. J Natl Cancer Inst 1988;80(6):432–8
8. Cancer facts and figures—1990. Atlanta: American Cancer Society, 1990:27
9. Balshem AM, Amsel Z, Workman S, et al. The experience of cancer warning signs in a general population and its implications for public education. Prog Clin Biol Res 1988;278:77–89
10. Baranovsky A, Myers MH. Cancer incidence and survival in patients 65 years of age and older. CA 1986;36(1):26–41
11. Holtedahl KA. The value of warning signals of cancer in general practice. Scand J Prim Health Care 1987;5(3):140–3
12. Greenwald HP. HMO membership, copayment, and initiation of care for cancer: a study of working adults. Am J Public Health 1987;77(4):461–6
13. Service FJ, Dale AJ, Elveback LR, et al. Insulinoma: clinical and diagnostic features of 60 consecutive cases. Mayo Clin Proc 1976;51(7):417–29
14. Shafer WG. Initial mismanagement and delay in diagnosis of oral cancer. J Am Dent Assoc 1975; 90(6):1262–4
15. Irvin TT, Creaney MG. Duration of symptoms and prognosis of carcinoma of the colon and rectum. Surg Gynecol Obstet 1977;144(6):883–6
16. Dent OF, Goulston KJ, Zubrzycki J, et al. Bowel symptoms in an apparently well population. Dis Colon Rectum 1986;29(4):243–7
17. Smith EM, Anderson B. The effects of symptoms and delay in seeking diagnosis on stage of disease at diagnosis among women with cancers of the ovary. Cancer 1985;56(11):2727–32
18. Chilvers CE, Saunders M, Bliss JM, et al. Influence of delay in diagnosis on prognosis in testicular teratoma. Br J Cancer 1989;59(1):126–8
19. MacArthur C, Smith A. Delay in breast cancer and the nature of presenting symptoms. Lancet 1981;1(8220 Pt 1):601–3
20. Robinson E, Mohilever J, Zidan J, et al. Delay in diagnosis of cancer: possible effects on the stage of disease and survival. Cancer 1984;54(7):1454–60
21. Wilkinson GS, Edgerton F, Wallace HJ Jr, et al. Delay, stage of disease and survival from breast cancer. J Chronic Dis 1979;32(5):365–73
22. Hill D, White V, Jolley D, et al. Self examination of the breast: is it beneficial? Meta-analysis of studies investigating breast self examination and extent of disease in patients with breast cancer. BMJ 1988;297(6643):271–5
23. Cassileth BR, Temoshok L, Frederick BE, et al. Patient and physician delay in melanoma diagnosis. J Am Acad Dermatol 1988;18(3):591–8
24. Temoshok L, DiClemente RJ, Sweet DM, et al. Factors related to patient delay in seeking medical attention for cutaneous malignant melanoma. Cancer 1984;54(12):3048–53
25. Cassileth BR, Lusk EJ, Guerry D 4th, et al. "Catalyst" symptoms in malignant melanoma. J Gen Intern Med 1987;2(1):1–4
26. Doherty VR, MacKie RM. Reasons for poor prognosis in British patients with cutaneous malignant melanoma. BMJ (Clin Res) 1986;292(6526):987–9
27. Williams PA, Williams M. Barriers and incentives for primary-care physicians and cancer prevention and detection. Cancer 1987;60(8 Suppl):1970–8

# PART TWO

## The Use of
## Health Services

This section addresses the use of health care services and its measurement. Two selections that focus on utilization are included. The first, by Charlotte Muller, reviews the twenty years of research on health care utilization up to the mid-1980s, a period which encompasses tremendous progress in the investigation and understanding of factors associated with the use of health care services. This excellent review article also raises many questions related to issues of measuring and understanding the use of health care services by consumers.

The second article in this section, by Mark R. Chassin and associates, addresses the very important issue of variations in the use of health care services by geography and other variables. A particularly challenging area of health services research has been the examination of geographic and other variations in utilization and attempts to explain such variation with regard to consumer and health services system variables. This article is an excellent illustration of this type of research. The inability of the authors to explain such variation readily is particularly disturbing.

# Chapter 3
# Review of Twenty Years of Research on Medical Care Utilization

Charlotte Muller

*A wide variety of issues in social distribution and system performance are approached through analysis of utilization, as shown by this review of twenty years of research. Utilization studies have been used to examine social norms with respect to dying and to geographical and class diffusion of access to the most useful diagnostic procedures. Prevention utilization is selected for special study but is difficult to analyze because both the boundary between prevention and treatment services and the unit of observation are ill defined. A series of studies of the class gradient in use of care under conditions of reduced barriers to care indicate that equity can be improved through program design even though deficits remain at this time. For health plans with social objectives, a stable low-user group presents a challenge to outreach rather than a source of financial comfort. Other work on utilization examines unnecessary care through study of interregional variation in surgical rates and the phenomenon of physician-induced demand; cost-sharing; the HMO model in its attempt theoretically to reconcile equity with cost-containment; the rule of sex differences in utilization; and the influence of women's social roles and traditional/contemporary cultural relationships on access.*

## ISSUES APPROACHED THROUGH UTILIZATION RESEARCH

The key to the sustained interest in utilization research over the past two decades is an appreciation of the power of statistics and the record of performance in public debate over what to do with the health care system. Explicitly or implicitly, utilization studies are policy-oriented. This is openly stated by Andersen[1] in modeling potential and realized access. Properties of the population at risk that are believed to be capable of alteration by health policies are separated from those that are not.[2] A wide variety of issues in social distribution and system performance are approached through analysis of utilization. Study of the rise of emergency room care has been based on normative expectations regarding the share of needs that should be met in the emergency room and the match of case type to emergency room capabilities. Such study has revealed use of the emergency room as a response to restricted availability of primary care for both affluent and nonaffluent groups. Location of physicians away from the inner-city poor, limited office hours, and low reimbursement rates for

Presented at the Twentieth Anniversary of Kaiser Permanente Health Services Research Center, Research Symposium, Portland, OR, September 30, 1984. Reprinted with permission from the Hospital Research and Educational Trust, June 1986. *Health Serv Res 1986;* 21 (Part I):129–144.

physicians treating the poor have contributed to the expansion of emergency room care.[3,4]

Another line of inquiry used the proportion of total utilization of hospital services taken up by the "catastrophic" and terminal patient as a basis for examining the social norm with respect to dying. Questions designed to establish an appropriate level of resource commitment and its setting[5] are significant in relation to trends in survival of the elderly and in development of life-prolonging techniques. Included in this type of inquiry is the study of criteria used in rationing intensive care by physicians when there is a constraint or shortage.[6] In pursuing this discussion, we should note that, realistically, the sickest in a given year are going to need more care than the others and that this was the original rationale for periodic payment systems in the report of the Committee on the Costs of Medical Care.

The application of utilization analysis to monitoring of the diffusion of technology is exemplified by national figures showing differences by race and geography in the performance of amniocentesis, and differences by community size in substitution of prenatal ultrasound for x-ray examination.[7] Interest in these is based on the issue of access to useful or safer procedures.

Much utilization research concerns the substitution of one form of care for another, as in research showing outpatient care to be a replacement for inpatient care, reflecting the economic influences of prices of the alternative types of care and the hospital occupancy rate.[8] An important implication of such work was the fact that decisions influencing hospitalization were not based solely on medical characteristics of a case, i.e., need.

As important as price-based substitution is indirect substitution through effect on health. One of the basic issues in evaluating HMOs, neighborhood centers for the elderly,[9] etc. is whether by providing ambulatory services it is possible to avert the need for hospital care. Again, substitution has been a criterion for appraising mental health benefits. Because of the marginal acceptance of mental health services in the insurance world, the likelihood that these services would pay for themselves by reducing utilization of general health care,[10] and the circumstances in which this reduction would occur, have been the subject of researchers' interest.

Measurement of utilization of preventive services is construed as an evaluation of the distribution of the most potent care as it is influenced by poverty, organizational forms, and other factors. Such measurement often puts on the same footing activities that may have very different payoffs in terms of health outcomes and ones that also differ according to the initiator—whether it is the patient or the physician. The measurement and analysis of preventive service utilization marks a shift of emphasis from the unified concept of medical care advanced by advocates of some type of national health

system within the public health movement. In their statements, the role of treatment services in preventing health deterioration was emphasized, and the separation of health department responsibility for immunizations and other preventive activities from the privately financed market for treatment services was considered a lag in adapting public health to the needs of modern society.[11] In the context of the present interest in prevention, prevalence of chronic disease means that the boundary between preventive and treatment services may be hard to find and, therefore, that total preventive services may not be measured. Furthermore, since the motivation for a treatment visit may include the patient's expectation of preventive services, we do not yet have a fully satisfactory unit of observation for the study of preventive utilization. Finally, with current interest focused on modification of personal health practices, we need more explicit measures of the quantitative and qualitative aspects of the preventive counseling or behavior modification provided.

## POVERTY AND UTILIZATION

One of the central themes of our current era is how the class gradient in utilization is affected by reduced financial barriers to care. Poverty is a persistent condition of our society. It is regenerated by the friction-full interplay of the labor market and the family system: low-wage jobs, long-lasting unemployment, homes without fathers, economic and educational discrimination, and chronic impairments contribute to poverty. The relation of personal health history to economic disability has long been known. So long as poverty remains, the issue of equity in health care is kept alive. The austerity applied to human services in the national budget and attempts to limit public and employer liability for health care costs have converted the interest of many in progress toward an ideal into anxiety about visible retrogression,[12] since methods of cost control do not always respect equity conceptually or administratively.

The legislation of 1965 setting up Medicare and Medicaid poured effective demand into the market, but it went for the most part into the mold of the conventional two-tier system. Private physicians were invited to take Medicaid patients, but fee schedules were often low. In contrast, when they took Medicare patients they could collect charges beyond the Medicare-allowed fee if they chose. Additional programs for the poor such as neighborhood health centers were established, but no universal scheme was adopted.

In Canada, however, a universal health insurance system was legislated. Utilization research was used to analyze its effects. Broyles et al. concluded that Canada's Medicare has resulted in equitable distribution of care, since medical needs and sociodemographic characteristics—not economic factors—have determined both probability and volume of physician care.[13] They noted that in various countries installation of more comprehensive insurance weakens the link between use of physician services and ability to pay. Yet United Kingdom data do show a continuation of less use by lower-income persons and more delay.

In the United States, the report of the Secretary of Health, Education and Welfare to the president and the Congress, entitled Health United States 1976–1977, assessed the equity of outcomes of the programs of the 1960s.[14] For all age groups, the user rate still remained higher for the nonpoor, although the number of visits per person was equal or greater for the poor. The user rate for children was more sensitive than the rate for adults to income, race, and place of residence. For the elderly, the gap between the poor and the nonpoor was narrowed as the user rate of the poor increased and the rate for the nonpoor declined, while the hospital discharge rates of the poor increased more than those of the nonpoor. The use of care by the elderly as a group was correlated with perception of poor health and presence of chronic conditions, and thus by implication represented a justifiable use of social resources. The fact that the bulk of ambulatory care was for follow-up and continuing care indicated the significance of Medicare in underwriting care of chronic conditions while suggesting a future problem as the number of aged in the population increased; prevention of chronic disease was not discussed. Surgical utilization statistics showing growth of cataract surgery and arthroplasty, for example, implied that financing could and did assist access to a more lively old age. While regional variations in discharge rate and length of stay overall and for given conditions suggested that styles of medical practice could influence resource use without benefit to patients, sex differences in hospital use rates were consistent with disease patterns reported.

Aday et al., from the Center for Health Administration Studies at the University of Chicago, analyzed the effect of the 1960s programs using special methods of measuring need. They stated that the position of the low-income population had greatly improved with regard to "reducing traditional utilization inequities" even when need for care was considered and found the contact rate for illness and the visits–disability ratio among the poor to be at parity with other income groups.

But they also reported that in the low-income group children were less likely to see a doctor and pregnant women to get early prenatal care, while the use of outpatient departments and longer waits for care indicated inferior access.

Kleinman et al., while acknowledging that access by the disadvantaged had improved, used data from the National Health Interview Survey of 1976–1978 to chal-

lenge the conclusion by Aday et al. that equity had been achieved.[15] The Kleinman group noted basic methodological differences between the studies. The Center for Health Administration Studies survey omitted telephone conversations, which are more likely to be part of the utilization of high-income and white persons, and used one-year recall for physician visits, thus biasing downward, because of memory losses, the measured total utilization of the affluent. Hence, class differences were underestimated. In contrast, the NHIS analysis included phone consultations and confined physician visit data to two-week recall. Also, Kleinman's research group, by adjusting income for family size, arrived at a markedly different distribution of the members of the population by income level. Kleinman et al., criticizing both the construction and the basic assumptions of the use–disability ratio employed by the Chicago group, came up with a modified form, and also used self-assessed health status to stratify people by need for care. Among children in fair or poor health, those in the lowest income group were found to have 47 percent fewer visits than those in the highest group, and at each level the number for blacks was 38 percent fewer than for whites. Other age groups for which there is an income–visit differential for those in fair or poor health are whites aged 17–44 years and both races at age 65 years and over. The comparisons based on visits per 100 bed-disability days also show substantial differences by income level and race, although the differentials vary by subgroups. In all age groups, however, there are substantial race and income differences in the type of visits. As Aday et al. had noted, the poor are more likely to get their care in clinics. This is considered important by health care analysts, because the quality of care received from private providers is believed to be better. While this is often said without documentation, it is known that the poor receive fewer preventive services—specifically, breast examinations, Pap tests, prenatal care, and immunization against childhood diseases. For children, Wolfe has found that use of private physicians is associated with receipt of preventive care.[16]

In 1981, 15.7 million children under 18, or 25.5 percent of all children in families, were living below 125 percent of poverty.[17] Orr and Miller assert that Medicaid's performance has not lived up to the hope of assuring access to care and specifically to mainstream care for the children of the poor.[18] Actually, Medicaid may have stimulated public service delivery through the WIC program for nutritional supplements, which motivated clinic attendance, and through the EPSDT program, which has been implemented by public providers. Orr and Miller note an actual decline in the proportion of children 1–5 years old with a private physician as their regular source of care—from 78 percent in 1963 to 69 percent in 1970. The fact that many poor children lack access to health services is taken to indicate that "reimbursement of existing providers appears an inadequate way of meeting their needs."

Efforts to place indigent families in Kaiser and other HMOs were designed as an economically feasible way of changing the source of care and utilization patterns of the poor. Greenlick et al. in 1972 evaluated the experience of the Portland plan with 1,500 families.[19] Poverty evidently left its mark, both in health effects and in style of care-seeking, for there was higher use of services by adult males for diseases with a strong emotional component, for chronic disease, and for injuries. More failure to keep appointments was also noted, and more use of unscheduled services. But the overall finding was that much of the reported difference in utilization between poverty groups and other parts of the general population seems to disappear when access barriers are removed.

Later analysis by Mullooley and Freeborn, using longitudinal data to study the low-income membership, shows higher overall use compared to the general membership, attributable to medical needs associated with poverty.[20] But poor as well as nonpoor new members had a drop in hospital utilization after enrollment. Mullooly and Freeborn concluded that the differences were not so large as to thwart integration of the poor into the program. Persistence of a stable low-user group was another research finding. This may have been a boon to a health organization with income-maximizing goals, but for a plan with social objectives it offered a challenge: how to use the opportunity presented by enrolling the poor to identify and meet needs that they were not themselves bringing to the system. It was established that outreach interventions in an HMO could alter both contact and volume rates for the medically indigent.

This experience with prepaid group practice formed part of a set of efforts to alter utilization by system or context changes. Riessman has reviewed the evidence supporting the efficacy of such changes and concludes that the structural rather than cultural explanation of utilization by the poor is supported.[21] While this conclusion makes for optimism regarding the potential for change, Reissman no longer considers working toward class homogeneity of utilization as a sufficient ideal but hopes to see changes, such as midwife deliveries, in the prevailing medical culture.

## UNNECESSARY SERVICES

The opening of doors to medical care—whether fully or only partially—came with incentives to provide more services; and concern over unnecessary services as a threat to the financial equilibrium of programs and a possible risk to health followed rather quickly. Research

on utilization of unnecessary services has followed two main tracks. One is the study of inter-area variations in rates of performance of surgery and in hospital use. Wennberg's work has delved extensively into this. He has noted that the variation was greater for conditions where there was less consensus on criteria for a firm diagnosis and for the treatment of choice. The inter-area variations for given procedures were associated with economic factors. While there was a strong implication of need to achieve greater convergence in physical knowledge and behavior,[22] it did not follow that the lowest rates were best. Differences shown in interregional comparisons of length of stay and hospital discharge rates under Medicare for specific diagnoses are suggestive of both under- and over-use.[23]

The other track for research on unnecessary care has been study of physician-induced demand. Much controversy was engendered by apparent demonstrations that quantity of services received per capita could not be explained by standard economic variables and the conclusion that was drawn from this—that physicians were able to control demand. As the focus of the argument shifted from doctors choosing interesting cases and preferring leisure to revenue, to doctors doing and earning too much, the theory was used to predict that increasing physician supply would not solve problems for the health care system but would cause them.

Several economists have been critical of both the conceptual and the empirical work of the promulgators of physician-induced demand.[24] The low information level of consumers is a theoretical precondition of willingness to go along with physicians' plans for more service, but Hay and Leahy found that medical families—presumably well informed—have a higher visit rate,[25] and Bunlar and Brown earlier found them to have a higher operative rate. Hay and Leahy also note that a statistical relation of physician density to physician-initiated visits may not show inappropriate services but may reflect the clustering of sicker patients around medical centers, the quality of care rendered by physicians in high-density areas, and the desire of physicians to locate where their services will be in demand. Wilensky and Rossiter used 1977 NMCES data to study physician-initiated ambulatory visits and[26] found that age, sex, and health status—i.e., need factors—are consistently important in explaining the variance, and that insurance and reimbursement are also consistently important. The physician–population ratio affects the chance of having a visit and the number of visits but not the likelihood of surgery. They conclude that our policy concern should be not the adverse effects of adding new medical graduates to our supply of doctors but the reimbursement design that would best keep utilization related to medical need.

# EFFECT OF HMOS

Analysis of utilization under HMOs is therefore critical to national policy. The theoretical model of HMOs reconciles goals of equity and accessibility with cost containment, since this organizational form covers all services including preventive services while avoiding the incentive under fee payment medicine to deliver "services of questionable necessity".[27] The prepaid group practice (PGP) form seems to be the one with the most leverage in these respects.

Luft reports that PGPs do in fact deliver fewer units of medical care per enrollee per year, compared to conventional insurance, largely because of reduced hospitalization. The utilization of 35 percent fewer hospital days per 1,000 enrollees is perhaps the best-known achievement of the PGP, and it is largely attributable to fewer admissions rather than shorter stays. There are no consistent differences in the proportion of surgical admissions that would explain the lighter uses of hospitals by PGP enrollees. HMOs do have an access effect in that there is more likelihood of having at least one physician visit per year. Some HMOs provide more preventive services than does the fee-for-service sector, and the receipt of more services by any group of consumers seems to depend on the range of services provided by the plan in which they are enrolled, whether it is an HMO or a conventional insurance plan.

Luft raises numerous unanswered questions for an HMO research agenda. They concern such matters as the effect of self-selection on utilization and cost outcomes, which HMO practices result in fewer admissions, and the content and true purposes of preventive visits in different settings. His book placed utilization in the context of efficiency, quality, enrollment and disenrollment, and satisfaction. Since costs of inputs are not under management control but are derived from the total economy, HMO ability to influence costs of care is dependent on ability to reduce utilization, especially of more expensive services.

# COST-SHARING

The effects of cost-sharing on utilization have been under scrutiny by a number of researchers. Most recently, Manning et al. have reported on a controlled trial of the effect of cost-sharing in prepaid group practice and in fee-for-service care. Group Health Cooperative (GHC) of Puget Sound was the PGP in the study.[28] Their study shows that GHC enrollees had 40 percent less hospitalization than fee-for-service (FFS) groups. This was not explained by the larger volume of preventive visits, which were largely well-child care and gynecological examinations unrelated to admissions; moreover,

FFS cost-sharing plans also had low admission rates despite having fewer preventive visits than GHC. Different reasons may explain the low rates in the different types of plans; as outpatient visits were the same for GHC and the free FFS group, ambulatory management of cases as a substitute for hospitalization is not an obvious explanation. While some mysteries remain, Enthoven[29] underscores the fact that the lower hospital use rate attributable to the set of practices referred to by Manning et al. as a "less hospital-intensive" style of care is not dependent on self-selection of health people into PGPs.

The other notable finding is that cost-sharing has reduced the percentage of enrollees seeking care and has had a marked effect on the volume of preventive visits (a measure that excludes prenatal care and vision and hearing services). The individual deductible group has .27 visits per person annually compared to .55 for the GHC experimental group. Proposals for cost-sharing as a solution to rising costs of Medicare should be evaluated in terms of effects on preventive services as well as access of the elderly poor to both ambulatory and hospital care.

# SEX

In Andersen's model of utilization, sex is an immutable factor. This means that unlike the price of care or the availability of physicians it is not likely to change in response to policy initiatives. The immutable designation leaves open the question of whether being female implies the need for a set of biologically related services or possession of a set of behavioral characteristics that are not captured in attitudes toward health represented in the model. Indeed, the attitude items are sex-neutral and would not capture beliefs about prenatal care, seriousness of female organ symptoms, and rating of contraceptive methods, or the frame of reference for decisions about health care of children.

While immutability is a rather strong block to inquiry, interest in gender did flower in utilization research. Verbrugge[30] posed the paradox that, despite a lower mortality rate, women reported more acute illnesses and used physician services by visit or telephone more often than men. Patient-oriented explanations by Verbrugge and others focused on sex differences in the response to illness. Women were hypothesized to be socialized toward ready acknowledgement of illness and toward seeking help, in conformity with dependency and with being in touch with their body signals. In contrast, sterner demands are placed on men for economic performance, and stoic denial would be a learned male stance toward illness. It was even argued that the sick role would appeal to persons of low social status, i.e., women.[1] However, the data themselves were suspected of gender bias.

Women might be more likely than men to recall their own illness-related events and more willing to report them, while in their capacity as informants concerning men, they might wish to minimize threats to family security or, indeed, not have been informed of husbands' conditions and care.

Other explanations focusing on the doctor as actor began to emerge as medical treatment began to be perceived as a form of male power. The influence of sex differences on services received, follow-up visits recommended, and prescribing of psychotropic drugs was reported.[31] At times, attitudes of doctors resulted in reduced utilization by women, as, for instance, when discomfort in pregnancy and other female complaints were attributed to psychogenic causes, and when medication replaced diagnostic investigation of presenting complaints. Among older persons, 60+ years, Haug finds that females are more likely to be underutilizers for serious complaints.[32]

Interaction between physician and patient is a likely model for explaining sex differences in utilization; in addition, the employment status of women should be taken into account. Hibbard and Pope have reported that the stereotype of greater female willingness to adopt the sick role when ill is not confirmed, but that women's perception of symptoms and interest in and concern with health are greater than men's and contribute to sex differences in utilization.[33] Readiness to adopt the sick role is not a factor in utilization for women with heavier role responsibilities, and in this they resemble men.

Muller has shown both similarities and differences in response of utilization by working men and women when confronted with marital dissolution, family illness, and being a single parent. Working men are more affected by a sick spouse than a sick child, and working men are more affected by a sick spouse than are working women.[34]

## THE GENDER AGENDA

Gender-related research has many tasks to address. First, the rise of single-parent families, the persistence of low-wage jobs for women with limited employer coverage for health benefits, and the loss of spouse-based benefits after divorce make it necessary for those concerned with equity to study the effects of the financial status of women in these familial and economic categories on their utilization of health care in the absence of a national health insurance system. Even if we were to achieve a universal scheme, effects of family- and job-related rules of eligibility, often drafted in previous proposals with male householders in mind, would have to be monitored. Meanwhile, and this is the second area, the rise of two-earner households has altered the meaning of private coverage. A spurious decline in the Blue Cross admission rate, due partly to duplication of cov-

erage and partly to the family size assumption used which affected the denominator for calculating use rates, led to excessive joy over effectiveness of cost-control efforts. [35,36] In current families, a husband and wife with two different kinds of coverage could have access both to comprehensive care and to second opinions and out-of-plan doctors. Utilization could take on different patterns given coverage choices, the value of time, and the demand for health in two-earner families. Today there are 23.2 million married-couple families with an employed wife. As their median income is $29,866, and as they make up well over half of the families with over $25,000,[37] analysis of utilization by income level should be disaggregated by wife's employment status to give a clearer picture.

Third, access to reproductive health services has been placed in question because of a combination of fiscal cutbacks with negative religious/political responses both to abortion and to contraceptive services. In the last decade, late abortion and out-of-state travel for abortion were reduced by legalization. Our concern with utilization as a measure of the impact of policies on health care should extend to all fertility-related services.

Fourth, awareness of the content and possible significance of female responsibilities and status should infuse utilization research that is not specifically focused on sex differences. Newachek and Butler,[38] studying utilization of care for chronic illness by the poor, omitted a breakdown of the chronically ill by sex—or age—thus missing differences in severity that might have led to interesting perceptions. Colle and Grossman,[39] following Andersen, put knowledge of signs of disease and taste for medical care into the set of variables used to analyze utilization of pediatric care, but the specific items asked had little to do with mothers' perceptions of danger signals for children or with the context of their rating of the value of child health services. As it turned out, the results for these two variables were insignificant or mixed.

## CULTURE

The relation of culture to utilization is an underdeveloped area of research. Qualitative studies of particular ethnic subgroups have been conducted separately and by investigators with different backgrounds from those focusing on quantitative studies using large national— or even smaller local—databases. The quantitative researchers have been incorporating attitudes and beliefs into decision models but rarely have they related these to ethnic cultures. They have also omitted interaction of practitioners and patients from two different cultures— the culture of medical care and that of the patient's family of origin. Moreover, the interplay of modernization and adaptation factors with traditional factors is not fully addressed. Information gaps on migrants and on changes in traditional behavior as new economic opportunities undercut the ecology of belief systems have not been widely incorporated into the thinking of the mainstream quantitative researchers.

The concept of utilization often implies that nonutilization of conventional care is a form of nonaction. Instead, it is a heterogeneous residual in which use of alternative healers is a definite and often preferred option for certain kinds of illness. And the fact that the United States continues to be a receiver for Asian, Hispanic, and East European migrant flows warns us that the implications of culture for health care will continue.

We should also be sensitized to the cultural changes in our majority population that influence the purposes served by medical care and expectations brought to the encounter as well as manifestations of ill health. These are exemplified but not exhausted by the gender theme. We should consider, for instance, product-related injuries as an important cause of emergency care. Stress on modernity and the probability of exposure to a diversity of products whose risks people are not familiar with, as well as salience of risk in people's decisions, are cultural features.

## CONCLUSION

Limitations of the collective utilization research endeavor come from several sources. Individual researchers' preferences and beliefs as well as prevailing cultural biases are reflected in the questions posed, the data sets employed, the selection and definition of variables, and the relationships hopefully asserted even when statistical significance is not obtained. Alternative explanations exist for some of the results that have been found, because the obtainable variable is only an approximation of some ideal variable in the author's model. Political forces may influence the kind of research questions that find support in a given year. The economist's orientation provides considerable power in dealing with substitution and other economic phenomena and, following Grossman, in placing the market for medical care in the context of the demand for health and the health production function.[40] The sociologist's orientation allows for the consideration of health beliefs as well as access factors. In actual empirical work, researchers from different backgrounds use many of the same variables and encounter similar difficulties. The debates over cost-sharing, unnecessary services and physician behavior, equity attainment, and the achievements of HMOs are indicative of this; but they also offer a basis for believing that flawed research can be identified and corrected. Sometimes this depends on creation of a better variable by a national data system as in the case of physician-initiated visits. Hence, we need to maintain and develop our data systems.

Our understanding of the utilization of health care based on past research needs to be brought in touch with social changes. To take just one example: under current budget constrains, public agencies delivering health care must look for all possible revenues and are thus more likely to use their capacities for sponsored clients rather than for no-pay patients at the low end of the sliding scale. Research skills can be used to assess the impact of such changes in agency practice on utilization and access.

Note—I am indebted to Marianne C. Fahs for sharing her literature review on women with me.

## References

1. Andersen, R. *A Behavioral Model of Families' Use of Health Services.* Research Series 25, University of Chicago, Center for Health Administration Studies, 1968.
2. Aday, L., R. Andersen, and G. V. Fleming. *Health Care in the United States, Equitable for Whom?* Denver: Sage Publications, Inc., 1980.
3. Steinmetz, N., and J. R. Hoey. Hospital emergency room utilization in Montreal before and after Medicare: The Quebec experience. *Medical Care* 16(2):133–39, February 1978.
4. Davidson, S. M. Understanding the growth of emergency department utilization. *Medical Care* 16(2):122–32, February 1978.
5. McCall, N. Utilization and costs of Medicare services by beneficiaries in their last year of life. *Medical Care* 22(4):329–42, April 1984.
6. Singer, D. E., et al. Rationing intensive care—physician response to a resource shortage. *New England Journal of Medicine* 309(19):1155–60, November 10, 1983.
7. National Center for Health Statistics. Health—United States and Prevention Profile 1983. Department of Health and Human Services, Publication No. (PHS)4–1232. Washington, DC: Government Printing Office, December 1983.
8. Davis, K., and L. B. Russell. The substitution of hospital outpatient care for inpatient care. *The Review of Economics and Statistics* 54(2):109–20, May 1972.
9. Inman, S. R., and I. R. Lawsen. Utilization of specialized ambulatory care by the elderly, a study of a clinic. *Medical Care* 20(3):331–38, March 1982.
10. Diehr, P., et al. Ambulatory mental health services utilization in three provider plans. *Medical Care* 22(1):1–13, January 1984.
11. Viseltear, A. J. Emergence of the medical care section of the American Public Health Association. *American Journal of Public Health* 63(1):986–1007, November 1973.
12. Inglehart, J. K. Federal policies and the poor. *New England Journal of Medicine* 307(13):836–40, September 23, 1982.
13. Broyles, R. W., et al. The use of physician services under a national health insurance scheme, an examination of the Canada Health Survey. *Medical Care* 21(11):1037–54, November 1983.
14. National Center for Health Statistics and National Center

for Health Services Research. *Health United States 1976–1977* Department of Health, Education and Welfare, Publication No. (HRA)77–1232. Washington, DC: Government Printing Office, 1977.

15. Kleinman, J. C., M. Gold, and D. Makuc. Use of ambulatory medical care by the poor, another look at equity. *Medical Care* 19(10):1011–29, October 1981.

16. Wolfe, B. L. Children's utilization of medical care. *Medical Care* 18(12):1196–1207, December 1980.

17. *Statistical Abstract of the United States, 1984.* Washington DC: U.S. Bureau of the Census, 1984, p. 473.

18. Orr, S. T., and C. A. Miller. Utilization of health services by poor children since advent of Medicaid. *Medical Care* 19(6):583–90, June 1981.

19. Greenlick, M. R., et al. Comparing the use of medical care services by a medically indigent and a general membership population in a comprehensive prepaid group practice program. *Medical Care* 10(3):187–200, May-June 1972.

20. Mullooly, J. P., and D. K. Freeborn. The effect of length of membership upon the utilization of ambulatory care services. *Medical Care* 17(9):922–36, September 1979.

21. Riessman, C. K. The use of health services by the poor: Are there any promising models? *Social Policy* 14(4):30–40, Spring 1984.

22. Wennberg, J. E., K. McPherson, and P. Caper. Will payment based on diagnosis-related groups control hospital costs? *New England Journal of Medicine* 311(5):295–300, August 2, 1984.

23. Gornick, M. Trends and regional variations in hospital use under Medicare. *Health Care Financing Review* 3(3):41–73, March 1982.

24. Public Health Service, Bureau of Health Manpower. The Target Income Hypothesis and Related Issues in Health Manpower Policy. U.S. Department of Health, Education and Welfare, Publication No. (HRA)80–27. Washington, DC: Government Printing Office, January 1980.

25. Hay, J., and M. Leahy. Physician-induced demand: An empirical analysis of the consumer information gap. *Journal of Health Economics* 1(3):231–44, December 1982.

26. Wilensky, G. R., and L. F. Rossiter. The relative importance of physician-induced demand in the demand for medical care. *Health and Society* 61(2):252–77, 1983.

27. Luft, H. S. *Health Maintenance Organizations: Dimensions of Performance.* New York: John Wiley and Sons, 1981.

28. Manning, W. G., et al. A controlled trial of the effect of a prepaid group practice on use of services. *New England Journal of Medicine* 310(23):1505–10, June 7, 1984.

29. Enthoven, A. C. The Rand experiment and economical health care. *New England Journal of Medicine* 310(23):1528–30, June 7, 1984.

30. Verbrugge, L. Sex differentials in health. *Public Health Reports* 97(5):417–37, September–October 1982.

31. Verbrugge, L., and R. P. Steiner. Physician treatment of men and women patients, sex bias or appropriate care? *Medical Care* 19(6):609–32, June 1981.

32. Haug, M. R. Age and medical care utilization patterns. *Journal of Gerontology* 36(1):103–11, January 1981.

33. Hibbard, J. H., and C. R. Pope. Gender roles, illness orientation and use of medical services. *Social Science and Medicine* 17(3):129–37, 1983.

34. Muller, C. Health and Health Care of Working Women, Blue Cross/Blue Shield of Greater New York, 1984.

35. Lerner, M. P., et al. The decline in the Blue Cross plan admission rate: Four explanations. *Inquiry* 20(2):103–13, Summer 1983.

36. Luft, H. S., Diverging trends in hospitalization: Fact or artifact? *Medical Care* 19(10):979–94, October 1981.

37. *Statistical Abstract of the United States, 1984.* Washington, DC: U.S. Bureau of the Census, 1984, p. 466.

38. Newachek, P. W., and L. H. Butler. Patterns of physician use among low-income, chronically ill persons. *Medical Care* 21(10):981–89, October 1983.

39. Colle, A. D., and M. Grossman. *Determinants of Pediatric Care Utilization.* NBER Reprint No. 14. Washington, DC: National Bureau of Economic Research, Inc., 1978.

40. Hadley, J. *More Medical Care: Better Health?* Washington, DC: The Urban Institute, 1982, p. 22.

# Chapter 4

# Variations in the Use of Medical and Surgical Services by the Medicare Population

Mark R. Chassin, M.D., M.P.P., M.P.H.; Robert H. Brook, M.D., Sc.D.; R.E. Park, Ph.D.; Joan Keesey; Arlene Fink, Ph.D.; Jacqueline Kosecoff, Ph.D.; Katherine Kahn, M.D.; Nancy Merrick, M.D.; and David H. Solomon, M.D.

**Abstract**  We measured geographic differences in the use of medical and surgical services during 1981 by Medicare beneficiaries (age ⩾65) in 13 large areas of the United States. The average number of Medicare beneficiaries per site was 340,000. We found large and significant differences in the use of services provided by all medical and surgical specialties. Of 123 procedures studied, 67 showed at least threefold differences between sites with the highest and lowest rates of use. Use rates were not consistently high in one site, but rates for procedures used to diagnose and treat a specific disease varied together, as did alternative treatments for the same condition.

These results cannot be explained by the actions of a small number of physicians. We do not know whether physicians in high-use areas performed too many procedures, whether physicians in low-use areas performed too few, or whether neither or both of these explanations are accurate. However, we do know that the differences are too large to ignore and that unless they are understood at a clinical level, uninformed policy decisions that have adverse effects on the health of the elderly may be made. (*N Engl J Med* 1986; 314:285–90.)

Nearly 50 years have passed since Glover reported a 10–fold difference in tonsillectomy rates among various geographic areas in England.[1] Since then, other researches have documented similar variations in hospital admissions, lengths of stay, and specific surgical procedures in many parts of the developed world.[2–24] Virtually all these studies, however, have been limited to a few procedures, to small geographic areas, or to foreign locations. In the United States, most work on variations has analyzed care provided in small hospital-service areas in three rural northeastern states.

The purpose of this paper is twofold. We will first present, for 18 percent of the population throughout the United States that is eligible for Medicare, age- and sex-adjusted population-based data on the use of selected specific medical and surgical services. We will also discuss the use of these data in establishing policies on health care.

## METHODS

To develop population-based use rates, we obtained a complete file of physician claims for the calendar year

Reprinted with permission from Mark R. Chassin, M.D., M.P.P.; Robert H. Brook, M.D., Sc.D.; R.E. Park, Ph.D.; Joan Keesey; Arlene Fink, Ph.D.; Jacqueline Kosecoff, Ph.D.; Katherine Kahn, M.D.; Nancy Merrick, M.D.; and David H. Solomon, M.D., Variations in the Use of Medical and Surgical Services by the Medicare Population, *The New England Journal of Medicine,* Vol. 314 No. 5, pp. 285–290, 1986. Supported in part by grants from the Commonwealth Fund (6137), The John A. Hartford Foundation (83172–2H), The Pew Memorial Trust (Glenmede Trust), and the Robert Wood Johnson Foundation (7309). The opinions, conclusions, and proposals in the text are those of the authors and do not necessarily represent the views of any of these Foundations or of The Rand Corporation.

1981 from the Medicare part B insurance carriers in Arkansas, Colorado, Iowa, Massachusetts, Montana, Pennsylvania, South Carolina, and northern California. These sites were selected because they represented the diversity of the population eligible for Medicare and of the medical system; they contained populations that did not often leave their own areas to obtain medical care; and their insurance carriers used sophisticated systems to process claims. All carriers also provided demographic data on patients from their eligibility files and data on physician specialty from their provider files.

The files of physician claims from these sites contained more than 75 million claims for all services, both inpatient and ambulatory (office-based), that were billed by physicians for elderly persons eligible for physician services under Medicare part B (97 percent of all elderly persons in all the areas). The only services provided to this population that were not reflected in those files were those rendered by the small number of salaried, hospital-based physicians whose services are not billed directly to Medicare part B—mainly hospital-based pathologists, although there were some anesthesiologists and radiologists.

We defined clinical procedures that were consistent across the different coding systems used by the eight insurance companies by combining detailed procedure codes into aggregates. For example, one carrier used six codes to describe various inguinal herniorrhaphies and another used five; we incorporated all these variations into a single procedure group. In this way, we derived 153 procedure groups, which together accounted for 87 percent of total physician charges under Medicare part B and which included all procedures that accounted for at least 0.1 percent of those charges.

We edited the data to ensure that even though bills from two or more physicians were received for a procedure, the procedure performed by them jointly was counted only once. We excluded claims from anesthesiologists and assistant surgeons and, when appropriate, counted a specific procedure performed on the same patient on the same day only once. Claims that were denied by the carrier and carrier adjustments to claims were not counted as separate procedures. To make the populations in the separate sites as comparable as possible, we excluded Medicare beneficiaries under the age of 65 (those eligible to receive Medicare benefits because of various disabilities, including chronic renal disease).

We report here the frequency with which physicians practicing in each of the 13 sites provided services to Medicare part B enrollees who resided in that site. On the basis of studies of the origins of Medicare patients[25] that delineate patterns of migration to obtain hospital care, we divided both northern California and Pennsylvania into three smaller areas and Massachusetts into two smaller areas. The boundaries were drawn so as to minimize the number of patients who crossed borders to receive hospital care.[26] We excluded claims for patients residing outside an area who came into it for services, primarily because we could not measure the population at risk from which these patients were drawn. We also excluded services performed for residents of an area by physicians practicing outside that area, because such services did not directly reflect medical practice within given areas, which was the primary focus of our study.

Using Medicare data,[25] we determined the proportion of hospitalized patients residing in each of our sites who received their hospital care outside the site. This proportion was small; it accounted for 10 percent in three sites, 6 to 8 percent in five sites, and 3 to 5 percent in five sites.

The denominator for calculating the rates for use of procedures was the number of persons 65 years of age or older eligible for Medicare part B who resided in each area. We adjusted the rates for age and sex differences among the 13 sites by calculating specific use rates for age and sex subgroups and applying these rates to a standard population distribution (the population of the United States that was over 65 in 1980). It should be noted, however, that the age and sex distributions among Medicare beneficiaries who were 65 or older in the 13 sites were similar enough so that this adjustment did not substantially change the unadjusted rate of any site.

We tested the statistical significance of the differences in rates across sites by use of a chi-square test. The null hypothesis was that the rate at each site was equal to the standardized rate for all the sites combined. The test statistic was compared with the critical value of chi-square with $S - 1$ degree of freedom (where $S$ = number of sites compared) to determine whether the observed differences in rates across sites were statistically significant.[26]

## RESULTS

Selected characteristics of the 13 sites are shown in Table 1. These sites which have an average Medicare population of 340,000, encompass a wide spectrum of geographic location and physician availability. If there are variations in the use of medical services in large populations—i.e., variations that are not produced by the behavior of a few physicians or groups of physicians—they should appear in these data.

Table 2 summarizes the variations among the 13 sites in the rates of use of 30 selected medical and surgical services. For each procedure, we present the highest, the mean, and the lowest age- and sex-adjusted rates. The mean rate is the total number of procedures performed in all sites, divided by the total number of beneficiaries of Medicare part B in all sites, adjusted for age

Table 1. Selected Characteristics of Geographic Sites.

| Site | 1981 Medicare Part B Enrollees | Physicians per 1000 Enrollees* | Enrollees per Square Mile |
|---|---|---|---|
| Arkansas | 296,000 | 9.9 | 6 |
| Coastal Calif. | 671,000 | 27.8 | 21 |
| Northern Calif. | 178,000 | 18.9 | 5 |
| Valley Calif. | 127,000 | 14.9 | 6 |
| Colorado | 236,000 | 25.4 | 2 |
| Iowa | 381,000 | 10.1 | 7 |
| Western Mass. | 182,000 | 15.7 | 43 |
| Eastern Mass. | 513,000 | 26.3 | 145 |
| Montana | 83,000 | 13.2 | 1 |
| Western Pa. | 549,000 | 12.6 | 26 |
| Central Pa. | 497,000 | 11.6 | 23 |
| Philadelphia | 437,000 | 24.4 | 201 |
| South Carolina | 270,000 | 16.1 | 9 |

*Source: American Medical Association.[27]

and sex. Table 2 also shows two summary measures of variation in the use rates. The ratio of the highest to the lowest rate has been widely used in previous studies and is not without interest, despite its statistical instability and unreliability. The more statistically appropriate coefficient of variation (standard deviation divided by the mean) is also presented. The standard deviation that we used in calculating the coefficient of variation was weighted to account for the unequal size of the 13 sites. Data from all 13 sites on all 123 procedures, including the precise definitions of procedure groups, are available elsewhere.[26] Laboratory procedures are excluded because of their high degree of incomplete representation in part B claims.

The data presented in Table 2 show large variations in use rates. Statistically, the probability that these dif-

Table 2. Rates of Use of Selected Medical and Surgical Procedures in 13 Sites by Medicare Beneficiaries 65 Years Old or Older during 1981.*

| Procedure | Rate of Use | | | Coefficient of Variation | Highest/Lowest Rate Ratio |
|---|---|---|---|---|---|
| | High | Mean | Low | | |
| | *per 10,000 beneficiaries* | | | | |
| **Greatest variation among sites** | | | | | |
| Injection of hemorrhoids | 17 | 7 | 0.7 | 0.79 | 26.0 |
| Hip arthroplasty (not total hip) | 18 | 9 | 2 | 0.69 | 11.4 |
| Destruction of benign skin lesion | 750 | 360 | 94 | 0.67 | 8.0 |
| Arthrocentesis | 1100 | 390 | 120 | 0.66 | 8.8 |
| Skin biopsy | 190 | 95 | 41 | 0.58 | 4.8 |
| Humeral fracture repair | 21 | 13 | 3 | 0.51 | 7.9 |
| Total knee replacement | 20 | 9 | 3 | 0.47 | 6.0 |
| Lumbar sympathectomy | 4 | 2 | 0.9 | 0.44 | 4.0 |
| Mediastinoscopy | 7 | 3 | 1 | 0.42 | 6.7 |
| Coronary-artery bypass surgery | 23 | 13 | 7 | 0.41 | 3.1 |
| **Moderate variation among sites** | | | | | |
| Carotid endarterectomy | 23 | 14 | 6 | 0.39 | 4.0 |
| Hiatus hernia repair | 5 | 2 | 0.8 | 0.38 | 5.9 |
| Excision of malignant skin lesion | 260 | 150 | 77 | 0.37 | 3.3 |
| Endoscopic retrograde cholangiopancreatography | 6 | 4 | 0.3 | 0.32 | 17.2 |
| Coronary angiography | 51 | 33 | 22 | 0.32 | 2.3 |
| Excision of benign breast lesion | 21 | 13 | 9 | 0.31 | 2.2 |
| Craniotomy | 8 | 5 | 3 | 0.31 | 2.6 |
| Total hip replacement | 24 | 15 | 8 | 0.31 | 3.0 |
| Arterial grafts of lower extremities | 19 | 13 | 6 | 0.28 | 3.5 |
| Colles' fracture repair | 34 | 26 | 15 | 0.25 | 2.3 |
| **Least variation among sites** | | | | | |
| Bronchoscopy | 78 | 50 | 35 | 0.21 | 2.2 |
| Appendectomy | 5 | 3 | 2 | 0.19 | 2.2 |
| Abdominal aortic aneurysm repair | 10 | 7 | 5 | 0.17 | 2.2 |
| Mastectomy | 21 | 17 | 8 | 0.17 | 2.7 |
| Diagnostic upper gastrointestinal endoscopy | 150 | 120 | 94 | 0.16 | 1.6 |
| Colectomy | 42 | 33 | 24 | 0.15 | 1.8 |
| Cholecystectomy | 52 | 41 | 34 | 0.14 | 1.6 |
| Prostatectomy | 97 | 82 | 57 | 0.12 | 1.7 |
| Lens extraction | 180 | 140 | 120 | 0.11 | 1.5 |
| Inguinal hernia repair | 53 | 45 | 38 | 0.10 | 1.4 |

*Rates are adjusted for age and sex. Chi-square tests are significant for all procedures at the 0.001 level. Rates greater than nine are rounded to two significant figures. Ratios and coefficients of variation are calculated from raw data.

Table 3. Rates of Use of Selected Cardiovascular Procedures by Medicare Beneficiaries 65 Years Old or Older during 1981.

| PROCEDURE | SITE* | | | | | | | | | | | | | MEAN |
|---|---|---|---|---|---|---|---|---|---|---|---|---|---|---|
| | A | B | C | D | E | F | G | H | I | J | K | L | M | |
| | rate per 10,000 beneficiaries ‡ | | | | | | | | | | | | | |
| Coronary-artery bypass | 15 | 14 | 15 | 9 | 7 | 9 | 10 | 11 | 16 | 8 | 16 | 19 | 23 | 13 |
| Coronary angiography | 39 | 37 | 38 | 23 | NA† | 26 | 26 | NA† | 51 | 22 | 33 | 41 | 50 | 33 |
| Electrocardiographic stress test | 148 | 94 | 77 | 49 | 46 | 43 | 69 | 62 | 182 | 63 | 57 | 141 | 99 | 75 |
| Implantation of transvenous pacemakers | 49 | 47 | 52 | 64 | 59 | 53 | 50 | 58 | 48 | 41 | 22 | 44 | 50 | 50 |
| Carotid endarterectomy | 11 | 14 | 20 | 6 | 11 | 10 | 12 | 12 | 20 | 9 | 16 | 15 | 23 | 14 |

*Sites are not necessarily given in the order in which they appear in Table 1.

†NA denotes data not available because procedure codes used in that site were nonspecific.

‡Adjusted for age and sex.

ferences were due to chance alone is very small—less than 0.001 in each case. Of 123 procedures studied, 76 had coefficients of variation greater than 0.30, and 67 had at least threefold differences between the highest and lowest rates. When we divided 117 procedures (physician visits were excluded) into 67 surgical procedures and 50 nonsurgical procedures, we found that the average coefficient of variation (0.44) for the nonsurgical procedures was greater ($P<0.001$) than that for the surgical procedures (0.31).

Tables 3 and 4 present the rates of use of selected cardiovascular and gastrointestinal procedures in all 13 sites. Several observations emerge from examination of these data. First, the differences summarized in Table 2 were not produced simply by one or two atypical sites: rather, for almost all the procedures, there was a distribution of rates that spanned the range between the sites with the highest rates of use and those with the lowest rates. Second, individual sites did not exhibit the highest or lowest rates with any degree of consistency. Instead, the same site often had a high rate for one procedure

and a low rate for another. For example, site D (Table 3) had low rates of use of coronary-artery bypass surgery and coronary angiography but the highest rate of transvenous pacemaker implantation. Similar examples can be seen in Table 4. We also observed these patterns in many other procedures.[26]

Third, the use of procedures employed to diagnose and treat the same disorder usually varied together. For example, the first three procedures listed in Table 3—electrocardiographic stress testing, coronary angiography, and coronary-artery bypass surgery—are all used primarily in the diagnosis or treatment of ischemic heart disease. Thus, geographic areas with high rates of coronary-artery bypass surgery generally also had high rates of the related diagnostic procedures, and vice versa. The same was true for cholecystography and cholecystectomy (Table 4). We found similar patterns for other combinations of diagnostic and therapeutic procedures, including colonoscopy and colectomy and skin biopsy and excision of a malignant skin lesion.[26]

The rates of use of procedures that can be employed

Table 4. Rates of Use of Selected Gastrointestinal Procedures by Medicare Beneficiaries 65 Years Old or Older during 1981.

| PROCEDURE | SITE* | | | | | | | | | | | | | MEAN |
|---|---|---|---|---|---|---|---|---|---|---|---|---|---|---|
| | A | B | C | D | E | F | G | H | I | J | K | L | M | |
| | rate per 10,000 beneficiaries † | | | | | | | | | | | | | |
| Diagnostic upper endoscopy | 149 | 153 | 100 | 144 | 100 | 139 | 129 | 111 | 94 | 117 | 114 | 107 | 102 | 122 |
| Colonoscopy | 62 | 70 | 81 | 104 | 71 | 72 | 95 | 84 | 43 | 50 | 76 | 52 | 70 | 76 |
| Oral cholecystography | 197 | 307 | 142 | 74 | 131 | 78 | 67 | 127 | 123 | 212 | 75 | 185 | 83 | 120 |
| Cholecystectomy | 48 | 50 | 37 | 36 | 40 | 40 | 43 | 40 | 45 | 42 | 52 | 50 | 34 | 41 |
| Hemorrhoidectomy | 21 | 13 | 16 | 31 | 17 | 23 | 17 | 15 | 18 | 13 | 17 | 20 | 20 | 19 |
| Injection of hemorrhoids | 14 | 8 | 2 | 17 | 2 | 9 | 2 | 1 | 2 | 0.7 | 16 | 4 | 8 | 7 |

*See footnote to Table 3.

†Adjusted for age and sex.

as alternative treatments for the same condition also varied together. Table 4 includes two such procedures— injection of hemorrhoids and hemorrhoidectomy. Geographic differences in the use of either of these procedures might be interpreted as a simple reflection of a preference for one of them by particular communities of physicians. In fact, however, areas with a high rate of use of either of these procedures also had a high rate of use of the other (r = 0.66, P<0.02). Our investigation of another alternative treatment combination—lower-extremity arterial reconstruction and amputation—also revealed the rates of use of these procedures to be positively correlated.[26]

In general, we found no significant relation between rates of use and the proportion of simple or complex procedures. Table 5 shows that neither the percentage of coronary-artery bypass operations in which one vessel was grafted nor the percentage in which more than one vessel was grafted was significantly related to the overall rate of bypass surgery. In fact, the likelihood of receiving more than one graft varied directly with the use rate (r = 0.44, P = 0.16). We expected the opposite result because we had hypothesized that people with less severe disease who required fewer grafts might have a relatively increased chance of undergoing coronary-artery bypass surgery in areas where the procedure had high rates of use.

Using similar reasoning, we looked for correlations between the rates of cholecystectomy and the proportion of cases that included exploration of the common bile duct, the rate of colonoscopy and the proportion of cases in which biopsies or polypectomies were done, and the rates of sigmoidoscopy and the proportion of

Table 5. Relation between Use Rate of Coronary-Artery Bypass Surgery and Number of Grafts Implanted, According to Geographic Site.

| SITE* | RATE PER 100,000† | NUMBER OF GRAFTS | | |
|---|---|---|---|---|
| | | 1 | 2 | ≥3 |
| | | | percent | |
| M | 231 | 12 | 20 | 68 |
| L | 189 | 4 | 22 | 74 |
| I | 164 | 8 | 22 | 70 |
| A | 151 | 7 | 17 | 76 |
| C | 146 | 7 | 11 | 82 |
| B | 139 | 7 | 15 | 78 |
| H | 108 | 18 | 19 | 62 |
| G | 100 | 7 | 19 | 74 |
| F | 87 | 17 | 32 | 51 |
| D | 87 | 12 | 19 | 69 |
| J | 75 | 9 | 11 | 80 |
| E | 74 | 16 | 23 | 60 |

*Site K is excluded because of the use of nonspecific procedure codes.
†Adjusted for age and sex.

those procedures that included biopsies or polypectomies. The correlations were not significant (P>0.05).

There was also no significant relation between use rates and the proportions of procedures done by physicians in particular specialties. Table 6 shows the proportion of patients who had diagnostic upper gastrointestinal endoscopy performed by physicians in various self-designated specialties. The proportion of all endoscopies done by gastroenterologists varied according to site, from 5 to 72 percent. The proportion performed by internists varied from 12 to 65 percent, and that done by general surgeons varied from 4 to 28 percent. There was, however, no relation between the overall rate of use of endoscopy in a site and the proportion of endoscopies performed by physicians in a particular specialty. For instance, the correlation between the rate of use and the

Table 6. Relation between Use Rate and Specialty of Physician Performing Upper Gastrointestinal Endoscopy.

| SITE* | RATE PER 100,000† | SPECIALTY OF PHYSICIAN | | | | | |
|---|---|---|---|---|---|---|---|
| | | GENERAL PRACTICE/ FAMILY PRACTICE | GENERAL SURGERY | INTERNAL MEDICINE | GASTROEN- TEROLOGY | UNSPECIFIED‡ | OTHER SPECIALTY |
| | | | | percent of procedures | | | |
| A | 1495 | 4 | 6 | 61 | 24 | 3 | 2 |
| D | 1435 | 0 | 4 | 19 | 72 | 1 | 4 |
| F | 1386 | 0 | 19 | 22 | 52 | 4 | 3 |
| G | 1292 | 0 | 9 | 18 | 66 | 5 | 2 |
| K | 1141 | 4 | 28 | 26 | 20 | 18 | 4 |
| H | 1107 | 0 | 7 | 23 | 44 | 20 | 6 |
| L | 1065 | 6 | 21 | 65 | 5 | 0 | 3 |
| M | 1021 | 0 | 4 | 32 | 44 | 18 | 3 |
| E | 1003 | 0 | 14 | 15 | 49 | 15 | 6 |
| C | 1002 | 1 | 6 | 28 | 35 | 27 | 3 |
| I | 935 | 0 | 12 | 12 | 52 | 21 | 2 |

*Sites B and J are excluded because of incomplete data on specialty.
†Adjusted for age and sex.
‡Procedures by physicians in group or clinic practice whose specialty was not specified.

percentage of endoscopies performed by gastroenter-ologists was 0.26 (P = 0.45); that between the rate of use and the percentage done by general surgeons was −0.19 (P = 0.57). We found similar results for colon-oscopy, cholecystectomy, coronary angiography, and carotid endarterectomy.[26]

## DISCUSSION

Our data document large geographic variations in the rates of use of many different medical and surgical services by Medicare beneficiaries during 1981. These differences involve procedures performed by physicians in almost all medical and surgical specialties and sub-specialties,[26] in both outpatient and inpatient settings. Because of the large size of the differences observed and of the geographic areas studied, the variations can-not have been due to the behavior of a few physicians or groups of physicians. For instance, if the site with the highest rate of use of upper gastrointestinal endoscopy had had the rate observed in the site with the lowest rate of use of that procedure, more than 1500 fewer proce-dures would have been performed on the elderly Medi-care beneficiaries in that area in 1981. Similarly, if the site with the lowest rate of electrocardiographic stress tests had experienced the rate found in the site with the highest rate of use of that procedure, more than 7000 additional people would have undergone such tests.

A small proportion of patients in each site did receive care elsewhere; 3 to 10 percent were hospitalized outside their areas. However, this low level of migration cannot begin to account for the differences we measured, many of which were 300 percent or greater.[26]

These differences in rates of use by the elderly pop-ulation in large geographic areas are difficult to compare with those found in other studies, because those inves-tigations involved only small geographic areas. For ex-ample, McPherson and his colleagues reported data on seven procedures from small areas of New England, Norway, and England.[18] The coefficients of variation we observed for the six procedures that we and McPherson et al. both studied were similar for hernia repair, appen-dectomy, and cholecystectomy, but were lower for pros-tatectomy, hysterectomy, and hemorrhoidectomy. We would expect to find less variation in our data because we intentionally studied large areas to avoid variations that were due solely to the actions of a few physicians. However, 62 percent of the procedures we studied had a coefficient of variation that was greater than 0.30, a level considered "highly variable" in the study by Mc-Pherson et al.

Studies of variations in small areas have suggested that the degree of variation observed for a particular procedure is linked directly to the degree of medical consensus concerning the indications for its use.[10,18] Our findings are partly consistent with such observations.

For example, the rates for appendectomy and inguinal hernia repair—procedures about which consensus ex-ists—have usually exhibited little variation in other stud-ies, and they followed a similar pattern in our study. However, some procedures for which a clear consensus about use is less well developed (such as bronchoscopy and endoscopy) also showed low variations in rates of use in our study. In addition, the large variations in use that we observed in other procedures (e.g., repair of humeral fracture) were surely not related to a lack of consensus regarding treatment but were presumably due to differences in the occurrence of the condition that required such treatment.

Our data do not provide evidence that variations can be explained by differences in physician preference for alternative procedures to treat the same clinical problem. We were able to study alternative treatment of two con-ditions—hemorrhoids and peripheral vascular disease. In each instance, the rates of use of the two alternative treatments varied together, with a positive correlation.

Our data provide no evidence that physicians in high-use areas perform procedures less appropriately than do those in low-use areas. If that were the case, the rate of use of less complex procedures, such as one-vessel coronary-artery bypasses or colonoscopy without biopsy or polypectomy, might be expected to be higher in high-use areas; however, our data did not reflect such a pattern. Similarly, a correlation might be expected be-tween the specialty of physicians performing a procedure and its rate of use. High rates of use might reflect performance of a procedure by less qualified physicians. Again, this was not the case in our study.

In summary, the available data do not allow us to explain the wide variations we have observed. In addition, we cannot establish the "correct" use rates from these data. For any given procedure, geographic differences may reflect substantial inappropriate overuse in the high-use areas with very little inappropriate use in the low-use areas. On the other hand, the variations may have occurred because physicians in the low-use areas were not providing enough services to those who needed them, whereas those in the high-use areas were meeting legitimate medical needs in an appropriate manner. A third possibility is that the rates of use of procedures were appropriate in both high- and low-use areas and that the differences in rates resulted from differences in the incidence of diseases. Finally, some combination of all three possibilities may have been responsible for our findings.

Whatever the actual explanation for our results, data like these will be employed increasingly by groups such as peer review organizations that are pursuing cost con-tainment. Policy makers seem ready to equate high use with inappropriate use. Such an assumption is both uninformed and dangerous. It is uninformed because at present we have no clinical data that would allow us to judge the difference in appropriateness of the use of any particular procedure between high-use and low-use areas. It is dangerous because such an assumption will surely result in policies that restrict access to care. Thus, if the assumption is wrong, patients will suffer.

Only a concerted effort by the medical community can bring rationality to the debate about geographic differences.[28] In particular, physicians must resolve the thorny issue of how to define appropriateness in both the presence and the absence of clinical studies that define the efficacy of a procedure. Better use of consensus techniques[29] and decision analysis will be necessary to address this question.

The best medical wisdom will be required to determine the indications for which services are provided to patients and to evaluate the appropriateness of performing procedures for these indications. Interpretation of the results of such an effort may be difficult and at times may not favor the medical profession. Nevertheless, if substantial inappropriate overuse of procedures is found, the medical profession will then be in a position to devise a strategy for correcting it. If underuse is demonstrated, the medical profession may constitute the most informed voice in helping to alleviate it. Perhaps this endeavor will lead not only to a fairer reimbursement system for physicians and hospitals but, more important, to one that protects the health of everyone in the United States, especially the elderly.

## References

1. Glover JA. The incidence of tonsillectomy in school children. *Proc R Soc Med* 1938; 31:1219–36.
2. Pearson RJC, Smedby B, Berfenstam R. Logan RFL, Burgess AM Jr, Peterson OL. Hospital caseloads in Liverpool, New England, and Uppsala. *Lancet* 1968; 2:559–66.
3. Bunker JP. Surgical manpower: a comparison of operations and surgeons in the United States and in England and Wales. *N Engl J Med* 1970; 282:135–44.
4. Lewis CE. Variations in the incidence of surgery. *N Engl J Med* 1969; 281:880–4.
5. Bunker JP, Brown BW Jr. The physician-patient as an informed consumer of surgical services. *N Engl J Med* 1974; 290:1051–5.
6. Lembcke PA. Measuring the quality of medical care through vital statistics based on hospital service areas. I. Comparative study of appendectomy rates. *Am J Public Health* 1952; 42:276–86.
7. Wennberg J, Gittelsohn A. Small area variations in health care delivery. *Science* 1973; 182:1102–8.
8. Stockwell H, Vayda E. Variations in surgery in Ontario. *Med Care* 1979; 17:390–6.
9. Lichtner S, Pflanz M. Appendectomy in the Federal Republic of Germany: epidemiology and medical care patterns. *Med Care* 1971; 9:311–30.
10. Vayda E. A comparison of surgical rates in Canada and in England and Wales. *N Engl J Med* 1973; 289:1224–9.
11. Bunker JP, Wennberg JE. Operation rates, mortality statistics and the quality of life. *N Engl J Med* 1973; 289:1249–51.
12. Roos NP, Henteleff PD, Roos LL Jr. A new audit procedure applied to an old question: is the frequency of T&A justified? *Med Care* 1977; 15:1–18.
13. Roos NP, Roos LL Jr, Henteleff PD. Elective surgical rates—do high rates mean lower standards?: tonsillectomy and adenoidectomy in Manitoba. *N Engl J Med* 1977; 297:360–5.
14. LoGerfo JP. Variation in surgical rates: fact vs. fantasy. *N Engl J Med* 1977; 297:387–9.
15. Roos NP, Roos LL. High and low surgical rates: risk factors for area residents. *Am J Public Health* 1981; 71:591–600.
16. Roos NP, Roos LL Jr. Surgical rate variations: do they reflect the health or socioeconomic characteristics of the population? *Med Care* 1982; 20:945–58.
17. Wennberg J, Gittelsohn A. Variations in medical care among small areas. *Sci Am* 1982; 246(4):120–35.
18. McPherson K, Wennberg JE, Hovind OB, Clifford P. Small-area variations in the use of common surgical procedures: an international comparison of New England, England, and Norway. *N Engl J Med* 1982; 307:1310–4.
19. National Center for Health Statistics. Utilization of short-stay hospitals; annual summary for the United States, 1980. (Series 13, No. 64). Hyattsville, Md.: Department of Health and Human Services, March 1982. (DHHS publication no. (PHS)82–1725).
20. Gornick M. Medicare patients: geographic differences in hospital discharge rates and multiple stays. *Soc Secur Bull* 1977; 40:22–41.
21. *Idem.* Trends and regional variations in hospital use under Medicare. *Health Care Financ Rev* 1982; 3(3):41–73.
22. Deacon R, Lubitz J, Gornick M, et al. Analysis of variations in hospital use by Medicare patients in PSRO areas, 1974–1977. *Health Care Financ Rev* 1979; 1(1):79–108.
23. Connell FA, Day RW, LoGerfo JP. Hospitalization of Medicaid children: analysis of small area variations in admission rates. *Am J Public Health* 1981; 71:606–13.
24. Chassin M. Variations in hospital length of stay: their relationship to health outcomes, Washington, D.C.: Government Printing Office, 1983. (Health Technology case study 24. OTA publication no. OTA-HCS-24.)
25. Office of Statistics and Data Management. Medicare patient origin and destination data by PSRO, 1979, Baltimore: Health Care Financing Administration, March 1981.
26. Chassin MR, Brook RH, Park RE, et al. Variations in the use of medical and surgical services by the Medicare population. Santa Monica, Calif.: Rand Corporation (in press).
27. Physical characteristics and distribution in the U.S. Chicago: American Medical Association, 1981.
28. Brook RH, Lohr KN, Chassin MR, Kosecoff J, Fink A, Solomon D. Geographic variations in the use of services; do they have any clinical significance? *Health Affairs* 1984; 3(2):63–73.
29. Fink A, Kosecoff J, Chassin M, Brook RH. Consensus methods: characteristics and guidelines for use. *Am J Public Health* 1984; 74:979–983.

# PART THREE
## Providers of Health Services

This section addresses the role of provider organizations in the health care system, focusing on hospital cost containment, on mental health, and on long-term care services. The first article, by William B. Schwartz and Daniel N. Mendelson, focuses on the hospital and suggests that hospital cost-containment efforts thus far, however successful, will likely not continue in the 1990s. This article suggests that hospital and health care cost pressures will continue to accelerate, raising substantial policy concerns regarding future decision making in the health care system.

Peter Kemper and Christopher M. Murtaugh address the use of nursing home care by examining lifetime risk for nursing home admissions and associated factors. The results of this study suggest the need for enhanced policy analysis and decision making regarding the continuum of long-term care.

Two fine articles addressing issues of mental illness are also included in this section. The first, by Chris Koyanagi and Howard H. Goldman, looks at national approaches and policy regarding the chronically mentally ill and highlights a number of successes as well as presents a number of suggestions for the future. H. Richard Lamb addresses the extremely important issue of the homeless and their need for mental health care. The problems associated with deinstitutionalization and many other complex factors are ably addressed in this second article on mental health services.

# Chapter 5

# Hospital Cost Containment in the 1980s

## Hard Lessons Learned and Prospects for the 1990s

William B. Schwartz, M.D., and Daniel N. Mendelson, M.P.P.

**Abstract** *Background.* A key strategy used to contain hospital costs during the 1980s was to reduce the total number of admissions and average lengths of stay. We assessed the magnitude of the savings achieved, the effect of the reductions on the rate of increase in costs, and the prospects for future savings through reductions in the number of days patients spend in the hospital (inpatient days).

*Methods.* Using data from the American Hospital Association and the Health Care Financing Administration, we calculated the savings in the total number of inpatient days as the deviation from the historical increase in the number of inpatient days per year. We then estimated the real increase in costs that would have been observed if the reduction in the number of inpatient days had not occurred; we defined this value as the "underlying" rate of increase in costs. Finally, we compared the rates of increase in hospital reimbursement for Medicare beneficiaries and patients not covered by Medicare (non-Medicare patients).

*Results.* The total number of inpatient days per year decreased by 28 percent, in aggregate, between 1981 and 1988. The annual reduction was greatest in 1984 and 1985 and became progressively smaller in each subsequent year; by 1988 there was virtually no further reduction in the total number of inpatient days. The brief slowing of the increase in costs in the mid-1980s can be attributed entirely to the reduction in the number of inpatient days per year. The underlying rate of increase in costs was thus unaffected by efforts to contain spending. An increased number of outpatient visits partially offset the savings that resulted from the reduction in the number of inpatient days. This increase persisted even when the savings due to the lower number of inpatient days dwindled, and it virtually eliminated any dollar savings during the latter part of the 1980s. Between 1976 and 1982, Medicare spending on services provided by acute care hospitals rose by 9.2 percent per year in real terms, whereas non-Medicare expenditures rose by only 4.6 percent. This pattern has been reversed in recent years; in 1987–1988, Medicare spending rose by only 0.6 percent per year, whereas non-Medicare spending rose by 9 percent.

*Conclusions.* Our findings suggest that the era of easy reductions in the number of inpatient days, with the associated attenuation of rising costs, is largely over. If further reductions in inpatient days are accompanied by an increase in the amount of ambulatory care similar to that during the past few years, the net savings will probably be negligible. Once the potential savings due to reductions in the number of inappropriate inpatient days has been exhausted, real hospital costs can be expected to rise, unless other effective measures to contain costs are implemented. (*N Engl J Med* 1991;324:1037–42.)

Throughout the 1980s, both the private sector and the federal government energetically attempted to contain the continuing increase in the costs of hospital care.

Reprinted with permission from William B. Schwartz, M.D., and Daniel N. Mendelson, M.P.P., Hospital Cost Containment in the 1980s: Hard Lessons Learned and Prospects for the 1990s, *The New England Journal of Medicine,* Vol. 324 No. 15, pp. 1037–1042, 1991.

A key part of their strategy has been to eliminate unnecessary hospital days and to shift as much care as possible from inpatient to outpatient settings. As a result of these efforts, the annual number of days patients spent in the hospital (inpatient days) fell, and the rate of increase in costs was slowed. On the basis of these findings, many observers believe that further efforts to eliminate inappropriate inpatient days, particularly through the use of new practice guidelines, can solve the problem of rising costs.

In the present study we used published and unpublished data from the American Hospital Association (AHA) and the Health Care Financing Administration (HCFA) to address these issues. First, we assessed the degree to which the total number of inpatient days per year was reduced during the 1980s and the effect of this reduction on the increase in hospital costs. Second, we estimated the rate of increase in costs that would have occurred had there been no reduction in the number of inpatient days. Third, we calculated the increase in hospital costs that should be attributed to the increased use of outpatient services. Fourth, we compared the changes over time in Medicare expenditures and all other (non-Medicare) expenditures for hospital care. Finally, we estimated the potential savings from a further reduction in the total number of inpatient days per year.

## THE NUMBER OF INPATIENT DAYS SAVED

We first examined the cumulative percentage of inpatient days saved during the 1980s. To calculate the savings, we measured the cumulative reduction in the total number of inpatient days per year between 1981, when admission peaked, and 1988, the most recent year for which data were available. The beginning of this period also marked the initiation of major cost-contain-

ment efforts, including prospective payment by Medicare and a variety of efforts in the private sector.

The reduction in the number of inpatient days in community hospitals between 1981 and 1988 was 18.6 percent (Table 1).[1] Although striking in itself, this percentage understates the actual reduction because it does not take into account the fact that the number of inpatient days in acute care hospitals had been increasing in previous years. Between 1976 and 1981, the total number of inpatient days in community hospitals rose at an annual rate of 1.3 percent.[1] About 1 percentage point per year of this increase can be attributed to the growth and aging of the population, with the small remainder accounted for by other factors, such as technological innovation. Because the most important forces responsible for the historical increase in the annual number of inpatient days were acting throughout the 1980s, it is reasonable to assume that without cost-containment efforts the number of inpatient days would have continued to grow at a rate of close to the historical rate.

The total effect of cost-containment programs as a percentage of the number of inpatient days in 1981 could thus be calculated as the difference between the actual cumulative reduction in the number of inpatient days since 1981 and the estimated cumulative increase in inpatient days that would otherwise have occurred during this period. Our calculations indicated that 28.1 percent of inpatient days had been eliminated by 1988 (Table 1). We call this sum the "imputed reduction" in days.

The annual savings in inpatient days, both observed and imputed, is shown in Figure 1. Each year from 1982 through 1985, the percentage of 1981 days saved increased dramatically; the largest savings occurred in 1985, when the imputed savings was 9.1 percent. In each of the following two years, the rate of savings slowed markedly, and by 1988 the imputed reduction in the number of inpatient days was only 1.5 percent.

Table 1. Cumulative Changes in the Number of Inpatient Days per Year and the Contribution of Changes in Admissions and Length of Stay, 1981 through 1988.*

| Category of Change | Admissions | Length of Stay | Inpatient Days |
|---|---|---|---|
| | *percent change* | | |
| Observed | −13.4 | −5.2 | −18.6 |
| Estimated | 10.2 | −0.6 | 9.5 |
| Imputed | −23.6 | −4.6 | −28.1 |

*"Estimated" percentages indicate the change in the number of inpatient days that we estimated would have occurred in the absence of cost-containment efforts. "Imputed" percentages are the deviation of the observed change in the number of days from the historical upward trend — i.e., the algebraic difference between "observed" and "estimated" numbers of days. The percentages listed for admissions and length of stay represent the change in total inpatient days attributable to each of these factors. Because of rounding, the percentages for inpatient days are not always exactly equal to the sum of those for admissions and length of stay.

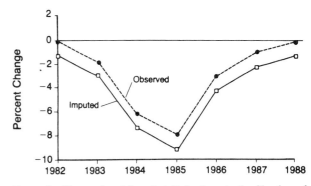

**Figure 1.** Observed and Imputed Reductions in the Number of Inpatient Days per Year, 1982 through 1988.
See the text for an explanation of the calculation of the imputed reduction in inpatient days. The solid circles indicate the observed reduction, and the open squares the imputed reduction.

## Contribution of Changes in the Number of Admissions

The total number of inpatient admissions fell by 13.4 percent between 1981 and 1988 but would have increased by 10.2 percent over this period if the historical trend had persisted (Table 1). The cumulative savings in the number of inpatient admissions during this period was thus 23.6 percent. To calculate the portion of the observed change in the number of inpatient days that was caused by the decrease in the number of inpatient admissions, we multiplied the cumulative change in admissions by the average length of stay over the period from 1981 through 1988 and divided the result by the number of inpatient days in 1981. The estimated reduction was calculated on the basis of the annualized change in the number of admissions from 1976 through 1981.

On an annual basis, the imputed savings in the number of inpatient days that was due to reductions in admissions peaked in 1985, with a reduction of 6.3 percent, and diminished during each subsequent year. Annual figures on the savings in inpatient days attributable to reductions in the number of admissions and the average length of stay are available elsewhere.*

## Contribution of Changes in the Average Length of Stay

About 4.6 percentage points of the reduction in the number of inpatient days was due to reductions in the average length of hospital stays. The observed reduction was 5.2 percent, but on the basis of historical trends, the length of stay would have been expected to drop by 0.6 percentage point without cost-containment efforts (Table 1). To calculate the portion of the change in the number of inpatient days caused by reductions in length of stay, we multiplied the cumulative change in length of stay by the average number of admissions between 1981 and 1988 and divided the result by the average length of stay in 1981. Nearly all of these reductions were achieved in 1984 and 1985, and there were no reductions after 1985. In fact, during subsequent years the average length of stay increased slightly.

## SAVINGS IN INPATIENT DAYS ACCORDING TO SECTOR

There were considerable differences in the savings in inpatient days used by Medicare beneficiaries and patients not covered by Medicare (non-Medicare patients).

*See NAPS document no. 04857 for two pages of supplementary material. Order from NAPS c/o Microfiche Publications, P.O. Box 3513, Grand Central Station, New York, NY 10163–3513. Remit in advance (in U.S. funds only) $7.75 for photocopies or $4 for microfiche. Outside the U.S. and Canada add postage of $4.50 ($1.50 for microfiche postage). There is an invoicing charge of $15 on orders not prepaid. This charge includes purchase order.

To obtain the number of inpatient hospital days used by Medicare beneficiaries, we used unpublished figures on admissions to short-stay acute care hospitals from the HCFA[2] and published figures on the average length of stay for Medicare beneficiaries in short-stay acute care hospitals.[3] The number of inpatient days used by Medicare patients was subtracted from the total number of days used in the United States to obtain data for non-Medicare patients.

Between 1982 and 1988, the number of inpatient days used by Medicare patients was reduced by 20.7 percent from the levels in 1982, the year before cuts began in that sector (Table 2). When we calculated the deviation from the historical upward trend between 1976 and 1982, the cumulative imputed savings in the number of inpatient days used by non-Medicare patients between 1982 and 1988 was only 15.4 percent. Because there was no increase in the number of inpatient days used in the non-Medicare sector between 1976 and 1982, the imputed reduction in the number of days was close to the observed figure (Table 2).

## OBSERVED AND UNDERLYING RATES OF INCREASE IN COSTS

The dramatic reductions in the number of inpatient days per year, documented above, raise a crucial question: Did these efforts have an effect on hospital costs? To answer this question, we first looked at what actually happened to hospital costs during the 1980s. We then estimated the increase in costs that would have occurred in the absence of reductions in the number of inpatient days.

### The Observed Increase in Costs

The annual real increase in community-hospital costs is shown in Figure 2.[1,4] During the five-year period immediately before 1982, the average annual increase in hospital costs was 6.1 percent. In 1982 costs rose by 8.7 percent, but by 1984 the annual increase in costs had fallen to a low of 2.2 percent. It then rose steadily, reaching 7.2 percent by 1988. All dollar figures reported

Table 2. Aggregate Changes in the Number of Inpatient Days Used by Medicare and Non-Medicare Patients between 1982 and 1988.*

| CATEGORY OF CHANGE | MEDICINE | NON-MEDICARE |
|---|---|---|
| | *percent change* | |
| Observed | − 20.7 | − 16.9 |
| Estimated | 20.4 | − 1.5 |
| Imputed | − 41.1 | − 15.4 |

*"Estimated" percentages indicate the change in the number of inpatient days that we estimated would have occurred in the absence of cost-containment efforts. "Imputed" percentages indicate the deviation of the observed change in the number of days from the historical upward trend—i.e., the algebraic difference between "observed" and "estimated" numbers of days. "Non-Medicare" days are defined as the number of hospital days used by patients not covered by Medicare.

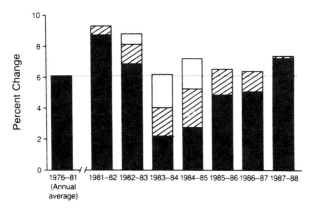

**Figure 2.** Observed and Underlying Annual Increases in Real Hospital Costs, 1976 through 1988.
The solid portion of each bar represents the observed rate of increase. The hatched and open portions represent the real savings due to the reduction in the number of inpatient days; the hatched portion shows the savings that resulted from a reduction in the number of admissions, and the open portion the savings that resulted from a reduction in the average length of stay. The full height of each bar indicates the underlying rate of increase in costs, as described in the text. The dotted line indicates the average annual increase from 1976 to 1981.

here have been adjusted to eliminate the influence of economy-wide inflation.[4]

### The Underlying Rate of Increase in Costs

To what degree can the attenuation in the rate of increase in costs in the mid-1980s be attributed to reductions in the number of inpatient days per year? To answer this question, we estimated the increase in costs that would have occurred if there had been no reduction in inpatient days. We call this value the "underlying" rate of increase in costs. This value was calculated by adding the dollar savings due to the reduced number of inpatient days to the observed increase in costs (Fig. 2).[1,4]

The dollar savings due to reductions in the number of inpatient days was calculated by multiplying the percent reduction in the number of days by an estimate of how much costs are reduced when inpatient days are eliminated. To measure the reduction in days, we used the number of "adjusted patient days"—a figure calculated by the AHA to take into account both inpatient days and outpatient visits. As discussed earlier, we estimated the savings in adjusted patient days as the deviation from the increase between 1976 and 1981. To measure the reduction in costs that resulted from a decrease in the number of hospital days, we started with an estimate of what the typical hospital might expect to save, after adjusting to the new level of occupancy (typically called the "long-run marginal cost"). Pauly and Wilson have estimated that the long-run marginal cost of a hospital day is 90 percent of the average cost[5]; the difference between this value and the average cost is

accounted for by fixed costs (such as those of administration, insurance, and heat), which persist in the face of small reductions in the occupancy rate. There are, however, two factors that probably caused the savings to hospitals to be lower during this period. First, it takes time for hospitals to adjust to operating efficiently after making reductions in the number of patient days. Second, it is possible that the cost of the patient days eliminated during this period was lower than that of the typical marginal hospital day, because the patients may have been less sick than average. For this reason, we assumed that the cost of the days saved was only 65 percent of the average patient day. We thus calculated the savings achieved by the reduction in the number of inpatient days by multiplying the percent reduction in adjusted patient days by 0.65.

The annual savings due to the reduced number of inpatient days is shown as the upper (hatched and open) portions of each bar in Figure 2 (the upper portion is divided into savings from reduced admissions and reduced length of stay). The total height of each bar represents the increase in costs that would have occurred if there had been no reduction in the number of adjusted patient days. In every year between 1982 and 1988, the underlying rate of increase exceeded 6 percent, the real increase in costs between 1976 and 1981. The attenuation of the rate of increase in costs in the mid-1980s can thus be attributed entirely to the reduction in the number of inpatient days.

### The Effect of Outpatient within The Hospital

As the number of inpatient days has fallen, the number of outpatient visits to the hospital has risen. Figure 3 shows the effect of this phenomenon on costs; the reduction in costs due to fewer inpatient days is plotted downward, whereas the offsetting increase in costs from increased visits for ambulatory care is plotted upward. We used annual data from the AHA[1] to calculate the increase in outpatient costs and adjusted for economy-wide inflation as described above.[4] As shown in Figure 3, the increase in costs due to the increase in outpatient visits remained at about 1.2 percentage points per year between 1984 and 1988.

### The Increase in Medicare and Non-Medicare Costs

The pattern of increases in costs for the Medicare and non-Medicare sectors over time has changed remarkably. To assess Medicare spending on hospital care, we obtained unpublished data on actual disbursements to acute care hospitals for inpatient care under Medicare Part A[6,7] and on spending for outpatient care for bene-

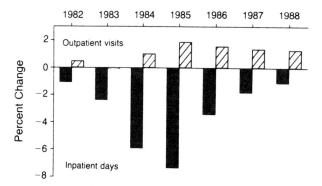

**Figure 3.** Impact on Hospital Costs of Reductions in the Number of Inpatient Days and Increases in the Number of Outpatient Visits, 1982 through 1988.
The solid bars show the reductions in costs due to fewer inpatient days, and the hatched bars the changes in costs due to increased outpatient visits.

ficiaries of Supplementary Medical Insurance (Medicare Part B).[8] We aggregated data on inpatient and outpatient care in order to make our figures compatible with the total expenditures for care at community hospitals reported by the AHA. We used actual disbursements to acute care hospitals rather than the standard time series on Medicare hospital spending published in the HCFA review, because the published data included spending on long-term care hospitals, home care, and other facilities not included in the AHA data.[9]

Table 3 shows the rates of increase in overall spending for hospital services by Medicare and by all payers other than Medicare. Between 1976 and 1982, Medicare expenditures rose by 9.2 percent per year, whereas non-Medicare expenditures rose by 4.6 percent per year. By 1987 and 1988, this pattern had been reversed: Medicare expenditures for hospital services rose by only 0.6 percent per year, whereas non-Medicare spending rose by about 9.0 percent per year.

Table 3. Observed Annual Increases in Real Hospital Costs in the Medicare and Non-Medicare Sectors, 1976 through 1988.*

| YEAR† | MEDICARE | NON-MEDICARE |
|---|---|---|
| | *percent change* | |
| 1976–1981 | 9.2 | 4.6 |
| 1982 | 10.0 | 8.2 |
| 1983 | 5.8 | 7.3 |
| 1984 | 5.0 | 0.8 |
| 1985 | 7.7 | 0.2 |
| 1986 | 3.0 | 5.8 |
| 1987 | −2.3 | 8.7 |
| 1988 | 3.5 | 8.9 |

*These figures include the costs of both inpatient and outpatient care, as explained in the text. Figures for non-Medicare costs were derived by subtracting Medicare costs from total costs.

†The 1976–1981 percentages are the annualized increases during this period. The percentages for 1982 through 1988 are the percent increases from the previous year.

## DISCUSSION

Between 1981 and 1988, a period of intense cost-containment efforts, there was an observed decrease of 19 percent in the total number of inpatient hospital days. This figure understates the real savings, however, because inpatient days have historically been increasing by more than 1 percent annually and would have been expected to continue increasing in the absence of cost-containment efforts. In terms of the deviation from the historical upward trend, we estimated that inpatient days were reduced by more than 28 percent between 1981 and 1988.

The year-by-year pattern of reductions is perhaps of even greater relevance, since it suggests that further savings will be difficult to achieve. After a steady increase in the percentage of days saved through 1985, the fraction of days saved shrank each year, so that by 1988 there was virtually no further savings (Fig. 1). This near-halt in the number of inpatient days saved merits particular attention, because it occurred in the face of continuous expansion of managed care and other initiatives designed to reduce the number of inpatient days overall.

Figure 2 shows the effect of the reduction in inpatient days on the increase in hospital costs. The solid bars, depicting the increase in real costs, indicate that the increase in costs slowed from a historical average of over 6 percent per year to about 2 percent per year by 1985. By 1988, the increase in costs had returned to a level above 6 percent.

A comparison with Figure 1 indicates that it was during the years in which the increase in costs was slowed that the bulk of the savings in the number of inpatient days was realized. The hatched bars quantify this observation by adding to the real increase the estimated additional increase in costs that would have occurred in the absence of reductions in the number of inpatient days.

The full height of each bar in Figure 2 thus represents our estimate of the increase in costs that would have occurred if there had been no reduction in the number of inpatient days. This value, which we call the "underlying" rate of increase in costs, exceeded 6 percent in each year throughout the 1980s. Because in the late 1980s this value was not appreciably different from that in the late 1970s and early 1980s, we conclude that efforts to contain costs did little to limit expenditures beyond decreasing the total number of inpatient days per year. Moreover, it seems likely that the upward pressure on costs will continue in the future, as a result of wage increases required to attract and hold personnel, a wave of expensive new forms of technology, a growing number of patients with the acquired immunodeficiency syndrome, and a new commitment to insurance coverage for the uninsured and underinsured.

Our calculations include only changes in expenditures for acute care in hospitals and do not indicate the overall effect of these changes on system-wide expenditures for health care. When care is transferred to free standing ambulatory care facilities and physicians' offices, the resulting costs partially offset the savings accomplished in hospital-based care. Because there are no readily available measures of care shifted to settings outside the hospital, we have been unable to calculate the net savings to society.

### Prospects for Future Savings in the Number of Inpatient Days

The sharp slowing in the number of inpatient days saved per year (Fig. 1) suggests that a further substantial reduction in inpatient days will be hard to achieve unless new practice guidelines are successfully implemented. We also believe that the data indicate that whatever further reductions are likely to be achieved will have only a limited and transient effect on costs.

To illustrate this point, we estimated the effect on costs of saving a total of 20 percent more inpatient days between 1989 and 1995, for a total reduction of nearly 50 percent of inpatient days since 1981. Assuming that each day eliminated saves 65 percent of the cost of an average day of inpatient care, the increase in expenditures would be reduced by 2 percentage points annually. But because a decrease in the number of inpatient days would almost inevitably be accompanied by an increase in visits for ambulatory care (Fig. 3), a reduction of this magnitude would probably not be observed. If the increase in the number of visits for ambulatory care were equal to that in 1987 and 1988, much or all of the savings from cutbacks in inpatient care would be offset.

Equally important, if by the mid-1990s we are successful in eliminating nearly all remaining inappropriate inpatient days, no further cutbacks will be available to mask the underlying rate of increase in costs. Only if other cost-containment measures are put in place will the control of costs be possible.

### Differences Between the Medicare and Non-Medicare Sectors

The aggregate figures just discussed conceal important differences between the rate of increase in Medicare and non-Medicare expenditures. Most notably, between 1982 and 1988 the number of inpatient days used by Medicare patients fell by 41 percent, whereas the number of days used by non-Medicare patients fell by only 15 percent (Table 2). This finding indicates either that most of whatever days remain to be saved are in the non-Medicare sector, or that the fraction of unnecessary days

originally present in the Medicare sector was substantially larger than that in the non-Medicare sector.

The pattern of increase in costs in the two sectors was also remarkably different. Between 1976 and 1982, real costs to Medicare rose at about twice the rate in the non-Medicare sector; between 1982 and 1988 the situation was completely reversed. Medicare expenditures under the prospective payment system fell steadily, so that by 1987 and 1988 the increase averaged only 0.6 percent per year. By contrast, the increase in non-Medicare expenditures accelerated to almost 9 percent per year during this period. It is important to note that the large increases in Medicare costs that have been reported in the popular press have been driven to a considerable extent by Medicare payments to physicians, which rose by more than 11 percent annually in 1987 and 1988.[10]

These data clearly indicate that the private sector is carrying a steadily increasing share of the responsibility for maintaining the quality of care for both Medicare and non-Medicare patients in the hospital. How long this burden will be accepted by private payers remains uncertain.

We are indebted to Joseph P. Newhouse, Ph.D., Harvard Medical School, and Peter W. Van Etten, University of Massachusetts Medical Center, for their helpful comments and criticisms and to Bernice M. Golder for valuable assistance in the preparation of the manuscript.

### References

1. Hospital statistics, 1976–1988 editions. Chicago: American Hospital Association, 1976–1988.
2. Bureau of Data Management and Strategy. Table AN-3A: number of admission notices processed since 7/1/66 by state and calendar year as of August 1989. Baltimore, Md: Health Care Financing Administration.
3. Idem. The Medicare decision support system: Medicare short-stay hospital utilization trends. Health care financing data compendium, 1989 update. Baltimore, Md: Health Care Financing Administration.
4. Department of Commerce, Bureau of Economic Analysis. Economic report of the President transmitted to the Congress, February 1990. Washington, D.C.: Government Printing Office, 1990:298.
5. Pauly MV, Wilson P. Hospital output forecast and the cost of empty hospital beds. Health Serv Res 1986:403–28.
6. Bureau of Data Management and Strategy. Annual Medicare program statistics reimbursement tables. Baltimore, Md: Health Care Financing Administration, 1986.
7. Idem. Table AA4-TOTAL: hospital insurance, number of inpatient hospital bills, total and covered days of care, total and covered charges and amount reimbursed by period, expense incurred, and type of hospital as of August 25, 1989. Baltimore, Md: Health Care Financing Administration.

8. *Idem.* SMI-1 Medicare: estimated supplementary medical insurance disbursements, calendar years 1966–1988. Baltimore, Md: Health Care Financing Administration, June 21, 1989.

9. Office of National Cost Estimates. National health expenditures, 1988. *Health Care Finance Rev* 1990; 11(4):20.

10. *Idem.* National health expenditures, 1988. *Health Care Finance Rev* 1990; 11(4):33.

# Chapter 6
## Lifetime Use of Nursing Home Care

Peter Kemper, Ph.D., and Christopher
M. Murtaugh, Ph.D.

**Abstract** *Background and Methods.* Despite the growth in the number of Americans in nursing homes, there are only limited data on the total amount of time that people spend in such facilities. We estimate the amount of time the average person spends in nursing homes over his or her lifetime (lifetime nursing home use), using data from the National Mortality Followback Survey of the next of kin of a sample of persons 25 years of age or older who died in 1986. On the basis of these data, we estimated the likelihood that Americans will use nursing home care during the course of their lifetimes and the total duration of such care. Current data on life expectancy were then used to reweight the sample to project lifetime nursing home use for those who became 65 years old in 1990.

*Results.* Of those who died in 1986 at 25 years of age or older, 29 percent had at some time been residents in a nursing home, and almost half of those who entered a nursing home spent a cumulative total of at least one year there. The probability of nursing home use increased sharply with age at death: 17 percent for age 65 to 74, 36 percent for age 75 to 84, and 60 percent for age 85 to 94. For persons who turned 65 in 1990, we project that 43 percent will enter a nursing home at some time before they die. Of those who enter nursing homes, 55 percent will have total lifetime use of at least one year, and 21 percent will have total lifetime use of five years or more. We also project that more women than men will enter nursing homes (52 percent vs. 33 percent), and among them, more women than men will have total lifetime nursing home use of five years or more (25 percent vs. 13 percent).

*Conclusions.* Our projections indicate that over a lifetime, the risk of entering a nursing home and spending a long time there is substantial. With the elderly population growing, this has important implications for both medical practice and the financing of long-term care. (*N Engl J Med* 1991; 324:595–600.)

In recent decades the nursing home population in the United States has increased substantially. A little over a half million people were residing in nursing homes or personal care facilities in 1964.[1] By 1985, after considerable growth in the elderly population and the establishment of the Medicaid program, which covers nursing home care for those without financial resources, the number of nursing home residents had almost tripled.[2] Total annual expenditures on nursing home care also rose dramatically during this period, from $4.2 billion[3] to $34.7 billion[4] after adjustment for inflation. Current

Reprinted with permission from Peter Kemper, Ph.D., and Christopher M. Murtaugh, Ph.D., Lifetime Use of Nursing Home Care, *The New England Journal of Medicine,* Vol. 324 No. 9, pp. 595–600, 1991.

Presented in abstract form at the annual meeting of the Gerontological Society of America, Minneapolis, November 18 through 21, 1989.

The views expressed in this paper are those of the authors. No official endorsement by either the Agency for Health Care Policy and Research or the Department of Health and Human Services is intended or should be inferred.

projections are for continued growth in the nursing home population.[5]

Health care providers, patients and their families, and public officials are now facing the consequences of this growth. Physicians are often called on to assist permanently disabled patients and their families with decisions about long-term care. At the same time, at least partly because of the system of prospective payment for hospital care, doctors and hospital discharge planners must seek care for elderly patients who are being discharged more rapidly, and nursing home personnel must care for patients who are sicker than in the past.[6] The elderly and their families worry about the potential cost of a lengthy nursing home stay. And public officials, responding in part to constituents' pressure for change and in part to the growing cost to the public of nursing home care, are searching for sensible policy reforms to spread the risk of catastrophic costs due to long stays in nursing homes.

Despite widespread concern about the expansion of nursing home care over the past several decades, information about how much care individual persons use over a lifetime has been limited. In this paper we present estimates of the total amount of time spent in nursing homes during a lifetime.

## METHODS

The data for this analysis were obtained from the 1986 National Mortality Followback Survey, a survey of the next of kin of a nationally representative sample of adults who died in 1986.[7] Death certificates of U.S. residents 25 years of age or older were drawn from the 1986 Current Mortality Sample; those from Oregon were excluded because of state requirements for the consent of survey respondents. In the survey, the next of kin or someone else familiar with each deceased person in the sample was asked about, among other things, the person's stays in nursing homes. Specifically, the respondent was asked whether the deceased person was ever admitted to a nursing home, how many nights were spent there in his or her last year of life, and the total amount of time spent in nursing homes over his or her entire lifetime (one day to less than three months, three months to less than one year, one year to less than five years, or five years or more). The answers to these questions, together with information on demographic characteristics and place of death obtained from questionnaires and death certificates, formed the basis of our analysis.

The overall rate of response to the questionnaire was 89 percent. The unweighted size of the sample of deceased subjects was 16,587. The estimates of the amount of time spent in nursing homes over a person's lifetime (lifetime nursing home use) by persons who died in

1986 have been weighted to adjust for nonresponse and the complex sample design. The resulting estimates are representative of all U.S. residents 25 years of age or older (excluding those in Oregon) who died in 1986.

All estimates presented for subjects who died in 1986 are expressed as proportions. In every instance the denominator for the proportion was at least 75 unweighted cases. Standard errors, included in parentheses in the tables, were estimated by a method developed by Shah for complex survey designs.[8] All estimates presented in this paper have relative standard errors of less than 30 percent. In addition, differences between reported estimates were tested for statistical significance. Unless otherwise indicated, we have discussed only differences that were significant at the 0.05 level, by two-tailed test.

After calculating estimates for subjects who died in 1986, we projected future nursing home use by persons who had their 65th birthday in 1990. Lifetime nursing home use by that cohort will differ from that of elderly people who died in 1986 either if patterns of nursing home use change (for example, as a result of changes in disease prevalence) or if the proportion dying at each age differs between the two groups. Our projections incorporate adjustments for expected differences in length of survival between the two groups that result from substantial gains in life expectancy[9] and the disproportionate number of deaths at younger ages among subjects who died in 1986 that was caused by the growth over the past 40 years in the size of the cohorts reaching the age of 65. To adjust for the effects of increased life expectancy and the differing composition of the cohorts, the sample was reweighted to reflect the Social Security Administration's projections of life expectancy for those who turned 65 in 1990. (Details of the methods are available from the National Auxiliary Publications Service.*)

## RESULTS

Lifetime Nursing Home Use
Among Persons Who Died in 1986

Residence in a nursing home at some point during a person's lifetime is far from rare. Almost 30 percent of those who died in 1986 were nursing home residents at some time during their lives (Table 1). Nursing home use increased sharply with age at death. Less than 5 percent of those who died before the age of 45 ever resided in a nursing home, as compared with 71 percent

*See NAPS document no. 04838 for 16 pages of supplementary material. Order from NAPS c/o Microfiche Publications, P.O. Box 3513, Grand Central Station, New York, NY 10163–3513. Remit in advance (in U.S. funds only) $7.75 for photocopies or $4 for microfiche. Outside the U.S. and Canada add postage of $4.50 ($1.50 for microfiche postage). There is an invoicing charge of $15 on orders not prepaid. This charge includes purchase order.

Table 1. Percentage of Persons Who Died in 1986 Who Spent Some Time in a Nursing Home.*

| AGE AT DEATH | MEN | WOMEN | ALL |
|---|---|---|---|
| yr | | percent (SE) | |
| 25–44 | 3 (<0.5) | 5 (1) | 3 (<0.5) |
| 45–64 | 7 (1) | 9 (1) | 8 (1) |
| 65–74 | 15 (1) | 21 (1) | 17 (1) |
| 75–84 | 30 (1) | 42 (1) | 36 (1) |
| 85–94 | 50 (2) | 65 (1) | 60 (1) |
| ≥95 | 52 (6) | 77 (3) | 71 (2) |
| <65 | 6 (1) | 8 (1) | 7 (<0.5) |
| ≥65 | 28 (1) | 46 (1) | 37 (1) |
| All | 21 (1) | 38 (1) | 29 (<0.5) |

*Data are from the 1986 National Mortality Followback Survey.[7]

of those who died at 95 years of age or older. Women were far more likely to enter nursing homes than men; some use was reported for 38 percent of women, as compared with 21 percent of men. Our estimate that 37 percent of those who died at 65 years of age or older spent some time in a nursing home is within the range reported in earlier studies (19 to 46 percent)[10–17] and is within one percentage point of the only estimate made with use of a similar method.[18]

Roughly half the persons who entered nursing homes spent at least a year of their lives there (Table 2). Just over one sixth had cumulative lifetime use of five years or more. For a minority, lifetime use was relatively brief; 30 percent used less than three months of nursing home care. Among elderly persons who died in 1986 who had ever spent time in a nursing home, the percentage with five or more years of lifetime use increased with age. (All comparisons were statistically significant except for that between the persons who were 65 to 74 years old at the time of death and those who were 75 to 84 years old.) Those who survived to very old age were particularly likely to have spent large amounts of time in nursing homes. For example, among persons who entered nursing homes, 42 percent of those who survived to the age of 95 resided in a nursing home for a total of five or more years, as compared with 9 percent of those who died at 65 to 74 years of age.

Lifetime nursing home use differs among sociodem-

Table 2. Distribution of Lifetime Use among Persons Who Died in 1986 Who Spent Time in Nursing Homes.*

| AGE AT DEATH | LIFETIME USE | | | |
|---|---|---|---|---|
| | <3 MO | 3–12 MO | 1–5 YR | ≥5 YR |
| yr | | percent (SE) | | |
| 25–44 | 47(5) | 22(4) | 13(3) | 18(4) |
| 45–64 | 42(4) | 28(3) | 17(3) | 13(3) |
| 65–74 | 45(2) | 24(2) | 21(2) | 9(1) |
| 75–84 | 35(1) | 23(1) | 31(1) | 12(1) |
| 85–94 | 22(1) | 20(1) | 38(1) | 20(1) |
| ≥95 | 14(2) | 10(2) | 35(3) | 42(3) |
| All | 30(1) | 21(1) | 31(1) | 17(1) |

*Data are from the 1986 National Mortality Followback Survey.[7] Because of rounding, percentages may not total 100.

ographic groups. Table 3 shows the percentage of persons who died in 1986 at 65 years of age or older who ever resided in nursing homes and the distribution of use among those subjects according to selected characteristics. The estimates have been standardized to adjust for differences among subgroups in longevity and sex. In a manner consistent with the unadjusted differences in Table 1, a much higher proportion of elderly women than men spent time in nursing homes (42 percent vs. 32 percent), even after we eliminated the effect of women's greater longevity. Moreover, women used more nursing home care than men. Among elderly persons who died in 1986 who had entered a nursing home, 19 percent of the women and 12 percent of the men received care for a total of five or more years.

A much higher percentage of whites than blacks used nursing homes (38 percent vs. 27 percent), after adjustment for differences between whites and blacks in longevity and sex. Among those who entered nursing homes, the amount of time spent there was slightly greater for whites than for blacks — 17 percent of whites who entered nursing homes spent a total of at least five years there, as compared with 14 percent of blacks, although this difference was not statistically significant.

Nursing home use varied little among educational groups. The percentage that ever used a nursing home did not differ significantly among the groups, and the percentage of users with five or more years of use differed significantly only between high-school graduates and those with less than an eighth-grade education.

Marital status was strongly associated with lifetime nursing home use, even after adjustment for differences

Table 3. Age- and Sex-Adjusted Estimates of Lifetime Nursing Home Use among Persons Who Died in 1986 at 65 Years of Age or Older, According to Sex, Race, Education, and Marital Status.*

| CHARACTERISTIC | PERCENTAGE USING NURSING HOMES | LIFETIME USE AMONG USERS | | | |
|---|---|---|---|---|---|
| | | <3 MO | 3–12 MO | 1–5 YR | ≥5 YR |
| | | percent (SE) | | | |
| All persons | 37 (1) | 30 (1) | 21 (1) | 31 (1) | 17 (1) |
| Sex | | | | | |
| Male | 32 (1) | 33 (1) | 24 (1) | 31 (2) | 12 (1) |
| Female | 42 (1) | 28 (1) | 20 (1) | 33 (1) | 19 (1) |
| Race | | | | | |
| Black | 27 (1) | 32 (2) | 22 (2) | 32 (2) | 14 (2) |
| White and other† | 38 (1) | 30 (1) | 21 (1) | 32 (1) | 17 (1) |
| Education | | | | | |
| <8 yr | 37 (1) | 30 (2) | 19 (2) | 31 (2) | 20 (2) |
| 8–11 yr | 38 (1) | 29 (1) | 21 (1) | 34 (1) | 16 (1) |
| High school | 38 (1) | 30 (2) | 22 (2) | 33 (2) | 15 (1) |
| Any college | 37 (1) | 27 (2) | 25 (2) | 30 (2) | 18 (2) |
| Marital status at death | | | | | |
| Married | 27 (2) | 40 (3) | 25 (3) | 28 (3) | 7 (2) |
| Widowed | 42 (1) | 27 (1) | 20 (1) | 36 (1) | 16 (1) |
| Divorced or separated | 46 (2) | 31 (3) | 23 (3) | 29 (3) | 17 (3) |
| Never married | 48 (2) | 19 (3) | 22 (3) | 30 (3) | 29 (3) |

*Data are from the 1986 National Mortality Followback Survey.[7] Estimates have been standardized for differences among groups in age at death and sex. Because of rounding, percentages may not total 100.

†"Other" includes Asians, Pacific Islanders, American Indians, and Alaska Natives.

in longevity and sex among marital-status groups. A little over one quarter of those who were married at the time of their deaths had used nursing homes, as compared with over two fifths of those who were widowed, divorced, or separated or who had never married. The association between the amount of time spent in nursing homes and marital status is even more striking. Among those who ever entered a nursing home, 7 percent of those who were married when they died spent five or more years in nursing homes, as compared with 16 percent of those who were widowed, 17 percent of those who were separated or divorced, and 29 percent of those who had never married.

Finally, the National Mortality Followback Survey also contains data on the timing of nursing home use during a person's life. The fraction of elderly nursing home residents who spent at least some time in a nursing home during the last year of life was a remarkably high 93 percent. Of those who used nursing homes in the last year of life, 55 percent died there, 42 percent died in or on the way to a hospital, and the remainder died at home or elsewhere (data not shown).

Projected Nursing Home Use Among Persons Who Turned 65 in 1990

Projections of the number of persons who reached the age of 65 in 1990 who will exceed various amounts of nursing home use during their lifetimes are presented in Table 4. Of the approximately 2.2 million persons who turned 65 in 1990,[19] more than 900,000 (43 percent) were expected to enter a nursing home at least once before they die. The greater number of women who reached the age of 65, combined with their higher likelihood of requiring nursing home care, means that according to our projections, almost two of every three persons who use nursing homes will be women.

We project that almost one third of all persons who reached 65 years of age in 1990 will spend at least three months in a nursing home during their lifetimes; 24 percent, at least a year; and 9 percent, at least five years. Women are more likely to spend large amounts of time in a nursing home than men; 13 percent of women are

projected to have lifetime nursing home use of five or more years, as compared with only 4 percent of men. Those who incur extremely high nursing home costs will be predominantly women. Almost 8 of 10 persons using at least five years of nursing home care will be women.

## DISCUSSION

The high likelihood of nursing home use projected for the elderly population has implications for medical practice over the next several decades. As the population continues to age, many physicians will receive more frequent requests for assistance with decisions about long-term care. The extent of the increase will depend not only on the clinical characteristics of their patients but also, as the demographic findings suggest, on their nonmedical characteristics (e.g., marital status, sex, and race or ethnic background). The need for physicians to be informed about the range of long-term care services available in their communities, including home care, has been noted previously.[20] Our projections suggest that this need will be even greater in the future.

Our projections also indicate that the likelihood of spending a large amount of time in a nursing home is substantial—a prospect that poses another challenge for medical practice. Physicians and other health care providers will need to be concerned not only with the needs of many patients recently transferred from hospitals for short-term rehabilitative services and skilled nursing care, but also with the routine health care needs of those who spend a substantial portion of their lives in nursing homes. In 1980, Vladeck reported that the ongoing care of chronically ill nursing home residents was deficient and that physicians were largely absent from nursing homes.[21] There is little evidence of substantial improvement in the quality of nursing home care since that time.[22] With more than 500,000 of the 2.2 million persons who turned 65 in 1990 projected to spend at least a year in a nursing home—and 195,000 projected to spend five or more years—the medical management of the chronic diseases of residents of nursing homes remains a major concern.

Inevitably, the projections of future nursing home use presented in this paper are subject to uncertainty. The reweighting procedure used in making the projections adjusted for changes in life expectancy and the composition of the cohorts, but not for possible future changes in the pattern of nursing home use. Many factors could affect future use. For example, because of the longer survival of spouses, the percentage of the very old who are married could increase in the future, reducing their reliance on nursing home care. The Social Security Administration's projections indicate, however, that the change in the percentage of persons 85 years of age or

Table 4. Projected Nursing Home Use for Persons Who Reached 65 Years of Age in 1990.*

| CATEGORY OF USE | MEN | | WOMEN | | TOTAL | |
|---|---|---|---|---|---|---|
| | NO. (THOUSANDS) | % | NO. (THOUSANDS) | % | NO. (THOUSANDS) | % |
| Size of cohort | 998 | 100 | 1175 | 100 | 2173 | 100 |
| Any use | 325 | 33 | 616 | 52 | 941 | 43 |
| ≥3 mo | 219 | 22 | 476 | 41 | 695 | 32 |
| ≥1 yr | 143 | 14 | 370 | 31 | 513 | 24 |
| ≥5 yr | 42 | 4 | 153 | 13 | 195 | 9 |

*The projections are based on data from the 1986 National Mortality Followback Survey.[7]

older who are married will be small—an increase from 54 to 57 percent for men and from 13 to 14 percent for women between 1990 and 2020.[23] Such a change is unlikely to have an important effect on future nursing home use.

Changes in the need for long-term care due to changes in medical knowledge and practice, lifestyle, or other factors also could affect future use. "Active life expectancy" is a measure of the amount of time persons are expected to be able to continue to function independently.[24] If the proportion of life spent without disability increases or decreases in the future, the projections of nursing home use presented here may be over- or underestimates. The extent to which changes in active life expectancy affect nursing home use depends in part on whether it is the proportion of life spent with serious as opposed to mild disability that changes.[25] Unfortunately, despite a growing number of studies, there remains considerable uncertainty about trends in active life expectancy.[26–29]

Other reasons why nursing home use may change in the future include the introduction of new financing methods for acute or long-term care. Prospective payment of hospitals, for example, appears to have increased the proportion of Medicare patients discharged from hospitals to nursing homes.[30,31] Limitations on the supply of nursing home beds, changes in the participation of women in the labor force, increases in coverage of long-term care by private insurers, and increases in the wealth and income of the elderly are yet other factors that could alert the use of nursing homes in the future. Because some of these changes would increase the use of nursing homes in the future whereas others would decrease it, their net effect is difficult to judge.

Possible errors in the survey responses that underlie our projections are another cause of uncertainty. The fact that information on the persons who died in 1986 was obtained from relatives is one potential source of error. Although the widely held belief among survey researchers is that proxy respondents generally underreport health events, carefully designed studies have found no evidence of a difference between reports by proxies and those by patients themselves.[32,33] A second potential cause of concern is the length of the recall period. Generally, research suggests that asking respondents to recall events after a long period leads to underreporting,[34,35] but few studies have recall periods of more than a year. A study with a longer recall period (2½ years) found that although there was underreporting overall, the most important determinant of error was salience (i.e., the importance of the event), not the length of the recall period.[36] Institutionalization is a salient event for most families, and over 80 percent of the respondents in the National Mortality Followback Survey were immediate family members (spouses, children, or siblings),

who should have been knowledgeable about the subjects' nursing home use. Thus, if there is error due to the use of proxy respondents or to the length of the recall period, it appears more likely to lead to underreporting, which would have caused us to underestimate lifetime nursing home use.

Although the projections are inevitably subject to some uncertainty, any errors are unlikely to be great enough to alter the conclusion that our findings on the distribution of lifetime use contrast sharply with information previously available. In the past, researchers have analyzed information on nursing home stays rather than cumulative use.[17,37–39] Lifetime use, however, is a very different concept from the length of a single nursing home stay. The former describes the total amount of time spent in nursing homes, including all of a person's separate stays, whereas the latter describes the duration of a single stay from admission to discharge. Since residents can have several stays, the average lifetime nursing home use is necessarily greater than the average length of single stays. In practice, this conceptual difference is exacerbated, because many nursing homes formally discharge residents when they go to a hospital and then readmit them when they return to the nursing home, thus artificially shortening the lengths of stay. Meiners and Trapnell[40] and Spence and Wiener[41] have tried to adjust for this effect by estimating the length of episodes of care, ignoring interruptions caused by hospitalization or transfers between nursing homes.

Table 5 compares the distribution of lengths of stay for a sample of discharged patients included in the 1985 National Nursing Home Survey, the duration of episodes as estimated by Meiners and Trapnell[40] and by Spence and Wiener,[41] and our projections of lifetime use on the basis of data from the National Mortality Followback Survey. Only 26 percent of those who turned 65 in 1990 who enter nursing homes are projected to use less than three months of care over their lifetimes. In contrast, over half of nursing home stays and roughly 45 percent of nursing home episodes last less than three months. At the other end of the distribution, we project that 21 percent of persons who enter nursing homes will have

**Table 5. Distributions of Use among Persons 65 Years of Age or Older Who Enter Nursing Homes.***

|  | DURATION OF USE | | | |
|---|---|---|---|---|
|  | <3 MO | 3–12 MO | 1–5 YR | ≥5 YR |
|  | *percent* | | | |
| Nursing home stay† | 51 | 22 | 21 | 6 |
| Episode of care |  |  |  |  |
| Meiners and Trapnell[40] | 44 | 23 | 26 | 7 |
| Spence and Wiener[41] | 45 | 20 | 26 | 10 |
| Lifetime use | 26 | 19 | 34 | 21 |

*The distribution of lifetime use is that projected for persons who turned 65 in 1990. Because of rounding, percentages may not total 100.

†Data are from National Center for Health Statistics et al.[2]

lifetime use of five or more years. In contrast, only 7 to 10 percent of episodes and only 6 percent of single stays last five or more years. Clearly, neither the nursing home stay nor the episode of care is a good substitute for lifetime nursing home use.

The highly skewed distribution of lifetime nursing home use has implications for the financing of nursing home care. If past patterns continue, a majority of those who reached 65 years of age in 1990 will not use any nursing home care. Yet, 1 in 11 can expect to spend at least five years in a nursing home, at an average cost in today's prices of $25,000 per year. Expenses of $125,000 or more are enough to exhaust the financial resources of all but the wealthiest elderly persons. Nursing home care is only partially covered under existing government health insurance programs. Medicare covers some post-acute care in nursing homes, but not long stays. Medicaid covers care for those who cannot afford to pay, but it requires that most assets and virtually all income be exhausted in order to meet eligibility criteria.[42-47] As a result, approximately half of all expenditures for nursing home care are private.[4]

Recognition of the unequal distribution of nursing home costs had led to the development of a private market for long-term care insurance that is small but growing rapidly.[48] The information presented here, however, arouses concern about the adequacy of private insurance coverage. Typically, benefits are limited to three to five years of care. Yet, as we have seen, many persons are expected to require more than five years of care. In addition, policies often have limited protection against inflation. Because the time between the purchase of insurance and the payment of benefits can be many years, the value of the benefits can be substantially eroded. Fortunately, coverage of long stays and protection against inflation are improving, but many policies will cover only a small fraction of the catastrophic expenses incurred late in life.

A variety of proposals have been made to expand public financing of long-term care, as either an alternative or a complement to private insurance.[49-53] The lifetime-use estimates presented here, however, suggest that congressional proposals currently under discussion will leave substantial gaps in the coverage of nursing home care. For example, a bipartisan congressional commission recently completed a yearlong study of options for financing long-term care. In addition to liberalizing coverage for low- and moderate-income families, it proposed covering the first three months of nursing home care through a public entitlement, regardless of a person's income.[54] Yet a third of those now turning 65—almost three quarters of those who will use nursing homes—can expect to exceed that amount of care. An alternative proposal would cover the costs of care after the first two years,[55] leaving uncovered the first $50,000

of nursing home costs—an amount that many could not afford to pay.

Changing financing mechanisms alone, however, is an inadequate response to the high projected likelihood of lengthy nursing home care. When one in seven men and one in three women who reached the age of 65 in 1990 are projected to spend at least one year in a nursing home, society needs to undertake a fundamental reassessment of long-term care, rather than simply paying for what has been done in the past. For example, innovations in the delivery of long-term care that reduce costs while maintaining or improving the quality of care should be strongly encouraged. In addition, research on extending the period of a person's life that is free of disability should be expanded. Extending active life expectancy has the potential both to improve the quality of life and to reduce the costs of long-term care.

The attention being directed toward long-term care by health professionals, the elderly and their families, and public officials is clearly warranted. The relatively high probability of use of large amounts of nursing home care that we report here, combined with the growth of the population surviving to the age of 65, will force society to make choices—either with forethought and debate or by default—about the delivery and financing of long-term care.

We are indebted to Judy Sangl for pointing out the information on nursing home use in the National Mortality Followback Survey; to Stephen Cohen, Ayah Johnson, and Nancy Mathiowetz for methodologic advice; to Alice Wade of the Office of the Actuary of the Social Security Administration for generating the cohort life-table data used in the analysis; to Judy Feder, Marc Frieman, Donald Goldstone, Korbin Liu, Marilyn Moon, Thomas Rice, Timothy Smeeding, William Spector, Brenda Spillman, Robyn Stone, and anonymous reviewers for helpful comments on an earlier draft of this paper; to Karen Pinkston of Social and Scientific Systems, Bethesda, Md., for programming support; and to Mary Seidenberg for assistance in the preparation of the manuscript.

## References

1. National Center for Health Statistics. Arrangements for physician services to residents in nursing and personal care homes. United States, May–June 1964. Vital and health statistics, Series 12. No. 13. Washington, D.C.: Government Printing Office, 1970. (PHS publication no. 1000–series 12–no. 13.)
2. National Center for Health Statistics, Hing E, Sekscenski E, Strahan G. The National Nursing Home Survey: 1985 summary for the United States. Vital and health statistics. Series 13. No. 97. Washington, D.C.: Government Printing Office, 1989. (DHHS publication no. (PHS) 89–1758.)
3. Reed LS, Hanft RS. National health expenditures, 1950–64. *Soc Secur Bull* 1966; 29(1):3–19.
4. Letsch SW, Levit KR, Waldo DR. National health expen-

ditures, 1987. *Health Care Finance Rev* 1988; 10(2):109–22.

5. Weissert WG. Estimating the long-term care population: prevalence rates and selected characteristics. *Health Care Finance Rev* 1985; 6(4):83–91.

6. Shaughnessy PW, Kramer AM. The increased needs of patients in nursing homes and patients receiving home health care. *N Engl J Med* 1990; 322:21–7.

7. Seeman I, Poe GS, McLaughlin JK. Design of the 1986 National Mortality Followback Survey: considerations on collecting data on decedents. *Public Health Rep* 1989; 104:183–8.

8. Shah BV. SESUDAAN: standard errors program for computing of standardized rates from sample survey data. Research Triangle Park, N.C.: Research Triangle Institute, 1981. (RTI document no. RTI/5250/99–O1S.)

9. Manton KG. Changing concepts of morbidity and mortality in the elderly population. *Milbank Mem Fund Q* 1982; 60:183–244.

10. Kastenbaum R, Candy S. The 4% fallacy: a methodological and empirical critique of extended care facility population statistics. *Int J Aging Hum Dev* 1973; 4:15–21.

11. Palmore E. Total chance of institutionalization among the aged. *Gerontologist* 1976; 16:504–7.

12. Ingram D, Barry J. National statistics on deaths in nursing homes: interpretations and implications. *Gerontologist* 1977; 17:303–8.

13. Lesnoff-Caravaglia G. The five per cent fallacy. *Int J Aging Hum Dev* 1978–79; 9:187–92.

14. Vicente L, Wiley JA, Carrington RA. The risk of institutionalization before death. *Gerontologist* 1979; 19:361–7.

15. National Center for Health Statistics. Zappolo A. Discharges from nursing homes: 1977 National Nursing Home Survey. Vital and health statistics. Series 13. No. 54. Washington, D.C.: Government Printing Office, 1981. (DHHS publication no. (PHS) 81–1715.)

16. Liang J, Tu EJ-C. Estimating lifetime risk of nursing home residency: a further note. *Gerontologist* 1986; 26:560–3.

17. Cohen MA, Tell EJ, Wallack SS. The lifetime risks and costs of nursing home use among the elderly. *Med Care* 1986; 24:1161–72.

18. Murtaugh C, Kemper P, Spillman B. The risk of nursing home use in later life. *Med Care* 1990; 28:952–62.

19. Bureau of the Census, Spencer G. Projections of the population of the United States, by age, sex, and race: 1988 to 2080. Current population reports. Series P-25 No. 1018. Washington, D.C.: Government Printing Office, 1989.

20. Committee on the Study on Aging and Medical Education, Institute of Medicine. Aging and medical education: report of a study. Washington, D.C.: National Academy of Sciences, 1978. (IOM publication no. IOM-78–04.)

21. Vladeck BC. Unloving care: the nursing home tragedy. New York: Basic Books, 1980.

22. Committee on Nursing Home Regulation, Institute of Medicine. Improving the quality of care in nursing homes. Washington, D.C.: National Academy Press, 1986.

23. Wade A. Social security area population projections, 1988. Baltimore: Social Security Administration, Office of the Actuary, 1988. (SSA publication no. 11–11549.)

24. Katz S, Branch LG, Branson MH, Papsidero JA, Beck JC, Greer DS. Active life expectancy. *N Engl J Med* 1983; 309:1218–24.

25. Rogers RG, Rogers A, Belanger A. Active life among the elderly in the United States: multistate life-table estimates and population projections. *Milbank Q* 1989; 67:370–411.

26. Gruenberg E. The failures of success. *Milbank Mem Fund Q* 1977; 55:3–24.

27. Fries J. The biological constraints on human aging: implications for health policy; position paper. In: Andreoli K, Musser L, Reiser S, eds. Health care for the elderly: regional responses to national policy issues. New York: Harworth Press, 1986:51–73.

28. Hayflick L. The biological constraints on human aging: implications for health policy; the human lifespan. In: Andreoli K, Musser L, Reiser S, eds. Health care for the elderly: regional responses to national policy issues. New York: Haworth Press, 1986:75–89.

29. Rogers A, Rogers RG, Belanger A. Longer life but worse health? Measurement and dynamics. *Gerontologist* 1990; 30:640–9.

30. Morrisey MA, Sloan FA, Valvona J. Medicare prospective payment and posthospital transfers to subacute care. *Med Care* 1988; 26:685–98.

31. Kahn KL, Keeler EB, Sherwood MJ, et al. Comparing outcomes of care before and after implementation of the DRG-based prospective payment system. *JAMA* 1990; 264:1964–8.

32. Moore JC. Self/proxy response status and survey response quality: a review of the literature. *J Off Stat* 1988; 4:155–72.

33. Mathiowetz NA, Groves R. The effects of respondent rules on health survey reports. *Am J Public Health* 1985; 75:639–44.

34. Marquis KH. Record check validity of survey responses: a reassessment of bias in reports of hospitalizations. Santa Monica, Calif.: Rand Corporation, 1978.

35. Cannell CF, Marquis KH, Laurent A. A summary of studies of interviewing methodology. Vital and health statistics. Series 2. No. 69. Washington, D.C.: Government Printing Office 1977, (DHEW publication no. (HRA) 77:1343.)

36. Mathiowetz NA, Duncan G. Out of work, out of mind: response errors in retrospective reports of unemployment. *J Bus Econ Stat* 1988; 6:221–9.

37. Keeler EB, Kane RL, Solomon DH. Short- and long-term residents of nursing homes. *Med Care* 1981; 19:363–70.

38. Liu K, Palesch Y. The nursing home population: different perspectives and implications for policy. *Health Care Finance Rev* 1981; 3(2):15–23.

39. Liu K, Manton KG. The length-of-stay pattern of nursing home admissions. *Med Care* 1983; 21:1211–22.

40. Meiners MR, Trapnell GR. Long-term care insurance: premium estimates for prototype policies. *Med Care* 1984; 22:901–11.

41. Spence DA, Wiener JM. Nursing home length of stay pattern: results from the 1985 National Nursing Home Survey. *Gerontologist* 1990; 30:16–20.

42. Branch LG, Friedman DJ, Cohen MA, Smith N, Socholitzky

E. Impoverishing the elderly: a case study of the financial risk of spend-down among Massachusetts elderly people. *Gerontologist* 1988; 28:648–52.

43. Carpenter L. Medicaid eligibility for persons in nursing homes. *Health Care Finance Rev* 1988; 10(2):67–77.

44. Liu K, Doty P, Manton K. Medicaid spenddown in nursing homes. *Gerontologist* 1990; 30:7–15.

45. Moses SA. The fallacy of impoverishment. *Gerontologist* 1990; 30:21–5.

46. Smeeding TM. Toward a knowledge base for long-term care finance. *Gerontologist* 1990; 30:5–6.

47. Burwell BO, Adams EK, Meiners MR. Spend-down of assets before Medicaid eligibility among elderly nursing-home recipients in Michigan. *Med Care* 1990; 28:349–62.

48. Van Gelder S, Johnson D. Long-term care insurance: a market update. Washington, D.C.: Health Insurance Association of America, 1991.

49. Somers AR. Long-term care for the elderly and disabled: a new health priority. *N Engl J Med* 1982; 307:221–6.

50. Davis K, Rowland D. Medicare policy: new directions for health and long-term care. Baltimore: Johns Hopkins University Press, 1986.

51. Harvard Medicare Project. The future of Medicare. In: Blumenthal D, Schlesinger M, Drumheller PB, eds. Renewing the promise: Medicare and its reform. New York: Oxford University Press, 1988:176–92.

52. Ball RM, Bethell TN: Because we're all in this together: the case for a national long term care insurance policy. Washington, D.C.: Families U.S.A. Foundation, 1989.

53. Himmelstein DU, Woolhandler S. Writing Committee of the Working Group on Program Design. A national health program for the United States: a physicians' proposal. N Engl J Med 1989; 320:102–8.

54. The Pepper Commission, Bipartisan Commission on Comprehensive Health Care. Recommendations to the Congress: access to health care and long-term care for all Americans. Washington, D.C.: Government Printing Office, 1990. (SUDOC no. Y4.Ag4:P39/recomm.)

55. U.S. Congress. Hearings on May 27 and June 17, 1988, before the Subcommittee on Health of the Committee on Finance, U.S. Senate, on the Long-Term Care Assistance Act of 1988. 100th Cong. 2nd Sess. Washington, D.C.: Government Printing Office, 1989.

# Chapter 7

## The Quiet Success of the National Plan for the Chronically Mentally Ill

Chris Koyanagi and Howard H. Goldman, M.D., Ph.D.

*In 1978 the President's Commission on Mental Health called for a national plan for the care of persons with chronic mental illness. The plan was completed and released in 1980, but was never adopted as the policy of the incoming Reagan Administration. Despite changes in attitudes in the 1980s toward the federal government's role in human services and an atmosphere of fiscal restraint, many of the plan's specific recommendations for changes in Supplemental Security Income, Social Security Disability Insurance, Medicaid, and Medicare have been implemented. In this paper, the implementation of these recommendations is analyzed. The authors discuss some of the strategies used by mental health advocacy groups to make gains in the 1980s. Recommendations for the 1990s are discussed.*

In 1978 the President's Commission on Mental Health called for the creation of a new partnership between the federal and state governments. After a major review of mental health in the nation, the commission released its report and recommendations, along with suggested legislation—a new Mental Health Systems Act to serve as the linchpin of the partnership. In addition, the commission called on the Department of Health and Human Services (DHHS) to develop a national plan for the care of persons with severe mental illness, focusing especially on Medicaid, Medicare, and Supplemental Security Disability Insurance (SSDI).[1]

The commission's legislative recommendations were favorably considered by Congress. By 1979 efforts were under way to dramatically reshape the Community Mental Health Centers Act, in particular to refocus federal support on the care of persons with severe mental illness. The Mental Health Systems Act (Public Law 96—398), which was passed in October 1980, called for a new approach to providing federal categorical mental health resources.[2] It focused on services, especially community support services, for individuals with severe mental illness, and it gave state mental health agencies a more important role in planning and allocating federal resources. The Mental Health Systems Act also authorized a major increase in federal categorical mental health expenditures, well above levels then being paid to the federally funded community mental health centers.

The national plan, also called for by the President's Commission on Mental Health, was produced in December 1980, after more than a year of study and deliberation involving various components of the DHHS and constituent participants. Unfortunately, this document

Chris Koyanagi and Howard H. Goldman, M.D., Ph.D., *The Quiet Success of the National Plan for the Chronically Mentally Ill,* Vol. 42 No. 9, pp. 899–905, 1991, Copyright 1992, The American Psychiatric Association. Reprinted by permission.

did not receive the immediate and positive attention accorded to the commission's legislative recommendations. Initially, only a few hundred copies were circulated, "to stimulate further public dialogue and comment," because the White House and senior officials in the administration were concerned about the cost of the recommendations.

After the election, despite the fact that a new administration was soon to be in office, the report was released, but it was issued without fanfare and was cautiously titled *Toward a National Plan for the Chronically Mentally Ill.*[3]

This paper reexamines the recommendations of the national plan of 1980 and assesses the strategies of mental health advocates for reform of the federal government's mainstream programs—Medicaid, Medicare, SSI, and SSDI. It is based on a report by the authors that assesses what has been accomplished in an environment of new social policies in the 1980s and what remains to be done.[4]

## THE NATIONAL PLAN IN THE 1980S

Despite official reservations, individuals involved in development of the national plan, especially advocates for persons with severe mental illness, were excited by the prospect for substantial incremental change reflected at the plan. Together with the Mental Health Systems Act, the national plan was believed to constitute an important blueprint for government action. The Mental Health Systems Act authorized additional federal categorical support for community mental health services. The national plan focused on federal mainstream resources, especially those available under the Social Security Act. The tentative nature of the release of the national plan however, foreshadowed a blow to the optimism of all those involved with the plan.

The change of presidential administrations in 1981 brought a change in attitude toward government's role in human services in general and mental health services in particular. The national plan, which had been tentative under President Carter, became an anathema under President Reagan. The Mental Health Systems Act, which had promised new resources, was repealed by the Omnibus Budget Reconciliation Act (OBRA) of 1981.

The conventional wisdom holds that mental health policy, especially at the federal level, went into a decline during the 1980s. The standard refrain is that fiscal conservatism, linked to a doctrine of new federalism and state responsibility for human services, meant sudden death for the infant national plan. According to the logic, the care of persons with serious mental illness was taken off the front burner of federal concerns, and a difficult decade began.

From one perspective, there is a great deal of truth in the conventional wisdom. Federal categorical resources, placed into a block grant, shrank dramatically following the passage of OBRA 1981. The Social Security rolls were purged of persons with mental disabilities.[5–7] There were a number of attempts to tighten Medicare and Medicaid restrictions, and low-income housing subsidies were slashed.

From another viewpoint, during the decade of the 1980s the care of persons with severe mental illness did become the highest priority for public mental health services policy across the nation. The National Institute of Mental Health's Community Support Program (CSP), a demonstration program for the care of persons with severe mental illness, which was repeatedly slated for elimination by the Reagan Administration, was saved by Congress throughout the decade. Through the CSP, states were assisted in making a radical nationwide shift in policy approaches to focus not only on persons with severe mental illness, but on the development of a system of care that went far beyond traditional mental health services. Under the CSP, ten essential services were fostered, including appropriate housing and rehabilitation, as well as traditional treatments.[8–9] The impact of the CSP and other federal mental health categorical programs is beyond the scope of this paper but is discussed more fully in the authors' report on progress made in federal mental health policy in the 1980s.[4]

Later in the decade, the State Comprehensive Mental Health Services Plan Act of 1986 (Public Law 99–660) built on the CSP base by calling for each state, working in concert with relevant state agencies, such as the Medicaid agency, to prepare a detailed plan for the care of individuals with serious mental illness that would involve consumers of mental health services as well as their families and advocates in the planning process.

At the federal level, changes in strategy emerged during the 1980s. Unable to reverse the block grant trend in categorical programming, advocacy groups pressured Congress to focus on changes in mainstream resources. Added costs for improved services were buried in omnibus budget reconciliation bills along with changes requested on behalf of non-mental-health interests. The national plan had been released, and it served as a blueprint for those who continued to push for incremental reform.

## ANALYSIS OF THE NATIONAL PLAN RECOMMENDATIONS

In this section we look at each of the four programs on which the plan focused—SSI, SSDI, Medicaid, and Medicare—and analyze the extent to which the national plan recommendations have been accepted and implemented. We discuss problems that remain in each area and new concerns that have arisen since the national

**Table 1**
Implementation of recommendations of the National Plan for the Chronically Mentally Ill, by program category

| Recommendation | Imple-mented | Comments |
|---|---|---|
| **Supplemental Security Income (SSI)** | | |
| Improve prerelease program for persons being discharged from state institutions | Yes | Some implementation problems remain but essentially achieved [1] |
| Eliminate substantial gainful activity test from definition of disability for people who return to work | Yes | An even broader provision was enacted as part of Section 1619 work incentive.[2] |
| Provide presumptive eligibility for persons discharged from mental institutions | In principle | An alternative prerelease system was implemented (see above). |
| Equate limits on monetary earnings with the break-even point when determining eligibility to eliminate work disincentives and allow individuals to retain income and Medicaid benefits | Yes | Enacted as part of Section 1619, but implementation still needs improvement |
| **Social Security Disability Insurance (SSDI)** | | |
| Eliminate substantial gainful activity test (similar to recommendation for SSI) | No | An improved work incentive program under SSDI is still needed. |
| Establish separate classification of eligibility for individuals with severe mental illnesses, dependent on diagnosis, functional disability, and duration of disability, measured by objective criteria | Yes | Although fully implemented, further refinements are needed to keep criteria up to date. [3] |
| **Medicaid** | | |
| Evaluate state plans to identify policies that discriminate against persons with mental illness | No | Not a priority |
| Study state disability processes to assess state adherence to SSI criteria and problems that the SSI eligibility criteria cause by restricting access to Medicaid | No | Action is still needed to ensure that all SSI recipients are covered by Medicaid and to expand Medicaid eligibility to more low-income persons. |
| Analyze state decision making that may lead to reimbursement policies rewarding inappropriate mental health services | No | Action still needed |
| Provide technical assistance to identify, document, and promote innovative ways to use Medicaid | Partly | Some activity occurred through efforts of private groups, foundations, and the National Institute of Mental Health, although not to the extent recommended. |
| Establish a resource management service for persons with chronic mental illness | Yes | A case management option that can be targeted to persons with mental illness was enacted.[4] |

plan was published. Table 1 summarizes the discussion.

Extensive changes in legislation and regulation in the direction suggested by the national plan have occurred in all four programs. However, many of the changes have not been fully effective, due to slow or incomplete implementation, and further changes, not identified in the national plan, are needed.

Supplemental Security Income

The main thrust of all the national plan's recommendations concerning SSI have been addressed. Recommendations to improve the pre-release program for persons being discharged from state institutions have been substantially adopted and in some ways strengthened. A major improvement in the SSI work incentives program addressed the issues relating to employment and receipt of SSI that were of concern to the national

plan's authors. Under the Section 1619 program, individuals may return to work and retain part of their cash benefit; even after their cash assistance is reduced to zero, the individual can still remain on SSI and thereby be eligible for Medicaid coverage.

However, implementation of these initiatives could be improved through more aggressive efforts by the Social Security Administration to work with institutions and to make the Section 1619 program operate more smoothly. There is a need for further legislative amendments to Section 1619 to correct technical and other problems that have arisen as the program has been implemented.

Since SSI is an important part of the safety net for low-income persons, it is not surprising that additional pressures have been placed on the program during the 1980s. Improvements are now needed in SSI outreach programs, with a focus on providing assistance to persons who are homeless and mentally ill.

| | | |
|---|---|---|
| Demonstrate and establish an intermediate care center benefit | No | No longer seen as a useful option by many |
| Expand psychosocial rehabilitation services | Yes | Implemented by states; law was later improved.[5] |
| Establish presumptive eligibility category | No | Recommendation not workable; alternative approaches to providing emergency benefits need to be devised. |
| Require reimbursement of mental health clinics under clinic option | Yes | Did not require legislative change; state policies now allow it. |
| Cover services of institutions for mental diseases, except for public hospitals | No | No longer viewed as appropriate; seen as a disincentive to community-based care |
| Develop and implement standards for nursing homes relating to persons with mental illness | Enacted | Enacted as part of nursing home reform law; extent of impact is not known, as regulations are still pending.[6] |
| Establish standards for intermediate care facilities for those both mentally retarded and mentally ill | No | Action still needed |
| Establish a respite care benefit | No | Action still needed |
| | | |
| Medicare | | |
| Increase Medicare coverage of physician's outpatient treatment to $750 a year | Exceeded | Even broader coverage was enacted.[7] |
| Provide for 20 percent coinsurance for mental health services provided by physicians | Partly | A 20 percent copayment applies to medical management services, but a 50 percent copayment is required for other services.[8] |

[1] The Drug Enforcement, Education, and Control Act of 1986 (Public Law 99–570) included provisions to improve the prerelease precedures to determine SSI eligibility and initiate payment of benefits to individuals being released from institutions. The Omnibus Budget Reconciliation Act of 1987 (Public Law 100–203) improved benefits for SSI recipients who are temporarily institutionalized.

[2] The Employment Opportunities for Disabled Americans Act, Amendments to Section 1619 of the Social Security Act (Public Law 99–643), as amended, 94 Stat 441

[3] Federal Old-Age, Survivors, and Disability Insurance; Listing of Impairments–Mental Disorders, Code of Federal Regulations, 20 CFR, Part 404, 1985

[4] Consolidated Omnibus Budget Reconciliation Act of 1985 (Public Law 99–272), Omnibus Budget Reconciliation Act of 1986 (Public Law 99–509), and Omnibus Budget Reconciliation Act of 1987

[5] Omnibus Budget Reconciliation Act of 1990 (Public Law 101–508)

[6] Omnibus Budget Reconciliation Act of 1987; Code of Federal Regulations, 42 CFR, Parts 405, 431, and 483 (Preadmission Screening); Code of Federal Regulations, 42 CFR, Parts 442 and 483 (Requirements for Long-Term Care Facilities); and Guidelines of the Health Care Financing Administration (see reference 19)

[7] This recommendation was enacted in stages. The Omnibus Budget Reconciliation Act of 1987 expanded mental health physician coverage from $250 to $1,100 a year and exempted medical management from the limit. It also expanded coverage of partial hospitalization services. The Omnibus Budget Reconciliation Act of 1989 (Public Law 101–239) removed the $1,100 limit on psychotherapy but retained the 50 percent copayment requirement.

[8] For a discussion of medical management, see Sharfstein and Goldman (13). The Omnibus Budget Reconciliation Act of 1987 set the 20 and 50 percent copayments.

## Social Security Disability Insurance

The major recommendation in the SSDI program, to improve the criteria for eligibility (the medical listings) for disability payments, which applies to both SSDI and SSI, has been implemented. However, implementation did not occur until after thousands of persons were terminated from the disability rolls inappropriately, and the Supreme Court and Congress found the Social Security Administration's policies to be invalid.[6,7] Although further refinements in the medical listings are needed, this single change has had a major impact on the number of persons with mental illness who are able to secure disability benefits, so that this group is now the fastest growing group on the rolls.[10]

On the other hand, the national plan's recommendation for an SSDI work incentives program to eliminate the substantial gainful activity test has not been imple-

mented, and extending the Section 1619 program to SSDI recipients remains a high priority of advocates for persons with disabilities.

## Medicaid

The national plan named Medicaid the highest-priority area, and 13 separate recommendations concerning the program were made. The most far reaching of these proposals have all been implemented. A number of those not implemented are either not relevant today or not seen as priorities by most mental health advocates.

The most important of the changes were the initiation of a case management option and the expansion of rehabilitation to include psychiatric rehabilitation services. New legislation was passed to create an optional benefit for case management services, which can be targeted by a state specifically to persons with mental illness. During the past few years, states have expanded their Medicaid plans to include psychosocial rehabilitation services, as recommended in the national plan.

In addition, the state option to reimburse clinics now clearly covers mental health clinics, and new rules have been promulgated relating to psychiatric care of residents in nursing homes as part of a major overhaul of nursing home standards.

The recommendation to provide technical assistance to states has been implemented in a small way as a result of action by private groups, foundations, and the National Institute of Mental Health, resulting in expanded use of Medicaid as a mental health care financing tool.[11,12]

Two eligibility expansions have also been instituted. Through Section 1619, persons with disabilities who return to work can continue to be covered by Medicaid under certain circumstances. Improvements in the prerelease program have made it easier for people to become eligible for SSI and thereby for Medicaid when they are about to be released from psychiatric inpatient facilities.

Several recommendations were not adopted. Medicaid continues not to reimburse care in freestanding "institutions for mental diseases" for individuals between the ages of 22 and 64, in part because of costs, but also because there is strong sentiment that such a change is a disincentive to community care. In addition, Medicaid still does not have a special category of intermediate care centers for persons with mental illness. An intermediate care center would provide housing, food, and treatment in a residence for 15 persons. The establishment of such centers is not seen as appropriate at this time because the mental health services that would be offered in the centers can be covered under other options. The special problems of persons with mental retardation who need mental health care is another area that has not been addressed. No action was taken to implement the national plan's recommendation for a respite care benefit under Medicaid.

In addition, nothing has been done to address the recommendations for a thorough review of the Medicaid program as a mental health financing tool, which include recommendations to examine allegations of discriminatory practice, state-to-state variation in eligibility, and incentives that favor costly services. This overall review is extremely critical, especially as Medicaid increases in importance as a payment system for individuals with severe mental disorders. In many states Medicaid payments are too low to attract a broad array of providers, and the financial incentives do not favor optimal psychiatric care and treatment.[11]

## Medicare

The national plan made a single recommendation to expand Medicare reimbursement for physician mental health services to $750 per year and to change the 50 percent copayment to 20 percent. At the time, this recommendation did not seem likely to be accepted. In fact, changes have exceeded the expectations of the plan's authors. Medical management services—short visits for a review of the patient's status and medication regimen[13]—are covered except for a 20 percent copayment. Other mental health services, furnished by physicians and under certain circumstances by clinical psychologists or social workers, are covered without limit and require a 50 percent copayment. Furthermore, coverage of partial hospitalization services has been expanded.

## DISCUSSION

### Change and Success

The 1980s were a time of significant fiscal constraint, particularly at the federal level, and a withdrawal of commitments to aid those who were not considered "truly needy." Yet in the 1980s, mental health advocates broke into four major federal financing programs and opened the door for significantly improved coverage of persons with mental illness in key federal programs. How did they do it?

There are probably many reasons for the outcomes, and often different reasons for the successes in different programs. However, some overall themes do emerge. First, the process of developing the national plan and its publication played a role. The document laid out a blueprint that was perfect for the climate of the 1980s. Incremental changes that were small in comparison to the total program were recommended in the very programs cited by many individuals—liberals, moderates, and many conservatives—as the vital safety net for the truly needy. Moreover, because the development of the plan involved not only mental health policymakers but also experts within the four financing programs, these insiders were educated about the importance of the changes.

A second broad reason for the gains made is that the mental health advocacy establishment was energized to pursue changes in these mainstream programs partly because the direct mental health categorical programs had been eliminated and the resulting block grant did not require or invite much attention. In addition, the Administration provoked the advocacy groups with its policy of terminating persons with severe mental illness from the disability programs.[5–7]

Third, the siege atmosphere of the early Reagan years brought together groups that had not worked in truly close alliances before. Mental health advocates positioned themselves as part of the disability community, working for changes in the financing programs that benefited all persons with disabilities, as well as working for specific changes on behalf of persons with mental illness. As a result, amendments always moved through Congress in concert, and the broader disability field was supporting the mental health amendments.

For example, the Disability Benefits Reform Act of 1984, which required the Social Security Administration to develop new mental health criteria, was supported by a very broad coalition of groups concerned about persons with a variety of disabilities who were being inappropriately terminated from the disability rolls. Another example was the enactment of a case management option under Medicaid, supported by advocates for persons with developmental disabilities as well as advocates for persons with mental illness. The diverse mental health community was also able to work well together, partly because of the exigencies of the times and partly because expanding financing programs was not as divisive as implementing policies that affected mental health treatment strategies.

Fourth, the Democratic Congress responded to the Reagan program cuts by developing a budget reconciliation bill strategy. This approach created multibillion-dollar packages of legislation touching on all domestic policy areas on which a single vote must be cast. Thus the mental health amendments did not attract critical attention from Congress or the President.

Finally, the budgetary impact of these changes was often obscure. For instance, the very dramatic changes in the criteria for disability benefits were given a zero cost estimate. It was assumed that the changes were merely a correction to return the program to the 1970 standard. In fact, the changes reversed policy errors of the 1970s and permitted the appropriate expansion of the number of individuals with mental illness receiving disability benefits. Eliminating the restrictions on outpatient mental health care under Medicare had been unthinkably expensive when the national plan was written. However, enactment took place in stages, and each stage was estimated to be relatively inexpensive. The total expense did not even approach the dire predictions made earlier. For each change made, there was a good reason for the low cost projection, but for each change to occur, that low cost projection was essential.

## Shortfalls and Problems

It is reasonable to ask why, when so many of the recommendations in the national plan have been ad-

dressed, the circumstances of the population of severely mentally disabled Americans still look so devastating. If one accepts that serious problems remain and conditions are no better—and for many perhaps are worse—than they were in 1980, there are several explanations for the apparent discrepancy between documented accomplishments and obvious shortfalls.

First, important as these four programs are for the well-being of persons with severe mental illness, it is not reasonable to expect that all problems can be solved through the provision of basic income support and mental health services. Other needs of this population were not as well met during the 1980s, particularly the need for housing and vocational services.[14]

Second, implementation of many of these changes has been slow and incomplete, as a consequence of both inadequate federal action and the states' failure to take advantage of the greater flexibility provided to them by federal law, particularly by Medicaid regulations. Federally, regulations were developed slowly or were confusing; for example, the medical management benefit in Medicare was widely misinterpreted. Administrative problems hampered the implementation of some provisions; for example, coordination between SSI staff and state hospital personnel for prerelease benefits presented difficulties, and outreach programs to potential SSI recipients were lacking.

Third, now that these structural changes have been accomplished, it will take money to fully implement them. To date, resources have been slow to develop. Overall financial limits on social program spending in the 1980s have made it difficult to implement the recommendations that have been adopted in principle and in regulation. For example, because of budgetary problems, states fail to select important new Medicaid options or limit their applicability.

Fourth, a whole set of problems has emerged, or grown significantly worse, since 1980. Foremost of these is the number of persons with severe mental illness who are now homeless, exacerbated in large part by loss of low-income housing and policies in the early 1980s to terminate individuals from the federal disability rolls.[15] Also, the decade saw increasing growth in the subgroup of individuals with severe mental illness who are hardest to serve—those who also abuse drugs or alcohol and who are more aggressively independent and alienated from the mental health system.[16,17]

In fact, the situation is indeed much better for many people, and overall it is much better than it might have been. The impact of the improvements is partly masked by the problems of homelessness and dually diagnosed and alienated consumers. The magnitude of the problems still faced makes even the substantial improvements resulting from implementation of so many of the national plan's recommendations seem minimally effective. While many people still do not have adequate incomes or access to the services theoretically provided through Medicaid and Medicare, the fact that the structure exists within these federal programs to meet the needs of these individuals represents a major step forward.

Perhaps most important for future planning, the four financing programs have bigger problems than just the exclusion of persons with mental illness or inappropriate application of the rules for persons with mental illness. Reading the national plan a decade after it was written points up how extremely inappropriate the rules of these four programs were in 1980 for persons with mental illness. As a result, the objectives of the plan, and of the advocates working to implement it, were focused on breaking into mainstream programs.

Now that the initial barriers to access are being dismantled, we see the shortfalls. For example, an individual may now be eligible to receive SSI, but the benefit received amounts to an income below the poverty level, which does not begin to meet the person's needs. Persons with mental illness may have gained full access to health and mental health care through Medicaid, but the program pays less than the true cost of services rendered, and few doctors will take Medicaid patients.

Policy Recommendations

Given the successful achievement of so many of the national plan's recommendations, we believe it is time for a new look at the goals of federal policy advocacy for persons with severe mental illness. Clearly, continued improvements need to be made in these four financing programs, but mental health concerns are now well incorporated in the structure at the federal level. Continued tinkering is needed,[18] such as full implementation of changes in entitlements, but that should not be our only objective.

Our analysis suggests a finished and unfinished agenda of the national plan. What is needed is the full implementation of changes in entitlements that were made in the past decade. In particular, outreach programs within the Social Security Administration are needed, as is assistance to individuals making disability benefits claims, a first step to gaining access to Medicaid and Medicare coverage. Mental health advocates must also become increasingly involved in the bigger problems of these entitlement programs, such as raising SSI benefit levels.

We need to move toward expanded advocacy at the state level. States must take advantage of the opportunities provided by federal law and must appropriate sufficient funds to fully implement the changes that have been made.

Our full report and analysis[4] assembles several rec-

ommendations from a number of different legislative and advocacy sources for improvements in the financing programs:

- Increase the SSI basic benefit level.
- Improve SSI outreach to ease bureaucratic barriers for homeless people to receive SSI.
- Continue improving standards for determining disability, including a study of changing the basic definition of disability.
- Permit families to set up trusts for the SSI recipient and improve the representative payee program.
- Enact an expanded work incentive program for SSDI and improve linkages with vocational rehabilitation programs.
- Eliminate the two-year waiting period for Medicare benefits for individuals receiving SSDI and create the option to secure Medicaid in place of Medicare.
- Implement in all states the federal options for case management and psychiatric rehabilitation under Medicaid.
- Improve eligibility for Medicaid to cover more low-income individuals with serious mental illness and to ensure that all SSI recipients are covered by Medicaid.
- Establish higher rates of payment for providers of Medicaid services.
- Expand Medicaid to cover respite care.

Finally, as federal policymakers move to address the pressing problems of the 1990s through consideration of national health care access bills and long-term-care proposals, we strongly caution the mental health field to ensure that persons with mental illness are appropriately covered under these new mainstream financing programs from the start. It has not been easy to redress the errors of the 1960s and 1970s, when Medicaid, Medicare, SSI, and SSDI were established without adequate consideration of the needs of persons with severe mental illness. It took substantial effort over the past decade to make incremental changes to correct structural defects in these key programs. To learn that positive changes occurred in the 1980s may be a pleasant shock, but before we become complacent, it is critical to remember that the full implementation and especially the funding of these programs remain an agenda for the immediate future.

The 1990s will have a new policy focus that is still evolving. One theme of that focus has already been set: individual consumer rights as reflected in the Americans With Disabilities Act. To move forward, the mental health field must work even better with others—with the disability community, with businesses, and with those involved in the mainstream programs. Most important of all, we must work better among ourselves. Divisiveness could so easily bring to an end the momentum built up in the 1980s by the national plan.

Acknowledgments
This paper is based on a report partially supported by the National Institute of Mental Health under purchase order 90MF45292101D. The opinions expressed are the authors' and do not represent official policy of NIMH. The authors acknowledge the contributions and editorial suggestions of

several individuals, in particular Irene Shifren-Levine, Fred Osher, Barry Blackwell, Susan Ridgely, Joe Manes, Stanley Platman, and Agnes Rupp.

## References

1. President's Commission on Mental Health: Report to the President, vol 1. Washington, DC, US Government Printing Office, 1978

2. Foley HA, Sharfstein SS: Madness and Government: Who Cares for the Mentally Ill? Washington, DC, American Psychiatric Press, 1983

3. US Department of Health and Human Services Steering Committee on the Chronically Mentally Ill: Toward a National Plan for the Chronically Mentally Ill. Washington, DC, Public Health Service, 1980

4. Koyanagi C, Goldman HH: Inching Forward: A Report on Progress Made in Federal Mental Health Policy in the 1980s. Alexandria, Va, National Mental Health Association, 1991

5. Anthony W, Jansen M: Predicting the vocational capacity of the chronically mentally ill: research and policy implications. *American Psychologist* 39:537–544, 1984

6. Goldman HH, Gattozzi AA: Murder in the cathedral revisited; President Reagan and the mentally disabled. Hospital and *Community Psychiatry* 39:505–509, 1988

7. Goldman HH, Gattozzi A: Balance of powers: Social Security and the mentally disabled, 1980–1985. *Millbank Quarterly* 66:531–551, 1988

8. Tessler R, Goldman HH: The Chronically Mentally Ill: Assessing Community Support Programs. Cambridge, Mass, Ballinger, 1982

9. Turner JC, Ten Hoor WJ: The NIMH Community Support Program: pilot approach to a needed social reform. *Schizophrenia Bulletin* 4:319–348, 1978

10. Task II: Federal Programs for Persons With Disabilities: Report to the Department of Health and Human Services, Office of the Assistant Secretary for Planning and Evaluation. Lexington, Mass, Systemetrics–McGraw-Hill, 1990

11. Taube CA, Goldman HH, Salkever D: Medicaid coverage for mental illness. *Health Affairs* 9:5–18, 1990

12. Koyanagi C: The missed opportunities of Medicaid. Hospital and *Community Psychiatry* 41:135–138, 1990

13. Sharfstein SS, Goldman HH: Financing and medical management of mental disorders. *American Journal of Psychiatry* 146:345–349, 1989

14. Mechanic D, Aiken LH: Improving the care of patients with chronic mental illness. *New England Journal of Medicine* 317:1634–1638, 1987

15. Lamb HR (ed): The Homeless Mentally Ill. Washington, DC, American Psychiatric Press, 1984

16. Ridgely MS, Goldman HH, Talbott JA: Chronic Mentally Ill Young Adults With Substance Abuse Problems: A Review of Relevant Literature and Creation of a Research Agenda, Baltimore, Department of Psychiatry, University of Maryland, 1986

17. Ridgely MS, Osher F, Talbott JA: Chronic Mentally Ill Young Adults With Substance Abuse Problems: Treatment and Training Issues, Baltimore, Department of Psychiatry, University of Maryland, 1987

18. Bloche MG, Cournos F: Mental health policy for the 1990s: tinkering in the interstices. *Journal of Health Politics, Policy, and Law* 15:387–398, 1990

19. Long-Term Care Facility Interpretive Guidelines, Survey Procedures, and Survey Forms. Baltimore, Health Care Financing Administration, 1989

# Chapter 8

# Will We Save the Homeless Mentally Ill?

## H. Richard Lamb, M.D.

*Progress in alleviating the plight of the homeless mentally ill has been very slow and disappointing. After reviewing the needs of the homeless mentally ill, the author makes recommendations for immediate action. Extensive case management services should be implemented rather than simply discussed. All incompetent and/or dangerous or gravely disabled homeless mentally ill persons should be brought to hospitals, involuntarily if necessary. Cost-effective alternatives to hospitals with varying degrees of structure should be provided. Involuntary mechanisms such as conservatorship and outpatient commitment should be used when needed. The emphasis should be on timely transfer to acceptable treatment and living situations rather than waiting for the ideal.*

*—(Am J Psychiatry 1990; 147:649–651)*

There has been much discussion about but very little definitive action on behalf of the homeless mentally ill, a problem whose very existence can only be considered incredible in a modern affluent nation. My purpose here is to advocate doing what is necessary to deal expeditiously and definitively with this problem.

## WHAT THE HOMELESS MENTALLY ILL NEED

The recommendations of APA's Task Force on the Homeless Mentally Ill,[1] if implemented, would probably greatly reduce the prevalence of homelessness among people with major mental illness. The task force saw homelessness as but one symptom of the problems besetting the chronically mentally ill generally in the United States and called for a comprehensive and integrated system of care for the chronically mentally ill to address the underlying problems that cause homelessness. Such a system would include an adequate number and range of supervised, supportive housing settings; a well-functioning system of case management; adequate, comprehensive, and accessible crisis intervention, both in the community and in hospitals; less restrictive laws on involuntary treatment; and ongoing treatment and rehabilitative services, all provided assertively through outreach when necessary.

Little has been done, however, to implement these recommendations since they were published in 1984. Some welcome exceptions are the current outreach services in New York City that include bringing patients to hospitals involuntarily, the implementation of case management strategies in some jurisdictions, and the broadening of civil commitment in some states, including outpatient commitment. Generally, when anything

*Will We Save the Homeless Mentally Ill?,* Vol. 147 No. 5, 649–651, May 1990, copyright 1990, the American Psychiatric Association. Reprinted by permission.

Received June 27, 1989; revision received Oct. 11, 1989; accepted Nov. 30, 1989. From the Department of Psychiatry, University of Southern California School of Medicine.

has been done, it has too often relied primarily on shelters. Although they are a necessary emergency resource, shelters address the symptom and do not get at the root of the problem; they are only temporary solutions from night to night.

The very fact that the homeless mentally ill are offered such facilities as shelters implies an acceptance by society of the principle that it is a basic right of the mentally ill, irrespective of their mental status and lack of competence, to refuse treatment and appropriate housing and live on the streets instead. There they live a life characterized by dysphoria and deprivation, can be victimized by any predator, and can develop life-threatening medical problems because of lack of medical intervention. Should the chronically and severely mentally ill have the right to "choose" such a life style without regard to their lack of competence to make such a decision? I think not. This is a cruel interpretation of the basic principles of civil rights that are so important to all of us in the United States.

Even a partial implementation of the recommendations of the APA task force would make a difference. Case management is an example. In a well-functioning system of case management, every chronically mentally ill person would be on the caseload of a mental health agency that would provide assertive outreach services, have sufficient staff to work intensively with these patients, take full responsibility for individualized treatment planning, link patients to needed resources, and monitor them so that they not only receive the services they need but are not lost to the system. It is reasonable to assume that such a system of case management would result in many more chronically mentally ill persons receiving services, including housing. Moreover, much of this could be accomplished on a voluntary basis. In such a situation, the number of homeless mentally ill would undoubtedly decrease.

Can we wait still longer for this to happen? Case management has been much discussed, but in too many jurisdictions little has been done to implement it. There is every indication, especially in our larger cities, where a high proportion of the homeless mentally ill are, that not only are there insufficient funds to do this but the bureaucracies are too ponderous and inefficient[2] to set up a comprehensive and competent case management system for the homeless mentally ill even if they had the funds.

Moreover, a large proportion of the homeless mentally ill tend to be resistant to taking psychotropic medications, to treatment generally, and to accepting any living situation. For instance, in funding a large-scale program designed to help the homeless mentally ill, the state legislature of California stipulated that services funded by this program could only be voluntary. An independent evaluation of this program[3] showed that, on average,

about 30% of the homeless mentally ill refused housing placements offered to them as a result of voluntary outreach case management, the primary modality of the program.

Because of their illness, many mentally ill individuals are unable to take advantage of living situations available to them. For instance, a recent study[4] found that some homeless mentally ill persons had places to live but were too paranoid to live there. The disabling functional deficits of major mental illness appear to be important contributing factors to homelessness among the mentally ill. These deficits include disorganized thinking and actions, poor problem-solving skills, and an inability to mobilize themselves due to depression. These are crucial deficits that should lead us to intervene, preferably with the patient's consent but without it if necessary. Still another major problem with a high proportion of the homeless mentally ill (probably two-thirds or more) is serious substance abuse problems over which these patients have little if any control.

## RECOMMENDATIONS

What then should we do? First of all, the chronically mentally ill must be our highest priority in public mental health. A large proportion of public mental health funding, now used for other activities, should be shifted to the care and treatment of the chronically mentally ill, which would, of course, include the homeless mentally ill.

We need to take action without waiting for the ideal to happen. We want to have comprehensive and coordinated mental health systems that would engage the homeless mentally ill and help many of them voluntarily accept treatment and suitable living arrangements. But the homeless mentally ill cannot wait decades for these systems to be established. Moreover, many homeless mentally ill persons will not accept services even with assertive outreach case management. In the meantime, if homeless persons with major mental illness are incompetent to make a decision with regard to accepting treatment and/or present a danger to themselves or others or are gravely disabled, then I believe that outreach teams including psychiatrists should bring all of these patients to hospitals, involuntarily if need be. No person meeting these criteria should be left living on the streets.

Do these persons have a right to live on the streets? It is my belief that the question should be phrased differently—Does society have the right to deny involuntary treatment to this population? I believe the answer is no and that these persons have a right to involuntary treatment.[5,6] Although being a danger to themselves or others or gravely disabled is a primary issue here and serves as legal and clinical grounds for depriving these persons of their "liberty," there are other fundamental questions. Are we physicians who care for the sick or are we not? Are we a caring society or are we not?

Although there has been hesitancy on the part of some professionals to use involuntary hospitalization, studies have shown that, after they have gone into remission, a large proportion of patients who had refused treatment state that their involuntary hospitalization was appropriate.[7,8]

If after a relatively brief hospitalization (a few weeks to a few months), mentally ill individuals can be placed voluntarily in a suitable living situation with built-in ongoing treatment, then we need to have these resources available. I believe that although we should have high standards for treatment and supportive housing, we cannot in good conscience leave the homeless mentally ill on the streets while we wait for such resources to be developed. In the short run we should settle for resources that are acceptable if not ideal. Moreover, cost has to be a consideration. We have to work within the limits of what society is willing to pay.

Many chronically mentally ill people also need such mechanisms as conservatorship, outpatient commitment, and payees to assist with money management, and these should be provided as long as the patient is in need of this kind of structure in the community. By giving up a little of their liberty, many patients can remain outside of hospitals and thus retain most of their liberty.

It is important that we recognize the needs of the homeless mentally ill. We need to recognize that the great majority need supervised housing; mainstream housing where persons live alone in their own apartments and have to manage by themselves is beyond the capability of the great majority of this population. Structure is a crucial concept; the needs of the homeless mentally ill fall on a continuum from modest amounts to moderate amounts to highly structured situations. It hardly needs to be stated that psychotropic medications are crucial, including neuroleptics, antidepressants, lithium, and others.

We are probably attempting to treat many patients in the community who cannot be managed in open community settings.[9] These persons have a need for structure in terms of a controlled living situation where their taking of medications is supervised and they are given as much freedom as they can handle but not more. For many, this will mean a locked setting. An active schedule of activities is for many patients another important way of providing structure.

Whether a patient needs a moderate or a high degree of structure should not be seen as an ideological issue but, rather, a clinical decision based on a pragmatic assessment of the needs of each individual patient. Does the patient have sufficient internal controls to organize himself or herself to cope with life's demands? To what degree do we need to add external structure to compensate for a lack of internal controls?

Some patients need more highly structured ongoing residential care in intermediate care facilities, such as California's locked skilled nursing facilities with special programs for psychiatric patients.[10] These private sector facilities have demonstrated that good-quality care can be provided at a relatively moderate cost, compared, for instance, with reopening state hospitals.

A relatively large group of patients who need highly structured 24–hour care are many of those with dual diagnoses—major mental illness and serious substance abuse problems. Probably no activity contributes more to staff burnout than trying to treat the more difficult patients with dual diagnoses in open settings.

A small but important minority of the homeless mentally ill need the highly structured setting that state hospitals provide. This should be high-quality care. But again there will be times when we cannot wait for the ideal. If funds are not available, it is more humane to place these patients in hospitals where the charts and even the staffing standards do not meet the standards of the Joint Commission on Accreditation of Healthcare Facilities than to leave these neglected human beings on the streets.

It is my belief that the time for endless (and fruitless) discussion is long past. There has been more than enough wringing of hands. The time for action is overdue. What needs to be done is abundantly clear. We need to be bold and strong of will. We must be prepared to mount a large-scale operation that will give relief to all of the homeless mentally ill. The fate of these persons with such great needs and at such great risk cannot be left in the hands of the fainthearted.

## References

1. Talbott JA, Lamb HR: Summary and recommendations, in The Homeless Mentally Ill: A Task Force Report of the American Psychiatric Association. Edited by Lamb HR. Washington, DC, APA, 1984
2. Keill SL: Politics and public psychiatric programs. *Hosp Community Psychiatry* 1985; 36:1143
3. Venez G, Burnam MA, McGlynn EA, et al: Review of California's Program for the Homeless Mentally Disabled. Santa Monica, Calif, Rand Corp, 1988
4. Lamb HR, Lamb DM: Factors contributing to homelessness among the chronically and severely mentally ill. *Hosp Commmunity Psychiatry* 1990; 41:301–304
5. Rachlin S: One right too many. *Bull Am Acad Psychiatry Law* 1975; 3:99–102
6. Lamb HR, Mills MJ: Needed changes in law and procedure for the chronically mentally ill. *Hosp Community Psychiatry* 1986; 37:475–480

7. Bradford B, McCann S, Merskey H: A survey of involuntary patients' attitudes towards their commitment. *Psychiatry J Univ Ottawa* 1986; 11:162–165

8. Srinivasan D, Soundarajan P, Hullin R: Attitudes of patients and relatives to compulsory admission. *Br J Psychiatry* 1980; 136:200–201

9. Lamb HR: Deinstitutionalization at the crossroads. *Hosp Community Psychiatry* 1988; 39:941–945

10. Lamb HR: Structure: the neglected ingredient of community treatment. *Arch Gen Psychiatry* 1980; 37:1224–1228

# PART FOUR
## Nonfinancial Resources

In the area of technology assessment, this section of the book includes an article by Mark B. Wenneker and Arnold M. Epstein examining inequitable distribution of technologies associated with ischemic heart disease in Massachusetts. This thought-provoking piece raises many questions associated with the diffusion of technology and equitable access to medical progress.

A number of important articles related to health care personnel are also included in this section. The first, by Beverley D. Rowley and associates, addresses characteristics of graduate medical education in the United States. This descriptive article provides an excellent overview of graduate medical education. The second article, by William B. Schwartz and Daniel N. Mendelson, challenges the widely held belief that there is an emerging physician surplus; key policy decisions hinge on a resolution of these controversies. Following these articles is one by Phillip R. Kletke, William D. Marder, and Anne B. Silberger on the changing sex composition of the physician work force in the United States and the significant implications of this change. This thought-provoking article examines the effect of underlying and dramatic changes in the types of physicians being trained and entering clinical practice. The final article related to health care personnel in this section, by Thomas E. Bittker, is a thoughtful policy-oriented assessment of the changing nature of American psychiatry and the role of the psychiatrist. The discussion reflects changes in the nation's health care system and the pressures that those changes exert on physicians.

# Chapter 9

# Racial Inequalities in the Use of Procedures for Patients With Ischemic Heart Disease in Massachusetts

Mark B. Wenneker, M.D., and Arnold M. Epstein, M.D., M.A.

*To examine interracial differences in the utilization of coronary angiography, coronary artery bypass grafting, and coronary angioplasty for white and black patients, we examined all admissions for circulatory diseases or chest pain to Massachusetts hospitals in 1985. After controlling for age, sex, payer, income, primary diagnoses, and the number of secondary diagnoses, whites underwent significantly more angiography and coronary artery bypass grafting procedures. Whites also underwent more angioplasty procedures, but the difference was not statistically significant. Although utilization differences may reflect patient preference or different levels of disease severity and socioeconomic status not adequately accounted for, this study suggests that substantial racial inequalities exist in the use of procedures for patients hospitalized with coronary heart disease.*
—(JAMA 1989;261:253–357)

Increasing competition in the medical marketplace and the advent of hospital prospective payment have increased concern about potential threats to patient access and quality of care.[1] At particular risk are likely to be disadvantaged groups, such as the poor, the uninsured, and racial minorities.

Previous studies have shown that interracial differences in utilization may be significant. Studies in ambulatory care settings have suggested that non-whites have greater barriers to access and lower use of services than whites.[2-6] Although the evidence on interracial differences in hospital use is equivocal,[7] some previous studies have suggested that blacks have lower use of surgery,[8] including coronary angiography and coronary artery bypass surgery.[9-11]

It seems particularly important to examine these cardiac procedures. They are relatively expensive and are commonly used to diagnose the extent of coronary artery disease and to relieve symptoms and prolong life for those with severe disease. Used appropriately, these procedures can have substantial health care benefits.[12-14] In 1985 approximately 200,000 coronary bypass operations were performed in the United States, a twofold increase since five years earlier.[15]

When we examined the existing studies of white-black differences in coronary procedure rates, we found several important limitations. In some instances[9] the investigations were population-based, providing information only on gross numbers of procedures per capita. This is an important limitation, since it does not allow one to determine whether differential procedure rates merely reflect different rates of physician contact, disease recognition, and hospitalization or whether there are also different procedure rates for black patients once they are hospitalized for serious cardiovascular conditions. Previous studies have also been based on single[11] or atypical settings[16] and have not controlled for clinical characteristics, insurance status, or socioeconomic status. Finally, the available studies predate the era of angioplasty. We have no information at all about black-white differences in this procedure, which may be an important substitute for coronary artery bypass surgery.

To better evaluate whether race is an important factor in cardiac procedure utilization, we procured data on hospitalizations in Massachusetts in fiscal year 1985. Information was included on comorbidity (secondary diagnoses), payer, zip code (which we used as a proxy for income), and admission type (referral or emergency). Among hospitalized patients we were able to determine whether racial differences in the utilization of cardiac procedures persisted after controlling for these potentially confounding variables.

## METHODS

We obtained discharge data from the Massachusetts Health Data Consortium on all patients discharged from hospitals in Massachusetts during fiscal year 1985 with principal diagnosis indicating diseases of the circulatory system (ICD-9–CM codes 390–459) or chest pain (ICD-9–CM codes 786.50–786.52 and 786.59) as well as all patients who underwent coronary arteriography (ICD-9–CM codes 37.21–37.23 and 88.55–88.57), coronary artery bypass graft surgery (ICD-9–CM codes 36.2 and 36.10–36.20), and coronary angioplasty (ICD-9–CM code 36.0), regardless of their diagnoses. All general short-term–care hospitals in Massachusetts are required to submit yearly case mix and charge data to the Massachusetts Rate Setting Commission on all patients regardless of payer. The data are edited by both the Rate Setting Commission and Health Data Consortium. In addition, summaries of data are reviewed by each hospital for accuracy in all of the key data variables. The discharge data included information on each patient's age, sex, primary payer, admission type, zip code, principal and secondary diagnoses, and procedures. Census data from 1980 were used to estimate median household income by zip code.

Patients not meeting the following criteria were excluded from the analysis: (1) zip code indicating Massachusetts residence, (2) age 30 through 89 years, (3) discharge from a nonfederal short-term–care hospital, and (4) race listed as white or black. We excluded patients with race listed as "unknown" or "other." This accounted for 8.8% and 0.4% of the population, respectively. Of the 140, 214 admissions for circulatory diseases or chest pain, 109, 575 (78.1%) were included in the analysis.

We pursued a two-pronged analytic approach, performing both population-based and hospital-based analyses. In the former analysis we calculated age- and sex-adjusted population-based admission and procedure rates for coronary angiography, coronary artery bypass surgery, and angioplasty. We calculated admission rates for two populations: those whose principal diagnosis was any circulatory disease or chest pain, and those whose principal diagnosis was myocardial infarction, unstable angina, chronic ischemia, angina, or chest pain. These represented the five most frequent principal discharge diagnoses for patients who underwent angiography. Angina, unstable angina, chronic ischemia, and myocardial infarction represented the four most frequent principal discharge diagnoses for bypass surgery and angioplasty. Patients admitted with these principal diagnoses accounted for 76.4% of all coronary catheterizations, 91.6% of all coronary artery bypass surgery procedures, and 96.2% of coronary angioplasty procedures performed on hospitalized patients in 1985. Population-based procedure rates were calculated from the total number of procedures per capita regardless of the primary diagnosis. Adjustment for age and sex was performed by direct standardization[17] using the Massachusetts population of blacks and whites aged 30 through 89 years as the standard.

Our hospital-based analysis was designed, of course, to assess whether patients had higher use of procedures once they were hospitalized for circulatory disease or chest pain. We were particularly interested in controlling for potential confounders. We first examined overall white-black odds ratios for hospitalized patients who underwent each of the three procedures. We then performed a series of analyses sequentially controlling for the following potential confounders: age, sex, principal diagnosis, disease severity (number of secondary diagnoses), admission type (emergency vs elective), payer, and income.

Principal diagnosis was grouped into six different conditions: (1) myocardial infarction, (2) unstable angina, (3) chronic ischemia, (4) angina, (5) chest pain, and (6) all other circulatory diseases. The number of secondary diagnoses was used as a proxy for disease severity. The payer was classified as one of five payer groups: (1) Blue Cross/Blue Shield, (2) Medicare, (3) Medicaid, (4) uninsured (self-pay or free care), or (5) "other," including those covered by worker's compensation, other government payment, commercial insurance, and health maintenance organization insurance and those whose insurer was unknown. We used residence as a proxy for income, assigning to each patient the median household income in his or her zip code. In each instance a Mantel-Haenszel summary estimate and confidence interval were calculated to assess the statistical significance of the relation between race and procedure use.[18]

Logistic regression was used to control simultaneously for age, sex, principal diagnosis, income, number of secondary diagnoses, and admission type in assessing

Table 1.—Unadjusted and Age- and Sex-Adjusted Admission and Procedured Rates for Massachusetts in 1985

| Group | Unadjusted Rate, per 10 000 Population | Rate Ratio Unadjusted (Whites per 10 000 Population/ Blacks per 10 000 Population) | Adjusted |
|---|---|---|---|
| Admission for any circulatory disease or chest pain | 378 | 1.25 (381/304) | 0.95 |
| Admission for ischemic heart disease | 159 | 1.49 (161/108) | 1.19 |
| Cardiac catheterization | 34.6 | 1.61 (35.0/21.7) | 1.38 |
| Coronary artery bypass surgery | 11.1 | 2.83 (11.3/4.0) | 2.26 |
| Angioplasty | 3.6 | 2.57 (3.6/1.4) | 2.52 |

interracial differences in whether a patient underwent a cardiac procedure.[19] Using this model, odds ratios were derived for differences in cardiac procedure utilization between blacks and whites, controlling for all other variables.

## RESULTS

As of 1980 there were 88,010 blacks and 2,806,310 whites in Massachusetts aged 30 through 89 years.[20] Women constituted 55.2% of the black population compared with 54.6% of the white population. The black population was also younger; 78.9% were below the age of 60 years compared with only 66.1% of the white population.

### Population-Based Analysis

Table 1 shows unadjusted and age- and sex-adjusted population-based admission rates for two groups: those whose principal diagnosis was any circulatory disease or

chest pain, and those whose principal diagnosis suggested ischemic heart disease (myocardial infarction, unstable angina, chronic ischemia, angina, or chest pain). Procedure rates for cardiac catheterization, coronary bypass surgery, and angioplasty are also displayed.

Adjusted white-black admission rate ratios are relatively close to 1.0; however, procedure rates differ substantially by race. Whereas whites are slightly less likely than blacks to be admitted with a circulatory disease or chest pain (rate ratio, 0.95), they are more likely to undergo angiography, coronary artery bypass grafting, and angioplasty, with adjusted rate ratios of 1.38, 2.26, and 2.52, respectively.

### Hospital-Based Analysis

Table 2 displays sociodemographic and clinical characteristics of patients hospitalized for a circulatory disease or chest pain at all 108 short-term-care hospitals. Black patients accounted for 2.4% of the cohort. White patients were older, more often male, and had a higher median income ($P<.05$).

Table 2.—Demographic, Socioeconomic, and Clinical Characteristics of Patients Hospitalized for Circulatory Diseases or Chest Pain in Massachusetts in 1985

| Item | Whites | Blacks |
|---|---|---|
| No. of patients | 106 902 | 2673 |
| Age, y (mean ± SD)* | 67.0 ± 12.9 | 59.7 ± 14.2 |
| Sex, % female* | 48.4 | 54.1 |
| Median income, $/y* | 18 067 | 13 040 |
| No. of diagnoses (mean ± SD)* | 3.8 ± 1.9 | 4.7 ± 2.3 |
| Diagnosis, No. (%)* | | |
| Unstable angina | 10 505 (9.8) | 146 (5.5) |
| Angina | 7542 (7.1) | 168 (6.3) |
| Chronic ischemia | 6189 (5.8) | 101 (3.8) |
| Chest pain | 6544 (6.1) | 287 (10.7) |
| Myocardial infarction | 14 414 (13.5) | 247 (9.2) |
| Other | 61 708 (57.7) | 1724 (64.5) |
| Payer, No. (%)* | | |
| Uninsured | 2827 (2.6) | 299 (11.2) |
| Medicare | 65 061 (60.9) | 1205 (45.1) |
| Medicaid | 2721 (2.5) | 332 (12.4) |
| Blue Cross/Blue Shield | 22 686 (21.2) | 429 (16.0) |
| Other | 13 607 (12.7) | 408 (15.3) |
| Type of admission, No. (%)* | | |
| Emergency | 83 969 (78.5) | 2207 (82.6) |
| Elective | 22 833 (21.4) | 463 (17.3) |

*$P<.05$.

The distribution of discharge diagnoses and payers differed significantly between the two races ($P<.001$). A much greater proportion of black patients was discharged with the diagnosis of chest pain, and lower proportions with diagnoses of unstable angina, myocardial infarction, and chronic ischemia. Relatively more whites were covered by Medicare or Blue Cross, and relatively fewer whites were uninsured or covered by Medicaid. A significantly higher percentage of blacks was admitted on an emergency basis ($P<.001$).

There were 9231 coronary catheterizations, 3131 coronary bypasses, and 1007 angioplasties performed on white patients compared with 156 catheterizations, 35 coronary bypasses, and 12 angioplasties for black patients. The white-black catheterization, bypass, and angioplasty rates were 1.52, 2.27, and 2.11, respectively ($P<.05$).

Analyses with potential confounders are displayed in Table 3. There are substantial differences in overall rates among different strata. Patients discharged with chronic ischemia had the highest likelihood of undergoing any of the three procedures, while patients with chest pain had the lowest likelihood. Being male, being admitted

electively, having Blue Cross insurance, and having a high income also increased the probability of undergoing procedures. Regardless of how we stratified the patients, the Mantel-Haenszel summary estimates reveal that interracial differences for all three procedures were in each instance statistically significant ($P<.05$), except for diagnosis stratification of angioplasty ($P = .23$).

As a final step, we performed logistic regression simultaneously, controlling for race and all of the potential confounders. For angiography and coronary artery bypass grafting there was a statistically significant interracial difference in utilization. The white-black odds ratios were 1.29 (95% confidence interval [CI], 1.07 to 1.56, $P<.01$) for angiography and 1.89 (95% CI, 1.30 to 2.74, $P<.001$) for bypass surgery. Seventy percent more whites than blacks underwent angioplasty, although this was not statistically significant (95% CI, 0.94 to 3.07, $P<.08$). Other significant ($P<.05$) predictors of utilization for all three procedures were payer, principal diagnosis, admission type, income, and number of secondary diagnoses. Sex was a significant predictor for angiography and coronary artery bypass grafting but not for angioplasty.

Table 3. Procedure Rate and White-Black Odds Ratios for Procedures Stratified by Potential Confounders

| Potential Confounder | No. of Patients | % White | CORONARY ANGIOGRAPHY Procedure Rate, % | CORONARY ANGIOGRAPHY White-Black Odds Ratio (95% Confidence Interval) | CORONARY BYPASS Procedure Rate, % | CORONARY BYPASS White-Black Odds Ratio (95% Confidence Interval) | ANGIOPLASTY Procedure Rate, % | ANGIOPLASTY White-Black Odds Ratio (95% Confidence Interval) |
|---|---|---|---|---|---|---|---|---|
| Diagnosis | | | | | | | | |
| Myocardial infarction | 14 661 | 98.3 | 7.3 | 0.73 (0.47–1.11) | 1.3 | 1.09 (0.34–3.42) | 0.9 | 2.15 (0.30–15.5) |
| Unstable angina | 10 651 | 98.6 | 12.3 | 1.22 (0.71–2.09) | 5.6 | 2.13 (0.79–5.78) | 2.0 | 0.71 (0.26–1.94) |
| Chronic ischemia | 6290 | 98.4 | 56.7 | 1.78 (1.20–2.65) | 30.2 | 1.25 (0.80–1.97) | 8.5 | 1.48 (0.65–3.40) |
| Angina | 7710 | 97.8 | 16.2 | 2.00 (1.17–3.42) | 3.2 | 5.58 (0.78–40.0) | 1.6 | 2.84 (0.39–20.42) |
| Chest pain | 6831 | 95.8 | 6.66 | 1.41 (0.82–2.43) | 0.0 | . . . | 0.0 | . . . |
| Other | 63 432 | 97.3 | 2.74 | 1.05 (0.78–1.42) | 0.4 | 6.36 (0.89–45.39) | 0.0 | . . . |
| Mantel-Haenszel summary | . . . | . . . | . . . | 1.26 (1.05–1.50) | . . . | 1.70 (1.18–2.45) | . . . | 1.42 (0.80–2.54) |
| Sex | | | | | | | | |
| M | 56 372 | 97.8 | 11.2 | 1.72 (1.37–2.14) | 4.3 | 2.73 (1.75–4.26) | 1.3 | 2.66 (1.19–5.94) |
| F | 53 176 | 97.3 | 5.7 | 1.19 (0.93–1.51) | 1.4 | 1.39 (0.83–2.33) | 0.6 | 1.38 (0.61–3.11) |
| Mantel-Haenszel summary | . . . | . . . | . . . | 1.47 (1.25–1.73) | . . . | 2.15 (1.54–3.01) | . . . | 2.02 (1.14–3.57) |
| Age, y | | | | | | | | |
| 31–50 | 13 088 | 94.3 | 14.5 | 1.99 (1.51–2.62) | 3.2 | 2.95 (1.46–5.96) | 2.4 | 2.53 (1.19–5.37) |
| 51–70 | 48 443 | 97.3 | 12.3 | 2.02 (1.62–2.52) | 4.4 | 2.61 (1.72–3.95) | 1.2 | 3.33 (1.38–8.04) |
| Mantel-Haenszel summary | . . . | . . . | . . . | 2.01 (1.69–2.39) | . . . | 2.69 (1.88–3.85) | . . . | 2.87 (1.62–5.09) |
| Payer | | | | | | | | |
| Blue Cross/Blue Shield | 23 115 | 98.1 | 15.2 | 1.11 (0.84–1.46) | 4.9 | 1.81 (1.01–3.22) | 1.9 | 2.78 (0.89–8.68) |
| Medicare | 66 266 | 98.2 | 5.1 | 1.42 (1.05–1.92) | 1.9 | 1.82 (1.05–3.15) | 0.4 | 2.42 (0.60–9.75) |
| Medicaid | 3053 | 89.1 | 7.9 | 3.00 (1.58–5.71) | 2.4 | 2.90 (0.91–9.25) | 0.6 | 2.08 (0.28–15.7) |
| Uninsured | 3126 | 90.4 | 7.8 | 1.36 (0.83–2.22) | 2.3 | 2.47 (0.77–7.89) | 1.0 | 0.71 (0.25–2.05) |
| Other | 14 015 | 97.1 | 14.4 | 2.73 (1.81–4.1) | 4.3 | 4.69 (1.75–12.60) | 1.9 | 4.06 (1.01–16.4) |
| Mantel-Haenszel summary | . . . | . . . | . . . | 1.59 (1.35–1.87) | . . . | 2.28 (1.63–3.19) | . . . | 2.22 (1.25–3.95) |
| Income, $ | | | | | | | | |
| Low (<15 000) | 30 298 | 93.6 | 7.1 | 1.26 (1.03–1.53) | 2.3 | 2.03 (1.33–3.08) | 0.8 | 1.72 (0.88–3.35) |
| High (≥15 000) | 78 642 | 99.1 | 9.1 | 1.56 (1.45–2.12) | 3.1 | 1.89 (1.06–3.34) | 1.0 | 2.36 (0.76–7.35) |
| Mantel-Haenszel summary | . . . | . . . | . . . | 1.34 (1.14–1.58) | . . . | 1.98 (1.41–2.77) | . . . | 1.89 (1.06–3.35) |
| No. of diagnoses | | | | | | | | |
| 1–3 | 51 435 | 98.2 | 9.9 | 1.52 (1.18–1.96) | 2.4 | 2.58 (1.33–4.98) | 1.0 | 2.35 (0.87–6.30) |
| 4–6 | 51 582 | 97.7 | 6.7 | 1.22 (0.95–1.57) | 2.8 | 2.84 (1.61–5.03) | 0.7 | 1.81 (0.75–4.38) |
| 7–9 | 6558 | 91.7 | 12.4 | 3.02 (2.02–4.51) | 7.6 | 3.31 (1.93–5.68) | 1.9 | 3.75 (1.19–11.83) |
| Mantel-Haenszel summary | . . . | . . . | . . . | 1.61 (1.37–1.90) | . . . | 2.94 (2.10–4.13) | . . . | 2.45 (1.38–4.34) |
| Admission type | | | | | | | | |
| Emergency | 86 176 | 97.4 | 4.7 | 1.22 (0.98–1.52) | 1.5 | 2.22 (1.33–3.70) | 0.6 | 1.12 (0.61–2.04) |
| Elective | 23 296 | 98.0 | 22.9 | 1.68 (1.30–2.17) | 8.1 | 1.98 (1.26–3.11) | 2.3 | 11.15 (1.56–79.5) |
| Mantel-Haenszel summary | . . . | . . . | . . . | 1.41 (1.19–1.66) | . . . | 2.09 (1.49–2.93) | . . . | 1.94 (1.10–3.34) |

## COMMENT

Our findings suggest that there are substantial inter-racial differences in cardiac procedure rates. Despite the fact that age- and sex-adjusted admission rates for whites and blacks were similar, our population-based analysis showed that whites underwent one third more coronary catheterizations and more than twice as many coronary artery bypass grafts and coronary angioplasties. These interracial inequalities were not merely a function of diminished physician contact and lower disease recognition for blacks. Rather, they were evident even among the cohort of individuals hospitalized for serious cardiovascular conditions.

Why do blacks undergo fewer cardiac procedures? One possible explanation is disease prevalence—white patients undergo more cardiac procedures because they are sicker than black patients and have a greater clinical need for intervention. Although one study from Evans County, Ga, noted a higher incidence of coronary heart disease among white men compared with black men,[21] the bulk of available evidence suggests that blacks may have equivalent if not greater rates of coronary disease.[22]

Blacks have a higher prevalence of cardiac risk factors, such as hypertension and diabetes,[23,24] and several studies have noted higher out-of-hospital cardiac fatality rates for blacks.[25–27] Overall mortality rates for ischemic heart disease also appear to be greater for blacks than for whites. For example, Sempos and colleagues[28] calculated that in 1985 the national age- and sex-adjusted rates for coronary heart disease mortality were 10% higher among black men than white men and 50% higher among black women than white women.

Another possible explanation relates to access, particularly the ability to pay for needed medical care. Bombardier and colleagues[8] studied the use of 11 noncardiac surgical procedures in 1970 and found that in aggregate, whites underwent significantly more procedures than blacks. When income was controlled for, however, the interracial differences became smaller and were no longer statistically significant. Other studies have noted that income influences utilization of primary-care[2,29,30] and hospital[7] services and choice of cancer treatment.[31]

In our study both of the proxy variables used to evaluate access and ability to pay, payer and median income by zip code, were significantly related to procedure utilization. Within strata defined by these variables the interracial differences in procedure use persisted. Our designation of income, however, was limited by the "ecological fallacy." Measurement for any single individual in our study is imprecise, and there is no way of ensuring that the distribution of incomes of the patients in our study is similar to the distribution of median incomes by zip code. It is possible that with a more precise designation of income, interracial differences would have decreased further.

Another explanation relates to sociocultural differences between blacks and whites and related preferences for different sorts of medical care. These may be true interracial differences or, in some instances, may merely reflect differences between different socioeconomic classes. Some studies have shown, for example, that blacks may be less likely to seek care or utilize health services even when they are available. Diehr and colleagues[4] noted that blacks in Seattle were at least 10% less likely than whites to use health services offered by Blue Cross/Blue Shield, a health maintenance organization, or an independent practice association. There is also evidence from the Coronary Artery Surgery Study,[16] which examined patterns of care for a nonrandomized group of patients who underwent angiography, that whites may prefer a more technological approach for the treatment of coronary disease. Among the subjects in the cohort for whom a bypass was recommended, more than 90% of the whites agreed to surgery compared with only 81% of the blacks. Of 100 blacks for whom medical therapy was initially recommended, only one had later surgery, whereas 11.6% of the 4652 whites for whom medical therapy was recommended had later bypass surgery.

Another explanation is that interracial differences may reflect differences in care provided, perhaps unintentionally, on the basis of race. Several studies[32–34] have noted large variations in the use of procedures. The reasons for such variation are complex, but, clearly, sociocultural factors influence physician and patient decision making.[35]

It is also possible that certain types of physicians, more academic and technologically oriented, may be more likely to care for black patients, and differences in procedure utilization may in part reflect different thresholds for intervention. Previous studies have shown that blacks undergoing surgery are more likely to receive care from a physician in training than from a senior staff surgeon.[36] Perhaps such differences in provision of services are reflected in the lower percentage of blacks who accept recommendations for surgery.

Several previous studies have evaluated interracial differences in coronary angiography and coronary bypass surgery, although none that we know of has examined coronary angioplasty. Gillum[9] used data from 1981 and found that in population-based analyses there were substantial age-adjusted interracial differences in rates for bypass surgery (relative white-black ratio, 3.6) and coronary angiography (relative white-black ratio, 1.4). Gillum did not control for diagnosis or adjust for any measure of severity, payer, or income.

Hospital-based analyses have also been used to evaluate racial differences in cardiac procedure rates once patients have been hospitalized. Ford and colleagues[10] analyzed a national discharge data set for patients hospitalized for acute myocardial infarction in 1984 and found that white rates for coronary angiography were twice those of blacks, and white rates were 50% higher for coronary bypass surgery. They did not, however, adjust for severity, payer, or income, and they only looked at one diagnosis. Oberman and Cutter[11] examined patients who underwent angiography at the University of Alabama, Birmingham, from 1970 through 1978 and found that being white significantly increased the probability of undergoing a bypass after controlling for age, history of cardiac disease, and cardiac risk factors as well as the number of diseased blood vessels. More recently, G. M. Ginsberg (unpublished results, 1987) examined procedures for patients hospitalized for cardiovascular disease in New York state and found similar interracial discrepancies in rates of angiography and bypass surgery.

The interpretation of our results is potentially limited by several factors. As with all hospital utilization data, the medical codes from the hospital discharge abstracts may not be completely reliable due to clinical disagreement and human error, and there may be coding "creep" as a means of increasing reimbursement.[37,38] Iezzoni and colleagues[39] have shown that coding for acute myocardial infarction may pose particular problems because of the inclusion of patients with chest pain who have been "ruled out" for myocardial infarction.

Nevertheless, we believe the quality of the data is suitable for our purposes. Since the accuracy of the information is key to the rate-setting process, Massachusetts edits the data to check items such as out-of-range values and inconsistencies among age, sex, and diagnosis. Similar data have been used successfully for numerous other investigations.[10,40,41] Although 9% of the patients did not have race coded, we have no reason to suspect that accuracy should be biased toward one racial group. The demographic and clinical characteristics of this cohort of unknown patients were similar to those of the overall population.

Angiography coding is another potential source of bias. Of our cohort, 56.5% were coded as undergoing "cardiac catheterization" (ICD-9–CM codes 37.21–37.23) only, 1.2% were coded as undergoing "coronary catheterization" (ICD-9–CM codes 88.55–88.57) only, and 42.2% were coded as undergoing both procedures. Coding practices in Massachusetts are variable for this procedure. Patients coded as undergoing "cardiac catheterization" had roughly the same distribution of ischemic diagnoses as those coded with "coronary catheterization" or both designations. Therefore, in our analysis, patients were included in the angiography cohort if they were coded in any one of the above categories. We also

analyzed white-black population-based age- and sex-adjusted rate ratios for angiography based on only the populations coded as undergoing "coronary catheterization" or both procedures. Using this cohort, the interracial differences actually increased to 1.52 from 1.38. We also repeated the logistic regression on this cohort; although whites underwent more angiography procedures, the difference was no longer statistically significant.

Since blacks are not randomly distributed into different regions and different hospitals, differences in rates among races may be due largely to regional or hospital variation rather than to deliberate differences in treatment of patient subgroups. Of the 108 short-term-care hospitals in Massachusetts, only 17 offered angiography, ten offered coronary bypass, and nine offered angioplasty in 1985. We therefore repeated our hospital-based analyses for each procedure for only the patients admitted to the hospitals that performed the procedure, but we found that in each instance the white-black differences increased and remained statistically significant. This study did not take into account utilization of angiography through outpatient cardiology clinics, an increasingly used option. If white patients have greater access to these clinics than blacks, our estimates of interracial differences are conservative. Finally, the exclusion of Veterans Administration (VA) hospitals could have also biased our results in favor of white patients if the proportion of blacks undergoing procedures at VA hospitals was greater than at non-VA hospitals. Unfortunately, discharge abstract coding for VA hospitals is not used for rate setting and is unreliable in Massachusetts.

It would be unwise to conclude from this study that black patients are underserved or directly harmed by undergoing fewer procedures. Higher procedure rates among the white population may be attributable to overutilization. If angioplasty was, in some sense, an "experimental" procedure in 1985, we found no evidence of increased use among blacks. Studies of the appropriateness of care by race certainly seem in order. Our study included data from only one state and cannot be generalized to the whole United States. Massachusetts is somewhat unusual in having a relatively small number of hospitals that offer bypass surgery and angioplasty.

This study suggests that racial inequalities exist in the provision of cardiac care in Massachusetts. These differences may not be due entirely to race per se; they may be due in part to differences in income or disease severity that have not been adequately accounted for in this study. Nevertheless, race does seem to be important. If medical decisions are being made on the basis of race we need to understand more about the complex interaction between physician and patient that leads to this inequality and the implications of these patterns for the appropriateness and efficiency of medical care.

## References

1. Stern RS, Epstein AM: Institutional responses to prospective payment based on diagnoses related group. *N Engl J Med* 1985;312:621–627.
2. Aday LA, Anderson RM: The national profile of access to medical care: Where do we stand? *Am J Public Health* 1984;74:1331–1339.
3. Davis K, Gold M, Makuc D: Access to health care for the poor: Does the gap remain? *Annu Rev Public Health* 1981;2:159–182.
4. Diehr P, Martin DP, Price KF, et al: Use of ambulatory care services in three provider plans. *Am J Public Health* 1984;74:47–51.
5. James SA, Wagner EH, Strogatz DS, et al: The Edgecombe County (NC) High Blood Pressure Control Program. *Am J Public Health* 1984;74:468–472.
6. Yergan J, Flood AB, LoGerfo JP, et al: Relationship between patient race and the intensity of hospital services. *Med Care* 1987;25:592–603.
7. Wilson PA, Griffith JR, Tedeschi PJ: Does race affect hospital use? *Am J Public Health* 1985;75:263–269.
8. Bombardier C, Fuchs VR, Lillard LE, et al: Socioeconomic factors affecting the utilization of surgical operations. *N Engl J Med* 1977;297:699–705.
9. Gillum RF: Coronary artery bypass surgery and coronary angiography in the United States, 1979–1983. *Am Heart J* 1987;113:1255–1260.
10. Ford E, Cooper R, Castaner A, et al: Coronary arteriography and coronary bypass surgery among whites and nonwhites relative to hospital-based incidence rates for coronary artery disease. *Am J Public Health,* in press.
11. Oberman A, Cutter G: Issues in the natural history and treatment of coronary heart disease in black populations: Surgical treatment. *Am Heart J* 1984;108:688–694.
12. CASS (Principal Investigators and Associates): Myocardial infarction and mortality in the Coronary Artery Surgery Study (CASS): Randomized trial. *N Engl J Med* 1984;310:750–758.
13. European Coronary Surgery Study Group: Long-term results of prospective randomized study of coronary artery bypass surgery in stable angina pectoris. *Lancet* 1982;2:1173–1180.
14. Peduzzi P, Hullgren HN: Effect of medical vs surgical treatment of symptoms in stable angina pectoris: The Veterans Administration Cooperative Study of Surgery for Coronary Arterial Occlusive Disease. *Circulation* 1979;60:888–900.
15. *Detailed Diagnosis and Procedures for Patients Discharged from Short-term Hospitals, US 1985,* US Dept of Health and Human Services publication (PHS) 87–1751. National Center for Health Statistics, 1985.
16. Maynard C, Fisher LD, Passamani ER, et al: Blacks in the Coronary Artery Surgery Study. *Circulation* 1986;74:64–71.
17. Colton T: *Statistics in Medicine.* Boston, Little Brown & Co Inc, 1974.
18. Robins J, Greenland S, Breslow NE: A general estimator for the variance of the Mantel-Haenszel odds ratio. *Am J Epidemiol* 1986;124:719–723.
19. *SUGI Supplemental Library User's Guide, version 5.* Cary, NC, SAS Institute, 1986.
20. *General Population Characteristics Massachusetts, US* Dept of Commerce publication PC80-1–B23. Bureau of the Census, 1982.
21. Cassel J, Heyden S, Bartel AG, et al: Incidence of coronary heart disease by ethnic group, social class and sex. *Arch Intern Med* 1971;128:901–906.
22. Gillum RF: Coronary heart disease in black populations: I. Mortality and morbidity. *Am Heart J* 1982;104:839–851.
23. Curry CL, Oliver J, Mumtaz FB: Coronary artery disease in blacks: Risk factors. *Am Heart J* 1984;108:653–657.
24. Gillum RF, Grant CT: Coronary heart disease in black populations: II. Risk factors. *Am Heart J* 1982;104:852–864.
25. Hagstrom RM, Federspiel CF, Ho YC: Incidence of myocardial infarction and sudden death from coronary heart disease in Nashville, Tennessee. *Circulation* 1971;44:844–890.
26. Keil JE, Saunders DE, Lackland DT, et al: Acute myocardial infarction: Period prevalence, case fatality, and comparison of black and white cases in urban and rural areas of South Carolina. *Am Heart J* 1985;109:776–784.
27. Weisse AB, Abiuso PD, Thind IS: Acute myocardial infarction in Newark, NJ: A study of racial incidence. *Arch Intern Med* 1977;137:1402–1405.
28. Sempos C, Cooper R, Kovar MG, et al: Divergence of the recent trends in coronary mortality for the four major race-sex groups in the United States. *Am J Public Health* 1988;78:1422–1427.
29. Dutton D: Explaining the low use of health services by the poor. *Am Soc Rev* 1978;43:348–368.
30. Hayward RA, Shapiro MF, Freeman HE, et al: Inequities in health services among insured Americans. *N Engl J Med* 1988;318:1507–1512.
31. Greenberg ER, Chute CG, Stukel T, et al: Social and economic factors in the choice of lung cancer treatment. *N Engl J Med* 1988;318:612–617.
32. Wennberg J, Gittelsohn A: Small-area variations in health care delivery. *Science* 1982;246:120–135.
33. Chassin MR, Brook RH, Park RE: Variations in the use of medical and surgical services by the Medicare population. *N Engl J Med* 1986;314:285–290.
34. Brook RH, Kosecoff JB, Park RE, et al: Diagnosis and treatment of coronary disease: Comparison of doctor's attitudes in the USA and UK. *Lancet* 1988;1:750–753.
35. Eisenberg JM: Sociologic influences on medical decision making by clinicians. *Ann Intern Med* 1979;90:957–964.
36. Egbert LD, Rothman IL: Relation between race and economic status of patients and who performs their surgery. *N Engl J Med* 1977;297:90–91.
37. Demlo LK, Campbell PM: Improving hospital discharge data. *Med Care* 1981;19:1030–1040.

38. Hsia DC, Krushat M, Fagan AB, et al: Accuracy of diagnostic coding for Medicare patients under the prospective-payment system. *N Engl J Med* 1988;318:352–355.

39. Iezzoni LI, Burnside S, Sickles L, et al: Coding of acute myocardial infarction: Clinical and policy implications. *Ann Intern Med* 1988;109:745–751.

40. Sloan FS, Valvona J, Mullner R: Identifying the issues: A statistical profile, in Sloan F, Blumenstein J, Perrin J (eds): *Uncompensated Hospital Care: Rights and Responsibilities.* Baltimore, Johns Hopkins University Press, 1986, pp 16–53.

41. Roos NP, Wennberg JE, McPherson K: Using diagnosis-related groups for studying variations in hospital admissions. *Health Care Financ Rev,* Summer 1988, p 53.

# Chapter 10
# Selected Characteristics of Graduate Medical Education in the United States

Beverley Davies Rowley, Ph.D.; DeWitt C. Baldwin, Jr. M.D.; and Mary B. McGuire, M.P.H.

*For the second year, the Department of Data Systems in the Medical Education Group of the American Medical Association gathered information on graduate medical education primarily by means of an electronic data collection system. Eighty-eight percent of 6622 programs surveyed responded, with 83% reporting detailed information on residents. Analysis of graduate medical education data shows that the number of residents increased by 34.9% from the academic years 1980–1981 to 1990–1991, while the number of graduate year 1 residents decreased by 2%. In the same decade, the proportion of women residents increased by 7.1%. The number of minorities in graduate medical education has grown, but their proportions within the total resident population have remained largely unchanged. The number of graduates from schools of osteopathic medicine has increased by 265% over the same 10–year period. Between 1989 and 1990, a 31.6% increase was recorded in the number of international medical graduates in graduate year 1 residency positions; most of this increase (63.4%) occurred among noncitizens of the United States*
*—(JAMA.1991; 266:933–943)*

Included in this report on graduate medical education in the United States for the 1990–1991 academic year are selected data for the academic years 1980–1981 and 1985–1986.[1,2] Data from programs accredited by the Accreditation Council for Graduate Medical Education (ACGME) are reported by specialty and by region; information on selected characteristics of the programs and on the residents in them is summarized.

In 1990, the ACGME began to accredit, through Residency Review Committees, programs in critical care pediatrics, adult reconstructive orthopedics, pediatric pulmonology, and trauma orthopedics. Recently, special requirements for programs in orthopedic spine surgery, pediatric neurological surgery, and vascular and interventional radiology were also approved.

For purposes of accreditation, all programs accredited by the ACGME are called *residency* programs, whether these are in a specialty or subspecialty. The term *resident* is used to refer to persons at all levels of graduate medical education (including fellows) in programs accredited by the ACGME. For the first time, data are provided on selected specialties that are certified by their own specialty boards, but are not part of the ACGME accreditation process.

## METHODS

Each fall the Department of Data Systems in the Medical Education Group of the American Medical Association (AMA) collects statistical information from all programs, institutions, and agencies that participate to a significant extent in graduate medical education in the

Reprinted with permission from *Journal of the American Medical Association,* August 21, 1991, Vol. 266 No. 7, pp. 933–943, copyright 1992, American Medical Association.

United States. The information is collected primarily by means of a computerized data collection system. In August 1990, preprogrammed computer diskettes were mailed to each ACGME-accredited program, each non-ACGME program (combined specialties and obstetrics and gynecology subspecialties), and each graduate medical education teaching institution in the United States. Printed survey forms were sent when requested. All surveys were returned to the AMA where the data were uploaded or manually entered into the computer system exactly as recorded by the programs. Information on residents and programs was later loaded into a database management system that allows for data analysis across a wide range of variables.

Response rates to different sections of the survey varied. Eighty-three percent of all programs accredited in the 1990–1991 academic year responded with resident information by December 31, 1990. Fifteen of the 66 specialty categories had response rates of 90% or above. Eighty-eight percent of programs reported general program data, including the number of positions.

## CHARACTERISTICS OF PROGRAMS AND POSITIONS BY SPECIALTY AND GEOGRAHPIC REGION

### Accredited Programs

The accreditation actions of the Residency Review Committees and of the ACGME are continuously updated. On January 1, 1991, there were 6664 accredited residency training programs in the United States, an increase of 73 (1.1%) over the previous year. This number includes programs no longer accredited as of June 30, 1991. Statistics from these programs, as well as from an additional 125 programs recognized in the combined training specialties and 149 programs recognized in the obstetrics and gynecology subspecialties, were included in the tabulations. Programs that received initial accreditation after the survey were not surveyed.

In the 1990–1991 academic year, internal medicine had the largest number of accredited programs (426), followed by family practice (383), general surgery (281), and obstetrics and gynecology (275). As of September 1, 1990, 38% of all residents were in training programs for internal medicine, family practice, or pediatrics. Table 1 lists the number and percentage of programs and residents in each specialty.

As in previous years, the densely populated areas of the Middle Atlantic region contain the largest percentages of residents (24.8%) and programs (23.6%) (Table 2. Outside the Eastern seaboard, California has the most programs (9.3%) and residents (8.3%).

### Positions Offered

In the annual survey conducted by the Department of Data Systems, program directors are asked to project the number of positions that will be offered on July 1 of the following year, often a difficult task. Some institutions make a determination of the total positions to be supported and individual program directors subtract from

Table 1.—Number and Percentage of Existing and Reporting Programs as of January 1, 1991, and Number and Percentage of Residents on Duty September 1, 1990, by Specialty

| Specialty | Existing Programs | | Programs Reporting Resident Data | Residents Reported | |
|---|---|---|---|---|---|
| | No. | % | | No. | % |
| Allergy and immunology | 86 | 1.2 | 72 | 322 | 0.4 |
| Anesthesiology | 155 | 2.2 | 143 | 4889 | 5.9 |
| Critical care | 38 | 0.5 | 18 | 37 | ...* |
| Colon and rectal surgery | 29 | 0.4 | 22 | 54 | 0.1 |
| Dermatology | 100 | 1.4 | 92 | 824 | 1.0 |
| Dermatopathology | 29 | 0.4 | 18 | 25 | ...* |
| Emergency medicine | 83 | 1.2 | 78 | 1781 | 2.1 |
| Family practice | 383 | 5.5 | 351 | 6680 | 8.1 |
| Geriatrics | 16 | 0.2 | 8 | 15 | ...* |
| Internal medicine | 426 | 6.1 | 400 | 18 734 | 22.6 |
| Cardiovascular disease | 217 | 3.1 | 168 | 1677 | 2.0 |
| Critical care | 91 | 1.3 | 41 | 190 | 0.2 |
| Endocrinology and metabolism | 137 | 2.0 | 90 | 295 | 0.4 |
| Gastroenterology | 183 | 2.6 | 145 | 764 | 0.9 |
| Geriatrics | 69 | 1.0 | 40 | 153 | 0.2 |
| Hematology (medicine) | 149 | 2.1 | 94 | 405 | 0.5 |
| Infectious diseases | 151 | 2.2 | 110 | 460 | 0.6 |
| Medical oncology | 154 | 2.2 | 87 | 534 | 0.6 |
| Nephrology | 146 | 2.1 | 110 | 417 | 0.5 |
| Pulmonary diseases | 176 | 2.5 | 138 | 725 | 0.9 |
| Rheumatology | 123 | 1.8 | 92 | 281 | 0.3 |

| | | | | | |
|---|---|---|---|---|---|
| Neurological surgery | 93 | 1.3 | 84 | 720 | 0.9 |
| Neurology | 118 | 1.7 | 100 | 1211 | 1.5 |
|   Child neurology | 68 | 1.0 | 40 | 101 | 0.1 |
| Nuclear medicine | 86 | 1.2 | 65 | 156 | 0.2 |
| Obstetrics and gynecology | 275 | 4.0 | 260 | 4315 | 5.2 |
|   Gynecologic oncology† | 29 | 0.4 | 15 | 40 | ...* |
|   Maternal and fetal medicine† | 77 | 1.1 | 40 | 135 | 0.2 |
|   Reproductive endocrinology† | 43 | 0.6 | 23 | 57 | 0.1 |
| Ophthalmology | 136 | 2.0 | 119 | 1446 | 1.7 |
| Orthopedic surgery | 163 | 2.3 | 144 | 2630 | 3.2 |
|   Adult reconstructive surgery‡ | 1 | ...* | ...‡ | ...‡ | ...‡ |
|   Hand surgery | 18 | 0.3 | 9 | 19 | ...* |
|   Musculoskeletal oncology | 6 | 0.1 | 4 | 5 | ...* |
|   Pediatric orthopedics | 18 | 0.3 | 6 | 15 | ...* |
|   Sports medicine | 18 | 0.3 | 8 | 10 | ...* |
|   Trauma orthopedics‡ | 1 | ...* | ...‡ | ...‡ | ...‡ |
| Otolaryngology | 107 | 1.5 | 97 | 1002 | 1.2 |
| Pathology | 208 | 3.0 | 185 | 2364 | 2.9 |
|   Blood banking | 35 | 0.5 | 22 | 32 | ...* |
|   Chemical pathology | 6 | 0.1 | 1 | 1 | ...* |
|   Forensic pathology | 40 | 0.6 | 17 | 28 | ...* |
|   Hematology (pathology) | 25 | 0.4 | 11 | 20 | ...* |
|   Immunopathology | 14 | 0.2 | 7 | 11 | ...* |
|   Medical microbiology | 3 | ...* | 1 | 1 | ...* |
|   Neuropathology | 50 | 0.7 | 24 | 38 | ...* |
| Pediatrics | 215 | 3.1 | 193 | 6115 | 7.4 |
|   Critical care‡ | 28 | 0.4 | ...‡ | ...‡ | ...‡ |
|   Neonatal-perinatal medicine | 103 | 1.5 | 73 | 304 | 0.4 |
|   Pediatric cardiology | 46 | 0.7 | 33 | 176 | 0.2 |
|   Pediatric endocrinology | 53 | 0.8 | 31 | 84 | 0.1 |
|   Pediatric hemato-oncology | 58 | 0.8 | 35 | 153 | 0.2 |
|   Pediatric nephrology | 42 | 0.6 | 28 | 64 | 0.1 |
|   Pediatric pulmonology‡ | 24 | 0.3 | ...‡ | ...‡ | ...‡ |
| Physical medicine and rehabilitation | 73 | 1.1 | 62 | 893 | 1.1 |
| Plastic surgery | 100 | 1.4 | 84 | 391 | 0.5 |
| Preventive medicine, general | 30 | 0.4 | 18 | 146 | 0.2 |
|   Aerospace medicine | 3 | ...* | 3 | 48 | 0.1 |
|   Combined general preventive medicine and public health | 6 | 0.1 | 4 | 56 | 0.1 |
|   Occupational medicine | 30 | 0.4 | 21 | 163 | 0.2 |
|   Public health | 9 | 0.1 | 6 | 19 | ...* |
| Psychiatry | 196 | 2.8 | 170 | 4673 | 5.6 |
|   Child psychiatry | 123 | 1.8 | 97 | 642 | 0.8 |
| Radiation oncology | 80 | 1.2 | 67 | 443 | 0.5 |
| Radiology, diagnostic | 210 | 3.0 | 201 | 3775 | 4.6 |
| Radiology, diagnostic (nuclear) | 38 | 0.5 | 17 | 32 | ...* |
| Surgery | 281 | 4.1 | 268 | 7644 | 9.2 |
|   Critical care | 12 | 0.2 | 4 | 10 | ...* |
|   Pediatric surgery | 22 | 0.3 | 19 | 37 | ...* |
|   Vascular surgery | 63 | 0.9 | 51 | 88 | 0.1 |
| Thoracic surgery | 92 | 1.3 | 83 | 305 | 0.4 |
| Urology | 126 | 1.8 | 114 | 963 | 1.2 |
| Transitional year | 171 | 2.5 | 156 | 1475 | 1.8 |
| **Combined Specialty Programs†** | | | | | |
| Internal medicine/pediatrics | 84 | 1.2 | 65 | 534 | 0.6 |
| Internal medicine/emergency medicine | 11 | 0.2 | 5 | 11 | ...* |
| Internal medicine/physical medicine and rehabilitation | 12 | 0.2 | 1 | 3 | ...* |
| Pediatrics/emergency medicine | 4 | 0.1 | 1 | 2 | ...* |
| Pediatrics/psychiatry/child psychiatry | 6 | 0.1 | 3 | 27 | ...* |
| Pediatrics/physical medicine and rehabilitation | 8 | 0.1 | 4 | 7 | ...* |
| **Total** | **6938** | **99.6** | **5516** | **82 902** | **99.9** |

*Less than 0.1%.
†Not accredited by the ACGME.
‡Programs in these subspecialties were accredited after the annual survey; resident data were not collected.

Table 2.—Number and Percentage of Programs and Residents on Duty September 1, 1990, by Region

| Region | Programs | | Residents | |
|---|---|---|---|---|
| | No. | % | No. | % |
| **New England, Subtotal** | **549** | **7.9** | **6146** | **7.5** |
| Connecticut | 146 | 2.1 | 1495 | 1.8 |
| Maine | 19 | 0.3 | 176 | 0.2 |
| Massachusetts | 291 | 4.2 | 3548 | 4.3 |
| New Hampshire | 23 | 0.3 | 229 | 0.3 |
| Rhode Island | 43 | 0.6 | 484 | 0.6 |
| Vermont | 27 | 0.4 | 214 | 0.3 |
| **Middle Atlantic, Subtotal** | **1636** | **23.5** | **20 523** | **24.7** |
| New Jersey | 182 | 2.6 | 2420 | 2.9 |
| New York | 979 | 14.1 | 12 673 | 15.3 |
| Pennsylvania | 475 | 6.8 | 5430 | 6.5 |
| **East North Central, Subtotal** | **1173** | **17.0** | **14 696** | **17.6** |
| Illinois | 357 | 5.1 | 4429 | 5.3 |
| Indiana | 81 | 1.2 | 1022 | 1.2 |
| Michigan | 276 | 4.0 | 3580 | 4.3 |
| Ohio | 344 | 5.0 | 4227 | 5.1 |
| Wisconsin | 115 | 1.7 | 1438 | 1.7 |
| **West North Central, Subtotal** | **462** | **6.7** | **5616** | **6.9** |
| Iowa | 67 | 1.0 | 818 | 1.0 |
| Kansas | 53 | 0.8 | 638 | 0.8 |
| Minnesota | 120 | 1.7 | 1875 | 2.3 |
| Missouri | 170 | 2.5 | 1670 | 2.0 |
| Nebraska | 37 | 0.5 | 457 | 0.6 |
| North Dakota | 9 | 0.1 | 82 | 0.1 |
| South Dakota | 6 | 0.1 | 76 | 0.1 |
| **South Atlantic, Subtotal** | **1061** | **15.3** | **12 391** | **14.8** |
| Delaware | 13 | 0.2 | 205 | 0.2 |
| District of Columbia | 177 | 2.6 | 1913 | 2.3 |
| Florida | 169 | 2.4 | 2342 | 2.8 |
| Georgia | 108 | 1.6 | 1496 | 1.8 |
| Maryland | 169 | 2.4 | 1868 | 2.3 |
| North Carolina | 163 | 2.3 | 2111 | 2.5 |
| South Carolina | 69 | 1.0 | 844 | 1.0 |
| Virginia | 144 | 2.1 | 1193 | 1.4 |
| West Virginia | 49 | 0.7 | 419 | 0.5 |
| **East South Central, Subtotal** | **329** | **4.8** | **3635** | **4.4** |
| Alabama | 84 | 1.2 | 907 | 1.1 |
| Kentucky | 80 | 1.2 | 875 | 1.1 |
| Mississippi | 36 | 0.5 | 366 | 0.4 |
| Tennessee | 129 | 1.9 | 1487 | 1.8 |
| **West South Central, Subtotal** | **608** | **8.7** | **7475** | **9.0** |
| Arkansas | 44 | 0.6 | 439 | 0.5 |
| Louisiana | 127 | 1.8 | 1257 | 1.5 |
| Oklahoma | 54 | 0.8 | 640 | 0.8 |
| Texas | 383 | 5.5 | 5139 | 6.2 |
| **Mountain, Subtotal** | **235** | **3.4** | **2546** | **3.1** |
| Arizona | 68 | 1.0 | 842 | 1.0 |
| Colorado | 82 | 1.2 | 845 | 1.0 |
| Montana | 0 | 0 | 0 | 0 |
| New Mexico | 32 | 0.5 | 335 | 0.4 |
| Utah | 51 | 0.7 | 482 | 0.6 |
| Wyoming | 2 | . . .* | 42 | 0.1 |
| **Pacific, Subtotal** | **812** | **11.6** | **9088** | **10.9** |
| Alaska | 0 | 0 | 0 | 0 |
| California | 646 | 9.3 | 6882 | 8.3 |
| Hawaii | 24 | 0.3 | 390 | 0.5 |
| Idaho | 2 | . . .* | 23 | . . .* |
| Nevada | 6 | 0.1 | 77 | 0.1 |
| Oregon | 49 | 0.7 | 537 | 0.6 |
| Washington | 85 | 1.2 | 1179 | 1.4 |
| **Territory, Subtotal** | **73** | **1.1** | **786** | **0.9** |
| Puerto Rico | 73 | 1.1 | 786 | 0.9 |
| **Total** | **6938** | **100.0** | **82 902** | **99.8** |

*Less than 0.1%.

that number as they fill positions with acceptable candidates. Because a small number of programs do not meet accreditation requirements, they are prohibited from filling any or all of the reported positions. Some new programs may obtain accreditation in time to accept candidates in July, but these positions are not included in the program directors' projections.

The number of reported resident positions offered for July 1991 is shown in Table 3, which also indicates the changes within each specialty from two prior periods. The number of positions projected for July 1991 was 89,566. Approximately 10,000 new positions have been added for 1980 to 1985 and again from 1985 to 1990. This increase can be explained by the accreditation of a number of subspecialties, growth in the number and size of programs, and the addition of one new specialty (emergency medicine) and the transitional year.

Table 3.—Number of Reported Residency Positions Offered July 1, by Specialty*

| Specialty | 1980 | 1985 | 1991 |
|---|---|---|---|
| Allergy and immunology | 209 | 288 | 337 |
| Anesthesiology | 2813 | 3940 | 5429 |
| Critical care | ... | ... | 89 |
| Colon and rectal surgery | 42 | 49 | 50 |
| Dermatology | 781 | 754 | 877 |
| Dermatopathology | 36 | 38 | 48 |
| Emergency medicine | ... | 1181 | 1597 |
| Family practice | 7004 | 7592 | 7713 |
| Geriatrics | ... | ... | 49 |
| Internal medicine | 16 576 | 18 377 | 19 705 |
| Cardiovascular disease | ... | ... | 1948 |
| Critical care | ... | ... | 375 |
| Endocrinology and metabolism | ... | ... | 456 |
| Gastroenterology | ... | ... | 896 |
| Geriatrics | ... | ... | 259 |
| Hematology (medicine) | ... | ... | 665 |
| Infectious diseases | ... | ... | 563 |
| Medical oncology | ... | ... | 779 |
| Nephrology | ... | ... | 639 |
| Pulmonary diseases | ... | ... | 918 |
| Rheumatology | ... | ... | 349 |
| Neurological surgery | 547 | 676 | 636 |
| Neurology | 1216 | 1452 | 1029 |
| Child neurology | ... | ... | 192 |
| Nuclear medicine | 226 | 250 | 215 |
| Obstetrics and gynecology | 4361 | 4611 | 4645 |
| Gynecologic oncology† | ... | ... | 67 |
| Maternal and fetal medicine† | ... | ... | 208 |
| Reproductive endocrinology† | ... | ... | 64 |
| Ophthalmology | 1518 | 1566 | 1003 |
| Orthopedic surgery | 2492 | 2832 | 2456 |
| Adult reconstructive surgery | ... | ... | ... |
| Hand surgery | ... | ... | 18 |
| Musculoskeletal oncology | ... | ... | 4 |
| Pediatric orthopedic | ... | ... | 55 |
| Sports medicine | ... | ... | 19 |
| Trauma orthopedics | ... | ... | ... |
| Otolaryngology | 981 | 1086 | 1167 |
| Pathology | 2522 | 2664 | 2478 |
| Blood banking | 39 | 49 | 60 |
| Chemical pathology | ... | ... | 9 |
| Forensic pathology | 31 | 60 | 53 |
| Hematology (pathology) | ... | ... | 37 |
| Immunopathology | ... | ... | 17 |
| Medical microbiology | ... | ... | 3 |
| Neuropathology | 74 | 87 | 80 |
| Pediatrics | 5505 | 6208 | 6950 |
| Critical care | ... | ... | ... |
| Neonatal-perinatal medicine | ... | 245 | 456 |
| Pediatric cardiology | 145 | 167 | 192 |
| Pediatric endocrinology | ... | ... | 139 |
| Pediatric hemato-oncology | ... | ... | 222 |
| Pediatric nephrology | ... | ... | 112 |
| Pediatric pulmonology | ... | ... | ... |
| Physical medicine and rehabilitation | 562 | 753 | 984 |
| Plastic surgery | 391 | 442 | 419 |
| Preventive medicine, general | 179 | 245 | 171 |
| Aerospace medicine | 43 | 68 | 29 |
| Combined general preventive medicine and public health | ... | 67 | 45 |
| Occupational medicine | 85 | 143 | 124 |
| Public health | 35 | 32 | 23 |
| Psychiatry | 4563 | 4875 | 5167 |
| Child psychiatry | 555 | 665 | 720 |
| Radiation oncology | 420 | 536 | 381 |
| Radiology, diagnostic | 2882 | 3197 | 3179 |
| Radiology, diagnostic (nuclear) | 61 | 102 | 71 |
| Surgery | 7846 | 8254 | 8213 |
| Critical care | ... | ... | 30 |
| Pediatric surgery | 30 | 25 | 37 |
| Vascular surgery | ... | 30 | 106 |
| Thoracic surgery | 260 | 293 | 304 |
| Urology | 1036 | 1049 | 868 |
| Transitional year | ... | 1463 | 1466 |
| **Combined Specialty Programs†** | | | |
| Internal medicine/pediatrics | | | 801 |
| Internal medicine/emergency medicine | | | 34 |
| Internal medicine/physical medicine and rehabilitation | | | 22 |
| Pediatrics/emergency medicine | | | 16 |
| Pediatrics/child psychiatry | | | 19 |
| Pediatrics/physical medicine and rehabilitation | | | 10 |
| Total | 66 066 | 76 411 | 89 566 |

*Number of positions offered as reported by program directors in the annual fall survey of residency programs. Newly accredited programs are not included. Ellipses indicate that there were no accredited programs or reported positions in the specialty or subspecialty at the time of the survey.
†Not accredited by the ACGME.

## Graduate Year 1 Positions Offered

First-year positions open to medical school graduates with no prior graduate medical education are identified as graduate year 1 (GY-1) positions. For the annual survey, program directors were asked to report the number of positions open to trainees seeking a first graduate year position. Several specialties have prerequisites for entry into their programs. For example, first-year positions in allergy and immunology are open only to those with at least 3 years of internal medicine or pediatrics. Table 4 shows that the number of GY-1 positions projected for July 1991 was 22,468, as estimated by the programs open to first-year residents after award of the MD degree. Data for 1981 and 1991 indicate that the number of projected GY-1 positions increased by 24.7%

Table 4.—Number of Graduate Year 1 Positions Offered July 1, by Specialty*

| Specialty | 1980 | 1985 | 1991 |
|---|---|---|---|
| Anesthesiology | 523 | 423 | 404 |
| Dermatology | 7 | 9 | 46 |
| Emergency medicine | † | 257 | 372 |
| Family practice | 2371 | 2521 | 2571 |
| Internal medicine | 5941 | 7047 | 8078 |
| Neurological surgery | 20 | 49 | 59 |
| Neurology | 81 | 81 | 74 |
| Obstetrics and gynecology | 1220 | 1113 | 1194 |
| Ophthalmology | 31 | 30 | 17 |
| Orthopedic surgery | 218 | 323 | 287 |
| Otolaryngology | 48 | 119 | 95 |
| Pathology | 642 | 603 | 527 |
| Pediatrics | 1864 | 2089 | 2333 |
| Physical medicine and rehabilitation | 129 | 111 | 91 |
| Preventive medicine, general | 15 | 22 | 21 |
| Occupational medicine | 8 | 0 | 32 |
| Public health | 4 | 0 | 6 |
| Psychiatry | 1063 | 1038 | 1168 |
| Radiation oncology | 87 | 62 | 19 |
| Radiology, diagnostic | 409 | 370 | 356 |
| Radiology, diagnostic (nuclear) | 10 | 0 | 8 |
| Surgery | 2539 | 2765 | 2938 |
| Urology | 65 | 78 | 67 |
| Transitional year | 718 | 1463 | 1466 |
| **Combined Specialty Programs†** | | | |
| Internal medicine/pediatrics | | | 215 |
| Internal medicine/emergency medicine | | | 10 |
| Internal medicine/physical medicine and rehabilitation | | | 8 |
| Pediatrics/emergency medicine | | | 2 |
| Pediatrics/psychiatry/child psychiatry | | | 2 |
| Pediatrics/physical medicine and rehabilitation | | | 2 |
| Total | 18 013 | 20 573 | 22 468 |

*Number of positions offered as reported by program directors in the annual fall survey of residency programs. Newly accredited programs are not included.
†Not accredited by the ACGME.

Table 5.—Number of Residents on Duty September 1, by Specialty*

| Specialty | 1980 | 1985 | 1990 |
|---|---|---|---|
| Allergy and immunology | 194 | 276 | 322 |
| Anesthesiology | 2490 | 4025 | 4889 |
| Critical care | ... | ... | 37 |
| Colon and rectal surgery | 37 | 45 | 54 |
| Dermatology | 755 | 745 | 824 |
| Dermatopathology | 30 | 27 | 25 |
| Emergency medicine | ... | 1122 | 1781 |
| Family practice | 6344 | 7276 | 6680 |
| Geriatrics | ... | ... | 15 |
| Internal medicine | 15 964 | 17 832 | 18 734 |
| Cardiovascular disease | ... | ... | 1677 |
| Critical care | ... | ... | 190 |
| Endocrinology and metabolism | ... | ... | 295 |
| Gastroenterology | ... | ... | 764 |
| Geriatrics | ... | ... | 153 |
| Hematology (medicine) | ... | ... | 405 |
| Infectious diseases | ... | ... | 460 |
| Medical oncology | ... | ... | 534 |
| Nephrology | ... | ... | 417 |
| Pulmonary diseases | ... | ... | 725 |
| Rheumatology | ... | ... | 281 |
| Neurological surgery | 511 | 704 | 720 |
| Neurology | 1114 | 1386 | 1211 |
| Child neurology | ... | ... | 101 |
| Nuclear medicine | 176 | 191 | 156 |
| Obstetrics and gynecology | 4221 | 4630 | 4315 |
| Gynecologic oncology† | ... | ... | 40 |
| Maternal and fetal medicine† | ... | ... | 135 |
| Reproductive endocrinology† | ... | ... | 57 |
| Ophthalmology | 1480 | 1561 | 1446 |
| Orthopedic surgery | 2418 | 2817 | 2630 |
| Adult reconstructive surgery | ... | ... | 0 |
| Hand surgery | ... | ... | 19 |
| Musculoskeletal oncology | ... | ... | 5 |
| Pediatric orthopedics | ... | ... | 15 |
| Sports medicine | ... | ... | 10 |
| Trauma orthopedics | ... | ... | 0 |
| Otolaryngology | 923 | 1094 | 1002 |
| Pathology | 2186 | 2358 | 2364 |
| Blood banking | 23 | 32 | 32 |
| Chemical pathology | ... | ... | 1 |
| Forensic pathology | 22 | 49 | 28 |
| Hematology (pathology) | ... | 8 | 20 |
| Immunopathology | ... | ... | 11 |
| Medical microbiology | ... | ... | 1 |
| Neuropathology | 52 | 41 | 38 |
| Pediatrics | 5171 | 6088 | 6115 |
| Critical care | ... | ... | 0 |
| Neonatal-perinatal medicine | ... | 325 | 304 |
| Pediatric cardiology | 130 | 140 | 176 |
| Pediatric endocrinology | ... | ... | 84 |
| Pediatric hemato-oncology | ... | ... | 153 |
| Pediatric nephrology | ... | ... | 64 |
| Pediatric pulmonology | ... | ... | 0 |
| Physical medicine and rehabilitation | 492 | 763 | 893 |
| Plastic surgery | 367 | 405 | 391 |
| Preventive medicine, general | 157 | 196 | 146 |
| Aerospace medicine | 25 | 62 | 48 |
| Combined general preventive medicine and public health | ... | 58 | 56 |
| Occupational medicine | 71 | 106 | 163 |
| Public health | 31 | 26 | 19 |
| Psychiatry | 3911 | 4809 | 4673 |
| Child psychiatry | 426 | 580 | 642 |
| Radiation oncology | 288 | 524 | 443 |

over the decade; the number of US medical school graduates increased 4.9% over the same decade.

## RESIDENTS IN TRAINING

Table 5 shows the total number of residents on duty September 1 for 1980, 1985, and 1990. The counts represent 97% of programs for 1980, 96% for 1985, and 8% for 1990. (The lower response rate in 1990 is partly as a result of the new electronic survey method and the low response rate from smaller subspecialty programs.) The number of residents has grown from 61,465 in 1989 to 82,902 in 1990, an increase of 34.9%. This increase can be explained by the accreditation of a number of subspecialties, growth in the number and size of programs, and the addition of one new specialty (emergency medicine) and the transitional year. The number of GY-1 residents on duty September 1, 1990, by specialty has remained remarkably stable since 1980 (Table 6). The number of GY-1 residents in 1990 was 18,322.

Differences between growth in the total number of

| | | | |
|---|---|---|---|
| Radiology, diagnostic | 2766 | 3132 | 3775 |
| Radiology, diagnostic (nuclear) | 48 | 74 | 32 |
| Surgery | 7440 | 8070 | 7644 |
| Critical care | ... | ... | 10 |
| Pediatric surgery | 29 | 24 | 37 |
| Vascular surgery | ... | 51 | 88 |
| Thoracic surgery | 256 | 285 | 305 |
| Urology | 917 | 1057 | 963 |
| Transitional year | ... | 1520 | 1475 |
| **Combined Specialty Programs†** | | | |
| Internal medicine/pediatrics | | | 534 |
| Internal medicine/emergency medicine | | | 11 |
| Internal medicine/physical medicine and rehabilitation | | | 3 |
| Pediatrics/emergency medicine | | | 2 |
| Pediatrics/psychiatry/child psychiatry | | | 27 |
| Pediatrics/physical medicine and rehabilitation | | | 7 |
| **Total** | **61 465** | **74 514** | **82 902** |

*Ellipses indicate that there were no accredited programs in the specialty or subspecialty at the time of the survey.
†Not accredited by the ACGME.

Table 6.—Number of Graduate Year 1 Residents on Duty September 1, in Specialties Open to Physicians with No Previous Postgraduate Medical Training*

| Specialty | 1980 | 1985 | 1990 |
|---|---|---|---|
| Anesthesiology | 523 | 378 | 358 |
| Dermatology | 0 | 7 | 14 |
| Emergency medicine | ... | 239 | 375 |
| Family practice | 2371 | 2346 | 1934 |
| Internal medicine | 5948 | 6557 | 6518 |
| Neurological surgery | 20 | 48 | 46 |
| Neurology | 81 | 66 | 59 |
| Obstetrics and gynecology | 1220 | 1064 | 1000 |
| Ophthalmology | 31 | 22 | 3 |
| Orthopedic surgery | 218 | 305 | 269 |
| Otolaryngology | 48 | 92 | 46 |
| Pathology | 642 | 451 | 449 |
| Pediatrics | 1864 | 2006 | 1937 |
| Physical medicine and rehabilitation | 129 | 86 | 79 |
| Preventive medicine, general | 15 | 4 | 10 |
| Aerospace medicine | 0 | 0 | 7 |
| Combined general preventive medicine and public health | ... | 0 | 2 |
| Occupational medicine | 8 | 0 | 1 |
| Public health | 4 | 0 | 0 |
| Psychiatry | 1063 | 982 | 874 |
| Radiation oncology | 87 | 39 | 19 |
| Radiology, diagnostic | 409 | 305 | 376 |
| Radiology, diagnostic (nuclear) | 10 | 0 | 7 |
| Surgery | 2539 | 2596 | 2408 |
| Urology | 65 | 75 | 46 |
| Transitional year | 1407 | 1500 | 1330 |
| **Combined Specialty Programs†** | | | |
| Internal medicine/pediatrics | | | 138 |
| Internal medicine/emergency medicine | | | 6 |
| Internal medicine/physical medicine and rehabilitation | | | 3 |
| Pediatrics/emergency medicine | | | 1 |
| Pediatrics/psychiatry/child psychiatry | | | 4 |
| Pediatrics/physical medicine and rehabilitation | | | 3 |
| **Total** | **18 702** | **19 168** | **18 322** |

*First-year positions open to physicians with no previous postgraduate medical training. Ellipses indicate that there were no accredited programs in the specialty at the time of the survey.
†Not accredited by the ACGME.

residents and stability in the number of GY-1 residents can be accounted for by the increased length of residency training and the accreditation of subspecialty programs.

## Women Residents

The number of women in residency programs has increased by 7.1% over the last decade (Table 7). In 1990, women accounted for 29.5% of the reported number of trainees; in 1980 they made up 22.4% of the total. The most women are found in internal medicine (5497), pediatrics (3321), and family practice (2362). Specialties with the largest proportion of women residents are public health (57.9%), combined internal medicine/emergency medicine (54.4%), pediatrics (54.3%), and forensic pathology (53.6%), followed by both child psychiatry and pediatric endocrinology (50%). The largest growth in the proportion of women residents during the decade from 1980 to 1990 occurred in preventive medicine-public health (22.4%), pediatric cardiology (21.3%), and dermatology (21.1%); the largest decrease occurred in physical medicine and rehabilitation (10.1%).

## Race, Ethnicity, and Citizenship of Residents

Information on the race and ethnic background of residents on duty as of September 1, 1990, shows that slightly more than 78% of residents were graduates of US or Canadian medical schools and 18% were graduates of foreign medical schools; 3.6% were graduates of schools of osteopathic medicine (Tables 8 through 10). Among international medical graduates (IMGs), 28.4% were Asian or Pacific Islander and 32.8% were white (non-Hispanic).

The number of both black and Hispanic residents has increased over the past 10 years, the latter by 63%. However, the percentage of black and Hispanic residents as a proportion of the entire resident population has not changed dramatically. The proportion of black residents decreased from 4.9% in 1980 to 4.7% in 1990; the proportion of Hispanic residents increased from 4.5% to 5.6% during this same period. Internal medicine is the most frequent specialty choice of both black (25.5%) and Hispanic (24.5%) residents (Table 10).

## International Medical School Graduates

Information on medical school of graduation was provided for 99.5% of all residents in the reporting programs. Table 11 indicates that the percentage of all IMG residents decreased by 3% from 1980 to 1985, but increased by 18% from 1985 to 1990. The increase in 1985 to 1990 is mostly accounted for by changes between 1989 and 1990, when the total number of IMG

Table 7.—Number of Women Residents on Duty September 1 and Percentage of Women Residents by Specialty*

| Specialty | No. (%) of Women | | |
|---|---|---|---|
| | 1980 | 1985 | 1990 |
| Allergy and immunology | 32 (16.5) | 76 (27.5) | 81 (25.2) |
| Anesthesiology | 600 (24.1) | 766 (19.0) | 1064 (21.8) |
|   Critical care | ... | ... | 6 (16.2) |
| Colon and rectal surgery | 1 (2.7) | 5 (11.1) | 7 (13.0) |
| Dermatology | 202 (26.8) | 297 (39.9) | 394 (47.8) |
| Dermatopathology | 5 (16.7) | 6 (22.2) | 7 (28.0) |
| Emergency medicine | ... | 242 (21.6) | 439 (24.6) |
| Family practice | 1235 (19.5) | 1891 (26.0) | 2362 (35.4) |
|   Geriatrics | ... | ... | 6 (40.0) |
| Internal medicine | 3342 (20.9) | 4605 (25.8) | 5497 (29.3) |
|   Cardiovascular disease | ... | ... | 174 (10.4) |
|   Critical care | ... | ... | 33 (17.4) |
|   Endocrinology and metabolism | ... | ... | 114 (38.6) |
|   Gastroenterology | ... | ... | 90 (11.8) |
|   Geriatrics | ... | ... | 58 (37.9) |
|   Hematology (medicine) | ... | ... | 105 (25.9) |
|   Infectious diseases | ... | ... | 178 (38.7) |
|   Medical oncology | ... | ... | 131 (24.5) |
|   Nephrology | ... | ... | 113 (27.1) |
|   Pulmonary diseases | ... | ... | 103 (14.2) |
|   Rheumatology | ... | ... | 128 (45.6) |
| Neurological surgery | 24 (4.7) | 45 (6.4) | 55 (7.6) |
| Neurology | 191 (17.1) | 339 (24.5) | 333 (27.5) |
|   Child neurology | ... | ... | 23 (22.8) |
| Nuclear medicine | 26 (14.8) | 45 (23.6) | 37 (23.7) |
| Obstetrics and gynecology | 1279 (30.3) | 1927 (41.6) | 2025 (46.9) |
|   Gynecologic oncology† | ... | ... | 10 (25.0) |
|   Maternal and fetal medicine† | ... | ... | 48 (35.6) |
|   Reproductive endocrinology† | ... | ... | 24 (42.1) |
| Ophthalmology | 185 (12.5) | 302 (19.3) | 345 (23.9) |
| Orthopedic surgery | 89 (3.7) | 119 (4.2) | 140 (5.3) |
|   Adult reconstructive surgery | ... | ... | 0 (0.0) |
|   Hand surgery | ... | ... | 0 (0.0) |
|   Musculoskeletal oncology | ... | ... | 1 (20.0) |
|   Pediatric orthopedics | ... | ... | 4 (26.7) |
|   Sports medicine | ... | ... | 2 (20.0) |
|   Trauma orthopedics | ... | ... | 0 (0.0) |
| Otolaryngology | 80 (8.7) | 128 (11.7) | 143 (14.3) |
| Pathology | 691 (31.6) | 847 (35.9) | 913 (38.6) |
|   Blood banking | 9 (39.1) | 16 (50.0) | 15 (46.9) |
|   Chemical pathology | ... | 0 (0.0) | 0 (0.0) |
|   Forensic pathology | 3 (13.6) | 8 (16.3) | 15 (53.6) |
|   Hematology (pathology) | ... | 2 (25.0) | 7 (35.0) |
|   Immunopathology | ... | 0 (0.0) | 4 (36.4) |
|   Medical microbiology | ... | ... | 0 (0.0) |
|   Neuropathology | 11 (21.2) | 13 (31.7) | 8 (21.1) |
| Pediatrics | 2432 (47.0) | 3002 (49.3) | 3321 (54.3) |
|   Critical care | ... | ... | 0 (0.0) |
|   Neonatal-perinatal medicine | ... | 126 (38.8) | 131 (43.1) |
|   Pediatric cardiology | 21 (16.2) | 31 (22.1) | 66 (37.5) |
|   Pediatric endocrinology | ... | ... | 42 (50.0) |
|   Pediatric hemato-oncology | ... | ... | 61 (39.9) |
|   Pediatric nephrology | ... | ... | 30 (46.9) |
|   Pediatric pulmonology | ... | ... | 0 (0.0) |
| Physical medicine and rehabilitation | 209 (42.5) | 204 (26.7) | 289 (32.4) |
| Plastic surgery | 33 (9.0) | 51 (12.6) | 54 (13.8) |
| Preventive medicine, general | 31 (19.7) | 65 (33.2) | 66 (45.2) |
|   Aerospace medicine | 1 (4.0) | 4 (6.5) | 5 (10.4) |
|   Combined general preventive medicine and public health | ... | 21 (36.2) | 20 (35.7) |
|   Occupational medicine | 16 (22.5) | 30 (28.3) | 29 (17.8) |
|   Public health | 11 (35.5) | 10 (38.5) | 11 (57.9) |

| | | | |
|---|---|---|---|
| Psychiatry | 1416 (36.2) | 1840 (38.3) | 2007 (42.9) |
| Child psychiatry | 185 (43.4) | 274 (47.2) | 321 (50.0) |
| Radiation oncology | 78 (27.1) | 121 (23.1) | 109 (24.6) |
| Radiology, diagnostic | 531 (19.2) | 691 (22.1) | 961 (25.5) |
| Radiology, diagnostic (nuclear) | 12 (25.0) | 24 (32.4) | 8 (25.0) |
| Surgery | 723 (9.7) | 954 (11.8) | 1079 (14.1) |
| Critical care | . . . | . . . | 2 (20.0) |
| Pediatric surgery | 5 (17.2) | 4 (16.7) | 7 (18.9) |
| Vascular surgery | . . . | 0 (0.0) | 4 (4.5) |
| Thoracic surgery | 8 (3.1) | 12 (4.2) | 12 (3.9) |
| Urology | 21 (2.3) | 49 (4.6) | 51 (5.3) |
| Transitional year | . . . | 370 (24.3) | 349 (23.7) |
| **Combined Specialty Programs†** | | | |
| Internal medicine/pediatrics | | | 188 (35.2) |
| Internal medicine/emergency medicine | | | 6 (54.5) |
| Internal medicine/physical medicine and rehabilitation | | | 0 (0.0) |
| Pediatrics/emergency medicine | | | 0 (0.0) |
| Pediatrics/psychiatry/child psychiatry | | | 17 (63.0) |
| Pediatrics/physical medicine and rehabilitation | | | 4 (57.1) |
| **Total** | **13 738** (22.4) | **19 562** (26.3) | **24 492** (29.5) |

*Ellipses indicate that there were no accredited programs in the specialty or subspecialty at the time of the survey.
†Not accredited by the ACGME.

Table 8.—Number of Residents on Duty September 1, 1990, by Type of Medical School and Race or Ethnic Background*

| Race or Ethnic Background | School of Medical Education | | | |
|---|---|---|---|---|
| | US and Canadian LCME | US Osteopathic | Foreign | Total |
| Black (non-Hispanic) | 3020 | 49 | 634 | 3703 |
| American Indian or Alaskan native | 124 | 4 | 21 | 149 |
| Mexican-American | 517 | 11 | 141 | 669 |
| Puerto Rican | 1131 | 4 | 270 | 1405 |
| Other Hispanic | 889 | 31 | 1472 | 2392 |
| Asian or Pacific Islander | 3619 | 88 | 4127 | 7834 |
| Indian subcontinent | 374 | 13 | 1707 | 2094 |
| Middle Eastern | 252 | 14 | 1119 | 1385 |
| Other | 168 | 7 | 260 | 435 |
| White (non-Hispanic) | 51 819 | 2586 | 4763 | 59 168 |
| **Total** | **61 913** | **2807** | **14 514** | **79 234** |

*Totals are less than those reported in other tables because some program directors omitted information on the race or ethnic background of residents. LCME indicates Liaison Committee for Medical Education. Totals in this table may be lower than those in Tables 9 and 10 because program directors failed to identify medical school of graduation.

Table 9.—Race or Ethnic Background of Residents on Duty September 1

| Race or Ethnic Background | 1980 | 1985 | 1990 |
|---|---|---|---|
| Black (non-Hispanic) | 3000 | 3322 | 3711 |
| American Indian or Alaskan native | 89 | 128 | 150 |
| Mexican-American | 574 | 731 | 669 |
| Puerto Rican | 997 | 1292 | 1407 |
| Other Hispanic | 1175 | 1519 | 2399 |
| Asian or Pacific Islander | 6560 | 5618 | 7869 |
| Indian subcontinent | * | * | 2143 |
| Middle Eastern | * | * | 1394 |
| Other | * | * | 439 |
| White (non-Hispanic) | 48 685 | 61 448 | 59 258 |
| **Total** | **61 080†** | **74 058†** | **79 439†** |

*The race or ethnic background category was added in 1990.
†Totals are less than those reported in other tables because some program directors omitted information on the race or ethnic background of residents.

Table 10.—Number of Black and Hispanic Residents on Duty September 1, 1990, by Specialty

| Specialty | Black | Hispanic |
|---|---|---|
| Allergy and immunology | 7 | 14 |
| Anesthesiology | 233 | 180 |
| Critical care | 1 | 0 |
| Colon and rectal surgery | 1 | 3 |
| Dermatology | 19 | 18 |
| Dermatopathology | 1 | 0 |
| Emergency medicine | 67 | 68 |
| Family practice | 291 | 428 |
| Geriatrics | 0 | 4 |
| Internal medicine | 948 | 1098 |
| Cardiovascular disease | 57 | 105 |
| Critical care | 10 | 11 |
| Endocrinology and metabolism | 12 | 16 |
| Gastroenterology | 26 | 30 |
| Geriatrics | 2 | 13 |
| Hematology (medicine) | 11 | 23 |
| Infectious diseases | 14 | 28 |
| Medical oncology | 18 | 29 |
| Nephrology | 30 | 20 |
| Pulmonary diseases | 29 | 41 |
| Rheumatology | 7 | 17 |
| Neurological surgery | 26 | 20 |
| Neurology | 38 | 73 |
| Child neurology | 1 | 8 |
| Nuclear medicine | 3 | 12 |
| Obstetrics and gynecology | 316 | 210 |
| Gynecologic oncology* | 3 | 2 |
| Maternal and fetal medicine* | 11 | 4 |
| Reproductive endocrinology* | 2 | 2 |
| Ophthalmology | 43 | 60 |
| Orthopedic surgery | 69 | 64 |
| Adult reconstructive surgery | † | † |
| Hand surgery | 0 | 1 |
| Musculoskeletal oncology | 0 | 0 |
| Pediatric orthopedics | 1 | 0 |
| Sports medicine | 0 | 0 |
| Trauma orthopedics | † | † |
| Otolaryngology | 28 | 22 |
| Pathology | 75 | 160 |
| Blood banking | 0 | 3 |
| Chemical pathology | 0 | 0 |
| Forensic pathology | 2 | 2 |
| Hematology (pathology) | 0 | 0 |
| Immunopathology | 0 | 0 |
| Medical microbiology | 0 | 0 |
| Neuropathology | 2 | 2 |
| Pediatrics | 363 | 546 |
| Critical care | † | † |
| Neonatal-perinatal medicine | 13 | 37 |
| Pediatric cardiology | 1 | 8 |
| Pediatric endocrinology | 4 | 10 |
| Pediatric hemato-oncology | 7 | 5 |
| Pediatric nephrology | 4 | 2 |
| Pediatric pulmonology | † | † |
| Physical medicine and rehabilitation | 43 | 51 |
| Plastic surgery | 11 | 5 |
| Preventive medicine, general | 9 | 6 |
| Aerospace medicine | 1 | 3 |
| Combined general preventive medicine and public health | 6 | 6 |
| Occupational medicine | 2 | 4 |
| Public health | 0 | 1 |
| Psychiatry | 202 | 322 |
| Child psychiatry | 31 | 49 |
| Radiology, diagnostic | 74 | 114 |
| Radiology, diagnostic (nuclear) | 0 | 2 |
| Radiation oncology | 19 | 8 |
| Surgery | 355 | 371 |
| Critical care | 2 | 1 |
| Pediatric surgery | 0 | 3 |
| Vascular surgery | 0 | 2 |
| Thoracic surgery | 7 | 10 |
| Urology | 37 | 25 |
| Transitional year | 82 | 81 |
| **Combined Specialty Programs*** | | |
| Internal medicine/pediatrics | 30 | 12 |
| Internal medicine/emergency medicine | 1 | 0 |
| Internal medicine/physical medicine and rehabilitation | 1 | 0 |
| Pediatrics/emergency medicine | 0 | 0 |
| Pediatrics/psychiatry/child psychiatry | 2 | 0 |
| Pediatrics/physical medicine and rehabilitation | 0 | 0 |
| **Total** | **3711** | **4475** |

*Not accredited by the ACGME.
†Programs in these new subspecialties were accredited after the annual survey; resident data were not collected.

residents grew from 12,259 to 14,914 (21.7%). (The response rate for resident data in 1989 was lower than in previous years. As a result, a regression model was used to calculate the number of residents that would have been expected if trends for previous years continued. In some instances, projected values were not used because these numbers were within a 5% variance of the reported figures. The figures on IMGs fall into this category; hence, no projected figures were used.)

In the period from 1989 to 1990, the number of GY-1 IMG residents increased by 31.6%. The number of GY-1 IMG residents who were not citizens rose by 63.4%, while the number of IMG GY-1 residents who were US citizens decreased by 14.9%. Twenty-six percent of IMG GY-1 residents on duty in 1990 were US citizens, a decrease from the 41% reported to be US citizens in 1989.

The citizenship or visa status of all IMG residents is shown in Table 13. The number and percentage of IMG residents who are native-born US citizens continue to decline. The number of IMGs who are naturalized US citizens increased by 24.5%. In the same period, the number and percentage of IMG residents who were exchange visitors increased 57.4%, from 2204 in 1989 to 3470 in 1990. Most of this growth occurred in IMG GY-1 residents.

## TRANSITIONAL YEAR PROGRAMS

A transitional year program must be sponsored by an institution and its affiliate conducting two or more ACGME-accredited residency programs. The objective of the 12–month curriculum is to provide a balanced medical education in multiple clinical disciplines. Responses from 156 of 171 transitional year programs indicated that they had 1475 trainees. Of these, 15.1% (223) were IMGs. Information on transitional year programs can be found in the tables showing statistics for specialty programs.

## AMA-FREIDA DATA

In 1987, the AMA medical student and resident physician sections proposed a computerized system of information that would provide more data on graduate medical education programs. The development of the AMA-Fellowship and Residency Electronic Interactive Database Access (AMA-FREIDA) system was the result of the proposal.

For every ACGME-accredited program, the AMA-FREIDA system lists the program name, program address, number of positions, and the person to whom an application should be addressed. For those programs listing detailed information in AMA-FREIDA, the system features 152 data elements on such program compo-

Table 11.—Number of International Medical Graduates (IMGs) on Duty September 1, and Percentage of All Residents Who Are IMGs by Specialty*

| Specialty | No. (%) of IMGs | | |
|---|---|---|---|
| | 1980 | 1985 | 1990 |
| Allergy and immunology | 42 (22.2) | 51 (18.5) | 76 (23.6) |
| Anesthesiology | 813 (32.7) | 554 (13.8) | 560 (11.5) |
| Critical care | . . . | . . . | 10 (27.0) |
| Colon and rectal surgery | 12 (32.4) | 10 (22.2) | 4 (7.4) |
| Dermatology | 37 (4.9) | 47 (6.3) | 19 (2.3) |
| Dermatopathology | 4 (26.6) | 3 (11.1) | 3 (12.0) |
| Emergency medicine | . . . | 47 (4.2) | 60 (3.4) |
| Family practice | 606 (9.9) | 938 (12.9) | 987 (14.8) |
| Geriatrics | . . . | . . . | 8 (53.3) |
| Internal medicine | 2954 (18.5) | 3803 (21.3) | 5351 (28.6) |
| Cardiovascular disease | . . . | . . . | 451 (26.9) |
| Critical care | . . . | . . . | 48 (25.3) |
| Endocrinology and metabolism | . . . | . . . | 78 (26.4) |
| Gastroenterology | . . . | . . . | 137 (17.9) |
| Geriatrics | . . . | . . . | 50 (32.7) |
| Hematology (medicine) | . . . | . . . | 128 (31.6) |
| Infectious diseases | . . . | . . . | 122 (26.5) |
| Medical oncology | . . . | . . . | 142 (26.6) |
| Nephrology | . . . | . . . | 156 (37.4) |
| Pulmonary diseases | . . . | . . . | 188 (25.9) |
| Rheumatology | . . . | . . . | 70 (24.9) |
| Neurological surgery | 87 (17.1) | 51 (7.2) | 49 (6.8) |
| Neurology | 224 (20.1) | 355 (25.6) | 313 (25.8) |
| Child neurology | . . . | . . . | 48 (47.5) |
| Nuclear medicine | 64 (37.6) | 74 (38.7) | 62 (39.7) |
| Obstetrics and gynecology | 743 (17.6) | 467 (10.1) | 344 (8.0) |
| Gynecologic oncology† | | | 5 (12.5) |
| Maternal and fetal medicine† | | | 13 (9.6) |
| Reproductive endocrinology† | | | 2 (3.5) |
| Ophthalmology | 100 (7.1) | 51 (3.3) | 53 (3.7) |
| Orthopedic surgery | 240 (9.9) | 46 (1.6) | 35 (1.3) |
| Adult reconstructive surgery | . . . | . . . | 0 (0.0) |
| Hand surgery | . . . | . . . | 1 (5.3) |
| Musculoskeletal oncology | . . . | . . . | 0 (0.0) |
| Pediatric orthopedics | . . . | . . . | 5 (33.3) |
| Sports medicine | . . . | . . . | 0 (0.0) |
| Trauma orthopedics | . . . | . . . | 0 (0.0) |
| Otolaryngology | 125 (13.6) | 43 (3.9) | 21 (2.1) |
| Pathology | 539 (24.7) | 670 (28.4) | 665 (28.1) |
| Blood banking | 8 (34.8) | 7 (21.9) | 10 (31.3) |
| Chemical pathology | . . . | . . . | 0 (0.0) |
| Forensic pathology | 3 (13.6) | 18 (36.7) | 3 (10.7) |
| Hematology (pathology) | . . . | 2 (25.0) | 6 (30.0) |
| Immunopathology | . . . | . . . | 6 (54.5) |
| Medical microbiology | 0 (0.0) | 0 (0.0) | 0 (0.0) |
| Neuropathology | 16 (30.8) | 13 (31.7) | 13 (34.2) |
| Pediatrics | 1294 (25.1) | 1709 (28.1) | 1922 (31.4) |
| Critical care | . . . | . . . | 0 (0.0) |
| Neonatal-perinatal medicine | . . . | 103 (31.7) | 115 (37.8) |
| Pediatric cardiology | 21 (20.4) | 33 (23.6) | 43 (24.4) |
| Pediatric endocrinology | . . . | . . . | 32 (38.1) |
| Pediatric hemato-oncology | . . . | . . . | 48 (31.4) |
| Pediatric nephrology | . . . | . . . | 23 (35.9) |
| Pediatric pulmonology | . . . | . . . | 0 (0.0) |
| Physical medicine and rehabilitation | 283 (57.5) | 227 (29.7) | 60 (6.7) |
| Plastic surgery | 78 (21.5) | 47 (11.6) | 23 (5.9) |
| Preventive medicine, general | 19 (12.1) | 15 (7.6) | 9 (6.2) |
| Aerospace medicine | 7 (28.0) | 4 (6.4) | 8 (16.7) |
| Combined general preventive medicine and public health | . . . | 9 (15.5) | 8 (14.3) |
| Occupational medicine | 7 (9.9) | 18 (17.0) | 11 (6.7) |
| Public health | 5 (16.1) | 5 (19.2) | 3 (15.8) |

| | | | |
|---|---|---|---|
| Psychiatry | 1104  (28.2) | 1370  (28.5) | 980  (21.0) |
| Child psychiatry | 135  (31.7) | 160  (27.6) | 141  (22.0) |
| Radiation oncology | 98  (34.0) | 88  (16.8) | 20  (4.5) |
| Radiology, diagnostic | 410  (14.8) | 236  (7.5) | 145  (3.8) |
| Radiology, diagnostic (nuclear) | 9  (18.8) | 12  (16.2) | 8  (25.0) |
| Surgery | 1661  (22.5) | 870  (10.8) | 649  (8.5) |
| Critical care | . . . | . . . | 2  (20.0) |
| Pediatric surgery | 2  (6.9) | 0  (0.0) | 2  (5.4) |
| Vascular surgery | . . . | 2  (3.9) | 10  (11.4) |
| Thoracic surgery | 54  (21.1) | 28  (9.8) | 24  (7.9) |
| Urology | 274  (29.9) | 130  (12.3) | 40  (4.2) |
| Transitional year | . . . | 193  (12.7) | 223  (15.1) |
| **Combined Specialty Programs†** | | | |
| Internal medicine/pediatrics | | | 61  (11.4) |
| Internal medicine/emergency medicine | | | 0  (0.0) |
| Internal medicine/physical medicine and rehabilitation | | | 0  (0.0) |
| Pediatrics/emergency medicine | | | 0  (0.0) |
| Pediatrics/psychiatry/child psychiatry | | | 0  (0.0) |
| Pediatrics/ physical medicine and rehabilitation | | | 2  (28.6) |
| **Total** | **12 078**  (19.8) | **12 509**  (16.8) | **14 914**  (18.0) |

*Ellipses indicate that there were no accredited programs in this specialty or subspecialty at the time of the survey.
†Not accredited by the ACGME.

Table·12.—Number of Graduate Year 1 IMG Residents on Duty September 1, 1990, by Citizenship and Specialty*

| Specialty | US Citizen | Non-US Citizen | Total |
|---|---|---|---|
| Anesthesiology | 9 | 28 | 37 |
| Dermatology | 0 | 1 | 1 |
| Emergency medicine | 7 | 2 | 9 |
| Family practice | 110 | 138 | 248 |
| Internal medicine | 441 | 1369 | 1810 |
| Neurological surgery | 0 | 4 | 4 |
| Neurology | 2 | 16 | 18 |
| Obstetrics and gynecology | 12 | 30 | 42 |
| Ophthalmology | 0 | 2 | 2 |
| Orthopedic surgery | 0 | 6 | 6 |
| Otolaryngology | 0 | 2 | 2 |
| Pathology | 25 | 109 | 134 |
| Pediatrics | 142 | 473 | 615 |
| Physical medicine and rehabilitation | 3 | 1 | 4 |
| Preventive medicine, general | 0 | 1 | 1 |
| Aerospace medicine | 0 | 2 | 2 |
| Combined general preventive | 1 | 0 | 1 |
| Occupational medicine | 0 | 0 | 0 |
| Public health | 0 | 0 | 0 |
| Psychiatry | 62 | 130 | 192 |
| Radiation oncology | 0 | 0 | 0 |
| Radiology, diagnostic | 1 | 16 | 17 |
| Surgery | 51 | 162 | 213 |
| Urology | 0 | 1 | 1 |
| Transitional year | 55 | 108 | 163 |
| **Combined Specialty Program†** | | | |
| Internal medicine/pediatrics | 8 | 10 | 18 |
| **Total** | **929** | **2611** | **3540** |

*First-year positions open to physicians with no previous postgraduate medical training; IMG indicates international medical graduate.
†Not accredited by the ACGME.

Table 13.—Citizenship/Visa Status of IMG Resident Physicians, 1989 and 1990*

| Citizenship/Visa Status | No. (%) of IMG Residents | |
| --- | --- | --- |
| | 1989 | 1990 |
| Native US citizen | 3040 (24.8) | 2817 (18.9) |
| Naturalized US citizen | 1774 (14.4) | 2209 (14.8) |
| Permanent US resident | 4107 (33.5) | 4974 (33.3) |
| Exchange visitor | 2204 (18.0) | 3470 (23.3) |
| Immigrant or refugee | 882 (7.2) | 904 (6.1) |
| Miscellaneous | 95 (0.8) | 145 (1.0) |
| Unknown | 157 (1.3) | 395 (2.6) |
| Total | 12 259 (100.0) | 14 914 (100.1) |

*IMG indicates international medical graduate. Detailed data on citizenship/visa status available only for last 2 years.

nents as educational environment, work environment, clinical resources, teaching staff, compensation and benefits, and community characteristics. In 1990, the first year of AMA-FREIDA operation, 70% of all graduate medical education programs submitted information and were listed; in 1991 the participation rate increased to 76.4%. Those specialty programs that accept first-year residency candidates after the award of the MD degree had a higher listing rate (83.9%) than did the subspecialties (68.6%). The first edition of the AMA-FREIDA software package was released in March 1990. Among other lessees, 124 medical schools or their primary teaching hospitals leased the system for use by medical students and residents. Feedback from students and administrators suggests that students' use of AMA-FREIDA during its first year was heavy at some locations and more limited at others. Student interest and use appear to depend on their familiarity with computers, accessibility of terminals, and the degree to which use is encouraged by administrators.

The following summarizes some of the information reported by the 5748 programs that responded to questions in the AMA-FREIDA portion of the survey.

## Research Activity

The AMA-FREIDA system contains questions on the research requirements and opportunities in graduate medical education programs. As shown in Table 14, more than three fourths of the reporting programs had research rotations available, with two thirds of the reporting programs requiring such rotations. A research project of some kind is required by almost half of the

responding programs. Research expectations varied by specialty, with the subspecialties more likely to require a research project (68.2%) than the specialties that accept GY-1 residents (37.6%).

## Maternity and Paternity Leave

Maternity leave was offered by 5513 (95.9%) of programs responding to the survey question. Of these programs, 2899 (52.5%) indicated that the number of days allowed for maternity leave was negotiable. Paternity leave was offered by 2795 (50%) of the 5540 programs responding. The number of days allowed for paternity leave was reported as negotiable by 1731 programs (61.9%).

## Learning Experiences in the Ambulatory Setting

The AMA-FREIDA system lists information provided by program directors on the number of weeks a resident is required to be on duty in both hospital ambulatory and nonhospital ambulatory settings over the length of the program. Across all reporting specialties, residents averaged 46 weeks of duty in hospital ambulatory settings and 18 weeks in nonhospital ambulatory settings. The average number of weeks varied across specialties for both settings. In the hospital ambulatory setting, ophthalmology required the most time on duty (110 weeks), followed by combined pediatrics/physical medicine and rehabilitation (108 weeks), dermatology (100 weeks), neurological surgery (80 weeks), urology (78 weeks), rheumatology (75 weeks), and medical oncology

Table 14.—Research Activity in Graduate Medical Education Programs as of September 1, 1990

| | Total Programs Responding | No. (%) of Affirmative Responses |
| --- | --- | --- |
| Research rotation available | 5696 | 4379 (76.9) |
| Research rotations optional | 3335 | 2502 (75.1) |
| Research rotations required | 2827 | 1891 (66.9) |
| Research project required | 5017 | 2451 (48.9) |

(73 weeks). In the nonhospital ambulatory setting, family practice geriatrics (56 weeks) reported requiring the highest average number of weeks on duty over the length of the program, followed by occupational medicine (49 weeks), family medicine (46 weeks), and dermatology (45 weeks).

## Resident Work Hours

The number of hours residents should be on duty continues to be a controversial issue. As reported by program directors, the average number of reported hours on duty on site in the first year of the program was highest for general surgery (84 hours per week) and thoracic surgery (81.5 hours per week). Internal medicine, obstetrics and gynecology, orthopedic surgery, pediatrics, combined internal medicine and pediatrics, and transitional year programs all averaged between 72 hours and 79 hours per week on duty in the first year of the program. Ten specialties (family medicine, neurology, neurological surgery, orthopedic surgery, orthopedic sports medicine, general preventive medicine, pediatric cardiology, vascular surgery, thoracic surgery, and urology) reported averages of between 30 and 34 continuous hours on duty.

The final question surrounding work hours concerns the number of 24–hour periods per month off duty. The average number of 24–hour periods per month off duty ranged from a low of 3.8 days in sports medicine to a high of 8.9 days in pediatric hemato-oncology. Most specialties averaged 6 days per month without any duty.

## Part-time Shared Positions

The number of programs offering part-time shared positions increased from 618 in 1980 to 744 in 1990. This represents 15.8% of responding programs. Specialties most likely to offer part-time shared positions are internal medicine (102), family medicine (70), pediatrics (68), psychiatry (63), and child psychiatry (50).

## OSTEOPATHIC PHYSICIANS IN ACGME-ACCREDITED PROGRAMS

The reported number of osteopathic physicians in ACGME-accredited programs increased from 787 in 1980 to 2872 in 1990. This increase is due in part to the greater number of graduates from schools of osteopathic medicine. Osteopathic physicians were most frequently found in family practice, internal medicine, anesthesiology, psychiatry, pediatrics, and obstetrics and gynecology, as shown in Table 15.

Table 15.—Number of Osteopathic Graduates on Duty September 1 in Residency Programs Accredited by the ACGME

| Specialty | 1980 | 1985 | 1990 |
|---|---|---|---|
| Allergy and immunology | 2 | 5 | 8 |
| Anesthesiology | 45 | 79 | 231 |
| Colon and rectal surgery | 1 | 0 | 0 |
| Dermatology | 14 | 16 | 6 |
| Emergency medicine | * | 48 | 116 |
| Family practice | 114 | 318 | 727 |
| Geriatrics | * | * | 1 |
| Internal medicine | 184 | 288 | 665 |
| Cardiovascular disease | * | * | 43 |
| Critical care | * | * | 13 |
| Endocrinology and metabolism | * | * | 4 |
| Gastroenterology | * | * | 13 |
| Geriatrics | * | * | 6 |
| Hematology (medicine) | * | * | 8 |
| Infectious diseases | * | * | 6 |
| Medical oncology | * | * | 14 |
| Nephrology | * | * | 12 |
| Pulmonary diseases | * | * | 25 |
| Rheumatology | * | * | 13 |
| Neurology | 26 | 37 | 68 |
| Nuclear medicine | 4 | 1 | 2 |
| Obstetrics and gynecology | 77 | 77 | 156 |
| Ophthalmology | 10 | 13 | 3 |
| Orthopedic surgery | 21 | 20 | 12 |
| Pediatric | * | * | 1 |
| Otolaryngology | 10 | 7 | 12 |
| Pathology | 23 | 28 | 52 |
| Blood banking | * | * | 1 |
| Forensic pathology | 1 | 0 | 1 |
| Neuropathology | 2 | 0 | 1 |
| Pediatrics | 46 | 73 | 170 |
| Neonatal-perinatal medicine | * | 2 | 8 |
| Cardiology | 0 | 0 | 2 |
| Hemato-oncology | * | * | 3 |
| Physical medicine and rehabilitation | 24 | 44 | 78 |
| Plastic surgery | 1 | 1 | 0 |
| Preventive medicine, general | 2 | 2 | 8 |
| Aerospace medicine | 2 | 8 | 10 |
| Combined general preventive medicine and public health | 0 | 3 | 0 |
| Occupational medicine | 0 | 2 | 10 |
| Public health | 1 | 2 | 1 |
| Psychiatry | 58 | 94 | 202 |
| Child psychiatry | 9 | 14 | 25 |
| Radiation oncology | 4 | 9 | 7 |
| Radiology, diagnostic | 37 | 27 | 40 |
| Radiology, diagnostic (nuclear) | 0 | 1 | 1 |
| Surgery | 15 | 6 | 46 |
| Thoracic Surgery | 0 | 2 | 0 |
| Urology | 8 | 12 | 4 |
| Transitional year | 46 | 38 | 37 |
| **Total** | **787** | **1277** | **2872** |

*No accredited programs in this specialty or subspecialty at the time of the survey.

## INSTITUTIONS AND AGENCIES PARTICIPATING IN GRADUATE MEDICAL EDUCATION

Institutions and agencies identified as offering a significant portion of training in graduate medical education programs numbered 1575. The 1990 survey elicited a response rate of 70% from the 945 institutions and agencies sponsoring graduate medical education and a 43% response rate from the 630 institutions affiliated with graduate medical education.

Hospitals are not the only institutions involved in graduate medical education. State medical examiners' of-

Table 16.—Sponsors and Affiliates Participating in Graduate Medical Education in 1990, by Type of Control

| Type of Control | Sponsor | Affiliate | Total |
|---|---|---|---|
| Local | 55 | 99 | 154 |
| State | 90 | 133 | 223 |
| Federal | 98 | 67 | 165 |
| Church | 89 | 125 | 214 |
| Other, nonprofit | 273 | 508 | 781 |
| Corporation, for profit | 25 | 13 | 38 |
| **Totals** | **630** | **945** | **1575** |

fices, blood banks, ambulatory clinics, and mental health agencies also regularly provide residency training.

Table 16 shows the sponsor or affiliate status and type of controlling agency for all graduate medical education institutions. Institutions under the control of local governments or hospital district authorities accounted for 10% of the respondents; 14% were state controlled; 11% were federal institutions; 14% were church-related institutions; and 50% were other nonprofit corporations or agencies. For-profit corporations made up 2% of the reporting institutions.

## CONCLUSION

The decade from 1980 to 1990 has been marked by the accreditation of one new specialty and many new subspecialty programs. As a result, the total number of residents has increased, while the number of first-year residents has remained stable. The actual numbers of minority and women residents have increased over the decade; however, their proportions relative to all residents have not changed dramatically. Women now account for 29.5% of all residents, but the number of women enrolled in medical school has increased from 26.5% to 37.3% in the last decade. Further research is needed to understand fully this finding; however, it appears to be due in part to the "pipeline phenomenon"— the accreditation of more subspecialties with higher proportions of men and the number of IMGs, with a slightly higher proportion of men, entering the system.

The number of IMGs has remained fairly stable between 1985 and 1989, with less than 6% variation for any year. During this same period, the proportion of IMGs as a percentage of the total number of residents has remained stable, varying between 15% and 17%. Thus, while some of the changes from 1989 to 1990 could be attributed to modest underreporting of IMGs in 1989, any underreporting does not account for all the increases seen in the 1990 data.

During the past year there has been a large increase in the number of GY-1 foreign visitors whose visa type implies they will return to their home country after completion of residency. This increase should be observed closely over the coming years to measure the impact on graduate medical education and on the supply in foreign countries of physicians trained in US residencies.

Finally, the ambulatory care data indicate that primary care residents may spend less time in ambulatory settings than those in some subspecialties. With the adjustment in special requirements for internal medicine residency programs calling for increased ambulatory learning experiences, these data also must be monitored over the next decade.

The authors wish to acknowledge the assistance of Maria Ferrara, Charles J. O'Leary, PhD, and Dwight Thompson, staff in the Department of Data Systems.

## References

1. Crowley AE, Etzel SI. Graduate medical education. *JAMA.* 1986;256:1585–1594.
2. Crowley AE. Graduate medical education, *JAMA.* 1981;246:2938–2944.

# Chapter 11

# No Evidence of an Emerging Physician Surplus

## An Analysis of Change in Physicians' Work Load and Income

**William B. Schwartz, M.D., and Daniel N. Mendelson**

*Analysis of physicians' work patterns and income between 1982 and 1987 provides strong evidence that the demand for physicians' services has risen at least as quickly as physician supply. Aggregate hours spent by US physicians who provide patient care rose by 21%, and aggregate real net income rose by more than 30% during a period in which the supply of physicians grew by only 16%. The aggregate number of visits rose by only 9%, indicating that the time spent per patient encounter rose sharply, presumably as a result of technological change and the increased complexity of care. Recently released data for 1988 are consistent with these trends. Our findings are inconsistent with the prediction by the Graduate Medical Education National Advisory Committee that there would be a large physician surplus by the year 1990. Moreover, if the upward trend in demand for physicians' services continues, as seems probable, a physician surplus should not develop in the foreseeable future. Only extensive rationing of beneficial services would be expected to alter this projection.*
*—(JAMA. 1990;263:557–560)*

In the late 1970s, the Graduate Medical Education National Advisory Committee predicted that there would be a surplus of approximately 70,000 physicians by 1990 and 150,000 or more by the year 2000.[1] Subsequently, other observers forecast an even larger surplus.[2,3] A more recent study, one that considered a number of factors neglected by previous analysts, reached the quite different conclusion that the supply of physicians and the demand for their services will remain in virtual balance between 1982 and 2000.[4]

Given these disparate conclusions, we have evaluated the experience of the last few years to see whether there is empirical evidence of an emerging surplus of physicians. According to standard economic theory, a falling work load and a decrease in physicians' income would indicate such a surplus. In the case of a physician deficit, the reverse would be anticipated. The present study, which has made use of this model and of data for the period 1982 through 1987, yields no evidence of an emerging surplus. In fact, the data suggest that demand for physicians' services may be rising faster than the supply.

## METHODS

The number of physicians who provide patient care is taken from the *Physician Characteristics and Distribution in the US*[5–7]; this figure includes only those who spent more than half of their time providing patient care. These physicians were also the source of survey data regarding the number of patient visits, hours of patient

Reprinted with permission from *Journal of the American Medical Association*, January 26, 1990, Vol. 263 No. 4, pp. 557–560, copyright 1990, American Medical Association. The opinions and conclusions expressed herein are solely those of the authors and should not be construed as representing the opinions or policies of The Robert Wood Johnson Foundation, Princeton, NJ.

care, and weeks of work, as reported in the *Socioeconomic Characteristics of Medical Practice, 1988*.[8] Our primary data regarding physicians' income are drawn from the survey of patient-care physicians and corrected for inflation using the consumer price index.[8] Our analysis is limited to the period between 1982 and 1987 because the American Medical Association (AMA) survey techniques were changed in 1982 and because several key questions concerning work patterns were not included in earlier surveys. Although data from earlier years might be of historical interest, they are not relevant to our determination of whether a surplus of physicians has emerged in recent years.

## RESULTS

### Changes in Work Patterns of Individual Physicians

Between 1982 and 1987, the number of hours of patient care per physician rose by 4% (Table 1 and Fig 1). The number of patient visits per physician fell by 8% between 1982 and 1984, but rose slightly during the next 3 years (Fig 1). These changes reflected a 12% increase in the average time spent with each patient during the 5–year period.

### Aggregate Changes in Work Load

To estimate aggregate changes in demand, it is necessary to account not only for changes in work load per physician but also for the increase in physician supply. The aggregate values are obtained by multiplying the supply of physicians by the average number of hours spent in patient care and the number of visits per year per physician. The total number of visits fell slightly between 1982 and 1984 but rose between 1985 and 1987, with a resulting increase of 9% for the 5–year period (Fig 2). The aggregate number of hours of patient care increased 21% during the same interval.

Between 1982 and 1987, physician supply rose 16%, 8 percentage points higher than the growth in visits and

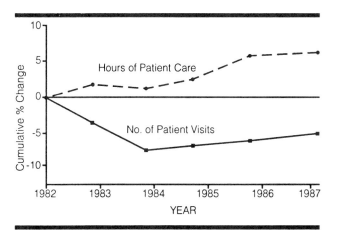

**Figure 1.** Changes in the number of patient visits and hours of patient care per physician between 1982 and 1987. Values are expressed as the cumulative percent change from 1982.

5 percentage points below the increase in hours. Some of the growth in the number of hours resulted from an increase in the amount of time physicians worked during weekends and evenings[9]; this trend may have represented a response to previously unmet demand or the desire of patients to avoid loss of time at work.

### Individual and Aggregate Changes in Physicians; Income

Real net income per physician, as determined by the AMA survey, increased 15% between 1982 and 1987. Aggregate net physician income, calculated by multiplying the AMA figures by the number of physicians who provided patient care for each year, rose by 34% during the 5–year period (Fig 3).

To verify the increase in physicians' income, we used yearly data regarding expenditures on physician's ser-

Table 1.—Changes in per-Physician and Aggregate Physician Work Load and Income Between 1982 and 1987

|  | Hours of Patient Care | No. of Patient Visits | Net Income |
|---|---|---|---|
| Per-physician changes | | | |
| Annualized | | | |
| % change | 0.8 | −1.4 | 2.8 |
| Total | | | |
| % change | 4.2 | −6.6 | 15.0 |
| Aggregate changes | | | |
| Annualized | | | |
| % change | 3.9 | 1.7 | 5.8 |
| Total | | | |
| % change | 21.3 | 8.7 | 33.9 |

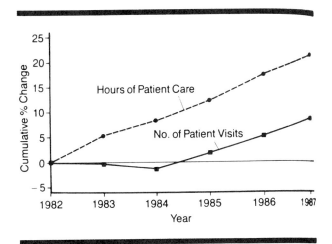

**Figure 2.** Changes in the aggregate number of patient visits and hours of patient care between 1982 and 1987. Values are expressed as the cumulative percent change from 1982.

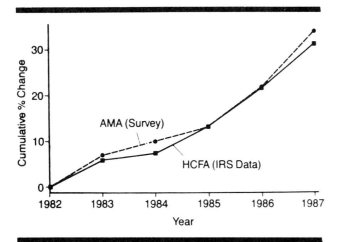

**Figure 3.** Changes in aggregate real net physician income between 1982 and 1987. Values are expressed as the .cumulative percent change from 1982. (See text for details of these calculations.) AMA indicates American Medical Association; HCFA, Health Care Financing Administration; and IRS, Internal Revenue Service.

Table 2. Changes in Real Physician Income by Specialty Between 1982 and 1987

| | % Change | | |
| --- | --- | --- | --- |
| | Income per Physician | No. of Physicians | Aggregate Physician Income |
| General/family practice | 8.9 | 9.4 | 19.1 |
| Internal medicine | 19.1 | 25.6 | 49.6 |
| Surgery/surgical specialties | 24.1 | 11.2 | 38.0 |
| Pediatrics | 2.8 | 24.0 | 27.5 |
| Obstetrics/gynecology | 23.4 | 13.9 | 40.6 |
| Radiology | 15.2 | 17.9 | 35.7 |
| Psychiatry | 15.1 | 11.2 | 28.0 |
| Anesthesiology | 5.0 | 30.4 | 37.0 |

vices that were calculated by the Health Care Financing Administration on the basis of Internal Revenue Service data[10,11]; the Health Care Financing Administration found that real expenditures on physicians' services increased by 41%, a figure closely similar to the 44% increase in gross real revenue in the AMA study (calculated by summing the AMA data regarding net revenues and expenses). To convert the Health Care Financing Administration figures into values for net income, we multiplied real expenditures as reported by the Health Care Financing Administration by the ratio of gross-to-net income as reported by the AMA for each year.[8] Expressed as net income, the cumulative increase seen in the Health Care Financing Administration data for the 5–year period was 31% as compared with 34% for the AMA data (Fig 3).

Changes in Income by Specialty

Is it possible that the aggregate increases in income masked decreases in income among some specialties? To address this question, we determined the changes in per capita and aggregate income for eight groups of specialties, which together comprises 89% of nonresident physicians who provide patient care (Table 2). As is apparent, there was a considerable amount of variation between specialties, but in no case did real income decrease during the 5–year period.

In addition, we used the specialty-specific data to estimate that change in average physician income that would have been expected if only the specialty mix had changed between 1982 and 1987. To do so, we first derived the change between 1982 and 1987 (expressed in percentage points) in the fraction of the physician

pool composed of each specialty, and then multiplied each of these values by average total income in that specialty in 1982. We then summed across all specialties and divided by the average physician income in 1982. This analysis indicated that the change in specialty mix had no effect on the overall change in per capita income observed during the study.

## COMMENT

Our analysis provides no empirical support for the view that a surplus of physicians has been developing in the United States during the 1980s. Indeed, the data suggest that the demand for physicians' services as measured by hours of patient care and real income, has been rising faster than physician supply. Although physician supply increased by 16% between 1982 and 1987, the aggregate number of hours worked by physicians rose even more (Fig 4). Further, aggregate net income of US physicians rose by more than 30%. Because income rose faster than number of hours in patient care, the financial return per hour increased substantially.

The aggregate number of hours increased more quickly

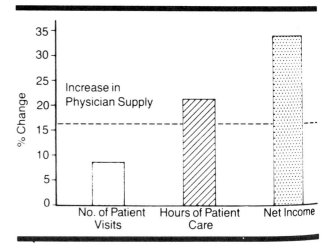

**Figure 4.** Cumulative changes in the aggregate number of patient visits, hours of patient care, and real net physician income between 1982 and 1987. Values are expressed as the cumulative percent change from 1982.

than the aggregate number of visits, reflecting increased time spent in each patient encounter. The greater amount of time spent per encounter would seem, on its face, most likely to be accounted for by technological change and increased physician specialization. This thesis is supported by a recent study that used regression analysis to control for a variety of factors that might have accounted for the increase in time spent per visit; the study concluded that the intensity of services provided during visits was largely responsible.[12]

The aggregate rise in demand for service was, of course, not solely caused by technological change but also was the consequence of other factors such as growth in the population, aging, and a rise in personal income.[13] Historically, the net effect of these changes has been to drive demand for physicians' services upward by more than 3% per year.[4] This figure is slightly lower than the 3.9% annual increase in overall demand between 1982 and 1987 as measured by the rise in the aggregate number of hours worked.

It is theoretically possible, of course, that some portion of the observed increase was caused by an increase in physician-induced demand for services that were medically unnecessary. However, because the increase in number of visits closely matches the growth that would be expected simply because of demographic changes during this period, any significant increase in induced demand could only have been expressed in increased intensity per visit. We doubt, however, that such a substantial steady growth in unnecessary care of this type could have been sustained in the face of the various cost-containment efforts implemented during the study period. Developments such as intensified competition and the spread of health maintenance organizations, preferred provider organizations, and managed care have made it increasingly difficult to provide unnecessary services.

Results of Physician Recruitment Studies

Our conclusion that the demand for physicians' services has equaled or exceeded the growing supply is supported by two recent surveys by a major physician-recruitment organization. The first, a study of 788 hospitals in 1988, indicated that 60% were actively recruiting physicians or planned to do so within the next 12 months.[14] The survey found demand to be strong across all geographic regions, city sizes, and hospital types. A second survey, carried out in 1989, showed that approximately half of medical groups with three or more physicians were looking for additional physicians or were planning to do so within the next year.[15] Furthermore, searches are said to be becoming more difficult to complete because physicians have so many opportuni-

ties to choose from (Bill J. Dismuke, written communication, November 6, 1989).

Relation of Present Findings to Previous Predictions

Until recently, it was widely accepted that a large surplus of physicians was emerging in the United States. The present study provides no empirical support for this conclusion. Instead, it shows that the rise in demand for physicians' services has equaled or exceeded the rise in supply and gives no evidence of the physician surplus of 70,000 predicted for 1990 by the Graduate Medical Education National Advisory Committee and other analysts.

Moreover, a variety of forces is likely to maintain the growth in demand for physicians' services, thus preventing the development of an appreciable surplus. A rapid rate of technological change, the growth and aging of the population, an increase in the number of cases of acquired immunodeficiency syndrome, and the likely extension of health insurance coverage to the uninsured are likely to maintain a rate of increase in demand of at least 2.2% per year,[4] the historical rate of growth in demand seen in health maintenance organizations, and, perhaps, a rate that is even higher. Indeed, a recent study concluded that the increase in demand between 1983 and 2000 was likely to roughly match the growth in the number of physicians, resulting in an appropriate balance between supply and demand during this period.[4]

This projection would, of course, be altered if the imposition of extensive rationing of health care caused a major change in patterns of care. However, even in the face of rigorous cost-containment efforts, demand is likely to rise appreciably because of the various factors mentioned earlier—eg, population growth, rapid technological change, and more widespread insurance coverage. Whether the current balance between supply and demand endures will thus depend largely on policy decisions concerning reimbursement of health care providers rather than on the anticipated growth in the supply of physicians.

Addendum

Recently released data for 1988 show a pattern similar to that reported between 1982 and 1987.[16] Mean net income of individual patient-care physicians rose by 5.0% in real terms, number of patient visits rose by 1.5%, and hours in patient care rose by 0.4%. On an aggregate level, there was an 8.4% increase in net income, a 4.8% rise in the number of patient visits, and a 3.6% increase in hours of patient care.

This study was supported in part by a grant from The Robert Wood Johnson Foundation.

We wish to express our appreciation to Bernice M. Golder for her valuable assistance in the preparation of the manuscript.

## References

1. *Report of the Graduate Medical Education National Advisory Committee to the Secretary, Department of Health and Human Services: Vol 1, GMENAC Summary Report.* Washington, DC: Government Printing Office; 1981. Publication 1980-0-721-748/266.

2. Ellwood PM Jr. Shaping the irreversible revolution: role of business in health care. In: The Florida Council of 100, Blue Cross and Blue Shield of Florida. *Financing Health Care: The Changing Scene.* 1985:28-32.

3. Tarlov AR. HMO enrollment growth and physicians: the third compartment. *Health Aff.* 1986:5(1):23-35.

4. Schwartz WB, Sloan FA, Mendelson DN. Why there will be little or no physician surplus between now and the year 2000. *N Engl J Med.* 1988;318:892-987.

5. Roback G, Randolph L, Mead D, Pasko T. *Physician Characteristics and Distribution in the US.* Chicago, Ill: American Medical Association; 1984.

6. Roback G, Mead D, Randolph L. *Physician Characteristics and Distribution in the US.* Chicago, Ill: American Medical Association; 1986.

7. Roback G, Randolph L, Seidman B, Mead D. *Physician Characteristics and Distribution in the US.* Chicago, Ill: American Medical Association; 1987.

8. Gonzalez ML, Emmons DW, Slora EJ, eds. *Socioeconomic Characteristics of Medical Practice, 1988.* Chicago, Ill: American Medical Association; 1987.

9. Emmons DW. Physician responses to competition, 1980-1987. In: Gonzalez ML, Emmons DW, eds. *Socioeconomic Characteristics of Medical Practice, 1987.* Chicago, Ill: American Medical Association; 1987:20-24.

10. Letsch SW, Levit KR, Waldo DR. National health expenditures, 1987. *Health Care Financing Rev.* 1988;10:109-129.

11. Lazenby H, Levit KR, Waldo DR. *National Health Expenditures, 1985.* Washington, DC: Dept of Health and Human Services; 1986. Publication 03232. Health Care Financing Notes.

12. Hurdle S, Pope GC. Physician productivity: trends and determinants. *Inquiry.* 1989;26:100-115.

13. Sloan FA, Schwartz WB. More doctors: what will they cost? physician income as supply expands. *JAMA.* 1983;249:766-769.

14. *Survey Shows 60% of Hospitals Recruiting Physicians, Despite Claims of Physician Glut: Physician Recruiting Trends.* Atlanta, Ga: Jackson & Coker; 1988.

15. *Survey Finds Most Medical Groups are Recruiting: Physician Recruiting Trends.* Atlanta, Ga: Jackson & Coker; 1989.

16. Gonzalez ML, Emmons DW, eds. *Socioeconomic Characteristics of Medical Practice, 1989.* Chicago, Ill: American Medical Association; 1989.

# Chapter 12

# The Growing Proportion of Female Physicians: Implications for US Physician Supply

Phillip R. Kletke, Ph.D.;
William D. Marder, A.M.; and
Anne B. Silberger, A.M.

**Abstract:** This study analyzes how the growing proportion of women in the United States physician population will affect the amount and type of physician services available to the US population. Female physicians work fewer hours per week, are slightly less likely to be in patient care, and tend to enter different specialties than male physicians. Female physicians also have higher retirement rates than male physicians, but due to their lower mortality rates, have work lives nearly as long as male physicians. We examined how the changing composition of the physician population will affect the availability of physician services by comparing historical and projected trends for the number of active post-residency physicians with comparable trends for a full-time-equivalent measure of physician supply. The full-time-equivalent measure takes into account the different labor supply behavior of key subpopulations (e.g., women and graduates of US versus foreign medical schools). The results suggest that the changing composition of the physician population will reduce the growth of effective physician supply between 1986 and 2010 but only by four percentage points. (*Am J Public Health* 1990; 80:300–304.)

## INTRODUCTION

The proportion of United States physicians who are women has grown rapidly since 1970 and, according to recent projections,[1] it will continue to rise until the year 2010. Since the practice characteristics of female physicians differ from those of male physicians, the growing representation of women in the medical profession is likely to have significant effects on the future supply of physicians.

In general, women physicians have been disproportionately represented in pediatrics and psychiatry and have been underrepresented in the surgical specialties.[2,3] Analyses of the most recent cohorts of new physicians, however, show that the specialty distributions of male and female physicians appear to be converging.[4] This convergence is much more pronounced among graduates of US medical schools (USMGs) than graduates of foreign medical schools (FMGs).[5] Nevertheless, there are still significant differences in the specialty choices of male and female US medical students.[6]

Phillip R. Kletke, Ph.D., William D. Marder, A.M., and Anne B. Silberger, A.M.; The Growing Proportion of Female Physicians: Implications for US Physician Supply, *American Journal of Public Health*, Vol. 80 No. 3, pp. 300–304, 1990, by permission of the American Public Health Association.

This paper, submitted to the Journal November 30, 1988, was revised and accepted for publication July 18, 1989. Work on this project was completed while the co-authors were members of the AMA Center for Health Policy Research. Mr. Marder is Director of Health Labor Market Research at Abt Associates, Inc.; Ms. Silberger is Policy Analyst in the AMA Department of Resident Physician Services. The opinions expressed in this paper are those of the authors and do not necessarily reflect the official position of the American Medical Association or Abt Associates.

Numerous studies have documented that female physicians work fewer hours per week than male physicians,[7-11] and several analyses have explored the extent to which this difference is attributable to marital status and household responsibilities.[12,13] Longitudinal data show that the differences in the number of hours male and female physicians work may be decreasing, although significant differences still remain.[14] Because women physicians work fewer hours per week than male physicians and are comprising an increasing proportion of the physician population, some analysts have concluded that current projections of the physician population overstate effective future physician supply.[15,16] Partly in response to this issue, a recent report of the US Council on Graduate Medical Education[17] indicated that the practice patterns of male and female physicians deserve greater research. This paper measures current differences between male and female physicians and traces their consequences for future physician supply.

## METHODS

We used the Physician Masterfile[2] of the American Medical Association (AMA) for both current and historical data on all US physicians (both AMA members and nonmembers). We used the Demographic Model of the Physician Population[1] to project the size and composition of the future physician population.

Our projection of the physician population assumed that:

- the proportion of women among graduates of US medical schools will increase 1 percent per year from 32 percent in 1986 until it reaches 40 percent and will remain constant thereafter;
- male and female physicians will chose specialties following patterns identical to the most recent cohorts of medical school graduates; and
- retirement and mortality rates for male and female physicians will remain constant at their current level.

We analyzed data from the AMA Socioeconomic Monitoring System[11] to examine practice differences of male and female physicians. These data come from a series of periodic telephone surveys of random samples of non-federal, post-resident, patient care physicians since 1982. We used data from the 1987 core survey, which has data on approximately 4,000 physicians.

## RESULTS

Demographic Characteristics

Table 1 shows that the proportion of women physicians increased from 7.1 percent to 15.3 percent between 1970 and 1986, and is projected to reach almost 30 percent by the year 2010. Consequently, women

**TABLE 1—Proportion of Active Physicians who are Female According to Age, Specialty, and Country of Graduation for Years 1970, 1986, 2000, and 2010**

| | Historical | | Projected | |
|---|---|---|---|---|
| | 1970 | 1986 | 2000 | 2010 |
| Total | 7.1% | 15.3% | 24.1% | 29.4% |
| Country of Graduation | | | | |
| USMG | 5.4 | 14.0 | 24.7 | 30.7 |
| FMG | 14.6 | 20.0 | 21.7 | 23.0 |
| USFMG | 4.2 | 10.7 | 13.0 | 14.0 |
| Foreign-born FMG | 16.0 | 21.7 | 24.0 | 25.9 |
| Age (years) | | | | |
| < 36 | 9.5 | 24.5 | 36.5 | 37.3 |
| 36–45 | 6.4 | 15.6 | 30.3 | 37.1 |
| 46–55 | 6.3 | 9.5 | 20.5 | 30.9 |
| 56–65 | 5.0 | 7.1 | 12.8 | 21.4 |
| > 65 | 5.4 | 5.9 | 8.8 | 13.8 |
| Specialty | | | | |
| General/Family Practice | 4.4 | 12.9 | 22.9 | 28.8 |
| General Internal Medicine | 5.8 | 17.4 | 26.5 | 31.5 |
| Medical Subspecialties | 5.0 | 10.2 | 18.4 | 22.8 |
| General Surgery | 1.1 | 5.8 | 10.6 | 14.0 |
| Surgical Subspecialties | 1.3 | 3.9 | 6.8 | 8.9 |
| Pediatrics | 21.4 | 35.3 | 47.5 | 54.1 |
| Obstetrics/Gynecology | 7.2 | 19.6 | 35.9 | 45.6 |
| Radiology | 5.3 | 12.1 | 19.7 | 24.4 |
| Psychiatry | 13.2 | 22.4 | 34.0 | 41.8 |
| Anesthesiology | 14.3 | 17.4 | 23.2 | 26.6 |
| Pathology | 12.9 | 21.8 | 29.2 | 34.7 |
| Emergency Medicine | —* | 12.9 | 20.5 | 24.3 |
| Other Specialties | 9.6 | 18.1 | 26.4 | 31.7 |

SOURCE: AMA Physician Masterfile, 1970–86, Department of Data Release Services, Division of Survey and Data Resources; AMA Demographic Model of the Physician Population, AMA Center for Health Policy Research, 1988.

physicians are concentrated in the younger age categories. In 1970 and 1986, female physicians were disproportionately represented among foreign medical graduates not born in the US, but the relationship between sex and country of graduation reverses during the projection period due to the growing number of females graduating from US medical schools. Female physicians are concentrated in pediatrics and psychiatry and are under-represented in general surgery and the surgical subspecialties. These patterns appear in both the 1970 and 1986 data as well as the projection estimates for 2000 and 2010.

Differences in the specialty distributions of male and female physicians persist but are gradually weakening, however. The index of dissimilarity for the specialty distributions of male and female post-resident physicians (i.e., the percent of female physicians who would have to change specialties so that their specialty distribution would match that of male physicians) dropped from 31.2 to 23.7 between 1970 and 1986, indicating that the concentration of female physicians in certain specialties has decreased. The index calculated only for physicians less than 35 years of age dropped from 28.5 to 18.4 during the same period.

The mortality, retirement, and accession (resumption of activity) rates for the projection model were estimated from an analysis of Masterfile data for years 1978 to 1986 from a set of logistic regression equations, based on the physician's age, sex, specialty, and country of

**TABLE 2—Expected Life and Work Life of Active USMG Physicians at Ages 35, 40, and 65 by Specialty and Sex**

| | Age (years) | | | | | |
| | 35 | | 50 | | 65 | |
| | Male | Female | Male | Female | Male | Female |
|---|---|---|---|---|---|---|
| **Expected Life** | | | | | | |
| Specialty General/Family Practice | 42.4 | 47.2 | 28.4 | 33.1 | 16.3 | 20.4 |
| General Internal Medicine | 43.8 | 48.4 | 29.7 | 34.2 | 17.3 | 21.3 |
| Medical Subspecialties | 45.0 | 49.6 | 30.8 | 35.3 | 18.2 | 22.2 |
| General Surgery | 43.7 | 48.4 | 29.6 | 34.1 | 17.2 | 21.2 |
| Surgical Subspecialties | 44.5 | 49.2 | 30.4 | 34.9 | 17.9 | 21.9 |
| Pediatrics | 44.9 | 49.6 | 30.8 | 35.3 | 18.2 | 22.2 |
| Obstetrics/Gynecology | 43.1 | 47.7 | 29.0 | 33.6 | 16.8 | 20.7 |
| Radiology | 44.4 | 49.2 | 30.2 | 34.9 | 17.8 | 21.9 |
| Psychiatry | 43.4 | 48.2 | 29.3 | 34.0 | 17.1 | 21.2 |
| Anesthesiology | 43.9 | 48.6 | 29.8 | 34.4 | 17.4 | 21.4 |
| Pathology | 43.6 | 48.6 | 29.6 | 34.4 | 17.3 | 21.5 |
| Emergency Medicine | 42.7 | 47.9 | 28.8 | 33.8 | 16.8 | 21.0 |
| Other Specialties | 43.7 | 48.6 | 29.6 | 34.4 | 17.4 | 21.5 |
| **Expected Work Life** | | | | | | |
| Specialty | | | | | | |
| General/Family Practice | 36.5 | 36.8 | 22.7 | 23.5 | 11.2 | 12.3 |
| General Internal Medicine | 37.6 | 37.8 | 23.6 | 24.3 | 11.8 | 13.0 |
| Medical Subspecialties | 39.1 | 39.7 | 25.1 | 26.1 | 13.0 | 14.3 |
| General Surgery | 37.1 | 37.0 | 23.1 | 23.7 | 11.5 | 12.5 |
| Surgical Subspecialties | 37.7 | 37.5 | 23.6 | 24.1 | 11.8 | 12.8 |
| Pediatrics | 37.8 | 37.6 | 23.7 | 24.2 | 11.9 | 12.9 |
| Obstetrics/Gynecology | 37.0 | 37.0 | 23.0 | 23.6 | 11.4 | 12.4 |
| Radiology | 36.5 | 36.0 | 22.6 | 22.8 | 11.0 | 11.9 |
| Psychiatry | 37.5 | 37.9 | 23.5 | 24.5 | 11.8 | 13.1 |
| Anesthsiology | 35.8 | 34.9 | 21.9 | 21.9 | 10.5 | 11.2 |
| Pathology | 36.3 | 35.9 | 22.4 | 22.8 | 10.9 | 11.9 |
| Emergency Medicine | 34.9 | 34.2 | 21.1 | 21.3 | 10.) | 10.8 |
| Other Specialties | 35.8 | 35.0 | 22.0 | 22.1 | 10.6 | 11.4 |

SOURCE: Marder, et al. Physician Supply and Utilization by Speciality: Trends and Projections. Table 3.1, p 42.

working hours treating patients in either an office-based or hospital-based practice). The proportion decreases somewhat for older physicians, and both USFMGs and foreign-born FMGs are slightly more likely than USMGs to be in patient care. (Data available upon request to author.) The probability of being in patient care was highest in general/family practice, the surgical subspecialties, and obstetrics/gynecology, and lowest in the medical subspecialties, pathology, and in the residual "other specialties" category. There are few differences by gender.

Table 3 shows that post-residency patient care physicians worked an average of 58.3 hours per week in 1987. On average, female physicians, older physicians and USMGs worked fewer hours than their counterparts. Physicians in general internal medicine, the medical subspecialties, pediatrics, obstetrics/gynecology, and emergency medicine worked several more hours per week than average, while physicians in psychiatry, pathology, and the other specialties worked fewer hours than average.

The findings reported for the proportion of physicians in patient care and their average hours of work per week were confirmed in a logistic regression analysis of whether a physician was in patient care and an ordinary least squares regression analysis of the log of hours worked per week by patient care physicians. (Analysis available on request to author.) Independent variables were: the physician's sex, country of graduation, specialty, physician's age and age-squared (since the relationships with

graduation. (Analyses available on request to author.) Female physicians had higher retirement rates and lower mortality rates than male physicians. By assuming that the schedules of transition rates remain constant, we estimated how much longer physicians of a given age, sex, specialty, and country of graduation are, on average, likely to live, and how much longer they are likely to be professionally active.

Table 2 presents the expected years of remaining life and the expected years of remaining work life for active male and female USMG physicians at ages 35, 50, and 65 in 13 different specialty groups. Physicians on average, live and work longer than the rest of the US population. Female physicians can expect to live approximately four to five years longer than male physicians, but their higher retirement rates mean that active female physicians at age 35 have approximately the same expected work life as male physicians at 35.

## Physician Time in Patient Care

Among the entire post-residency physician population, 89.7 percent of male physicians and 88.0 percent of female physicians are classified as being in direct patient care (i.e., spending the plurality of their professional

**TABLE 3—Average Hours Worked per Week by Male and Female Non-Federal Post-residency Patient Care Physicians According to Age, Specialty, and Country of Graduation, 1987**

| | Total | Male | Female |
|---|---|---|---|
| Total | 58.3 | 59.0 | 52.3 |
| Country of Graduation | | | |
| USMG | 58.1 | 58.6 | 52.3 |
| FMG | 59.3 | 60.6 | 52.2 |
| USFMG | 59.1 | 59.3 | 55.0 |
| Foreign-born FMG | 59.3 | 60.9 | 52.1 |
| Age (years) | | | |
| < 36 | 60.3 | 61.7 | 53.9 |
| 36–45 | 60.2 | 61.4 | 50.6 |
| 46–55 | 58.8 | 59.2 | 54.3 |
| 56–65 | 55.6 | 55.8 | 51.9 |
| > 65 | 49.0 | 49.1 | 45.7 |
| Specialty | | | |
| General/Family Practice | 58.2 | 59.3 | 48.0 |
| General Internal Medicine | 60.6 | 62.0 | 50.5 |
| Medicine Subspecialties | 62.1 | 62.4 | 56.1 |
| General Surgery | 59.7 | 59.7 | 53.7 |
| Surgical Subspecialties | 57.8 | 57.9 | 52.5 |
| Pediatrics | 59.8 | 62.2 | 53.3 |
| Obstetrics/Gynecology | 60.9 | 61.7 | 56.2 |
| Radiology | 57.2 | 57.3 | 54.8 |
| Psychiatry | 50.4 | 51.1 | 46.5 |
| Anesthesiology | 58.8 | 60.3 | 49.7 |
| Pathology | 52.9 | 52.5 | 56.1 |
| Emergency Medicine | 60.7 | 60.2 | 64.3 |
| Other Specialties | 54.6 | 54.7 | 54.4 |

SOURCE: Marder, et al. Physician Supply and Utilization by Specialty: Trends and Projections. Table 2.6, p 18.

the dependent variables did not appear to be linear with respect to age), and interaction terms for sex with age and age-squared.

In each analysis, the coefficients for sex and the age-sex interactions were jointly significant at the .001 level. Plots of the age-specific regression estimates for male and female physicians indicated that female physicians are slightly less likely to be in patient care than male physicians for all ages. The hours worked per week by patient care physicians peak at age 37 for male physicians and at age 43 for female physicians. Male physicians generally work more hours than female physicians, but the differential decreases with age.

### Alternate Measures of Physician Supply

Some researchers have speculated that because female physicians work fewer hours per week than male physicians and because the proportion of female physicians is increasing, projections of the total physician population may overestimate effective physician supply. We investigated this issue by estimating the *aggregate time worked by patient care physicians,* measured in terms of full-time-equivalent physicians. This measure includes only physicians in direct patient care and weights each physician and the amount of time spent in professional activities. This adjusted measure of physician supply takes into account the changing composition of the physician population. We compared this measure of the effective physician supply with the simple number of physicians.

We considered the population of post-resident physicians—physicians who have completed specialty training—because we wanted to analyze how the changing composition of physician supply will affect the specialty distribution of physician services. Our projection estimates did not indicate how many physicians have completed residency training, so we estimated the future number of post-resident physicians based on the available information—the projected age, sex, country of graduation, and specialty distributions of the future physician population. We used a logistic regression analysis of the 1986 AMA Physician Masterfile data to estimate $q_{i,j,k,l}$, the proportion of physicians of age i, sex j, specialty k, and country of graduation l who have completed residency training. (Analyses available upon request to author.) Assuming that these proportions remain constant throughout the projection, we estimated P, the projected size of the active post-resident physician population, as follows:

$$P = \Sigma P_{i,j,k,l}$$
$$= \Sigma [q_{i,j,k,l} A_{i,j,k,l}]$$

where $A_{i,j,k,l}$ represents the projected number of active physicians in the corresponding age-sex-specialty-country of graduation category.

We estimated F, the future number of full-time equivalent patient care physicians, as follows:

$$F = \Sigma F_{i,j,k,l}$$
$$= \Sigma [c_{i,j,k,l} h_{i,j,k,l} P_{i,j,k,l} \frac{1}{58.0}]$$

where $c_{i,j,k,l}$ is the estimated proportion of physicians in each sex-age-specialty-country of graduation category who are in patient care, derived from our logistic regression analysis of the 1986 Masterfile data; $h_{i,j,k,l}$ is the estimated number of hours worked by patient care physicians, derived from the ordinary least squares analysis of the SMS data; and 58.0 is the average hours per week worked by patient care physicians in 1987.

Table 4 presents historical and projected data for the number of active post-residency physicians, and the number of full-time-equivalent post-residency patient care physicians. Both measures show that physician supply is growing rapidly. Projected growth is slightly slower for the full-time-equivalent measure.

The bottom line of Table 5 presents the number of full-time-equivalent patient care post-residency physicians divided by the total number of post-residency physicians. This ratio describes how effectively the projected physician population will provide time to patient care in terms of 1986 full-time-equivalent patient care physicians. During the 1970–86 historical period, the ratio increased slightly from .888 to .896. Despite the growing proportion of female physicians throughout this time period, the average physician provided more patient care because: the proportion of patient care physicians increased; and a greater proportion of physicians were entering the middle parts of their careers, during which they provide the most patient care.

Between 1986 and 2010, the ratio is projected to decrease from .896 to .854, representing more than a 4

TABLE 4—The Number of Active Post-residency Physicians and the Number of Full-Time-Equivalent Post-residency Patient Care Physicians by Age, Specialty, and Country of Graduation, for Years 1970, 1986, 2000, and 2010

|  | Historical | | Projected | |
|---|---|---|---|---|
|  | 1970 | 1986 | 2000 | 2010 |
| Active Post-residency Physicians | 262,694 | 438,935 | 567,300 | 611,100 |
| Full-Time-Equivalent Post-residency Patient Care Physicians | 233,400 | 393,500 | 495,700 | 522,100 |
| Ratio of Full-Time-Equivalent Post-residency Patient Care Physicians to Active Post-residency Physicians | .888 | .896 | .873 | .854 |

SOURCE: AMA Physician Masterfile, 1970–86, Department of Data Release Services, Division of Survey and Data Resources; AMA Demographic Model of the Physician Population, AMA Center for Health Policy Research, 1988.

**TABLE 5—Percent Change in the Number of Active Post-residency Physicians and the Number of Full-Time-Equivalent Post-residency Patient Care Physicians, 1986–2000 and 1986–2010**

| | Percent Change in Post-residency Population | | | |
|---|---|---|---|---|
| | 1986–2000 | | 1986–2010 | |
| | All Active | Full-Time-Equivalent Patient Care | All Active | Full-Time-Equivalent Patient Care |
| Total | 29.2 | 26.0 | 39.2 | 32.7 |
| **Sex** | | | | |
| Male | 15.6 | 13.8 | 15.1 | 11.5 |
| Female | 120.0 | 120.7 | 199.3 | 197.4 |
| **Country of Graduation** | | | | |
| USMG | 34.7 | 32.0 | 49.5 | 43.6 |
| FMG | 11.6 | 6.8 | 5.9 | -2.1 |
| USFMG | 64.3 | 62.1 | 92.4 | 85.5 |
| Foreign-born FMG | 3.7 | -1.7 | -7.1 | -15.7 |
| **Age (years)** | | | | |
| < 36 | -19.5 | -21.3 | -21.1 | -23.0 |
| 36–45 | 16.0 | 13.8 | 2.6 | -1.3 |
| 46–55 | 76.0 | 73.0 | 71.8 | 67.1 |
| 56–65 | 30.6 | 30.0 | 100.2 | 97.2 |
| > 65 | 71.2 | 67.9 | 121.1 | 115.5 |
| **Specialty** | | | | |
| General/Family Practice | 11.8 | 10.7 | 17.0 | 14.4 |
| General Internal Medicine | 54.1 | 51.1 | 72.5 | 64.6 |
| Medical Subspecialties | 38.4 | 32.7 | 58.7 | 47.4 |
| General Surgery | 25.7 | 24.0 | 25.5 | 21.5 |
| Surgical Subspecialties | 18.4 | 15.2 | 21.2 | 15.8 |
| Pediatrics | 47.1 | 41.3 | 67.9 | 56.5 |
| Obstetrics/Gynecology | 26.6 | 21.2 | 37.6 | 28.4 |
| Radiology | 30.9 | 26.3 | 41.5 | 33.9 |
| Psychiatry | 13.8 | 8.9 | 15. | 7.8 |
| Anesthesiology | 41.5 | 37.9 | 58.9 | 51.9 |
| Pathology | 14.4 | 8.5 | 12.0 | 3.2 |
| Emergency Medicine | 57.6 | 53.0 | 87.4 | 77.4 |
| Other Specialties | 20.0 | 15.8 | 22.4 | 14.4 |

SOURCE: AMA Physician Masterfile, 1970–86, Department of Data Release Services, Division of Survey and Data Resources, AMA Demographic Model of the Physician Population, AMA Center for Health Policy Research, 1988.

percent decrease in the amount of patient care provided by the average physician. This finding is attributable to the growing proportion of women physicians who, on average, work fewer hours per week and are somewhat less likely to be in patient care; and to the growing proportion of older physicians, who work fewer hours per week.

Table 5 shows the percent growth in the two supply measures for the various components of the physician population in 1970–86 and 1986–2010. Both measures indicate that the physician population is growing rapidly, although the growth rate is gradually diminishing. Both indicate that: the percent growth is substantially larger for female physicians than for male physicians; growth rates for emergency medicine, general internal medicine, and pediatrics are greater than for other specialties; and the number of physicians over age 65 will grow faster than the physician population as a whole.

More important for this analysis are the subtle differences between the two measures attributable to changes in the composition of the physician population. In both time periods, the percent increase of active post-resi-

dency physicians is several percentage points greater than their full-time equivalents, i.e., the growth of the physician population is slightly faster than the growth of effective physician supply.

For almost all the components of the physician population, the percent increase in active physicians exceeds the percent increase in full-time-equivalent patient care physicians. Female physicians are an important exception. Between 1986 and 2000, disproportionate numbers of female physicians will enter the middle age categories when they spend the most time in patient care. On the other hand, male physicians will be entering the older age categories and thus are expected to work fewer hours per week. Due to this difference, the sex differential in the rate at which physicians provide patient care will decrease in the future.

## DISCUSSION

If current patterns persist, the rapidly growing proportion of female physicians will affect both the amount and type of health care available in the future. We have presented data on several important past differences between male and female physicians. The projected growth of the physician population slightly overstates projected growth in the effective supply of physician hours worked. However, the actual magnitude of this difference is small, especially when compared to the rapid growth projected for the physician population.

It is quite likely that, as the number of female physicians increases over time, their practices will more closely resemble those of male physicians. Several factors suggest that some of the differences between male and female physicians may be declining. The specialty distributions of male and female physicians appear to be becoming more similar, especially among the young age groups. Female physicians are no longer disproportionately represented among foreign-born FMGs. Even though female physicians have higher retirement rates than male physicians, their expected work lives are just as long as male physicians due to their lower mortality rates. As career patterns of male and female physicians become more similar, the classic measures of physician supply will be more reliable indicators of long-term growth.

Acknowledgments
An earlier draft of this paper was presented at the 1988 annual meeting of the Population Association of America.

## References

1. Marder WD, Kletke PR, Silberger AB, Willke RJ: Physician Supply and Utilization by Specialty: Trends and Projections. Chicago: American Medical Association, 1988.
2. Roback G, Randolph L, Seidman B, Mead D: Physician

Characteristics and Distribution in the US, 1986. Chicago: American Medical Association, 1987.

3. Crowley AE, Etzel SI: Graduate medical education in the United States, *JAMA* 1988; 260:1093–1101.

4. Weisman CS, Levine DM, Steinwachs DM, Chase GA: Male and female physician career patterns: Specialty choices and graduate training. *J Med Educ* 1980; 55:813–825.

5. Mick SS, Worobey JL: Impact of women and foreign medical graduates on specialty distribution of US house officers. *J Med Educ* 1984; 59:921–927.

6. Babbott D, Baldwin DC, Killian CD, Weaver SO: Trends in evolution of specialty choice: Comparison of US medical school graduates in 1983 and 1987. *JAMA* 1989; 261:2367–2373.

7. Powers L, Parmelle RD, Wiesenfelder H: Practice patterns of women and men physicians. *J Med Educ* 1969; 44:481–491.

8. Jussim J, Muller C: Medical education for women: How good an investment? *J Med Educ* 1975; 50:571–580.

9. Williams PB: Recent trends in the productivity of women and men physicians. *J Med Educ* 1978; 53:420–422.

10. Bobula JD: Work patterns, practice characteristics and incomes of male and female physicians. *J Med Educ* 1980; 55:826–833.

11. Gonzalez ML, Emmons DW (eds): Socioeconomic Characteristics of Medical Practice, 1986. Chicago: American Medical Association, 1987.

12. Mitchell JB: Why do women physicians work fewer hours than men physicians? *Inquiry* 1984; 21:361–368.

13. Weisman CS, Teitelbaum MA: The work-family role system and physician productivity. *J Health Soc Behav* 1987; 28:247–257.

14. Freiman MP, Marder WD: Changes in the hours worked by physicians, 1970–80. *Am J Public Health* 1984; 74:1348–1352.

15. Lanska MJ, Lanska DJ, Rimm AA: Effect of rising percentage of female physicians on projections of physician supply. *J Med Educ* 1984; 59:849–855.

16. Jacobsen SJ, Rimm AA: The projected physician surplus reevaluated. *Health Affairs* 1987; 6:48–56.

17. US Council on Graduate Medical Education: Report to Congress, 1988.

# Chapter 13

# The Industrialization of American Psychiatry

Thomas E. Bittker, M.D.

*Physician surpluses and escalating medical care costs have fostered an alliance among government, corporate America, and health insurers that has inspired medicine's industrialization. These same forces will transform psychiatry into an industry where prospective payment, automation, salaried employment, and central control of clinical activities threaten to become the dominant form of medical practice. Emerging trends suggest that both patients and health professionals will gravitate to various forms of alternative provider organizations in an effort to shield themselves from the economic uncertainties of seeking and providing care. The chronically mentally ill and others requiring extensive treatment risk exclusion from this new system, where cost consciousness may supplant compassion.*

(Am J Psychiatry 142:149–164, 1985)

Many of the economic problems confronting psychiatry today have sprung from changes that have influenced the entirety of American medicine. Two of the most important changes have been the expanding supply of physicians and the enormous increase in the cost of health care.

In his comprehensive review, Tarlov[1] chronicled the development of the social consensus that will lead to a projected doubling of the supply of actively practicing physicians between 1970 and 2000. During this period the physician-to-population ratio will have climbed from 152 per 100,000 to 240 per 100,000. This latter figure is estimated by most students of health economics to far exceed the need. Physician excesses will have been reached in most specialties by 1990, according to the Graduate Medical Education National Advisory Committee.[2,3] Psychiatric patients in general and child psychiatric patients in particular will be among the few underserved populations in an era of physician abundance.

From 1965 to 1981 health expenditures grew from 6% to 9.8% of the gross national product, and per capita expenditures exploded from $211 to $1,225 per year, a 580% increase in 16 years.[4] The trend is likely to continue. Economists from both the public and private sectors have predicted that by 1987, total annual health expenditures will exceed $550 billion and will consume 12% of the gross national product.[5]

Government has responded to this cost explosion by legislating an end to the cost-reimbursement system for Medicare providers and establishing that federal payment will be based on payer-determined prices.[6–8] In addition to regulations directly limiting medical care

*The Industrialization of American Psychiatry,* Vol. 142 No. 2, 149–154, February 1985, copyright 1985, the American Psychiatric Association. Reprinted by permission.

Adapted from a paper presented at the 137th annual meeting of the American Psychiatric Association, Los Angeles, May 5–11, 1984. Received March 12, 1984; revised July 6, 1984; accepted July 23, 1984. Copyright © 1985 American Psychiatric Association.

expenditures, both government and industry have fostered a climate encouraging competition among organized providers of care. Federal legislation has overturned state laws discriminating against closed-panel prepaid practice, established regulations to permit federal certification of health maintenance organizations HMOs), and provided mandating mechanisms wherein employers of 25 or more employees are obliged, on written request, to offer federally qualified prepaid plans as a health insurance option.

HMOs have emerged as powerful competitors to traditional indemnity-based, fee-for-service practice. In 1978 HMOs served 7.8 million members, two-thirds of whom were concentrated in the Pacific coast states. It was predicted that by 1984, membership would grow to include 15.4 million people, distributed throughout the United States.[5] Abramowitz has estimated that by 1988, HMO membership will grow to include 25.6 million people and that publicly held HMOs may prove to be among the most profitable service industries on Wall Street.[5] In an effort to maintain their flow of patients, hospitals and fee-for-service practitioners have collaborated with insurers and employers to form various preferred provider organizations PPOs) and exclusive provider organizations EPOs) intended to offer care at a discounted rate.

## THE GROWTH OF CORPORATE MEDICINE

Several observers[6–9] have warned of the implications in the transition of medicine from a cottage industry to a "medical-industrial complex". In coining this term, Relman[6,7] was referring to the growing influence on the health economy of large, national, diversified, multidimensional corporations that sell health services for profit. In addition to providing hospital and nursing care, dialysis centers, and general laboratory services, such corporations are monitoring psychotropic drugs, as well as providing psychological testing, alcoholism treatment, and a comprehensive array of inpatient and outpatient psychiatric treatment services.[10] Any doubts that the corporation has penetrated the private psychiatric sector ought to have been dispelled by a review of a recent survey of private psychiatric hospitals.[11] As of 1980 there were 184 private psychiatric hospitals in the United States, two-thirds of which were for profit. Of these for-profit hospitals, 109 of 121 were owned by corporations.

Starr[8] has outlined five dimensions distinguishing the growth of corporate medicine, as follows.

1. Change in the type of ownership and control: the shift from nonprofit and governmental organizations to for-profit companies in health care.
2. Horizontal integration: the decline of free-standing institutions and rise of multi-institutional systems and the con-

sequent shift in the locus of control from community boards to regional and national health care corporations.
3. Diversification and corporate restructuring: the shift from single-unit organizations operating in one market to conglomerates, often organized as holding companies, sometimes with both nonprofit and for-profit subsidiaries involved in a variety of difference health care markets.
4. Vertical integration: the shift from single-level-of care organizations, such as acute care hospitals, to organizations, such as HMOs, that embrace the various phases and levels of care.
5. Industry concentration: the increasing concentration of ownership and control of health services in regional markets and the nation as a whole.

Currently, three species of national corporation are vying for control of this new, highly profitable industry:[5] integrated hospital chains, for-profit HMOs, and older, multiline insurance companies. The emergence of these national corporations has conspired with four previously mentioned trends—industrial coalitions organized to control health care costs; various forms of EPOs and PPOs, intended to reward patients who use lower-cost health care providers; the government-led effort to alter reimbursement from a retrospective, provider-determined cost basis to a prospective, payer-determined price basis; and the burgeoning supply of physicians—to produce a climate ideal for greater integration and centralization of control.

Cost efficiency will fuel this move to integrate and centralize. The employer corporations demanding a cap on health cost exposure will select only the most cost-conscious health insurers. Health insurers will turn away from cost-reimbursement forms of insurance toward prospective payment systems, e.g., EPOs, PPOs, or HMOs. Physicians, in an effort to increase their market share, are more likely to accept prospective payment as a necessary evil. But prospective payment is too risky for solo and small group practices; a few very sick patients can produce economic ruin for the physician who shares the financial risk of care. Consequently, physicians will either coalesce in large-risk pools or seek "safety nets" through secondary insurers. Neither the risk pools nor the umbrella insurance schemes will work unless the utilization patterns of physicians are tightly controlled. Thus, doctors will be forced to choose a more cost-efficient manner of practice in order to survive.

## THE INDUSTRIALIZATION OF PSYCHIATRY

How will psychiatry be affected by medicine's economic transformation? In considering this question, I will extract from several authors[6,8,9] four features fundamental to industrialization: economic determinants of supply and demand; centralization of financing, management review, and control; division of labor; and automation and computerization.

## Economic Determinants of Supply and Demand

The demand for psychiatric services reflects the interaction of four factors: the effectiveness of psychiatric services, the prevalence of mental disorder, the financing of services, and manpower.

Psychiatric services have been deemed responsible for saving the United States an estimated $4 billion over a 10–year period by promoting the management of manic-depressive disease through the use of lithium,[12] accelerating the recovery of heart attack and heart surgery patients,[13] and, in fee-for-service settings, providing sufficient cost offsets in other medical care utilization to defray the cost of more than 21 outpatient visits while improving the appropriateness of medical care utilization.[14] In addition, as Strupp[15] and Marmor[16] have suggested, although it is difficult to assess global outcome, psychotherapy in well-motivated patients yields an apparent improvement in the perceived quality of life.

Conservative estimates indicate the prevalence of mental disorder in this country as approximately 15% of the population. The Graduate Medical Education National Advisory Committee (GMENAC) panel on psychiatry estimated the prevalence to be 18%, two-thirds of which (12% of the total population) consisted of persons requiring at least one visit annually for mental health care.[17] Only 25% of this potential patient group were determined to need the attention of a psychiatrist. The panel then assumed that the average psychiatrist worked 46 weeks per year, 36 hours per week, performing patient care activities. On the basis of these assumptions and adjusting for population projections, the panel predicted a need for 38,500 general psychiatrists by 1990; the supply will approximate 30,500, a shortfall of 8,500 or 20%. For child psychiatry, using a similar model, GMENAC foresaw a need for 9,000 practitioners, an availability of 4,100, and a shortfall of 4,900 or 55%.

On first impression the data on both the effectiveness of psychiatric services and the prevalence of mental disorder might reassure the psychiatrist concerned about future employability. However, competition from other mental health disciplines clouds this optimism. In 1975–1976, for every 100,000 U.S. citizens there were only 12.4 psychiatrists, but there were 19.5 psychologists and 32.2 social workers.[18] At the time of this 1975–1976 analysis, psychologists had not yet been granted hospital admission privileges,[19] nor had they been emboldened by court endorsement of direct payment for psychotherapy.[20] If current trends continue, these professionals will increasingly challenge psychiatry's status as the preeminent provider of reimbursable psychotherapy services. Furthermore, internists, family practitioners, and neurologists—all specialties in modest surplus in 1990—may encroach on psychiatric territory in the management of structurally and biochemically based emotional disturbances. Pediatrics, a specialty likely to see a surplus of 7,500 or 25% of the required number in 1990, may nurture the subspecialty of behavioral pediatrics, thus filling some of the needs unmet by child psychiatry. In short, we are likely to see other disciplines invade the mental health service sector to fill the manpower vacuum left by psychiatry.

Admittedly, this leaves open the question of how well these other professions will do the job when compared with psychiatry. Emphasis on quality, however, will likely be overshadowed by preoccupation with cost control. The measure of effective service may become more heavily weighted toward answering the question of "How cheap?" rather than "How well?"

Although private psychiatric insurance coverage grew in tandem with the expansion of coverage for all medical services between 1965 and 1981,[21] substantial barriers remain. Coinsurance for psychiatric services is typically higher than that required for general medical services; in addition, there are unique ceilings on the duration and costs of psychiatric services that are not present for other specialties. Thirteen percent of plans fail to cover emotional disorders at all.[22] In the face of preoccupation with cost control, this situation is unlikely to improve. Indeed, some health economists have suggested that increased cost sharing by consumers may substantially reduce medical costs while having only minimal effect on health outcomes.[23–25] If this thinking prevails, patients can anticipate paying even higher coinsurance fees for indemnity sector psychiatric services.

The psychiatric service consumer faces three options to finance care in the private sector. First, choose a relatively expensive indemnity insurance program and expect close scrutiny on service utilization and substantial out-of-pocket costs, approximately 20% of the total cost of care in the most richly endowed programs. Second, choose basic insurance coverage, at a lower premium, and expect to finance most mental health care by direct payment. Third, affiliate with one of several alternative provider organizations (e.g., HMOs, EPOs, PPOs) and expect very modest coinsurance payments but strict limits on the duration of services, e.g., 20 outpatient visits and 30–45 inpatient days in most federally qualified HMOs.[26] Under the market assumptions discussed earlier, "pro-competitive" economists[5] are betting that the rational consumer will more likely suffer the limitations of freedom imposed by the prospective payment option in exchange for access to affordable services.

Prepaid psychiatry assumes a fundamentally different form than its fee-for-service counterpart. Heavy emphasis is placed on outpatient crisis intervention, time-limited and group psychotherapy, and collaboration with other mental health professionals.[27,28] Since physicians are at risk for all service costs, every reasonable and ethically sound effort is made to avoid long-term treatment and hospitalization. Under these circumstances, psychiatrists make up about 30% of mental health staffs, with psychiatrist-to-patient ratios ranging from 5 per 100,000[29,30] to 10 per 100,000.[26] If translated into the needs of prepaid settings, the GMENAC estimates of 34,600 general and child psychiatrists per 250,000,000 population in 1990 (13.8 per 100,000) would be more than sufficient.

Centralization

Comprehensive prospective payment systems will enjoy a robust future. Indeed, examples of psychiatric practice in HMOs, currently the most common model of prospective payment, have been shown to be cost effective. Jones and Vischi[29] reviewed 25 studies to determine whether treatment for alcoholism, drug abuse, and mental illness would reduce subsequent general medical care utilization. In 11 of 13 studies in which there were comparison groups followed for a period of at least 1 year, treatment for alcoholism, drug abuse, and mental illness yielded a decrease in other medical care used; reductions ranged from 26% to 69%, with a median of 40% of the cost of the treatment for these three conditions. For mental health patients, 12 of 13 studies showed reductions in medical care utilization in the year following treatment for alcoholism, drug abuse, and mental illness, with the cost offsets ranging from 5% to 85% of the cost of the treatment provided (the median saving was 20%).

In order to sustain a flow of patient referrals and ensure their incomes, psychiatrists will affiliate with the growing numbers of alternative provider organizations (e.g., HMOs, EPOs, PPOs, and independent physicians associations). Like other physicians,[1] a growing proportion of psychiatrists will assume full-time salaried positions within these organizations. To ensure the lowest premium to their enrollees and thus to maintain their competitive position, these organizations will demand that each participating provider undergo close scrutiny by utilization reviewers. Hospitalization for problems that *might* be managed in an outpatient setting, psychotherapy beyond 10 visits, and treatment of masochistic or ill-motivated patients are all practices warranting review in such settings.[27,28]

Utilization control ensures the financial survival of prepaid systems; a strong quality assurance program ensures the integrity of its professionals. As cost-based reimbursement systems risk overutilization in search of fees, so there is a complementary risk in prepaid systems—the provision of fewer and cheaper services than the patient requires. To protect against the provision of marginal or poor quality care, health plan managers must select mental health professionals who are as thoroughly committed to the quality of care as they are to cost control.

Determining the values of the HMO mental health system emerges as the first quality assurance task of the professional staff. The next is to define these values— e.g., quality of care and service, a population rather than an individual focus, and affordability—in a manner that confers operational meaning on them. How long should a patient be required to wait between indicating a need for noncrisis treatment and the first visit? How long should he wait between intake and follow-up visits? Should the health plan permit a waiting list for mental health visits? What should be the criteria for hospitalization? For individual or group therapy? How many individual, couple, or family visits should be permitted before a case is considered for utilization review? How many new cases per week can the full-time mental health professional assume? Once standards have been defined, measurement of results may be readily achieved assuming the existence of effective and accurate medical/psychiatric record and management information systems.

Annual performance appraisals assessing factors such as productivity, proper utilization of resources, teamwork, and peer and patient estimates of practice quality will become key determinants of the psychiatrist's salary and sense of accomplishment in such settings.[28] Success, then, will be determined not only by professional skills but also by the psychiatrist's effectiveness in adapting to the values, the goals, and the procedures of the health care organization.

Division of Labor

Psychiatry enjoys a tradition of collaborating with other medical disciplines and other mental health professions. A generation ago, however, psychiatrists retained leadership in psychiatric hospitals and outpatient settings. Labor was divided according to the direction of that psychiatric leadership. With the growing importance of cost consciousness, institutions are reluctant to squander relatively expensive psychiatric time in institutional management roles. Furthermore, many psychiatrists lack formal administrative training and perceive themselves or are perceived as less suitable for these roles. Consequently, institutional leadership positions have been abdicated or lost to other disciplines more attuned to financial management and public administration. Often the determinants of the division of labor are directed by cost rather than by the clinical needs of patients. A disturbing illustration of this phenomenon occurs in some community mental health centers and state hospitals where "medical direction" of patient care has gradually been transformed into the directing of medications. Psychotherapy in these settings, and in some multidisiplinary groups, has been delegated to psychologists, social workers, and psychiatric nurses.

We can anticipate further subspecialization; each discipline will concentrate on its own core skills. Unfortunately, what core skills belong to which discipline has not been determined impartially. Who knows the most about treating schizophrenia? Phobias? Families of children with anorexia nervosa? Alcoholism? Which discipline trains the best psychodiagnosticians? How essential will the psychologist be in an era of computerized diagnostic testing? Can a skilled and compassionate internist successfully manage the bipolar patient with lithium? All of these questions provoke turf disputes that are beyond the scope of this paper. It becomes apparent, however, that whatever boundaries exist among the mental health professions and between psychiatry and her sister medical specialties are both uncertain and permeable.

## Automation and Computerization

Of all the trends associated with industrialization, automation may provoke the most fear for some while offering the most promise for others. Computerized systems for psychiatric diagnosis and testing, medical records stored on hard disks, and computer-facilitated psychotherapy all present opportunities for abuse as well as benefit. The computer threatens to dehumanize communication. If mishandled, computerized records threaten the confidentiality of medical communications. Like other forms of automation, the computer can expand the power of an effective procedure, but it can stifle intuition and innovation.

On the other hand, automation compels the innovator to carefully analyze the effectiveness of each procedural step before committing to replicating the process. Furthermore, once translated to its automated form, a procedure can be readily tested because of the accuracy in its replication. The computerization of diagnostic testing systems has forced and will continue to force rigor on the diagnostician, who must carefully define phenomena before employing the system. Interactive computers also permit replication of the professional's instructions and facilitating responses, thereby enhancing the patient-user's ability to complete a diagnostic test accurately at his or her own pace.

Distinguishing specific factors, e.g., replicable techniques, from nonspecific factors, e.g., warmth, empathy, and positive therapist and patient expectations, has been a fundamental issue in the research on psychotherapy.[15,16,30,31] Computer facilitation permits the patient to analyze cognitive distortion and develop action plans for personal growth according to previously tested principles of psychotherapy. Gould[32] has developed a Therapeutic Learning Program, reflecting a psychodynamically based theory of growth-inhibiting and growth-promoting fac-

tors in adult development, that he has incorporated into an interactive computer program. The Therapeutic Learning Program encourages the user to analyze the origin and impact of cognitive distortions on subsequent thoughts, feelings, and interpersonal interactions. Since the program encourages the use of a common therapeutic framework and replicable interventions, it can be adapted readily to psychotherapy research.

The computer also will facilitate retrieval of current scientific knowledge by connecting the clinical psychiatrist to a telecommunications network fed by state-of-the-art research. It will permit pharmacists to assess the possibility of adverse drug interactions. Finally, because access to such technology has become so broad, the computer will promote, eventually, the decentralization of the psychiatric industry. The industrial transformation of psychiatry, then, does not compel geographical consolidation; rather, many psychiatrists will participate in large, decentralized but integrated networks. From the tree of industrialization, then, could come the seeds of the postindustrial age described by Toffler[33] and Naisbitt.[34]

## CONCLUSIONS

In medicine's new industrial age, psychiatry will compete with other disciplines for resources that will be growing leaner. Both patients and psychiatrists will affiliate with prospective payment systems that should provide reasonable access to time-limited and cost-efficient treatment approaches. The chronically mentally ill, the disturbed adolescent requiring time to build a trusting treatment relationship, and the characterologically disordered patient requiring intensive, long-term psychotherapy are all likely to be orphaned by such a prospective payment system. Cost efficiency may occur by exclusion.

Hegel argued that within every historical era there exist conflicts which fuel a creative synthesis that energizes and sustains a new age. Medicine is among the last enterprises to industrialize. Its industrialization grew from the assumption that an individualistic cottage industry which served the middle class so well could be adapted to serve every citizen. The experiment is not yet a failure, but it has indeed been costly. If Toffler and Naisbitt are correct, the postindustrial age in medicine will contrast sharply with the industrial age from which it will emerge. This new age will emphasize the patient-physician partnership, decentralization of resources, wide access to technical information, human contact, and network rather than isolation. To adapt to the values of this postindustrial age and at the same time conserve finances, medicine must become oriented more toward prevention rather than cure, toward behavioral rather than surgical transformation, and toward patient engagement in rather than domination by the treatment process. The synergy between these postindustrial values and the traditions of psychiatry is fortuitous. Should psychiatry survive its current stresses, it may become a most suitable ambassador to the new age.

# References

1. Tarlov AR: Shattuck lecture—the increasing supply of physicians, the changing structure of the health-services system, and the future practice of medicine. *N Engl J Med* 308:1235–1244, 1983

2. Graduate Medical Education National Advisory Committee: Report to the Secretary: US Department of Health and Human Services Publication (HRA) 81–651–657. Hyattsville, Md, Health Resources Administration, Office of Graduate Medical Education, 1989

3. Report of the Graduate Medical Education National Advisory Committee, vol 2. US Department of Health and Human Services Publication (HRA) 81–652. Hyattsville, Md, Modeling, Research and Data Technical Panel, Health Resources Administration, Office of Graduate Medical Education, 1980

4. Gibson RM, Waldo DR: National health expenditures, 1981. *Health Care Financing Review* 4:1–35, 1982

5. Abramowitz K: Health Maintenance Organizations. New York, Sanford C Bernstein & Co, 1984

6. Relman AS: The new medical-industrial complex. *N Engl J Med* 303:963–970, 1980

7. Relman AS: Investor-owned hospitals and health-care costs. *N Engl J Med* 309:370–372, 1983

8. Star P: The Social Transformation of American Medicine. New York, Basic Books, 1983

9. Kormos HR: The industrialization of medicine. *Psychiatr Annals* 13:464–472, 1983

10. Levenson AI: The growth of investor-owned psychiatric hospitals. *Am J Psychiatry* 139:902–907, 1982

11. Trends in number of psychiatric hospitals, services, costs, staffing uncovered by NIMH survey, *Psychiatr News*, Feb 3, 1984, pp 24–25

12. Reifman A. Wyatt RJ: Lithium: A brake in the rising cost of mental illness. *Arch Gen Psychiatry* 37:385–388, 1980

13. Mumford E, Schlesinger HJ, Glass GV: The effects of psychological intervention on recovery from surgery and heart attacks: an analysis of the literature. *Am J Public Health* 72:141–151, 1982

14. Schlesinger HJ, Mumford E, Glass G, et al: Mental health treatment and medical care utilization in a fee-for-service system: outpatient mental health treatment following the onset of a chronic disease. *Am J Public Health* 73:422–429, 1983

15. Strupp HH: Success and failure in time-limited psychotherapy. *Arch Gen Psychiatry* 37:595–603, 1980

16. Marmor J: Short-term dynamic psychotherapy. *Am J Psychiatry* 136:149–155, 1979

17. Pardes H, Pincus HA: Report of the Graduate Medical Education National Advisory Committee and Health Manpower Development: implications for psychiatry. *Arch Gen Psychiatry* 40:97–102, 1983

18. Langsley DG, Robinowitz CB: Psychiatric manpower: an overview. *Hosp Community Psychiatry* 30:749–755, 1979

19. New JCAH standards allow nonphysician admitting privileges. *Psychiatr News,* Jan 20, 1984, pp 1, 25

20. *Blue Shield of Virginia v McCready,* 102 Supreme Ct 2540 (1982)

21. Sharfstein SS, Muszynski S, Gattozzi A: Maintaining and Improving Psychiatric Insurance Coverage: An Annotated Bibliography. Washington, DC, American Psychiatric Press, 1983

22. American Psychiatric Association: Economic Fact Book for Psychiatry. Washington, DC, American Psychiatric Press, 1983

23. Newhouse JP, Manning SG, Morris CN, et al: Some interim results from a controlled trial of cost sharing in health insurance. *N Engl J Med* 305:1501–1507, 1981

24. Brook RH, Ware JE, Rogers WH: Does free care improve adults' health? Results from a randomized controlled trial. *N Engl J Med* 309:1426–1434, 1983

25. Manning WG, Leibowitz A, Goldberg GA, et al: A controlled trial of the effect of a prepaid group practice on use of services. *N Engl J Med* 310:1505–1510, 1984

26. Levin BL: Mental health coverage within health maintenance organizations (HMOs) (doctoral dissertation). Houston, University of Texas, 1978

27. Bittker TE, Idzorek S: The evolution of psychiatric services in a health maintenance organization. *Am J Psychiatry* 135:339–342, 1978

28. Bittker TE, George J: Psychiatric service options within a health maintenance organization. *J Clin Psychiatry* 41:192–198, 1980

29. Jones KR, Vischi TR: Impact of Alcohol, Drug Abuse and Mental Health Treatment on Medical Care Utilization: A Review of the Research Literature. *Med Care* (Suppl) 17, 1979

30. Greenspan SI, Sharfstein SS: Efficacy of psychotherapy: asking the right questions. *Arch Gen Psychiatry* 38:1213–1219, 1981

31. Hine FR, Werman DS, Simpson DM: Effectiveness of psychotherapy: problems of research on complex phenomena. *Am J Psychiatry* 139:204–208, 1982

32. Gould RL: Developmental Stress Profile. Santa Monica, Calif, Interactive Health Systems, 1982

33. Toffler A: The Third Wave. New York, William Morrow, 1980

34. Naisbitt J: Megatrends, New York, Warner, 1982

# PART FIVE
## Financial Resources

This section addresses the issues of national health care expenditures and financial reimbursement alternatives, particularly health insurance and entitlement programs. The first article in this section, by Katharine R. Levit and associates, is a comprehensive overview of national health expenditures, with valuable detail concerning where the dollars come from and how they are spent. The article also includes important historical trends in national health expenditures. Following up on this report is an article by Sally T. Sonnefeld and associates projecting national expenditures through the year 2000; these projections raise fundamental policy and fiscal concerns that are quite serious.

The next article in this section, by Peter Ries, again addresses issues of health care financing by examining the characteristics of individuals who have, and those who do not have, health care coverage either through insurance or entitlement programs. This article highlights the extent of the uninsured problem in our society.

The traditional or conventional health insurance industry is described and analyzed in the article by Steven DiCarlo and John Gabel. Conventional insurance remains an important aspect of our nation's health care system.

The next two articles address issues associated with the nation's Medicare program. The first, by Louise B. Russell and Carrie Lynn Manning, examines the effect of the prospective payment system, which was implemented in 1983 for Medicare expenditures in the United States. Addressed are important issues related to health policy, which forms the subject of a later section of this book.

The second article, by William C. Hsiao and associates, presents the physician resource-based relative-value scale approach to physician reimbursement now being implemented under Medicare. In both describing and analyzing this approach to physician reimbursement, the authors provide a better understanding of the design, operation, and objectives of Medicare's current effort to change the way in which physicians are paid.

The final article in this section, by Robert A. Dorwart, describes managed care, a rapidly growing form of reimbursement, with an emphasis on its effect on mental health care. Managed health services have expanded greatly and raise very complex and important questions, which are addressed in this article.

# Chapter 14

## National Health Expenditures, 1990

Katharine R. Levit, Helen C. Lazenby, Cathy A. Cowan, and Suzanne W. Letsch

*During 1990, health expenditures as a share of gross national product rose to 12.2 percent, up from 11.6 percent in 1989. This dramatic increase is the second largest increase in the past three decades. The national health expenditure estimates presented in this article document rapidly rising health care costs and provide a context for understanding the health care financing crisis facing the Nation today.*

*The 1990 national health expenditures incorporate the most recently available data. . . . The length of time and complicated process of producing projections required use of 1989 national health expenditures—data available prior to the completion of the 1990 estimates presented here.*

### HIGHLIGHTS

Health care expenditures reached $666.2 billion in 1990. During the last three decades, health care expenditures grew at a substantially faster pace than did the overall economy, consuming an increasing percentage of gross national product (GNP). Following are several highlights from the 1990 numbers:

- National health expenditures (NHE) rose 10.5 percent from 1989 to 1990, approximately the same growth rate as for the prior 2 years.
- In 1990, NHE absorbed 12.2 percent of GNP, compared with 11.6 percent for the preceding year. The abnormally high increase in the share of GNP spent for health care in 1990, the second largest jump since 1960, is the result of a slowdown in the general economy rather than an acceleration in the growth of health care costs.
- Per capita expenditures of $2,566 in 1990 were almost 1.5 times as great as expenditures 10 years earlier. Personal health care expenditures accounted for 88 percent of that amount, or $2,255 per person.
- In 1990, spending for hospital services returned to the double-digit growth experienced in 1982 and earlier, prior to the advent of the prospective payment system (PPS). Expenditures for this category increased 10.1 percent from 1989 to $256.0 billion in 1990. Hospital spending, 38.4 percent of total health expenditures, is the largest category in NHE (Figure 1).
- Expenditures for professional services, which consist of physician services, dental services, and services of other professionals, totaled $191.3 billion for 1990, 28.7 percent of all health spending. This is an increase of 11.0 percent from 1989.
- Public programs contributed 42.4 percent of the funding for health care, with private payments funding the other 57.6 percent. Public programs funded a larger share of NHE in 1990 than in any previous year. Medicaid was the single largest contributor to the rising public share. Medicaid payments grew 20.7 percent from 1989 through 1990, the highest growth since the mid-1970s.
- Medicaid and Medicare combined paid for 28.0 percent of NHE in 1889, up from 27.3 percent during 1989. These two

Reprinted from *Health Care Financing Review,* Fall 1991, Vol 13, No. 1.

**Where it came from**

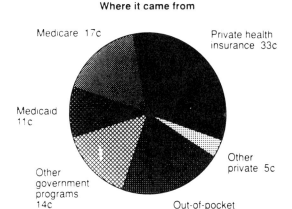

**Where it went**

NOTES: Other private includes industrial inplant health services. non-patient revenues, and privately financed construction. Other personal health care includes dental, other professional services, home health care, drugs and other non-durable medical products, and vision products and other durable medical products. Other spending covers program administration and the net cost of private health insurance, government public health, and research and construction.

SOURCE: Health Care Financing Administration, Office of the Actuary: Data from the Office of National Cost Estimates

**Figure 1.** The Nation's health dollar: 1980

programs financed 37.8 percent of hospital care and approximately one-third of physician services.

• Consumers continued paying for a little more than one-half of all health care expenditures through private health insurance and out-of-pocket payments, a share that has changed very little during the past 16 years. The private health insurance share remained relatively constant for the last 2 years, after steadily increasing since 1960. Out-of-pocket payments dropped slightly as a percent of total expenditures in 1989 and 1990.

Health care costs continue to rise faster than GNP, a measure of total output of the United States. Despite an increasing share of GNP devoted to health care, a large and increasing number of people (33.4 million in 1989) remain uninsured by private health insurance or by public programs; additional persons are underinsured. Without sufficient insurance coverage, many Americans find access to the health care system limited for many services.

Extensive debate on various proposals that attempt to address the questions of access and rising health care costs is under way. The NHE estimates provide a backdrop for understanding health care financing issues and the factors that account for cost increases during the past three decades.

Detailed Tables 8–13 at the end of this article show expenditures for health care for selected years 1960 through 1990, both by type of service and by source of funds. Data figures from the detailed tables are highlighted throughout this article.

## NATIONAL HEALTH EXPENDITURES

NHE reached a level of $666.2 billion in 1990. Spending grew 10.5 percent, the third consecutive year of similar growth. In 1990, health expenditures absorbed 12.2 percent of GNP, compared with 11.6 percent of GNP in 1989. The 0.6–percentage-point change in the ratio from 1989 to 1990 was the largest increase since 1982 and the second largest increase since 1960. The increase in the proportion of the Nation's output going for health care can be attributed to rising health care costs and, more importantly, to the recession that began at the end of 1990. As GNP growth slowed in 1990 and health care cost growth remained strong, health care consumed an even greater incremental share of GNP than in the recent past.

In the United States, the average expenditure per person for health care reached $2,566 during 1990, an increase of 9.4 percent from 1989. Public expenditures accounted for $1,089 per capita (42.4 percent of the total expenditures for health care), and private funds paid for the remaining $1,478 (57.6 percent).

NHE is divided into two broad categories. The first category, health services and supplies (expenditures related to current health care), increased 10.5 percent to $643.4 billion in 1990, accounting for 96.6 percent of health expenditures. Health services and supplies, in turn, consists of personal health care (the direct provision of care), program administration and the net cost of private health insurance, and government public health activities.

The second category, research and construction of medical facilities (expenditures related to future health care), accounted for 3.4 percent of total expenditures, or $22.8 billion.

Personal Health Care Expenditures

Personal health care expenditures (PHCE) reached $585.3 billion in 1990, accounting for 87.9 percent of all NHE. PHCE includes all spending for health services received by individuals and health products purchased in retail outlets. The proportion of NHE that is PHCE

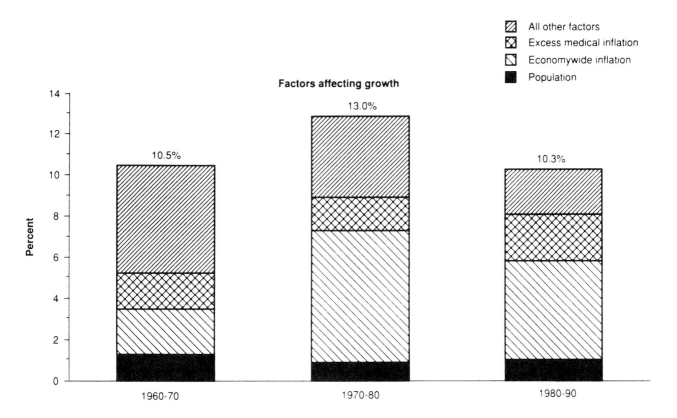

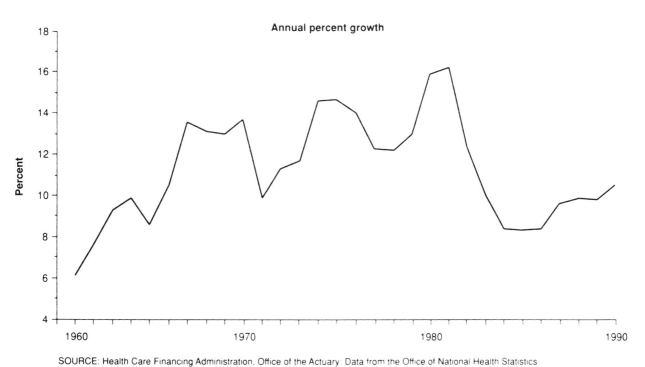

SOURCE: Health Care Financing Administration, Office of the Actuary. Data from the Office of National Health Statistics

**Figure 2.**  Annual percent growth in personal health care expenditures (PHCE) and factors affecting average annual growth in PHCE for selected periods: 1960–90

has been fairly constant since 1960. The amount spent per person averaged $2,255 in 1990. Spending for personal health care increased 10.5 percent from 1989 to 1990. This rate of growth is equal to growth in NHE for the same period and about the same as the average growth in PHCE for the 1980s.

The factors that cause growth in PHCE have changed during the past three decades. Factors affecting growth are economywide inflation, medical price inflation in excess of economywide inflation, population, and all other factors. Other factors include any increases in use and intensity of health care services delivered per capita. The average annual growth in PHCE from 1960 to 1970 was 10.5 percent. One-half of this growth was caused by increases in use and intensity of health care services (Figure 2), primarily as a result of the implementation of the Medicare and Medicaid programs that increased access to health care by the elderly and poor beginning in 1966. Increases in population caused a larger portion (12 percent) of this increase than in later decades as the last spurt in the post-war baby boom occurred in the early 1960s.

During the period 1970–80, growth in PHCE was the highest, averaging 13.0 percent per year. The entire economy experienced high inflation causing one-half of this growth. Although population growth during this period was stable, the share of growth attributable to population increases was the lowest in three decades because population growth was small relative to the large growth in PHCE.

During the 1980s, economywide inflation remained a major factor, responsible for nearly one-half of the growth in PHCE. PHCE grew at an average annual rate of 10.3 percent, somewhat lower than it had in the 1970s. Increases in medical-specific prices affected health expenditures more during the 1980s than in the previous two decades. Medical price inflation in excess of economywide inflation caused 22 percent of the growth. Excess medical inflation caused 16 percent of the growth in the 1960s and only 12 percent in the 1970s.

During the last three decades, the components of personal health care have grown at different rates, changing the distribution among the different types of spending. In the 1960s and 1970s, spending for hospital care grew more rapidly than spending for other types of care. As a result, hospital care as a share of total PHCE increased. During the 1980s, cost-containment efforts of public and private insurers were focused on hospital

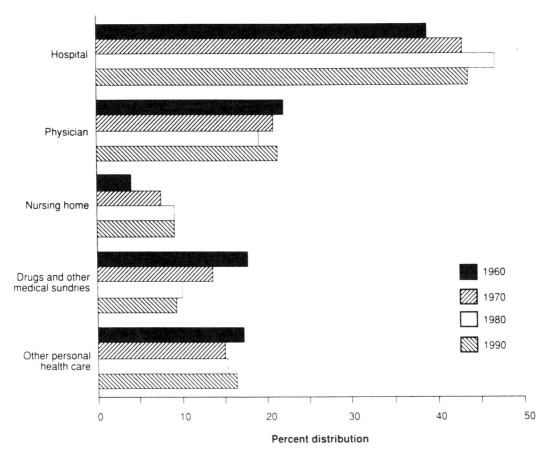

SOURCE: Health Care Financing Administration, Office of the Actuary: Data from the Office of National Health Statistics.

**Figure 3.** Distribution of personal health care expenditures: Selected years 1960–90

care spending. These efforts were effective in slowing the growth of hospital spending and, as a result, its share of PHCE decreased (Figure 3). At the same time, expenditures for physician services were growing more rapidly than other types of spending. In 1980, 19.1 percent of PHCE was for physician services. By 1990, this share rose to 21.5 percent. In the past 30 years, expenditures for drugs and other medical non-durables have not grown as rapidly as other types of health care spending, causing drugs and medical non-durables' share of PHCE to decrease by one-half from 17.8 percent in 1960 to 9.3 percent in 1990.

Hospital Care

The largest category of health care spending is hospital care, amounting to 43.7 percent of PHCE. In 1990, $256.0 billion was spent for hospital care. Hospital care in NHE includes spending for services delivered to inpatients and outpatients, for physician services billed through hospitals (mainly for the services of anesthesiologists, radiologists, and pathologists, but also medical residents), for drugs dispensed during hospitalization, and for services rendered through hospital-based home health agencies. Nursing home-type care provided in a hospital facility is also included in this category. Hospital care is measured by net revenues received from all sources. These net revenues are the sum of net revenue from patients (charges to patients less bad debt, charity, contractual and other adjustments), other operating revenue (tax appropriations and philanthropy), and non-operating revenue (from cafeterias, parking lots, gift shops).

During the 17–year period that followed the implementation of Medicare and Medicaid, hospitals experienced a period of tremendous revenue growth. From 1966 to 1983, the average annual rate of growth in hospital revenues was 14.0 percent. By about 1983, both private and public payers were straining to pay these spiraling costs and had initiated efforts to contain them. By 1984, the annual rate of growth for hospital care was cut in half to 7.0 percent—a result, in part, of the implementation of Medicare's PPS. After several years of steady low growth, hospital costs began to rise once again in 1987. Accelerating growth in hospital revenues continued through 1990. From 1989 to 1990, hospital revenues increased 10.1 percent, marking the fourth year of accelerated growth.

Throughout the 1960s and 1970s, public funding played an increasing role in funding of hospital care, the most expensive of all types of health care. Public funding rose from 42.5 percent in 1960 to 53.3 percent in 1980. The government's share of hospital financing increased slightly during the 1980s, to 54.7 percent in 1990. This increase offsets a falling share of hospital expenditures

paid by private health insurance. The share of hospital care paid for out of pocket fell during the last 30 years, from 20.7 percent in 1960 to 5.2 percent in 1980, where it has remained since.

Short-term acute care community hospitals delivered 86 percent of all hospital care (Table 1). The cost-containment efforts of the 1980s caused a shift to more care being delivered in less costly outpatient settings. In 1980, 13 percent of care in community hospitals was delivered in outpatient settings, and by 1990, this share increased to 24 percent. Non-community non-Federal hospitals accounted for 7 percent of all hospital revenues in 1990. These hospitals include long-term care hospitals (where the average length of stay is 30 days or longer), psychiatric hospitals, alcohol and chemical-dependency hospitals, units of institutions such as prison hospitals or college infirmaries, chronic disease hospitals, and some institutions for the mentally retarded. This share remained unchanged during the 1980s. Federal hospitals received the remaining 7 percent of hospital revenues in 1990, most of which came from the Federal Government.

Physician Services

Expenditures for physician services reached $125.7 billion in 1990, up 10.7 percent from 1989. Physician services account for 21.5 percent of PHCE, but physicians direct or prescribe the provision of services that account for more than 70 percent of PHCE.

Physician services are funded predominantly by consumer payments (private health insurance and out-of-pocket payments), although this share has dropped considerably during the past three decades. In 1960, consumers paid for 92.8 percent of physician services; by 1990, that share fell to 65.0 percent. Out-of-pocket payments account fully for the falling off of financing by consumer payments over the last 30 years, from 62.7 percent in 1960 to 18.7 percent in 1990. That decrease is somewhat offset by private health insurance coverage, the share of which has increased from 30.2 percent in 1960 to 46.3 percent in 1990.

The share of physician services funded by public programs has also been increasing during the past 30 years. In 1990, public funding accounted for $43.9 billion or 35.0 percent of physician service expenditures, compared with 7.1 percent in 1960. The majority of the increase in public funding comes from the Medicare program that began in 1966. Medicaid and Medicare comprised the bulk of public funding in 1990, with $35.2 billion or 80 percent of public expenditures for physician services.

The 1989 estimates for physician services have been revised downward by 3.5 percent. This revision is the result of additional information from the U.S. Bureau of

## Table 1
## Hospital revenues, percent distribution, and annual percent growth: 1980-90

| Type of hospital | 1980 | 1981 | 1982 | 1983 | 1984 | 1985 | 1986 | 1987 | 1988 | 1989 | 1990 |
|---|---|---|---|---|---|---|---|---|---|---|---|
| | | | | | Amount in millions | | | | | | |
| Total | $102,399 | $119,563 | $135,866 | $147,161 | $157,486 | $168,264 | $179,789 | $194,237 | $212,030 | $232,557 | $256,009 |
| Non-Federal | 93,707 | 109,967 | 125,383 | 136,102 | 145,212 | 154,953 | 165,764 | 179,354 | 196,696 | 215,965 | 238,097 |
| Community | 85,601 | 100,929 | 115,532 | 125,903 | 134,362 | 143,293 | 153,189 | 165,685 | 181,733 | 199,866 | 220,452 |
| Inpatient | 74,404 | 87,477 | 99,916 | 108,247 | 114,082 | 119,104 | 125,133 | 133,335 | 143,613 | 155,642 | 168,341 |
| Outpatient | 11,197 | 13,452 | 15,616 | 17,656 | 20,280 | 24,189 | 28,056 | 32,350 | 38,120 | 44,224 | 52,111 |
| Non-community | 8,106 | 9,038 | 9,851 | 10,199 | 10,850 | 11,660 | 12,575 | 13,669 | 14,963 | 16,099 | 17,644 |
| Federal | 8,692 | 9,596 | 10,483 | 11,059 | 12,274 | 13,311 | 14,025 | 14,883 | 15,334 | 16,592 | 17,913 |
| | | | | | Percent distribution | | | | | | |
| Total | 100 | 100 | 100 | 100 | 100 | 100 | 100 | 100 | 100 | 100 | 100 |
| Non-Federal | 92 | 92 | 92 | 92 | 92 | 92 | 92 | 92 | 93 | 93 | 93 |
| Community | 84 | 84 | 85 | 86 | 85 | 85 | 85 | 85 | 86 | 86 | 86 |
| Inpatient | 73 | 73 | 74 | 74 | 72 | 71 | 70 | 69 | 68 | 67 | 66 |
| Outpatient | 11 | 11 | 11 | 12 | 13 | 14 | 16 | 17 | 18 | 19 | 20 |
| Non-community | 8 | 8 | 7 | 7 | 7 | 7 | 7 | 7 | 7 | 7 | 7 |
| Federal | 8 | 8 | 8 | 8 | 8 | 8 | 8 | 8 | 7 | 7 | 7 |
| | | | | | Annual percent growth | | | | | | |
| Total | — | 16.8 | 13.6 | 8.3 | 7.0 | 6.8 | 6.8 | 8.0 | 9.2 | 9.7 | 10.1 |
| Non-Federal | — | 17.4 | 14.0 | 8.5 | 6.7 | 6.7 | 7.0 | 8.2 | 9.7 | 9.8 | 10.2 |
| Community | — | 17.9 | 14.5 | 9.0 | 6.7 | 6.6 | 6.9 | 8.2 | 9.7 | 10.0 | 10.3 |
| Inpatient | — | 17.6 | 14.2 | 8.3 | 5.4 | 4.4 | 5.1 | 6.6 | 7.7 | 8.4 | 8.2 |
| Outpatient | — | 20.1 | 16.1 | 13.1 | 14.9 | 19.3 | 16.0 | 15.3 | 17.8 | 16.0 | 17.8 |
| Non-community | — | 11.5 | 9.0 | 3.5 | 6.4 | 7.5 | 7.8 | 8.7 | 9.5 | 7.6 | 9.6 |
| Federal | — | 10.4 | 9.2 | 5.5 | 11.0 | 8.5 | 5.4 | 6.1 | 3.0 | 8.2 | 8.0 |

NOTE: Non-community non-Federal hospitals include long-term care hospitals (where the average length of stay is 30 days or longer) psychiatric hospitals, alcoholism and chemical dependency hospitals, units of institutions such as prison hospitals or college infirmaries, chronic disease hospitals, and some institutions for the mentally retarded.

SOURCE: Health Care Financing Administration, Office of the Actuary: Data from the Office of National Health Statistics.

the Census that was not available when the previous estimates were completed. The U.S. Bureau of the Census (1990) estimated the 1989 growth for business receipts from physician offices at a lower rate than did estimates developed from the American Medical Association's (AMA) Socioeconomic Monitoring System Survey (American Medical Association, 1991). Other information from Medicare and from the U.S. Bureau of Labor Statistics measures of employment and average weekly hours (Letsch et al., 1991) are consistent with a higher growth rate derived from AMA statistics. As 1990 data become available from the U.S. Bureau of the Census and from other data sources, the estimates for physician expenditures for 1989 will be re-examined.

### Dental Services

Expenditures for dental services rose by 7.6 percent in 1990 to $34.0 billion. This category of NHE includes expenditures for visits to dental offices, dental laboratory costs, and salaries for dentists in staff-model health maintenance organizations (HMOs). In 1990, dental service expenditures accounted for 5.8 percent of PHCE, down from 8.2 percent in 1960. This decline in share reflects the fact that dental expenditures typically grow at a slower rate than NHE.

In 1990, dental visits continued to be funded primarily (97.5 percent) by out-of-pocket payments and private health insurance. Out-of-pocket payments experienced a deceleration in growth rate from 6.1 percent in 1989 to 3.8 percent in 1990. One reason for this deceleration is that the purchase of dental services by consumers tends to be more sensitive to changes in overall economic conditions than are many other types of health care services. As the United States entered into a recession in 1990, individuals may have become more concerned about the general economic outlook and delayed discretionary purchases. Generally, non-emergency dental visits are considered discretionary on the part of the dental care consumer because the services delivered are frequently for prevention or maintenance, rather than to treat a life-threatening problem. Because out-of-pocket payments account for more than one-half of all dental expenditures, a slowdown in economic activity and associated concerns about job retention and future income are likely to have an effect on dental expenditures not covered by third-party payments.

### Other Professional Services

The category of other professional services includes spending for services of licensed health practitioners other than physicians and dentists and expenditures for services rendered in outpatient clinics. In 1990, spending for other professional services reached $31.6 billion, 5.4 percent of PHCE. These services grew 16.6 percent from

1989 and are one of the fastest growing segments of NHE.

Funding for other professional care is provided primarily through consumer payments, which account for 68.1 percent of expenditures. However, within this source of funds, there has been a switch from out-of-pocket to private health insurance payments. More and more health insurance plans are providing coverage for additional services such as those provided by optometrists and by drug and alcohol rehabilitation outpatient clinics (Levit and Cowan, 1990).

Public funds pay for 20.4 percent or $6.4 billion of other professional services, with Medicaid and Medicare providing the bulk of the funding. Expenditures for these two programs grew 18.3 percent, from $4.3 billion to $5.1 billion from 1989 to 1990.

### Home Health Care

The NHE category of home health care includes expenditures for services and supplies furnished by non-facility-based home health agencies (HHAs). Spending for home health care included in NHE reached $6.9 billion in 1990. An additional $1.6 billion, not included in the NHE home health care category, was spent for

care furnished by facility-based (primarily hospital-based) HHAs (included with hospital care in this article). Including the hospital share, $8.5 billion was spent for home health care services in 1990 (Figure 4).

Spending for home health care grew faster than spending for any other category of personal health care in 1989 and 1990. Growth in spending for home health care increased 22.5 percent in 1990, almost as fast as the 24.9 percent growth in 1989. After 4 years of slower growth, spending for home health care accelerated in 1989 primarily because of increased funding by the Medicare and Medicaid programs. Medicare clarified its home health care coverage criteria in 1988 and fewer of these claims are being denied.

Public sources financed three-fourths of the home health care services described here. More than one-half of public spending was paid by Medicare and almost all of the residual by Medicaid. Out-of-pocket payments accounted for 12.1 percent of home health care spending and the residual private share, 14.4 percent, was split between private health insurance and non-patient revenue.

The home health care segment of NHE measures a portion of the Nation's annual expenditures for medical care services delivered in the home. These estimates

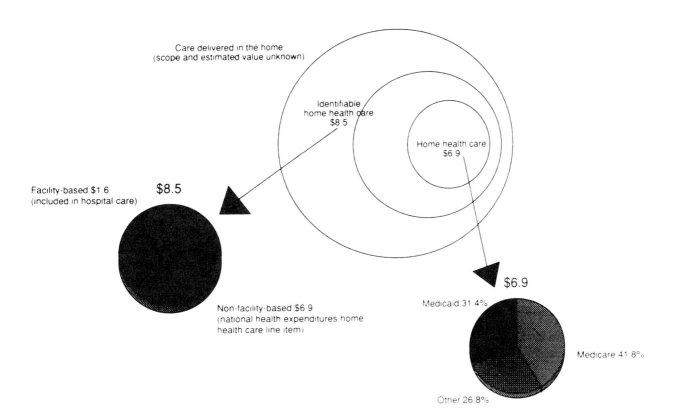

' Amounts shown are billions of dollars

SOURCE: Health Care Financing Administration. Office of the Actuary: Data from the Office of National Statistics

**Figure 4.** Scope and source of funds for home health care spending:[1] 1990

are constructed from information reported to the Health Care Financing Administration (HCFA) by HHAs participating in the Medicare and Medicaid programs. A broader definition of home health care would include services delivered by facility-based agencies (counted in the NHE hospital category) and by non-Medicare providers, unpaid caregivers, and services currently beyond the scope of NHE.

## Drugs and Other Medical Non-Durables

In NHE, this class of expenditure is limited to spending for drugs and over-the-counter (OTC) products purchased from retail outlets. The value of drugs dispensed in hospitals, nursing homes, or in offices of health professionals is included implicitly in the estimates of spending for those providers' services. Retail purchases of drugs and other non-durable medical products reached $54.6 billion in 1990, an increase of 7.9 percent from the previous year.

Estimates of spending for prescription drugs includes retail sales of human-use dosage-form drugs. Transactions may occur in locations such as community or HMO pharmacies, grocery store pharmacies and mail-order establishments. Retail sales of prescription drugs amounted to $32.3 billion in 1990, up 8.0 percent from 1989. This represents 59.2 percent of the non-durable medical product category.

Non-prescription drugs and other medical non-durables are estimated separately from prescription drugs and include a long list of products. The estimate is based on personal consumption expenditures (PCE) for drug preparations and sundries, which is a component of GNP. That portion of the PCE category that matches the NHE definition was established in each of several GNP benchmark years, using detailed PCE tables for 1963, 1967, 1972, 1977, and 1982. Published PCE estimates, based on annual and periodic surveys of retail trade, were used to develop estimates between and beyond benchmark years. The PCE detail for 1982 recently became available. A higher portion of the PCE category matched the NHE definition in 1982 than it did in 1977. Therefore, current estimates for non-prescription drugs and other medical non-durables differ from previously published NHE estimates, with those changes beginning in 1978. In 1990, $22.3 billion was spent by consumers for non-prescription drugs and other medical non-durables, an increase of 7.7 percent from 1989.

Typically, third parties cover prescription drug purchases but not OTC medicines and sundries. For that reason, all third-party financing is assumed to be for prescription drugs only. Under that assumption, consumers paid the entire $22.3 billion spent on non-prescription items from out-of-pocket sources. In addition to this amount, consumers paid another $17.9

billion out of pocket for prescription drugs. This includes amounts spent by people without third-party coverage or for copayments and deductibles for persons with third-party coverage. Out-of-pocket spending accounts for 55.4 percent of prescription drug purchases. Private health insurance, the second most common source of payment, covered 25.8 percent of all prescription drug purchases. Public programs, mostly Medicaid, covered the remaining 18.8 percent.

During the past 10 years, expenditures for drugs and other medical non-durables grew less rapidly than did other types of health spending. After removing the effects of price and population increases, there is almost no real growth in these expenditures.

## Vision Products and Other Medical Durables

This category includes retail purchases of eyeglasses and contact lenses and the purchase or rental of other durable medical equipment such as hearing aids, crutches, wheelchairs, and artificial limbs. Spending for these items reached $12.1 billion in 1990, an increase of 6.1 percent from 1989. Estimates are calculated based on PCE in the same way as for non-prescription drugs. The PCE category of ophthalmic and orthopedic appliances is adjusted to match the NHE definition in the GNP benchmark years mentioned earlier. Published PCE estimates, based on annual and periodic surveys of retail trade, are used to move the adjusted levels between and beyond benchmark years. As a result of the recent availability of the 1982 benchmark detail, revisions to durable medical equipment, as with non-prescription drugs, begin in 1978.

Vision products, including eyeglasses and contact lenses, are the largest component of durable medical equipment. GNP benchmark years provide the only detailed breakdown of this category. Data from the latest year available, 1982, indicate that nearly two-thirds of the $5.1 billion spent in that year was for vision products.

Third-party coverage of durable medical products is limited. Private insurance paid for only 10.4 percent of all spending in 1990. Government payments, mostly through the Medicare program, financed another 22.3 percent. The remainder, 67.3 percent, was paid by consumers out of pocket.

## Nursing Home Care

In 1990, spending for nursing home care reached $53.1 billion, an increase of 11.4 percent from 1989. Expenditures for nursing home care grew faster than expenditures for aggregate personal health care, hospital care, or physician services for the second consecutive year. From 1960 to 1970, spending for nursing home care as a share of PHCE grew from 4.1 percent to 7.5

percent. By 1980, nursing home care accounted for 19.1 percent of PHCE, a share maintained through 1990.

Nursing home expenditures are estimated in three parts: revenues of non-Federal facilities primarily providing some level of inpatient nursing care; Medicaid funding of intermediate care facilities for the mentally retarded (ICFs/MR); and funding for nursing care in U.S. Department of Veteran Affairs nursing homes.

Growth in spending for nursing home care other than in ICFs/MR (91 percent of total estimated spending for nursing home care) slowed from 11.4 percent in 1989 to 10.9 percent in 1990. Data from the U.S. Bureau of Labor Statistics show that growth in aggregate hours worked by non-supervisory personnel in nursing and related care facilities accelerated from 4.6 percent in 1989 to 4.9 percent in 1990, consistent with the continued strong growth in nursing home expenditures. Growth in nursing home employment showed a similar trend (Letsch et al., 1991).

These nursing home estimates imply that the average charge per day for care in nursing home facilities reached $86 in 1990, more than double the charge per day in 1980.

The relative importance of factors contributing to the growth in spending for nursing home care other than for ICFs/MR has changed in the decades since 1960. From 1960 to 1970, only 13.1 percent of the increase in expenditures for nursing home care was attributable to general price inflation, with 15.8 percent resulting from nursing home-specific inflation, 11.7 percent from growth in the aged population, and 59.5 percent from changes in the amount and mix of nursing home goods and services per capita. From 1970 to 1980 and from 1980 to 1990, general price inflation accounted for 45.2 percent of the growth in nursing home expenditures. During these two decades, the share attributable to nursing home price inflation rose from 10.8 percent to 11.4 percent; the population share rose from 16.5 percent to 21.2 percent; and the residual share declined in importance from 27.6 percent to 19.5 percent.

ICF/MR care is a Medicaid benefit first offered in 1973. In 1990, $4.9 billion (60 percent of all ICF/MR expenditures) was spent for ICF/MR services in nursing homes; the remaining 40 percent was spent in facilities classified as hospitals in NHE. The average annual rate of growth in ICF/MR spending for nursing home care was 11.4 percent during the 8-year period from 1982 to 90, slightly higher than the 9.3-percent rate of growth in total nursing home spending. This compares with the 44.5-percent annual growth from 1973 to 1981 when, despite the relatively small size of ICF/MR spending, these payments raised the growth rate for total nursing home spending in almost every year. During this period of high growth in spending for ICF/MR services, States made efforts to discharge mentally retarded patients

from institutions not qualifying for Federal financial participation (FFP) to smaller, more expensive nursing homes that were in compliance with Medicaid FFP standards. Both the number of recipients and cost per recipient contributed to program growth during this period (Lakin et al., 1990).

In 1990, public programs, mainly Medicaid, financed 52.1 percent of nursing home care. In 1970, prior to Medicaid's coverage of ICFs/MR, Medicaid accounted for 60.1 percent of the public share. Since the early 1970s, Medicaid has funded about 90 percent of public spending for nursing home care.

Most nursing home care financed from private sources is paid directly by patients or their families. These out-of-pocket expenditures totaled $23.9 billion in 1990.

## Other Personal Health Care

In 1990, expenditures of $11.3 billion for other personal health care came from a variety of public programs (80.1 percent) and from industrial inplant health care services (19.9 percent) offered by employers at the work site. These expenditures account for less than 2 percent of all PHCE.

Responsibility for approximately one-third of these expenditures fell to Medicaid for health screening services, certain home and community waivered services, case management, and other unspecified services. Other public expenditures came through State and local school health and maternal and child health programs, and through Federal agency programs targeting veterans, military personnel, native Americans, and persons with drug abuse, alcoholism, and mental health-related problems.

## Administration and Net Cost of Insurance

The administrative costs borne by public financers of health care, the administrative costs of philanthropic organizations, and the net cost of private health insurance amounted to $38.7 billion or 5.8 percent of NHE in 1990. Excluded from this category are health care providers' administrative costs that are associated with the filing of insurance claims and maintenance of information to support those claims. These costs are included with the provider expenditure estimate.

In 1990, the net cost of private health insurance accounted for 79.2 percent of expenditures for this category. Of the remainder, 1.4 percent represented the fund-raising costs of philanthropic health organizations and 19.3 percent the administrative costs of public programs.

The net cost of private health insurance amounted to 14.2 percent of private health insurance premiums earned in 1990. In contrast, the Medicare program spend 2.1

percent of total expenditures to administer the program, and Medicaid spent 5.1 percent. Private health insurance's net cost share of total premiums exceeded the administrative cost share of government programs by a wide margin. Part of the reason for this difference is the clientele served by each third party. For Medicare, beneficiaries establish their eligibility once to participate in this entitlement program. The remaining costs for Medicare are primarily in the processing and paying of health care claims. In addition to these costs, Medicaid incurs additional costs of establishing eligibility because of income limitations for coverage. Private health insurers have more diverse expenses in addition to claims processing. They have extensive costs associated with advertising and marketing of their product to companies as well as individuals. These insurers must pay commissions to salespersons and premium taxes to States as well as incur expenses in meeting licensing and reserve requirements for each State in which they operate. Because many private health insurers are for-profit, they must allocate funds for profits and dividends to shareholders.

### Public Health Activity

Governments spent $19.3 billion for public health activities in 1990, up 5.6 percent from 1989. The Federal Government, funding 12.1 percent of all public health activity, provided substantial increases in funding for the Centers for Disease Control for measles immunizations and acquired immunodeficiency syndrome (AIDS) in fiscal year 1990. State and local public health activities conducted through State and local health departments accounted for 87.9 percent of all public health activity.

### Research

Non-commercial research and development consumed 1.9 percent of NHE in 1990. Funded mostly through Federal Government expenditures, spending amounted to $12.4 billion, increasing 11.9 percent from 1989 levels. This category excludes commercial research expenditures of drug and medical supply companies, because the value of this expenditure is recaptured through the sale of goods and services counted elsewhere in NHE. Philanthropy's role in funding research has dropped considerably during the past three decades, falling from 20.1 percent of all research funding in 1960 to 6.7 percent in 1990. During the same period, the Federal Government share of spending rose from 72.7 percent in 1960 to 81.1 percent in 1990, mostly through the National Institutes of Health; the share funded by State and local governments almost doubled, up from 7.2 percent in 1960 to 12.2 percent in 1990.

### Construction

Medical facility construction put in place in 1990—including new construction and renovation of existing hospitals, nursing homes, medical clinics, and medical research facilities-was valued at $10.4 billion in 1990. Construction spending experienced a surge in growth in 1987 and 1988, as construction of hospital facilities that had been held in abeyance during the initial implementation of PPS in the mid-1980s was undertaken. In 1990, construction expenditure increases of 8.3 percent indicate a return to moderate growth in health care facility construction.

Construction growth for inpatient hospital beds will likely remain moderate at best until hospital occupancy rates begin to stabilize or increase. Contractions in the number of available non-Federal hospital beds, down 9.1 percent from 1983 to 1989, did not keep pace with the decline in the number of inpatient days of care provided at these facilities, resulting in a decline in occupancy rate from 76.1 percent in 1983 to 69.6 percent in 1989 for all hospitals (American Hospital Association, 1990).

## SOURCES OF FUNDS

During the past three decades, the system for funding of health care services was transformed from one mostly relying on private sources to one relying heavily on government programs (Figure 5). In 1960, 75.5 percent of health care financing came from private payers, including out-of-pocket payments directly by individuals, private health insurance, and other private funds. By 1990, 57.6 percent was privately financed. This transition occurred in two phases: First, the introduction of Medicaid and Medicare in 1965 caused the private share to fall from 75.3 percent in 1965 to 62.9 percent in 1967; second, a more gradual decline in the share of privately funded health expenditures occurred between 1970 and 1974 (62.8 percent to 59.8 percent), as Medicare expanded to cover the disabled, and Medicaid picked up coverage for institutionalization of the mentally retarded population. During the next 15 years, the share of privately funded health expenditures dropped slowly, only 2 percentage points during the entire 1975–90 period.

### Out-of-Pocket Expenditures

More dramatic, however, has been the change in the share of health care costs funded by one private-payer source—out-of-pocket expenditures. The rapid rise in health care costs has increased Americans' concern about large out-of-pocket payments at the time services are purchased. Employers, who sponsor a significant portion of private health insurance coverage, address

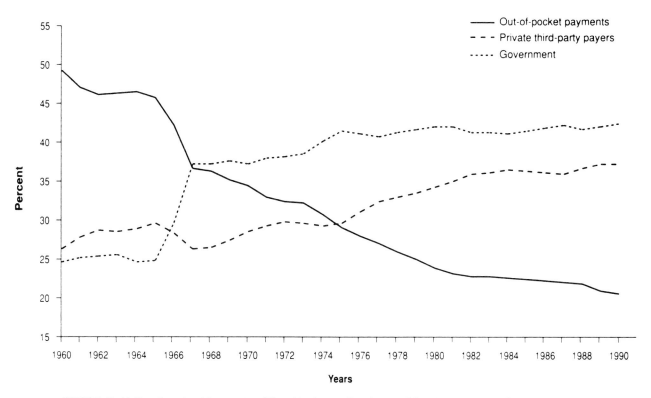

SOURCE: Health Care Financing Administration. Office of the Actuary. Data from the Office of National Health Statistics.

**Figure 5.** Distribution of national health expenditures, by source of financing: 1960–90

this concern by offering policies with low out-of-pocket costs. At the urging of employees, employers also increase the breadth of health insurance coverage, including services formerly paid directly by the employee. Employers can do so with pre-tax dollars. In this manner, they pass along to employees a richer post-tax compensation package than they could if an equivalent wage increase were offered.

From 1960 to 1990, out-of-pocket expenditures fell from 49.2 percent of all health expenditures to 20.4 percent. Out-of-pocket spending rose to $136.1 billion in 1990, 7.9 percent higher than the 1989 level. These expenditures, amounting to $524 per person, include co-payments and deductibles, fees for non-covered services and goods, and the portion of payments that insurers determine exceeds the usual, customary, and reasonable charges for these services. Out-of-pocket spending does not include individual's expenditures for private or public health insurance premiums. These amounts are counted as part of third-party payments, because the third party (private health insurance or Medicare) is responsible for paying the benefit. Given this definition, Americans, on average, spent approximately the same proportion of disposable income on out-of-pocket health care in 1990 (3.4 percent) as they did in 1960 (3.7 percent). The amount of out-of-pocket expenditures (including premiums) that is the respon-

sibility of individuals amounted to 5.1 percent of adjusted personal income in 1989 (Levit and Cowan, 1990). . . .

Private Health Insurance

Private health insurance, the largest source-of-financing category in NHE, paid for almost one-third of all health care costs in 1990. Americans paid $216.8 billion in private health insurance premiums and received $186.1 billion in benefits. The difference of $30.7 billion, the net cost of private health insurance, covers administrative costs of insurers, net additions to reserves, rate credits and dividends, premium taxes, and profits or losses of insurance companies.

The role of private health insurance in financing health care has steadily increased during the past three decades. Private health insurance funded 21.7 percent of all health care in 1960, 22.5 percent in 1970, 29.3 percent in 1980, and 32.5 percent in 1990.

According to the 1990 Current Population Survey (CPS), 183.5 million Americans, 74.5 percent of the total non-institutionalized population, are covered by private health insurance. Almost 39 percent of these people, 70.9 million, obtain health insurance coverage as an employment benefit. These workers cover an additional 69.0 million persons as dependents under their employer-sponsored policies. The remaining 43.6 million people acquire coverage through individually purchased policies, including Medicare supplemental policies purchased by the elderly. (CPS tabulations are by Fu Associates of Arlington, Va., under HCFA Basic Ordering Agreement No. 500–90–0010.)

## Other Private Funds

In 1990, other private funds financed 4.6 percent of all health care costs, the same share as it did in 1960. Of the $30.6 billion in other private funds expended in 1990, $2.3 billion came from businesses for work-site health services provided directly to employees, $7.5 billion funded medical facility construction projects, and $20.9 billion came from philanthropic sources and from non-patient revenue sources (revenues from gift shops, parking lots, cafeteria sales, etc.) of hospitals, nursing homes, and HHAs.

## Government Spending

Government spending for health care accounted for 42.4 percent of NHE in 1990. In 1960, only 24.5 percent of NHE was funded by public programs. With the enactment of the Medicare and Medicaid programs, this share increased to 37.2 percent by 1970. From 1970 to 1980, coverage was expanded by Medicare to include disabled people and by Medicaid to include the mentally retarded. As a result, by 1980, 42.0 percent of NHE was funded by public programs.

More than four-fifths of all public spending for health care is for personal health care. The remainder is spent on public health activities, research and construction, and administrative expenses of public programs.

Although government's share of total health expenditures has remained relatively constant since the mid-1970s, public spending for health care is consuming an increasing share of both Federal and State and local government expenditures (Table 2). In 1960, only 3.1 percent of Federal expenditures and 7.4 percent of State and local spending were allocated to health care. In 1990, spending for health care accounted for 15.3 percent of total Federal expenditures and 11.4 percent of State and local government expenditures.

The government share of expenditures for personal health care varies by type of care. For example, public programs financed more than one-half of all hospital and nursing home care in 1990, but only 2.5 percent of dental services.

Medicare and Medicaid are the two largest government programs financing health care. Between them, they funded 30.8 percent of all spending for personal health care in 1990 and accounted for 74.5 percent of the public share. From 1970 to 1980, their share increased from 18.9 percent to 27.9 percent of total PHCE

### Table 2
### Government health expenditures as a percent of total government expenditures: Selected years 1960-90

| Year | Federal | State and local |
|------|---------|-----------------|
|      | Percent |                 |
| 1960 | 3.1  | 7.4  |
| 1970 | 8.5  | 7.4  |
| 1980 | 11.7 | 9.1  |
| 1981 | 11.9 | 9.7  |
| 1982 | 11.9 | 10.0 |
| 1983 | 12.3 | 10.1 |
| 1984 | 12.6 | 9.9  |
| 1985 | 12.5 | 9.9  |
| 1986 | 12.9 | 10.2 |
| 1987 | 13.4 | 10.7 |
| 1988 | 14.1 | 10.8 |
| 1989 | 14.7 | 11.0 |
| 1990 | 15.3 | 11.4 |

SOURCES: Health Care Financing Administration. Office of the Actuary. Office of National Health Statistics and Department of Commerce. Bureau of Economic Analysis.

and from 54.8 percent to 70.3 percent of the public share of PHCE.

## Medicare

Medicare, a Federal insurance program created by title XVIII of the Social Security Act of 1965, was originally designed to protect people 65 years of age or over from the high cost of health care. In 1972, the program was expanded to cover permanently disabled workers eligible for old age, survivors, and disability insurance benefits and their dependents, as well as people with end stage renal disease.

Medicare has two parts, each with its own trust fund. The hospital insurance (HI) program pays for inpatient hospital services, post-hospital skilled nursing services, home health care services, and hospice care. The supplementary medical insurance (SMI) program covers physician services, outpatient hospital services and therapy, and a few other services.

Unlike other Federal health programs, Medicare is not financed solely by general revenue (appropriations from general tax receipts). In 1990, 89 percent of the income for the HI program (Figure 6) came from a 1.45–percent payroll tax levied on employers and on employees for the first $51,300 of wages. (Self-employed people were required to contribute 2.9 percent, the equivalent of both the employer's and the employee's share of the HI tax.)

The SMI program was financed by monthly premium payments of $28.60 per enrollee in 1990 and by general revenue. The general revenue share of SMI receipts grew from about 50 percent in the early 1970s to approximately 70 percent in 1980 and later. In 1990, the general revenue share accounted for 72 percent of SMI program income.

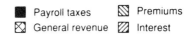

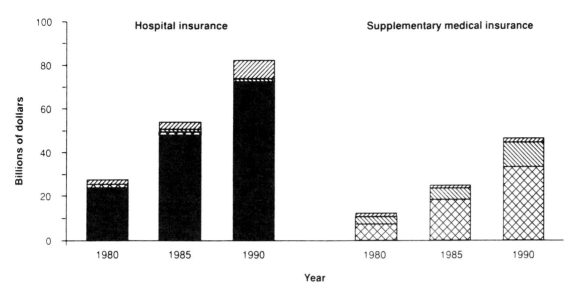

SOURCE: Health Care Financing Administration. Office of the Actuary: Data from the Office of National Health Statistics.

**Figure 6.** Payments into Medicare trust funds: 1980, 1985, and 1990

More than 34 million aged and disabled people were enrolled in Medicare on July 1, 1990. The program spent $108.9 billion in personal health care (benefit) payments for expenses incurred in 1990 by the 26.6 million enrollees who received benefits (Table 3). Growth in Medicare spending for personal health care slowed to 8.6 percent in 1990 from the 13.4 percent growth experienced in 1989.

During the past two decades, Medicare has accounted for increasing shares of spending for personal health care. In 1990, Medicare financed 45.0 percent of the public share of PHCE and 18.6 percent of total spending for personal health care. From 1970 to 1980, these shares grew from 32.2 percent to 41.8 percent of the public share and 11.1 percent to 16.6 percent of total spending for personal health care.

Almost 63 percent of Medicare benefits were for hospital care and another 27.5 percent for physician services in 1990. Prior to implementation of various hospital cost-containment measures starting in 1983, the distribution of Medicare spending was relatively stable at approximately 72 percent for hospital care and 22 percent for physician services.

Medicare expenditures for hospital care reached $68.3 billion in 1990, an increase of 9.9 percent from 1989. Medicare's PPS, other cost-containment measures, and a slowdown in growth of general and medical prices caused growth in Medicare spending for hospital care to decelerate from a high of 21.4 percent in 1980 to a low of 5.1 percent in 1986. Since then, growth in Med-

icare spending for hospital care services including inpatient, outpatient, and hospital-based HHA services has accelerated, almost returning to the double digits observed through the early-1980s. Current efforts to control the growth in Medicare spending for hospital care include reductions in payments for outpatient hospital services.

Medicare spending for physician services increased 9.5 percent from 1989, reaching $30.0 billion in 1990. Medicare's share of total spending for physician services grew from 11.8 percent in 1970 to 19.0 percent in 1980 and 23.9 percent in 1990. Efforts to restrain the growth in spending for physician services included incentives to encourage physician participation in the Medicare program, a temporary freeze on physician fees for Medicare services, reductions in payments to certain physicians, and reductions in payments for diagnostic laboratory tests and some overpriced surgical procedures.

The Federal Government is currently attempting to control the growth in Medicare spending for physician services through reductions in Medicare payments for additional overpriced procedures, volume performance standards, and other restrictions that limit the growth of Medicare payments to physicians, and increased beneficiary cost-sharing through higher Part B deductibles. Fee schedules based on resource-based relative value scales are scheduled to be phased in over a 3-year period starting in 1992.

Medicare paid $2.5 billion for skilled nursing facility care in 1990, 35 percent less than in 1989. Provisions

## Table 3

**Personal health care expenditures under Medicare and Medicaid and sources of Medicare financing: 1966–90**

| Year | Personal health care expenditures | | | Population | | | Medicare financing | | | |
|------|-----------------------------------|---------|----------|------------|-------|----------------------|--------------------|--------------------------------------------|------------------|-------------------|
| | Medicare and Medicaid[2] | Medicare | Medicaid | Medicare[1] | | Medicaid recipients[5] | Inpatient hospital deductible[6] | Supplementary medical insurance monthly premium[7] | Annual maximum taxable earnings | Contribution rate[8,9] |
| | | | | Enrollees[3] | Users[4] | | | | | |
| | Amount in billions | | | Number in million | | | Amount in dollars | | | Percent |
| 1966 | $2.9 | $1.6 | $1.3 | 19.1 | 3.7 | – | $40 | $3.00 | $6,600 | 0.35 |
| 1967 | 7.9 | 4.9 | 3.0 | 19.5 | 7.2 | — | 40 | 3.00 | 6,600 | 0.50 |
| 1968 | 9.3 | 5.9 | 3.4 | 19.8 | 7.9 | — | 40 | 4.00 | 7,800 | 0.60 |
| 1969 | 10.8 | 6.8 | 4.0 | 20.1 | 8.6 | — | 44 | 4.00 | 7,800 | 0.60 |
| 1970 | 12.3 | 7.2 | 5.1 | 20.5 | — | — | 52 | 5.30 | 7,800 | 0.60 |
| 1971 | 14.5 | 8.1 | 6.4 | 20.9 | 9.4 | — | 60 | 5.60 | 7,800 | 0.60 |
| 1972 | 16.8 | 8.8 | 8.0 | 21.3 | 10.0 | 17.6 | 68 | 5.80 | 9,000 | 0.60 |
| 1973 | 19.2 | 10.2 | 9.1 | 23.5 | 10.2 | 19.6 | 72 | [10]6.30 | 10,800 | 1.00 |
| 1974 | 23.4 | 12.8 | 10.6 | 24.2 | 11.8 | 21.5 | 84 | 6.70 | 13,200 | 0.90 |
| 1975 | 28.6 | 15.7 | 12.9 | 25.0 | 13.0 | 22.0 | 92 | 6.70 | 14,100 | 0.90 |
| 1976 | 33.4 | 18.9 | 14.5 | 25.7 | 14.1 | 22.8 | 104 | 7.20 | 15,300 | 0.90 |
| 1977 | 38.6 | 22.1 | 16.6 | 26.5 | 14.9 | 22.8 | 124 | 7.70 | 16,500 | 0.90 |
| 1978 | 44.3 | 25.8 | 18.5 | 27.2 | 15.9 | 22.0 | 144 | 8.20 | 17,700 | 1.00 |
| 1979 | 51.3 | 30.1 | 21.2 | 27.9 | 16.9 | 21.5 | 160 | 8.70 | 22,900 | 1.05 |
| 1980 | 61.2 | 36.4 | 24.8 | 28.5 | 18.0 | 21.6 | 180 | 9.60 | 25,900 | 1.05 |
| 1981 | 72.7 | 43.9 | 28.9 | 29.0 | 18.9 | 22.0 | 204 | 11.00 | 29,700 | 1.30 |
| 1982 | 81.9 | 51.4 | 30.6 | 29.5 | 18.8 | 21.6 | 260 | 12.20 | 32,400 | 1.30 |
| 1983 | 92.1 | 58.5 | 33.6 | 30.0 | 19.7 | 21.6 | 304 | 12.20 | 35,700 | 1.30 |
| 1984 | 100.4 | 64.4 | 36.0 | 30.5 | 20.7 | 21.6 | 356 | 14.60 | 37,800 | 1.30 |
| 1985 | 110.1 | 70.4 | 39.7 | 31.1 | 22.3 | 21.8 | 400 | 15.50 | 39,600 | 1.35 |
| 1986 | 118.6 | 75.7 | 42.9 | 31.7 | 23.1 | 22.5 | 492 | 15.50 | 42,000 | 1.45 |
| 1987 | 129.9 | 81.7 | 48.2 | 32.4 | 24.3 | 23.1 | 520 | 17.90 | 43,800 | 1.45 |
| 1988 | 140.5 | 88.5 | 52.1 | 33.0 | 25.1 | 22.9 | 540 | 24.80 | 45,000 | 1.45 |
| 1989 | 159.5 | 100.3 | 59.2 | 33.6 | 26.2 | 23.5 | 560 | [11]31.90 | 48,900 | 1.45 |
| 1990 | 180.2 | 108.9 | 71.3 | 34.2 | [12]26.6 | 25.3 | 592 | 28.60 | 51,300 | 1.45 |

[1] Hospital insurance (HI) and/or supplementary medical insurance (SMI).
[2] Excludes "buy-in" premiums paid by Medicaid for SMI coverage of aged and disabled Medicaid recipients eligible for coverage.
[3] Enrollees as of July 1 of specified year.
[4] Enrollees with some reimbursement under Medicare during calendar year. Data through 1973 reflect aged users only. Data for 1974 and later include aged and disabled users.
[5] Unduplicated count of Medicaid recipients during fiscal year.
[6] As of January of specified year with the exception of 1966, for which July data are used.
[7] As of July for 1966-83 and as of January for 1984 and later.
[8] Employer and employee (each) and self-employed people through 1983.
[9] Effective in 1984, self-employed people pay double this rate, the equivalent of both the employer and the employee share.
[10] Monthly premium for July and August 1973 was reduced to $5.80 and $6.10, respectively, by the Cost of Living Council.
[11] Includes $27.90 SMI monthly premium and $4.00 catastrophic coverage monthly premium.
[12] Estimated.

SOURCE: Health Care Financing Administration, Office of the Actuary and the Bureau of Data Management and Strategy.

of the Medicare Catastrophic Coverage Act of 1988 that affected the Medicare nursing home benefit became effective in 1989. In December 1989, the Act was repealed, but Medicare beneficiaries who were entitled to nursing home benefits under the less restrictive provisions of the Act continued to receive benefits. Effects of the Act lingered but are now diminishing. As a result, Medicare's share of total spending for nursing home care declined from 8.0 percent in 1989 to 4.7 percent in 1990. This compares with Medicare's share of total spending for nursing home care of 5.0 percent in 1970 and 2.1 percent in 1980.

Because Medicare clarified its conditions for payment in 1988, it seems likely that Medicare will maintain its current share of total spending for nursing home care at 4–5 percent.

### Medicaid

Medicaid spent $71.3 billion of combined Federal and State funds for personal health care in 1990. Growth in program spending for personal health care accelerated from 13.6 percent in 1989 to 20.6 percent in 1990, the fastest annual rate of growth in Medicaid spending since 1975. As a result, Medicaid's share of PHCE grew from 11.2 percent in 1989 to 12.2 percent in 1990.

Medicaid expenditures are largely institutional, with 39.9 percent spent on hospital care and 33.8 percent spent on nursing home care in 1990. Medicaid continues to be the largest third-party payer of long-term care expenditures, financing 45.4 percent of nursing home care in 1990. Growth in Medicaid benefit expenditures accelerated in 1990 for almost all categories of service. In 1990, growth in Medicaid spending accelerated from 14.5 percent in 1989 to 24.1 percent for hospitals, and from 8.6 percent to 17.0 percent for nursing homes.

Medicaid is funded jointly by Federal and State and local governments. The Federal Government sets minimum requirements for eligibility and services, allowing State governments considerable flexibility in designing the total scope of the program within the constraints of the State budgetary process. The Federal Government requires that all people receiving income benefits under the Supplementary Security Income (SSI) program (covering aged, blind, and disabled individuals) and families qualifying for Aid to Families with Dependent Children (AFDC) automatically qualify for Medicaid benefits. Certain individuals (pregnant women, children under age 6, Medicare enrollees, and Social Security Title IV-E recipients of foster care and adoption assistance) with income too high to qualify for SSI or AFDC cash benefits are also mandatorily eligible for Medicaid. Mandatory coverage of certain children ages 7–18 will be phased in as children born after September 30, 1983, attain age 7. State governments may, at their option, extend the program to cover "medically indigent" individuals or families, recipients of State supplementary payments, and other people with income or resources below specified levels.

Aged and disabled Medicare enrollees with incomes below certain levels were mandatorily covered by Medicaid under the Medicare Catastrophic Coverage Act of 1988. These Medicaid recipients are not eligible for full Medicaid benefits; Medicaid is required to pay only the Medicare premiums, deductibles, and coinsurance amounts. Legislation in 1989 required Medicaid to pay a portion of the Medicare HI premium for certain low-income disabled people. These are Medicare enrollees who qualified for Medicare because they were disabled but who, through rehabilitation and retraining, were able to return to work. Previously, after a specified number of months, these enrollees would have lost their eligibility for Medicare coverage. So that these working disabled people are not penalized for returning to work, they are allowed to retain Medicare coverage by paying the monthly HI and SMI premiums. (Medicaid is not required to pay the SMI premium.)

The Federal Government also defines minimum services that must be provided to all or specified groups of Medicaid recipients. These services include inpatient and outpatient hospital services; physician care; rural health clinic services; laboratory and X-ray services; nursing

home and home health care; and services of selected other health professionals. States may elect to provide additional services such as prescribed drugs, eyeglasses, dental care, and ICFs/MR.

Through State "buy-in" agreements, Medicaid purchases Medicare supplementary medical insurance (Part B) coverage for people who are eligible for both programs. For these "dual-eligibles," Medicare is the primary payer for Medicare-covered services, and Medicaid pays deductibles and coinsurance amounts and provides additional Medicaid-covered health care services. To avoid double counting, the Medicaid estimates presented here do not include the $1.1 billion paid to Medicare by Medicaid in 1990 for buy-in premiums. Therefore, actual Medicaid program expenditures were $72.5 billion in 1990.

Although more than two-thirds of Medicaid recipients in fiscal year 1990 qualified because they were members of an AFDC family, the consumed only one-fourth of program benefits. Conversely, the aged, blind, and disabled, who represent less than one-third of Medicaid recipients, consumed nearly three-fourths of Medicaid benefits.

In fiscal year 1990, there were 25.3 million people who received some type of Medicaid benefit. The number of Medicaid recipients has increased rapidly in recent years. In fiscal year 1990, an additional 1.7 million people received Medicaid benefits. With recent legislation phasing in various expansions to the Medicaid program and limited revenues available to finance the program, States are being pressured to control program costs (*The Nation's Health,* 1991). Tactics in use or proposed by some States include reallocation of available funds from high-cost services provided to selected recipients to lower cost services furnished to broader groups of recipients (Mayer and Kimball, 1991), creative techniques to generate additional financing such as provider-specific taxes and "voluntary donations" from hospitals and physicians (Kimball, 1991) and overall spending cuts.

## METHODOLOGY AND REVISIONS

Revisions introduced in this article began in 1978, incorporating the best and most current data available at this time. In the past, efforts have been made to consolidate revisions and to introduce them periodically. With the growing intensity of the health care policy debate, the decision was made to incorporate new information as soon as it becomes available. In this manner, the health care policy debate will include the best historical background information on NHE.

In aggregate, the 1989 estimates presented in this article are 0.2 percent lower than those reported earlier (Lazenby and Letsch, 1990). Revisions began in 1978 for two types of services—non-durable and durable medical products—and for the private sources of funding that finance the purchases of these goods. The remaining changes to the national health accounts began in 1982 or later, with the largest changes concentrated in the most recent years.

These revisions to estimates for 1989 and earlier result primarily from the availability of additional years of data from sources traditionally used to estimate NHE (Office of National Health Statistics, 1990). Other revisions originate from methodological changes.

The largest revision to the 1989 estimates of health care expenditures occurs in non-durable medical products, up $6.0 billion from estimates previously reported. Almost all of this revision ($5.1 billion) is concentrated in the non-prescription drug and sundry portion of this estimate and is paid from out-of-pocket resources; the remaining $0.9 billion is a revision to the prescription drug portion of the non-durable medical product estimates.

Estimates for non-durable medical products and their companion category, durable medical products, are benchmarked periodically, coinciding with GNP benchmark years. These estimates are based on PCE, a component of the GNP. Detailed information on the composition of each component of PCE is available only periodically, at benchmarks occurring every 5 years. Using this detail, PCE levels are adjusted to match NHE definitions for durable and non-durable medical products. Recently, the 1982 PCE information became available, updating the detail from 1963, 1967, 1972, and 1977 benchmark years. As a result, revisions were made to the two categories of health spending beginning in 1978.

The second largest change occurred in physician services estimates for 1989, revised downward by $4.1 billion from previously reported 1989 estimates. Since the late 1970s, estimates for all professional service categories (physician services, dental services, and other

professional services) that were based solely on Internal Revenue Service (IRS) business receipts were modified to incorporate information from both the U.S. Bureau of the Census' Services Annual Survey (SAS) and the IRS. For 1989, all professional service category estimates rely solely upon expenditure growth reported by the SAS (U.S. Bureau of Census, 1990). This change closely aligns methodology used in NHE with methods used by the U.S. Department of Commerce's national income and product accounts to produce similar estimates. The reason for this switch is the gradual deterioration in size of the IRS Statistics of Income samples, and the use by IRS of a different establishment coding scheme than the Standard Industrial Classification (SIC) codes used by most other Federal Government statistical agencies. The use of a different coding scheme by IRS may be the cause of increasing divergence between the IRS and SAS of estimates of business receipts for physicians. Classification of physician services has become obscured, as the difference between offices and clinics of physicians (SIC 801 and 803) and outpatient care facilities (SIC 808) become less distinct. IRS coding is less able to distinguish subtle differences in establishment type.

Despite the modification in data source used for physician expenditure estimates beginning in 1989, we remain concerned about the level of physician services expenditures for 1989 reported in this article. Estimates of physician business receipts from the AMA imply stronger growth for 1989 than that reported by SAS. Stronger growth is more consistent with separately estimated Medicare physician revenues and would produce a more moderate increase in Medicare's share of total physician revenues for 1989 than that reported here. Analysts will re-examine this issue when the 1990 estimates of physician business receipts and net income become available from the U.S. Bureau of the Census and the AMA. . . .

## Table 4
### Personal health care expenditures (PHCE) per capita: Selected years 1960-90

| Item | 1960 | 1970 | 1980 | 1982 | 1990 |
|---|---|---|---|---|---|
| Current (nominal) PHCE per capita | $126 | $302 | $933 | $1,193 | $2,255 |
| PHCE per capita deflated by gross national product fixed-weight price index (GNP-FWPI) | 330 | 640 | 1,083 | 1,193 | 1,665 |
| PHCE per capita deflated by PHCE fixed-weight price index (PHCE-FWPI) | 474 | 779 | 1,132 | 1,193 | 1,402 |
| **Addenda** | | | Prices indexes | | |
| GNP-FWPI | 38.1 | 47.2 | 86.1 | 100.0 | 135.4 |
| PHCE-FWPI | 26.5 | 38.8 | 82.4 | 100.0 | 160.9 |

SOURCES: Health Care Financing Administration, Office of the Actuary, Office of National Health Statistics and Department of Commerce, Bureau of Economic Analysis.

# DEFLATING PERSONAL HEALTH CARE EXPENDITURES

Health care spending has grown more rapidly than other sectors of the economy. This is not necessarily a problem, if the value obtained for the expenditure meets societal priorities in terms of additional quantity and quality of services purchased. In health care, price inflation plays a major role in rapidly increasing costs. Deflating health care spending separates the effects of price growth from growth attributable to all other factors. However, the index used to deflate health expenditures determines the growth attributable to all other factors and its meaning.

One approach to removing the effects of price growth from health spending is to deflate health care expenditures by a measure of medical-specific price inflation (Table 4).[1] The resulting measure of "real" growth gauges growth in quantity of health services delivered per capita devoid of medical care price changes. Quantity changes are generated by technological developments, changes in the age and sex composition of the population, or changes in the intensity and quantity of health care services delivered per person. Also, this residual would include the net effect of any error in the measurement of medical prices or medical expenditures. The Office of the Actuary in HCFA develops a personal health care expenditure fixed-weight price index.

An alternate approach to deflating health spending is to remove the effects of economywide inflation alone. The most appropriate deflator for economywide prices for our purposes is the gross national product fixed-weight price index (GNP-FWPI). The GNP-FWPI is the most comprehensive measure of pure price inflation for the economy as a whole. Personal health care expenditures per capita deflated by the GNP-FWPI can be interpreted as the opportunity cost of health care. These constant-dollar health care costs per capita measure the value of the other goods and services that society could have purchased instead of health care. This measure eliminates the cause of growth over which the health sector has little control—economywide inflation. The remainder measures change in medical-specific price inflation in excess of economywide inflation, and intensity and use per capita of health care services. These are factors over which the health sector has at least some control.

The decision made in choosing an index to deflate health care costs determines the size of real health spending growth as well as its interpretation. From 1980 to 1990, nominal (current-dollar) personal health spend-

**Table 5**

**Average annual percent change in personal health care expenditures (PHCE) per capita: Selected years 1960-90**

| Item | 1960-70 | 1970-80 | 1980-90 |
|------|---------|---------|---------|
| | | Percent | |
| Current (nominal) PHCE per capita | 9.2 | 11.9 | 9.2 |
| PHCE per capita deflated by gross national product fixed-weight price index (GNP-FWPI) | 6.9 | 5.4 | 4.4 |
| PHCE per capita deflated by PHCE fixed-weight price index (PHCE-FWPI) | 5.1 | 3.8 | 2.2 |
| **Addenda** | | | |
| GNP-FWPI | 2.2 | 6.2 | 4.6 |
| PHCE-FWPI | 3.9 | 7.8 | 6.9 |
| Difference between PHCE-FWPI and GNP-FWPI | 1.7 | 1.6 | 2.3 |

SOURCES: Health Care Financing Administration. Office of the Actuary. Office of National Health Statistics and Department of Commerce. Bureau of Economic Analysis

ing per capita increased at an average rate of 9.2 percent per year (Table 5). Economywide prices grew at an average annual rate of 4.6 percent during this period. Deflating personal health care expenditures per capita by the GNP-FWPI removes the effects of economywide inflation and indicates growth in real output and real price change (medical inflation in excess of economywide inflation) of 4.4 percent per year. This means that about one-half of the growth in per capita health spending from 1980 to 1990 can be attributed to economywide inflation.[2]

From 1980 to 1990, medical prices grew at an average annual rate of 6.9 percent. Deflating personal health care expenditures per capita by PHCE-FWPI removes the effects of medical-specific inflation (which includes economywide inflation), resulting in an average annual growth in real health care output of 2.2 percent. This measure of deflated personal health spending per capita identifies the change in quantity of health care services per capita. During the 1980s, three-quarters of the growth in per capita health spending was attributable to medical-specific price increases.[3] During the past three decades, increases in overall medical prices have become a progressively more important factor in the growth of per capita health care spending.

During the past two decades, the gap between medical care prices and economywide prices has widened. One cause of the widening gap is imperfections within the health care marketplace that interfere with competition.

[1] Growth in population has remained fairly constant at about 1 percent per year since 1960. Therefore, per capita spending has been used to simplify this discussion.

[2] Calculated by dividing growth in economywide prices by growth in the sum of growth in prices and in real output per capita. In this case, 4.6/(4.6 + 4.4) = .51.

[3] Calculated as 6.9/(6.9 + 2.2) = .76.

Most of this interference comes from private and public insurance. These third-party payers insulate consumers from the full price of health care goods and services at the time of purchase. Additional interference comes from the lack of consumer knowledge about the appropriateness of quality and quantity of health services and about competing provider prices for the same service. Medical care procedures and services have become increasingly complex, and it becomes more difficult for consumers to assess the reasonableness of practitioners' recommendations and of prices charged. Beyond marketplace imperfections, health care is a service industry. Service industries typically are less able to take advantage of labor-saving and cost-cutting efficiencies than are non-service industries.

Personal Health Care Price Index

The PHCE-FWPI is a Laspeyres index with 1982 as a base year. Table 6 lists price proxies assigned to each component of PHCE, along with a weight that is equal to the proportion of PHCE that component represented in the base year 1982. For each year, PHCE-FWPI is the summation of each index multiplied by its 1982 weight.

In our judgment, this PHCE-FWPI is a more appropriate measure of medical price inflation associated with PHCE than two other available indexes—the Consumer Price Index (CPI) or the personal consumption expenditure fixed-weight price index. First, the medical care component of the CPI is weighted based on consumer out-of-pocket expenditures. Because a large proportion of health care is paid for by third parties, certain health care services are assigned weights that under- or overrepresent their shares if all payers were considered. For example, out-of-pocket expenditures for hospital care, representing only 9 percent of all out-of-pocket expenditures, are undervalued in the CPI, because hospital spending comprises 39 percent of PHCE. Second, the medical care component of the personal consumption expenditure fixed-weight price index, estimated and published as part of the national income and product accounts, excludes portions of public expenditures when its weights are determined. Expenses of government-owned and -operated facilities are not included in the personal consumption expenditures portion of the GNP, but rather in government purchases of goods and services.

Each component of PHCE can be deflated by its assigned price index to produce a constant-dollar estimate of that component. Summing all of the deflated components yields a constant-dollar estimate of PHCE. This estimate differs from PHCE deflated by PHCE-FWPI in that it reflects any change in quantity purchased of each of the components. From 1980 to 1990, constant-dollar PHCE grew at an average annual rate of 3.2 percent (Table 7). From 1960 to 1970, constant-dollar PHCE grew at twice that rate (6.4 percent), and from 1970 to 1980, 1.5 times (4.8 percent).

[Tables 7 through 13 follow]

Acknowledgments—The national health expenditures are prepared in the Office of National Health Statistics within the Health Care Financing Administration's Office of the Actuary, under the general supervision of Mark Freeland. In addition to the authors, Madie Stewart and Sue Donham prepared selected source-of-funds estimates. Sally Sonnefeld and Patricia McDonnell supplied estimates of the net cost of private health insurance.

**Table 6**
**Derivation of the personal health care expenditure fixed-weight price index**

| Commodity or service | Price proxy | 1982 weight |
|---|---|---|
| All personal health care | — | 100.0 |
| Hospital care | Hospital Input Price Index[1] | 47.4 |
| Physician services | CPI[2], physician services | 18.8 |
| Dental services | CPI[2], dental services | 6.4 |
| Other professional services and home health care[3] | CPI[2], professional services | 4.9 |
| Drugs and other medical non-durables | CPI[2], medical care commodities | 9.6 |
| Vision products and other medical durables | CPI[2], eye care | 1.8 |
| Nursing home care | National Nursing Home Input Price Index | 9.1 |
| Other personal care | CPI[2], medical care | 1.9 |

[1] The specific hospital input price index is All Hospitals with Capital and Medical Fees (Wages = AHE806NS, Fringes = PanelFB).
[2] Consumer Price Index for all urban consumers, U.S. Bureau of Labor Statistics, U.S. Department of Labor. Indexes are scaled so that the 1982 value is 100.0.
[3] Two categories combined because no price proxy is available for home health care for the entire time period.

SOURCE: Health Care Financing Administration, Office of the Actuary: Data from the Office of National Health Statistics.

## References

American Hospital Association: *Hospital Statistics: A Comprehensive Summary of U.S. Hospitals, 1990–1991.* Chicago, 1990.

American Medical Association: *Socioeconomic Characteristics of Medical Practice, 1990/1991.* Chicago, 1991.

Kimball, M.C.: States outfox feds for Medicaid cash. *HealthWeek* 5(10):1,59, May 20, 1991.

Lakin, K.C., Prouty, R.W., White, C.C., et al.: *Intermediate Care Facilities for Persons with Mental Retardation (ICFs/MR): Program Utilization and Resident Characteristics.* Center for Residential and Community Services, University of Minnesota, Minneapolis, Mar. 1990.

Lazenby, H.C., and Letsch, S.W.: National health expenditures, 1989. *Health Care Financing Review* 12(2):1–26. HCFA

**Table 7**

**Personal health care expenditures in current and constant dollars and associated price indexes, by type of spending: Selected years 1960-90**

| Type of spending | 1960 | 1970 | 1980 | 1982 | 1990 |
|---|---|---|---|---|---|
| | Current dollars in billions | | | | |
| Personal health care | $23.9 | $64.9 | $219.4 | $286.4 | $585.3 |
| Hospital care | 9.3 | 27.9 | 102.4 | 135.9 | 256.0 |
| Physician services | 5.3 | 13.6 | 41.9 | 53.8 | 125.7 |
| Dental services | 2.0 | 4.7 | 14.4 | 18.4 | 34.0 |
| Other professional services and home health care | 0.6 | 1.7 | 10.0 | 14.0 | 38.5 |
| Drugs and other medical non-durables | 4.2 | 8.8 | 21.6 | 27.6 | 54.6 |
| Vision products and other medical durables | 0.8 | 2.0 | 4.6 | 5.1 | 12.1 |
| Nursing home care | 1.0 | 4.9 | 20.0 | 26.1 | 53.1 |
| Other personal health care | 0.7 | 1.4 | 4.6 | 5.6 | 11.3 |
| | Price indexes | | | | |
| Hospital care | 22.7 | 36.2 | 81.7 | 100.0 | 153.8 |
| Physician services | 23.5 | 37.1 | 82.3 | 100.0 | 173.2 |
| Dental services | 29.0 | 42.1 | 84.7 | 100.0 | 167.2 |
| Other professional services and home health care | 25.5 | 39.7 | 83.6 | 100.0 | 167.4 |
| Drugs and other medical non-durables | 50.8 | 50.3 | 81.7 | 100.0 | 177.2 |
| Vision products and other medical durables | 34.8 | 46.4 | 86.7 | 100.0 | 143.6 |
| Nursing home care | 24.8 | 39.7 | 83.9 | 100.0 | 147.3 |
| Other personal health care | 24.1 | 36.7 | 80.9 | 100.0 | 176.0 |
| | Constant 1982 dollars in billions | | | | |
| Personal health care | 90.1 | 166.9 | 266.3 | 286.4 | 364.1 |
| Hospital care | 40.8 | 77.2 | 125.3 | 135.9 | 166.5 |
| Physician services | 22.4 | 36.6 | 50.9 | 53.8 | 72.6 |
| Dental services | 6.8 | 11.1 | 17.0 | 18.4 | 20.3 |
| Other professional services and home health care | 2.5 | 4.2 | 12.0 | 14.0 | 23.0 |
| Drugs and other medical non-durables | 8.4 | 17.5 | 26.5 | 27.6 | 30.8 |
| Vision products and other medical durables | 2.3 | 4.4 | 5.3 | 5.1 | 8.5 |
| Nursing home care | 4.0 | 12.3 | 23.8 | 26.1 | 36.1 |
| Other personal health care | 2.9 | 3.7 | 5.6 | 5.6 | 6.4 |

SOURCE: Health Care Financing Administration. Office of the Actuary. Data from the Office of National Health Statistics.

No. 03316. Office of Research and Demonstration, Health Care Financing Administration. Washington. U.S. Government Printing Office, Winter 1990.

Letsch, S.W., Maple, B.M., Cowan, C.A., and Donham, C.S.: Health Care Indicators. *Health Care Financing Review* 13(1):129–153. HCFA Pub. No. 03321. Office of Research and Demonstrations, Health Care Financing Administration. Washington, U.S. Government Printing Office, Fall 1991.

Levit, K.R., and Cowan, C.A.: The burden of health care costs: Business, households, and governments. *Health Care Financing Review* 12(2):127–137. HCFA Pub. No. 03298. Office of Research and Demonstrations. Health Care Financing Administration. Washington, U.S. Government Printing Office, Winter 1990.

Mayer, D., and Kimball, M.C.: Ore. commission OKs Medicaid pecking order. *HealthWeek* 5(4):1,36, Feb. 25, 1991.

Office of National Cost Estimates: Revisions to the national health accounts and methodology. *Health Care Financing Review* 11(4):42–54. HCFA Pub. No. 03298. Office of Research and Demonstrations. Health Care Financing Administration. Washington, U.S. Government Printing Office, Summer 1990.

*The Nation's Health:* Outlays for Medicaid Mandates Strapping Budgets, say States. 21(2):5. American Public Health Association, Washington, Feb. 1991.

U.S. Bureau of Census: *Services Annual Survey.* U.S. Department of Commerce. Washington, U.S. Government Printing Office, 1990.

## Table 8

### National health expenditures aggregate and per capita amounts, percent distribution, and average annual percent growth, by source of funds: Selected years 1960-90

| Item | 1960 | 1970 | 1980 | 1985 | 1986 | 1987 | 1988 | 1989 | 1990 |
|---|---|---|---|---|---|---|---|---|---|
| | | | | | Amount in billions | | | | |
| National health expenditures | $27.1 | $74.4 | $250.1 | $422.6 | $454.8 | $494.1 | $546.0 | $602.8 | $666.2 |
| Private | 20.5 | 46.7 | 145.0 | 247.9 | 264.6 | 285.7 | 318.9 | 350.2 | 383.6 |
| Public | 6.7 | 27.7 | 105.2 | 174.8 | 190.2 | 208.4 | 227.1 | 252.6 | 282.6 |
| Federal | 2.9 | 17.7 | 72.0 | 123.6 | 133.1 | 144.0 | 156.7 | 175.0 | 195.4 |
| State and local | 3.7 | 9.9 | 33.2 | 51.2 | 57.2 | 64.4 | 70.5 | 77.6 | 87.3 |
| | | | | | Number in millions | | | | |
| U.S. population[1] | 190.1 | 214.9 | 235.3 | 247.2 | 249.6 | 252.0 | 254.5 | 257.0 | 259.6 |
| | | | | | Amount in billions | | | | |
| Gross national product | $515 | $1,015 | $2,732 | $4,015 | $4,232 | $4,516 | $4,874 | $5,201 | $5,465 |
| | | | | | Per capita amount | | | | |
| National health expenditures | $143 | $346 | $1,063 | $1,710 | $1,822 | $1,961 | $2,146 | $2,346 | $2,566 |
| Private | 108 | 217 | 616 | 1,003 | 1,060 | 1,134 | 1,253 | 1,363 | 1,478 |
| Public | 35 | 129 | 447 | 707 | 762 | 827 | 893 | 983 | 1,089 |
| Federal | 15 | 83 | 306 | 500 | 533 | 571 | 616 | 681 | 753 |
| State and local | 20 | 46 | 141 | 207 | 229 | 255 | 277 | 302 | 336 |
| | | | | | Percent distribution | | | | |
| National health expenditures | 100.0 | 100.0 | 100.0 | 100.0 | 100.0 | 100.0 | 100.0 | 100.0 | 100.0 |
| Private | 75.5 | 62.8 | 58.0 | 58.6 | 58.2 | 57.8 | 58.4 | 58.1 | 57.6 |
| Public | 24.5 | 37.2 | 42.0 | 41.4 | 41.8 | 42.2 | 41.6 | 41.9 | 42.4 |
| Federal | 10.7 | 23.9 | 28.8 | 29.2 | 29.3 | 29.1 | 28.7 | 29.0 | 29.3 |
| State and local | 13.8 | 13.3 | 13.3 | 12.1 | 12.6 | 13.0 | 12.9 | 12.9 | 13.1 |
| | | | | | Percent of gross national product | | | | |
| National health expenditures | 5.3 | 7.3 | 9.2 | 10.5 | 10.7 | 10.9 | 11.2 | 11.6 | 12.2 |
| | | | | | Average annual percent growth from previous year shown | | | | |
| National health expenditures | — | 10.6 | 12.9 | 11.1 | 7.6 | 8.6 | 10.5 | 10.4 | 10.5 |
| Private | — | 8.6 | 12.0 | 11.3 | 6.8 | 8.0 | 11.6 | 9.8 | 9.5 |
| Public | — | 15.3 | 14.3 | 10.7 | 8.8 | 9.5 | 9.0 | 11.2 | 11.9 |
| Federal | — | 19.8 | 15.0 | 11.4 | 7.6 | 8.2 | 8.8 | 11.7 | 11.7 |
| State and local | — | 10.2 | 12.8 | 9.0 | 11.8 | 12.6 | 9.5 | 10.1 | 12.5 |
| U.S. population | — | 1.2 | 0.9 | 1.0 | 1.0 | 1.0 | 1.0 | 1.0 | 1.0 |
| Gross national product | — | 7.0 | 10.4 | 8.0 | 5.4 | 6.7 | 7.9 | 6.7 | 5.1 |

[1] July 1 Social Security area population estimates

NOTE: Numbers and percents may not add to totals because of rounding

SOURCE: Health Care Financing Administration, Office of the Actuary. Data from the Office of National Health Statistics.

## Table 9
### National health expenditures aggregate amounts and average annual percent change, by type of expenditure: Selected years 1960-90

| Type of expenditure | 1960 | 1970 | 1980 | 1985 | 1986 | 1987 | 1988 | 1989 | 1990 |
|---|---|---|---|---|---|---|---|---|---|
| | Amount in billions | | | | | | | | |
| National health expenditures | $27.1 | $74.4 | $250.1 | $422.6 | $454.8 | $494.1 | $546.0 | $602.8 | $666.2 |
| Health services and supplies | 25.4 | 69.1 | 238.9 | 407.2 | 438.9 | 476.8 | 526.2 | 582.1 | 643.4 |
| Personal health care | 23.9 | 64.9 | 219.4 | 369.7 | 400.8 | 439.3 | 482.8 | 529.9 | 585.3 |
| Hospital care | 9.3 | 27.9 | 102.4 | 168.3 | 179.8 | 194.2 | 212.0 | 232.6 | 256.0 |
| Physician services | 5.3 | 13.6 | 41.9 | 74.0 | 82.1 | 93.0 | 105.1 | 113.6 | 125.7 |
| Dental services | 2.0 | 4.7 | 14.4 | 23.3 | 24.7 | 27.1 | 29.4 | 31.6 | 34.0 |
| Other professional services | 0.6 | 1.5 | 8.7 | 16.6 | 18.6 | 21.1 | 23.8 | 27.1 | 31.6 |
| Home health care | 0.0 | 0.1 | 1.3 | 3.8 | 4.0 | 4.1 | 4.5 | 5.6 | 6.9 |
| Drugs and other medical non-durables | 4.2 | 8.8 | 21.6 | 36.2 | 39.7 | 43.2 | 46.3 | 50.6 | 54.6 |
| Vision products and other medical durables | 0.8 | 2.0 | 4.6 | 7.1 | 8.1 | 9.1 | 10.1 | 11.4 | 12.1 |
| Nursing home care | 1.0 | 4.9 | 20.0 | 34.1 | 36.7 | 39.7 | 42.8 | 47.7 | 53.1 |
| Other personal health care | 0.7 | 1.4 | 4.6 | 6.4 | 7.1 | 7.8 | 8.7 | 9.7 | 11.3 |
| Program administration and net cost of private health insurance | 1.2 | 2.8 | 12.2 | 25.2 | 24.6 | 22.9 | 26.8 | 33.9 | 38.7 |
| Government public health activities | 0.4 | 1.4 | 7.2 | 12.3 | 13.5 | 14.6 | 16.6 | 18.3 | 19.3 |
| Research and construction | 1.7 | 5.3 | 11.3 | 15.4 | 16.0 | 17.3 | 19.8 | 20.7 | 22.8 |
| Research[1] | 0.7 | 2.0 | 5.4 | 7.8 | 8.5 | 9.0 | 10.3 | 11.0 | 12.4 |
| Construction | 1.0 | 3.4 | 5.8 | 7.6 | 7.4 | 8.2 | 9.5 | 9.6 | 10.4 |
| | Average annual percent change from previous year shown | | | | | | | | |
| National health expenditures | — | 10.6 | 12.9 | 11.1 | 7.6 | 8.6 | 10.5 | 10.4 | 10.5 |
| Health services and supplies | — | 10.5 | 13.2 | 11.3 | 7.8 | 8.7 | 10.3 | 10.6 | 10.5 |
| Personal health care | — | 10.5 | 13.0 | 11.0 | 8.4 | 9.6 | 9.9 | 9.8 | 10.5 |
| Hospital care | — | 11.7 | 13.9 | 10.4 | 6.8 | 8.0 | 9.2 | 9.7 | 10.1 |
| Physician services | — | 9.9 | 11.9 | 12.1 | 10.9 | 13.3 | 13.1 | 8.0 | 10.7 |
| Dental services | — | 9.1 | 11.9 | 10.1 | 6.4 | 9.6 | 8.5 | 7.3 | 7.6 |
| Other professional services | — | 9.6 | 19.1 | 13.8 | 12.0 | 13.6 | 12.4 | 14.0 | 16.6 |
| Home health care | — | 14.5 | 25.2 | 23.3 | 3.6 | 3.6 | 9.6 | 24.9 | 22.5 |
| Drugs and other medical non-durables | — | 7.6 | 9.4 | 10.8 | 9.9 | 8.6 | 7.2 | 9.3 | 7.9 |
| Vision products and other medical durables | — | 9.6 | 8.5 | 9.4 | 13.0 | 12.3 | 11.8 | 12.9 | 6.1 |
| Nursing home care | — | 17.4 | 15.2 | 11.3 | 7.6 | 8.0 | 7.8 | 11.5 | 11.4 |
| Other personal health care | — | 7.1 | 12.8 | 6.9 | 11.1 | 10.0 | 12.1 | 11.2 | 16.4 |
| Program administration and net cost of private health insurance | — | 9.0 | 16.0 | 15.5 | -2.5 | -6.6 | 16.9 | 26.6 | 14.1 |
| Government public health activities | — | 13.9 | 18.0 | 11.3 | 9.6 | 8.3 | 13.5 | 10.4 | 5.6 |
| Research and construction | — | 12.1 | 7.8 | 6.4 | 3.7 | 8.2 | 14.9 | 4.3 | 10.2 |
| Research[1] | — | 10.9 | 10.8 | 7.4 | 9.5 | 5.7 | 14.5 | 6.8 | 11.9 |
| Construction | — | 12.8 | 5.6 | 5.4 | -2.4 | 11.1 | 15.3 | 1.5 | 8.3 |

[1] Research and development expenditures of drug companies and other manufacturers and providers of medical equipment and supplies are excluded from "research expenditures," but they are included in the expenditure class in which the product falls

NOTE: Numbers may not add to totals because of rounding.

SOURCE: Health Care Financing Administration, Office of the Actuary; Data from the Office of National Health Statistics

# Table 10

## National health expenditures, by source of funds and type of expenditure: Selected years 1980-90

| Year and type of expenditure | Total | All private funds | Private Consumer Total | Out-of-pocket | Private insurance | Other | Government Total | Federal | State and local |
|---|---|---|---|---|---|---|---|---|---|
| **1980** | | | | | Amount in billions | | | | |
| National health expenditures | $250.1 | $145.0 | $132.9 | $59.5 | $73.4 | $12.1 | $105.2 | $72.0 | $33.2 |
| Health services and supplies | 238.9 | 140.7 | 132.9 | 59.5 | 73.4 | 7.8 | 98.1 | 66.8 | 31.4 |
| Personal health care | 219.4 | 132.3 | 124.8 | 59.5 | 65.3 | 7.6 | 87.1 | 63.5 | 23.6 |
| Hospital care | 102.4 | 47.8 | 42.8 | 5.3 | 37.5 | 5.0 | 54.6 | 41.3 | 13.3 |
| Physician services | 41.9 | 29.2 | 29.2 | 11.3 | 18.0 | 0.0 | 12.6 | 9.7 | 3.0 |
| Dental services | 14.4 | 13.7 | 13.7 | 9.4 | 4.4 | — | 0.6 | 0.4 | 0.3 |
| Other professional services | 8.7 | 6.9 | 6.0 | 3.8 | 2.2 | 0.9 | 1.7 | 1.3 | 0.4 |
| Home health care | 1.3 | 0.4 | 0.2 | 0.1 | 0.1 | 0.1 | 1.0 | 0.8 | 0.1 |
| Drugs and other medical non-durables | 21.6 | 20.0 | 20.0 | 17.5 | 2.5 | — | 1.7 | 0.8 | 0.8 |
| Vision products and other medical durables | 4.6 | 4.0 | 4.0 | 3.5 | 0.4 | — | 0.6 | 0.5 | 0.1 |
| Nursing home care | 20.0 | 9.5 | 8.8 | 8.7 | 0.2 | 0.6 | 10.5 | 6.1 | 4.4 |
| Other personal health care | 4.6 | 0.9 | — | — | — | 0.9 | 3.7 | 2.5 | 1.2 |
| Program administration and net cost of private health insurance | 12.2 | 8.4 | 8.1 | — | 8.1 | 0.2 | 3.8 | 2.1 | 1.8 |
| Government public health activities | 7.2 | — | — | — | — | — | 7.2 | 1.2 | 6.0 |
| Research and construction | 11.3 | 4.2 | — | — | — | 4.2 | 7.0 | 5.2 | 1.8 |
| Research | 5.4 | 0.3 | — | — | — | 0.3 | 5.2 | 4.7 | 0.5 |
| Construction | 5.8 | 4.0 | — | — | — | 4.0 | 1.9 | 0.6 | 1.3 |
| **1985** | | | | | | | | | |
| National health expenditures | 422.6 | 247.9 | 228.5 | 94.4 | 134.1 | 19.4 | 174.8 | 123.6 | 51.2 |
| Health services and supplies | 407.2 | 241.9 | 228.5 | 94.4 | 134.1 | 13.4 | 165.4 | 116.4 | 48.9 |
| Personal health care | 369.7 | 221.3 | 208.4 | 94.4 | 114.0 | 12.9 | 148.4 | 111.8 | 36.6 |
| Hospital care | 168.3 | 76.5 | 68.3 | 8.8 | 59.5 | 8.3 | 91.7 | 72.0 | 19.7 |
| Physician services | 74.0 | 49.8 | 49.8 | 16.1 | 33.7 | 0.0 | 24.1 | 19.2 | 4.9 |
| Dental services | 23.3 | 22.7 | 22.7 | 13.5 | 9.1 | — | 0.6 | 0.3 | 0.3 |
| Other professional services | 16.6 | 13.5 | 11.3 | 6.1 | 5.2 | 2.2 | 3.2 | 2.4 | 0.8 |
| Home health care | 3.8 | 1.1 | 0.7 | 0.5 | 0.3 | 0.4 | 2.7 | 2.3 | 0.5 |
| Drugs and other medical non-durables | 36.2 | 33.1 | 33.1 | 28.0 | 5.2 | — | 3.0 | 1.5 | 1.5 |
| Vision products and other medical durables | 7.1 | 5.6 | 5.6 | 4.8 | 0.7 | — | 1.6 | 1.4 | 0.2 |
| Nursing home care | 34.1 | 17.6 | 16.9 | 16.6 | 0.3 | 0.7 | 16.5 | 9.7 | 6.8 |
| Other personal health care | 6.4 | 1.4 | — | — | — | 1.4 | 4.9 | 3.0 | 1.9 |
| Program administration and net cost of private health insurance | 25.2 | 20.5 | 20.0 | — | 20.0 | 0.5 | 4.7 | 3.2 | 1.4 |
| Government public health activities | 12.3 | — | — | — | — | — | 12.3 | 1.4 | 10.9 |
| Research and construction | 15.4 | 6.0 | — | — | — | 6.0 | 9.4 | 7.2 | 2.2 |
| Research | 7.8 | 0.5 | — | — | — | 0.5 | 7.3 | 6.4 | 0.9 |
| Construction | 7.6 | 5.5 | — | — | — | 5.5 | 2.1 | 0.8 | 1.3 |
| **1988** | | | | | | | | | |
| National health expenditures | 546.0 | 318.9 | 293.7 | 119.3 | 174.4 | 25.2 | 227.1 | 156.7 | 70.5 |
| Health services and supplies | 526.2 | 311.0 | 293.7 | 119.3 | 174.4 | 17.3 | 215.1 | 147.5 | 67.6 |
| Personal health care | 482.8 | 290.2 | 273.4 | 119.3 | 154.1 | 16.8 | 192.6 | 141.7 | 50.9 |
| Hospital care | 212.0 | 97.7 | 86.6 | 11.2 | 75.4 | 11.1 | 114.3 | 86.2 | 28.1 |
| Physician services | 105.1 | 70.0 | 70.0 | 20.9 | 49.1 | 0.0 | 35.1 | 28.1 | 7.0 |
| Dental services | 29.4 | 28.7 | 28.7 | 16.3 | 12.4 | — | 0.7 | 0.4 | 0.3 |
| Other professional services | 23.8 | 19.2 | 16.6 | 7.6 | 8.9 | 2.6 | 4.6 | 3.5 | 1.1 |
| Home health care | 4.5 | 1.2 | 0.8 | 0.5 | 0.3 | 0.3 | 3.4 | 2.6 | 0.7 |
| Drugs and other medical non-durables | 46.3 | 41.8 | 41.8 | 35.3 | 6.5 | — | 4.5 | 2.2 | 2.3 |
| Vision products and other medical durables | 10.1 | 7.9 | 7.9 | 6.8 | 1.0 | — | 2.2 | 2.0 | 0.3 |
| Nursing home care | 42.8 | 21.9 | 21.0 | 20.6 | 0.5 | 0.8 | 20.9 | 12.6 | 8.3 |
| Other personal health care | 8.7 | 1.9 | — | — | — | 1.9 | 6.9 | 4.2 | 2.7 |
| Program administration and net cost of private health insurance | 26.8 | 20.8 | 20.3 | — | 20.3 | 0.5 | 6.0 | 3.9 | 2.1 |
| Government public health activities | 16.6 | — | — | — | — | — | 16.6 | 1.9 | 14.7 |
| Research and construction | 19.8 | 7.8 | — | — | — | 7.8 | 12.0 | 9.2 | 2.8 |
| Research | 10.3 | 0.7 | — | — | — | 0.7 | 9.6 | 8.3 | 1.3 |
| Construction | 9.5 | 7.1 | — | — | — | 7.1 | 2.4 | 0.9 | 1.5 |

Table 10—Continued

| Year and type of expenditure | Total | Private | | | | | Government | | |
|---|---|---|---|---|---|---|---|---|---|
| | | All private funds | Consumer | | | Other | Total | Federal | State and local |
| | | | Total | Out-of-pocket | Private insurance | | | | |
| **1989** | | | | | | | | | |
| National health expenditures | $602.8 | $350.2 | $322.5 | $126.1 | $196.4 | $27.7 | $252.6 | $175.0 | $77.6 |
| Health services and supplies | 582.1 | 342.1 | 322.5 | 126.1 | 196.4 | 19.6 | 240.0 | 165.2 | 74.8 |
| Personal health care | 529.9 | 314.7 | 295.7 | 126.1 | 169.6 | 19.0 | 215.2 | 158.8 | 56.3 |
| Hospital care | 232.6 | 107.9 | 95.3 | 12.1 | 83.2 | 12.6 | 124.6 | 93.7 | 30.9 |
| Physician services | 113.6 | 74.2 | 74.1 | 21.3 | 52.8 | 0.0 | 39.4 | 31.6 | 7.8 |
| Dental services | 31.6 | 30.8 | 30.8 | 17.3 | 13.5 | — | 0.7 | 0.4 | 0.3 |
| Other professional services | 27.1 | 21.5 | 18.6 | 7.9 | 10.6 | 3.0 | 5.6 | 4.2 | 1.3 |
| Home health care | 5.6 | 1.4 | 1.0 | 0.7 | 0.4 | 0.4 | 4.2 | 3.3 | 0.9 |
| Drugs and other medical non-durables | 50.6 | 45.5 | 45.5 | 38.1 | 7.3 | — | 5.1 | 2.5 | 2.6 |
| Vision products and other medical durables | 11.4 | 9.0 | 9.0 | 7.8 | 1.2 | — | 2.4 | 2.1 | 0.3 |
| Nursing home care | 47.7 | 22.3 | 21.4 | 20.8 | 0.5 | 0.9 | 25.4 | 16.4 | 9.0 |
| Other personal health care | 9.7 | 2.1 | — | — | — | 2.1 | 7.7 | 4.5 | 3.2 |
| Program administration and net cost of private health insurance | 33.9 | 27.3 | 26.8 | — | 26.8 | 0.5 | 6.6 | 4.3 | 2.3 |
| Government public health activities | 18.3 | — | — | — | — | — | 18.3 | 2.1 | 16.2 |
| Research and construction | 20.7 | 8.2 | — | — | — | 8.2 | 12.5 | 9.7 | 2.8 |
| Research | 11.0 | 0.8 | — | — | — | 0.8 | 10.3 | 8.9 | 1.4 |
| Construction | 9.6 | 7.4 | — | — | — | 7.4 | 2.2 | 0.8 | 1.4 |
| **1990** | | | | | | | | | |
| National health expenditures | 666.2 | 383.6 | 352.9 | 136.1 | 216.8 | 30.6 | 282.6 | 195.4 | 87.3 |
| Health services and supplies | 643.4 | 374.8 | 352.9 | 136.1 | 216.8 | 21.8 | 268.6 | 184.3 | 84.3 |
| Personal health care | 585.3 | 343.5 | 322.2 | 136.1 | 186.1 | 21.3 | 241.8 | 177.2 | 64.6 |
| Hospital care | 256.0 | 116.0 | 102.2 | 12.8 | 89.4 | 13.8 | 140.0 | 104.6 | 35.3 |
| Physician services | 125.7 | 81.7 | 81.7 | 23.5 | 58.2 | 0.0 | 43.9 | 35.1 | 8.8 |
| Dental services | 34.0 | 33.1 | 33.1 | 18.0 | 15.1 | — | 0.9 | 0.5 | 0.4 |
| Other professional services | 31.6 | 25.2 | 21.5 | 8.8 | 12.8 | 3.6 | 6.4 | 4.9 | 1.6 |
| Home health care | 6.9 | 1.8 | 1.3 | 0.8 | 0.5 | 0.5 | 5.1 | 4.1 | 1.0 |
| Drugs and other medical non-durables | 54.6 | 48.5 | 48.5 | 40.2 | 8.3 | — | 6.1 | 3.0 | 3.1 |
| Vision products and other medical durables | 12.1 | 9.4 | 9.4 | 8.2 | 1.3 | — | 2.7 | 2.4 | 0.3 |
| Nursing home care | 53.1 | 25.5 | 24.4 | 23.9 | 0.6 | 1.0 | 27.7 | 17.2 | 10.5 |
| Other personal health care | 11.3 | 2.2 | — | — | — | 2.2 | 9.1 | 5.5 | 3.5 |
| Program administration and net cost of private health insurance | 38.7 | 31.2 | 30.7 | — | 30.7 | 0.6 | 7.5 | 4.8 | 2.7 |
| Government public health activities | 19.3 | — | — | — | — | — | 19.3 | 2.3 | 17.0 |
| Research and construction | 22.8 | 8.8 | — | — | — | 8.8 | 14.0 | 11.0 | 3.0 |
| Research | 12.4 | 0.8 | — | — | — | 0.8 | 11.5 | 10.0 | 1.5 |
| Construction | 10.4 | 8.0 | — | — | — | 8.0 | 2.5 | 1.0 | 1.5 |

NOTES: 0.0 denotes amounts less than $50 million. Research and development expenditures of drug companies and other manufacturers and providers of medical equipment and supplies are excluded from research expenditures, but are included in the expenditure class in which the product falls. Numbers may not add to totals because of rounding.

SOURCE: Health Care Financing Administration, Office of the Actuary; Data from the Office of National Health Statistics.

## Table 11

### Personal health care expenditures aggregate and per capita amounts and percent distribution, by source of funds: Selected years 1960-90

| Year | Total | Out-of-pocket payments | Third-party payments Total | Private health insurance | Other private funds | Government Total | Federal | State and local | Medicare[1] | Medicaid[2] |
|---|---|---|---|---|---|---|---|---|---|---|
| | | | | | | | | | | |
| | | | | Amount in billions | | | | | | |
| 1960 | $23.9 | $13.3 | $10.5 | $5.0 | $0.4 | $5.1 | $2.1 | $3.0 | — | — |
| 1970 | 64.9 | 25.6 | 39.3 | 15.2 | 1.7 | 22.4 | 14.6 | 7.8 | $7.2 | $5.1 |
| 1980 | 219.4 | 59.5 | 159.9 | 65.3 | 7.6 | 87.1 | 63.5 | 23.6 | 36.4 | 24.8 |
| 1981 | 254.8 | 67.2 | 187.7 | 77.1 | 8.9 | 101.6 | 74.9 | 26.7 | 43.9 | 28.9 |
| 1982 | 286.4 | 74.2 | 212.2 | 88.5 | 10.2 | 113.5 | 84.0 | 29.5 | 51.4 | 30.6 |
| 1983 | 314.9 | 81.4 | 233.5 | 97.3 | 11.0 | 125.3 | 93.4 | 31.8 | 58.5 | 33.6 |
| 1984 | 341.2 | 87.7 | 253.5 | 106.3 | 11.4 | 135.7 | 101.8 | 33.9 | 64.4 | 36.0 |
| 1985 | 369.7 | 94.4 | 275.3 | 114.0 | 12.9 | 148.4 | 111.8 | 36.6 | 70.4 | 39.7 |
| 1986 | 400.8 | 100.9 | 299.9 | 123.8 | 14.0 | 162.1 | 120.7 | 41.4 | 75.7 | 42.9 |
| 1987 | 439.3 | 108.8 | 330.5 | 137.7 | 15.0 | 177.8 | 130.8 | 46.9 | 81.7 | 48.2 |
| 1988 | 482.8 | 119.3 | 363.5 | 154.1 | 16.8 | 192.6 | 141.7 | 50.9 | 88.5 | 52.1 |
| 1989 | 529.9 | 126.1 | 403.8 | 169.6 | 19.0 | 215.2 | 158.8 | 56.3 | 100.3 | 59.2 |
| 1990 | 585.3 | 136.1 | 449.2 | 186.1 | 21.3 | 241.8 | 177.2 | 64.6 | 108.9 | 71.3 |
| | | | | Per capita amount | | | | | | |
| 1960 | $126 | $70 | $55 | $26 | $2 | $27 | $11 | $16 | — | — |
| 1970 | 302 | 119 | 183 | 71 | 8 | 104 | 68 | 36 | (3) | (3) |
| 1980 | 933 | 253 | 680 | 277 | 32 | 370 | 270 | 100 | (3) | (3) |
| 1981 | 1,073 | 283 | 790 | 325 | 38 | 428 | 315 | 112 | (3) | (3) |
| 1982 | 1,193 | 309 | 884 | 368 | 43 | 473 | 350 | 123 | (3) | (3) |
| 1983 | 1,299 | 336 | 963 | 401 | 45 | 517 | 385 | 131 | (3) | (3) |
| 1984 | 1,394 | 358 | 1,036 | 434 | 47 | 555 | 416 | 139 | (3) | (3) |
| 1985 | 1,496 | 382 | 1,114 | 461 | 52 | 600 | 452 | 148 | (3) | (3) |
| 1986 | 1,606 | 404 | 1,202 | 496 | 56 | 650 | 484 | 166 | (3) | (3) |
| 1987 | 1,743 | 432 | 1,311 | 546 | 60 | 705 | 519 | 186 | (3) | (3) |
| 1988 | 1,897 | 469 | 1,428 | 606 | 66 | 757 | 557 | 200 | (3) | (3) |
| 1989 | 2,062 | 491 | 1,571 | 660 | 74 | 837 | 618 | 219 | (3) | (3) |
| 1990 | 2,255 | 524 | 1,731 | 717 | 82 | 932 | 683 | 249 | (3) | (3) |
| | | | | Percent distribution | | | | | | |
| 1960 | 100.0 | 55.9 | 44.1 | 21.0 | 1.7 | 21.4 | 8.9 | 12.5 | — | — |
| 1970 | 100.0 | 39.5 | 60.5 | 23.4 | 2.6 | 34.6 | 22.6 | 12.0 | 11.1 | 7.8 |
| 1980 | 100.0 | 27.1 | 72.9 | 29.7 | 3.5 | 39.7 | 28.9 | 10.8 | 16.6 | 11.3 |
| 1981 | 100.0 | 26.4 | 73.6 | 30.3 | 3.5 | 39.9 | 29.4 | 10.5 | 17.2 | 11.3 |
| 1982 | 100.0 | 25.9 | 74.1 | 30.9 | 3.6 | 39.6 | 29.3 | 10.3 | 17.9 | 10.7 |
| 1983 | 100.0 | 25.8 | 74.2 | 30.9 | 3.5 | 39.8 | 29.7 | 10.1 | 18.6 | 10.7 |
| 1984 | 100.0 | 25.7 | 74.3 | 31.2 | 3.4 | 39.8 | 29.8 | 9.9 | 18.9 | 10.6 |
| 1985 | 100.0 | 25.5 | 74.5 | 30.8 | 3.5 | 40.1 | 30.2 | 9.9 | 19.0 | 10.7 |
| 1986 | 100.0 | 25.2 | 74.8 | 30.9 | 3.5 | 40.5 | 30.1 | 10.3 | 18.9 | 10.7 |
| 1987 | 100.0 | 24.8 | 75.2 | 31.3 | 3.4 | 40.5 | 29.8 | 10.7 | 18.6 | 11.0 |
| 1988 | 100.0 | 24.7 | 75.3 | 31.9 | 3.5 | 39.9 | 29.4 | 10.5 | 18.3 | 10.8 |
| 1989 | 100.0 | 23.8 | 76.2 | 32.0 | 3.6 | 40.6 | 30.0 | 10.6 | 18.9 | 11.2 |
| 1990 | 100.0 | 23.3 | 76.7 | 31.8 | 3.6 | 41.3 | 30.3 | 11.0 | 18.6 | 12.2 |

[1] Subset of Federal funds.
[2] Subset of Federal and State and local funds.
[3] Calculation of per capita estimates is inappropriate.

NOTES: Per capita amounts based on July 1 Social Security area population estimates. Numbers and percents may not add to totals because of rounding.

SOURCE: Health Care Financing Administration. Office of the Actuary: Data from the Office of National Health Statistics.

## Table 12
## Personal health care expenditures, by type of expenditure and selected sources of payment:
## Selected years 1960-90

| Source of payment | Total | Hospital care | Physician services | Dental services | Other professional services | Home health care | Drugs and other medical non-durables | Vision products and other medical durables | Nursing home care | Other personal care |
|---|---|---|---|---|---|---|---|---|---|---|
| **1960** | | | | | | Amount in billions | | | | |
| Personal health care expenditures | $23.9 | $9.3 | $5.3 | $2.0 | $0.6 | $0.0 | $4.2 | $0.8 | $1.0 | $0.7 |
| Out-of-pocket payments | 13.3 | 1.9 | 3.3 | 1.9 | 0.5 | 0.0 | 4.1 | 0.8 | 0.8 | — |
| Third-party payments | 10.5 | 7.4 | 2.0 | 0.1 | 0.1 | 0.0 | 0.1 | 0.1 | 0.2 | 0.7 |
| Private health insurance | 5.0 | 3.3 | 1.6 | 0.0 | 0.0 | 0.0 | 0.0 | 0.0 | 0.0 | — |
| Other private | 0.4 | 0.1 | 0.0 | — | 0.0 | 0.0 | — | — | 0.1 | 0.2 |
| Government | 5.1 | 3.9 | 0.4 | 0.0 | 0.0 | 0.0 | 0.1 | 0.0 | 0.1 | 0.5 |
| Federal | 2.1 | 1.6 | 0.1 | 0.0 | 0.0 | — | 0.0 | 0.0 | 0.1 | 0.3 |
| Medicare | — | — | — | — | — | — | — | — | — | — |
| Medicaid | — | — | — | — | — | — | — | — | — | — |
| Other | 2.1 | 1.6 | 0.1 | 0.0 | 0.0 | 0.0 | 0.0 | 0.0 | 0.1 | 0.3 |
| State and local | 3.0 | 2.3 | 0.3 | 0.0 | 0.0 | 0.0 | 0.0 | 0.0 | 0.1 | 0.2 |
| Medicaid | — | — | — | — | — | — | — | — | — | — |
| Other | 3.0 | 2.3 | 0.3 | 0.0 | 0.0 | 0.0 | 0.0 | 0.0 | 0.1 | 0.2 |
| Total Medicaid | — | — | — | — | — | — | — | — | — | — |
| **1970** | | | | | | | | | | |
| Personal health care expenditures | 64.9 | 27.9 | 13.6 | 4.7 | 1.5 | 0.1 | 8.8 | 2.0 | 4.9 | 1.4 |
| Out-of-pocket payments | 25.6 | 2.5 | 5.8 | 4.2 | 0.9 | 0.0 | 8.0 | 1.8 | 2.3 | — |
| Third-party payments | 39.3 | 25.4 | 7.8 | 0.4 | 0.7 | 0.1 | 0.8 | 0.2 | 2.5 | 1.4 |
| Private health insurance | 15.2 | 9.6 | 4.8 | 0.2 | 0.1 | 0.0 | 0.3 | 0.1 | 0.0 | — |
| Other private | 1.7 | 0.9 | 0.0 | — | 0.1 | 0.1 | — | — | 0.2 | 0.3 |
| Government | 22.4 | 14.9 | 3.0 | 0.2 | 0.4 | 0.1 | 0.5 | 0.1 | 2.3 | 1.1 |
| Federal | 14.6 | 9.8 | 2.1 | 0.1 | 0.2 | 0.1 | 0.2 | 0.1 | 1.4 | 0.6 |
| Medicare | 7.2 | 5.3 | 1.6 | — | 0.0 | 0.1 | — | 0.0 | 0.2 | — |
| Medicaid | 2.7 | 1.2 | 0.3 | 0.1 | 0.0 | 0.0 | 0.2 | — | 0.7 | 0.1 |
| Other | 4.7 | 3.3 | 0.2 | 0.0 | 0.2 | — | 0.0 | 0.0 | 0.4 | 0.5 |
| State and local | 7.8 | 5.1 | 0.8 | 0.1 | 0.1 | 0.0 | 0.2 | 0.0 | 0.9 | 0.5 |
| Medicaid | 2.3 | 1.0 | 0.3 | 0.1 | 0.0 | 0.0 | 0.2 | — | 0.6 | 0.1 |
| Other | 5.5 | 4.1 | 0.5 | 0.0 | 0.1 | 0.0 | 0.1 | 0.0 | 0.3 | 0.4 |
| Total Medicaid | 5.1 | 2.2 | 0.6 | 0.2 | 0.1 | 0.0 | 0.4 | — | 1.4 | 0.2 |
| **1988** | | | | | | | | | | |
| Personal health care expenditures | 482.8 | 212.0 | 105.1 | 29.4 | 23.8 | 4.5 | 46.3 | 10.1 | 42.8 | 8.7 |
| Out-of-pocket payments | 119.3 | 11.2 | 20.9 | 16.3 | 7.6 | 0.5 | 35.3 | 6.8 | 20.6 | — |
| Third-party payments | 363.5 | 200.8 | 84.3 | 13.1 | 16.1 | 4.0 | 11.0 | 3.3 | 22.2 | 8.7 |
| Private health insurance | 154.1 | 75.4 | 49.1 | 12.4 | 8.9 | 0.3 | 6.5 | 1.0 | 0.5 | — |
| Other private | 16.8 | 11.1 | 0.0 | — | 2.6 | 0.3 | — | — | 0.8 | 1.9 |
| Government | 192.6 | 114.3 | 35.1 | 0.7 | 4.6 | 3.4 | 4.5 | 2.2 | 20.9 | 6.9 |
| Federal | 141.7 | 86.2 | 28.1 | 0.4 | 3.5 | 2.6 | 2.2 | 2.0 | 12.6 | 4.2 |
| Medicare | 88.5 | 57.5 | 24.2 | — | 2.1 | 1.8 | — | 1.8 | 1.0 | — |
| Medicaid | 29.4 | 11.2 | 2.2 | 0.3 | 0.8 | 0.8 | 2.1 | — | 10.7 | 1.3 |
| Other | 23.9 | 17.5 | 1.7 | 0.1 | 0.6 | — | 0.1 | 0.2 | 1.0 | 2.9 |
| State and local | 50.9 | 28.1 | 7.0 | 0.3 | 1.1 | 0.7 | 2.3 | 0.3 | 8.3 | 2.7 |
| Medicaid | 22.7 | 8.8 | 1.5 | 0.3 | 0.6 | 0.7 | 1.5 | — | 8.3 | 1.0 |
| Other | 28.2 | 19.3 | 5.5 | 0.1 | 0.5 | 0.0 | 0.8 | 0.3 | 0.0 | 1.7 |
| Total Medicaid | 52.1 | 20.0 | 3.7 | 0.6 | 1.4 | 1.5 | 3.6 | — | 19.0 | 2.2 |

## Table 12—Continued

| Source of payment | Total | Hospital care | Physician services | Dental services | Other professional services | Home health care | Drugs and other medical non-durables | Vision products and other medical durables | Nursing home care | Other personal care |
|---|---|---|---|---|---|---|---|---|---|---|
| **1989** | | | | | | | | | | |
| Personal health care expenditures | $529.9 | $232.6 | $113.6 | $31.6 | $27.1 | $5.6 | $50.6 | $11.4 | $47.7 | $9.7 |
| Out-of-pocket payments | 126.1 | 12.1 | 21.3 | 17.3 | 7.9 | 0.7 | 38.1 | 7.8 | 20.8 | — |
| Third-party payments | 403.8 | 220.5 | 92.2 | 14.2 | 19.2 | 5.0 | 12.4 | 3.6 | 26.9 | 9.7 |
| Private health insurance | 169.6 | 83.2 | 52.8 | 13.5 | 10.6 | 0.4 | 7.3 | 1.2 | 0.5 | — |
| Other private | 19.0 | 12.6 | 0.0 | — | 3.0 | 0.4 | — | — | 0.9 | 2.1 |
| Government | 215.2 | 124.6 | 39.4 | 0.7 | 5.6 | 4.2 | 5.1 | 2.4 | 25.4 | 7.7 |
| Federal | 158.8 | 93.7 | 31.6 | 0.4 | 4.2 | 3.3 | 2.5 | 2.1 | 16.4 | 4.5 |
| Medicare | 100.3 | 62.2 | 27.4 | — | 2.6 | 2.3 | — | 2.0 | 3.8 | — |
| Medicaid | 33.6 | 13.0 | 2.5 | 0.4 | 1.0 | 1.0 | 2.4 | — | 11.7 | 1.7 |
| Other | 24.9 | 18.6 | 1.7 | 0.1 | 0.6 | — | 0.1 | 0.2 | 0.9 | 2.7 |
| State and local | 56.3 | 30.9 | 7.8 | 0.3 | 1.3 | 0.9 | 2.6 | 0.3 | 9.0 | 3.2 |
| Medicaid | 25.6 | 10.0 | 1.7 | 0.3 | 0.7 | 0.9 | 1.7 | — | 8.9 | 1.3 |
| Other | 30.8 | 20.9 | 6.0 | 0.1 | 0.6 | 0.0 | 0.9 | 0.3 | 0.0 | 1.9 |
| Total Medicaid | 59.2 | 22.9 | 4.3 | 0.6 | 1.7 | 1.9 | 4.1 | — | 20.6 | 3.1 |
| **1990** | | | | | | | | | | |
| Personal health care expenditures | 585.3 | 256.0 | 125.7 | 34.0 | 31.6 | 6.9 | 54.6 | 12.1 | 53.1 | 11.3 |
| Out-of-pocket payments | 136.1 | 12.8 | 23.5 | 18.0 | 8.8 | 0.8 | 40.2 | 8.2 | 23.9 | — |
| Third-party payments | 449.2 | 243.2 | 102.2 | 16.0 | 22.8 | 6.1 | 14.4 | 4.0 | 29.3 | 11.3 |
| Private health insurance | 186.1 | 89.4 | 58.2 | 15.1 | 12.8 | 0.5 | 8.3 | 1.3 | 0.6 | — |
| Other private | 21.3 | 13.8 | 0.0 | — | 3.6 | 0.5 | — | — | 1.0 | 2.2 |
| Government | 241.8 | 140.0 | 43.9 | 0.9 | 6.4 | 5.1 | 6.1 | 2.7 | 27.7 | 9.1 |
| Federal | 177.2 | 104.6 | 35.1 | 0.5 | 4.9 | 4.1 | 3.0 | 2.4 | 17.2 | 5.5 |
| Medicare | 108.9 | 68.3 | 30.0 | — | 3.1 | 2.9 | — | 2.2 | 2.5 | — |
| Medicaid | 40.6 | 16.2 | 3.1 | 0.4 | 1.2 | 1.2 | 2.9 | — | 13.7 | 2.0 |
| Other | 27.7 | 20.1 | 2.0 | 0.1 | 0.7 | — | 0.1 | 0.2 | 1.0 | 3.5 |
| State and local | 64.6 | 35.3 | 8.8 | 0.4 | 1.6 | 1.0 | 3.1 | 0.3 | 10.5 | 3.5 |
| Medicaid | 30.7 | 12.3 | 2.1 | 0.3 | 0.9 | 1.0 | 2.1 | — | 10.5 | 1.6 |
| Other | 33.9 | 23.0 | 6.7 | 0.1 | 0.7 | 0.0 | 1.0 | 0.3 | 0.1 | 2.0 |
| Total Medicaid | 71.3 | 28.5 | 5.2 | 0.7 | 2.0 | 2.2 | 4.9 | — | 24.1 | 3.6 |

NOTES: 0.0 denotes amounts less than $50 million. Medicaid expenditures exclude Part B premium payments to Medicare by States under buy-in agreements to cover premiums for eligible Medicaid recipients. Numbers may not add to totals because of rounding

SOURCE: Health Care Financing Administration, Office of the Actuary: Data from the Office of National Health Statistics

# Table 13

## Expenditures for health services and supplies under public programs, by type of expenditure and program: 1990

| Program area | All expenditures | Personal health care Total | Hospital care | Physician services | Dental services | Other professional services | Home health care | Drugs and other medical non-durables | Vision products and other medical durables | Nursing home care | Other | Administration | Public health activities |
|---|---|---|---|---|---|---|---|---|---|---|---|---|---|
| | | | | | | Amount in billions | | | | | | | |
| Public and private spending | $643.4 | $585.3 | $256.0 | $125.7 | $34.0 | $31.6 | $6.9 | $54.6 | $12.1 | $53.1 | $11.3 | $38.7 | $19.3 |
| All public programs | 268.6 | 241.8 | 140.0 | 43.9 | 0.9 | 6.4 | 5.1 | 6.1 | 2.7 | 27.7 | 9.1 | 7.5 | 19.3 |
| Federal funds | 184.3 | 177.2 | 104.6 | 35.1 | 0.5 | 4.9 | 4.1 | 3.0 | 2.4 | 17.2 | 5.5 | 4.8 | 2.3 |
| State and local funds | 84.3 | 64.6 | 35.3 | 8.8 | 0.4 | 1.6 | 1.0 | 3.1 | 0.3 | 10.5 | 3.5 | 2.7 | 17.0 |
| Medicare | 111.2 | 108.9 | 68.3 | 30.0 | — | 3.1 | 2.9 | — | 2.2 | 2.5 | — | 2.3 | — |
| Medicaid[1] | 75.2 | 71.3 | 28.5 | 5.2 | 0.7 | 2.0 | 2.2 | 4.9 | — | 24.1 | 3.6 | 3.8 | — |
| Federal | 42.9 | 40.6 | 16.2 | 3.1 | 0.4 | 1.2 | 1.2 | 2.9 | — | 13.7 | 2.0 | 2.2 | — |
| State and local | 32.3 | 30.7 | 12.3 | 2.1 | 0.3 | 0.9 | 1.0 | 2.1 | — | 10.5 | 1.6 | 1.6 | — |
| Other State and local public assistance programs | 4.2 | 4.2 | 2.7 | 0.5 | 0.0 | 0.1 | 0.0 | 0.7 | 0.1 | 0.1 | 0.1 | 0.0 | — |
| Department of Veterans Affairs[2] | 11.4 | 11.4 | 9.5 | 0.1 | 0.0 | — | — | 0.0 | 0.1 | 1.0 | 0.5 | 0.0 | — |
| Department of Defense[2] | 11.5 | 11.3 | 9.1 | 1.4 | 0.0 | — | — | 0.1 | — | — | 0.7 | 0.2 | — |
| Workers' compensation | 15.6 | 14.6 | 7.4 | 6.2 | — | 0.4 | — | 0.3 | 0.3 | — | — | 1.0 | — |
| Federal | 0.5 | 0.4 | 0.3 | 0.1 | — | 0.0 | — | 0.0 | 0.0 | — | — | 0.0 | — |
| State and local | 15.1 | 14.1 | 7.1 | 6.0 | — | 0.4 | — | 0.3 | 0.3 | — | — | 1.0 | — |
| State and local hospitals[3] | 14.1 | 14.1 | 13.0 | — | — | — | — | — | — | — | — | — | — |
| Other public programs for personal health care[4] | 6.2 | 6.0 | 1.5 | 0.5 | 0.0 | 0.8 | — | 0.0 | 0.1 | — | 3.1 | 0.2 | — |
| Federal | 4.6 | 4.5 | 1.2 | 0.3 | 0.0 | 0.6 | — | 0.0 | 0.1 | — | 2.3 | 0.1 | — |
| State and local | 1.6 | 1.5 | 0.3 | 0.2 | 0.0 | 0.2 | — | 0.0 | 0.0 | — | 0.8 | 0.1 | — |
| Government public health activities | 19.3 | — | — | — | — | — | — | — | — | — | — | — | 19.3 |
| Federal | 2.3 | — | — | — | — | — | — | — | — | — | — | — | 2.3 |
| State and local | 17.0 | — | — | — | — | — | — | — | — | — | — | — | 17.0 |
| Medicare and Medicaid | 186.4 | 180.2 | 96.8 | 35.2 | 0.7 | 5.1 | 5.1 | 4.9 | 2.2 | 26.6 | 3.6 | 6.1 | — |

[1] Excludes funds paid into the Medicare trust funds by States under "buy-in" agreements to cover premiums for public assistance recipients and for people who are medically indigent.

[2] Includes care for retirees and military dependents.

[3] Expenditures not offset by revenues.

[4] Includes program spending for maternal and child health; vocational rehabilitation medical payments; temporary disability insurance medical payments; Public Health Service and other Federal hospitals; Indian health services; alcoholism, drug abuse, and mental health; and school health.

NOTES: 0.0 denotes amounts less than $50 million. Numbers may not add to totals because of rounding.

SOURCE: Health Care Financing Administration, Office of the Actuary: Data from the Office of National Health Statistics.

# Chapter 15

# Projections of National Health Expenditures through the Year 2000

Sally T. Sonnefeld, Daniel R. Waldo, Jeffrey A. Lemieux, and David R. McKusick

*In this article, the authors present a scenario for health expenditures during the 1990s. Assuming that current laws and practices remain unchanged, the Nation will spend $1.6 trillion for health care in the year 2000, an amount equal to 16.4 percent of that year's gross national product. Medicare and Medicaid will foot an increasing share of the Nation's health bill, rising to more than one-third of the total. The factors accounting for growth in national health spending are described as well as the effects of those factors on spending by type of service and by source of funds.*

## INTRODUCTION

Concern over rapid increases in health care spending is reaching a fevered pitch. Rapid growth in expenditures is not new: Spending for health care has grown faster than the overall economy in almost every one of the last 30 years. As a direct result of differential growth, health expenditures have risen as a share of our Nation's gross national product (GNP), from 5.3 percent in 1960 to 11.6 percent in 1989. This percentage is widely perceived as a measure of the impact of health expenditures on the Nation's ability to finance health care. Therefore, a flurry of renewed concern resulted when the combination of economic stagnation and "business as usual" in the health care sector drove health expenditures as a percent of the GNP to a projected 12.3 percent in 1990.

This concern has been heightened by two additional factors. First, government health programs are in serious financial difficulty. The trust fund for the Federal hospital insurance (HI) program (better known as Medicare Part A), which derives most of its income from payroll taxes, is currently projected to be exhausted in 2005. Unless additional sources of revenue are tapped, benefits would need to be reduced by $46 billion in that year. Ultimately, the program would need to be cut by more than 50 percent. In addition, State-operated Medicaid programs, which are financed through a combination of State and Federal taxes, are in generally dire financial straits. State income taxes dwindle during economic slowdowns, but program demands increase with the cost of health care in general and with the number of unemployed and low-income residents of the State.

Second, private financing of health care is reaching a watershed. Employer payments for health care (including health-related payroll taxes), which amounted to 14 percent of aggregate after-tax profits in 1965, today

Reprinted from *Health Care Financing Review*, Fall 1991, Vol 13, No. 1.

exceed after-tax profits (Levit et al., 1991a). The distribution of that burden is uneven across employers, further disadvantaging some. Yet, despite the large private expenditure for health care insurance, as many as 15 percent of Americans lack even the most rudimentary health insurance. Between 33 and 38 million people have—either by choice or not—neither private nor public insurance. And many Americans have little insurance protection against truly catastrophic medical expenses.

Given these factors, an unusual chorus of voices is calling for reform of the U.S. health care system. Some large employers and conservative policymakers, traditionally leery of government intervention in private matters, see national reform as a way to relieve themselves of a fringe benefit that is uncontrollable as well as being a source of contract dispute. Liberal policymakers see reform as necessary to extend health care coverage to the uninsured and underinsured population. Even provider organizations, some of which have traditionally been hostile to government attempts to change market rules, have recently offered proposals for reform of the system.

In light of the clamor for reform, it is instructive to speculate on what health expenditures might look like in the next 10 years in the absence of any such reform. To do so can yield insights regarding which services and goods will experience more demand than others. In addition, a projection scenario can provide a "big picture" for the various parties paying for health care.

In this article, we have used an actuarial projection model of the health care sector to project national health expenditures (NHE) through the end of the century. The scenario is tied to the assumptions and conclusions of the Medicare actuaries concerning progress of that program, providing the context for discussion of the future of Medicare. Use of the projection model also facilitates a discussion of the trends in the use, intensity, and price of various types of health goods and services.

Of course, such a model does not predict the future. Macroeconomic shocks, reforms in health care financing and delivery, technological breakthroughs, and unexpected changes in morbidity and mortality all affect what will happen. What the model does show is what might plausibly happen if current mechanisms, laws, and programs continue in existence through the end of the century. Thus, the model provides a "base case" against which the advantages and disadvantages of proposed reforms can be measured.

Detailed Tables 6–10 at the end of this article show expenditures for health for selected years 1966 through 2000, both by type of service and by source of funds. Data figures from the detailed tables are highlighted throughout this article.

## PROJECTION MODEL

The model used to develop the scenario we discuss is built upon actuarial models described in previous articles on projections of expenditure (Arnett et al., 1986; Division of National Cost Estimates, 1987). It is actuarial in nature, relying on trend analysis rather than econometric fitting of dependent to independent variables, and consists of a series of identities, the factors of which are projected and reconciled.

The projections are based on historical estimates of NHE. Estimates of annual expenditure by type of service and by source of fund comprise the overall framework within which the model operates. The scenario we present was developed using historical figures through 1989 (Lazenby and Letsch, 1990); elsewhere . . . , colleagues present updated figures for the last several years, along with a preliminary figure for 1990 (Levit et al., 1991b). To the extent that these newer figures differ from those used to prepare our projections, particularly for professional services, the level of the projected expenditures (especially in 1991) may not be strictly comparable with the newest history, but the longrun trends we discuss are not significantly affected by the revisions.

The projection scenario incorporates several exogenous factors. As already mentioned, it is tied to the assumptions and conclusions of the Medicare trustees' reports for 1991. Projected values of hospital insurance and supplementary medical insurance benefits are built into the projection model.

Similarly, the scenario takes as given the macroeconomic assumptions used to prepare the Medicare and Social Security trust fund reports. Those reports contain three different sets of assumptions: optimistic, intermediate, and pessimistic. We used Alternative II assumptions (the intermediate scenario) to prepare our projections. In theory, differential growth of health care spending should affect macroeconomic activity as well as sector-specific activity, but at present, the former effects are not explicitly modeled. We are working to incorporate the projection model with a model of the general macroeconomy, but results of that effort are not yet available. However, because our scenario assumes the continuation of current practices and mechanisms, we expect that the projection results are quite consistent with what would have resulted from a fully integrated model.

In addition to exogenous macroeconomic assumptions, our model incorporates projections of provider manpower. Projections of the number of physicians and dentists made by the Health Resources and Services Administration (Bureau of Health Professions, 1990) have been used when projecting expenditures for the services of those professionals.

As mentioned earlier, the model used for our projections consists of a series of identity equations. The typical equation consists of seven factors that describe expenditure for a good or service:

$$E = \text{Pop} \times \text{PGNP} \times \frac{\text{Price}}{\text{PGNP}} \times \text{Ua} \times \frac{\text{Util}}{\text{Pop} \times \text{Ua}}$$

$$\times \text{Ra} \times \frac{E}{\text{Price} \times \text{Util} \times \text{Ra}}$$

where the factors are defined as follows:

*Pop*—This is the number of people in the United States as of July 1. Projections are made by Social Security Administration actuaries and are exogenous to the model (Board of Trustees of the Old Age, Survivors, and Disability Trust Fund, 1991).

*PGNP*—This represents the GNP implicit price deflator, which is a measure of economywide price inflation. It is exogenous to the model, having been projected by the Social Security and Medicare trustees (Board of Trustees of the Old Age, Survivors, and Disability Trust Fund, 1991).

$\dfrac{\text{Price}}{\text{PGNP}}$—This measure compares the price of the health good or service to general inflation, that is, it reflects sector-specific price inflation. It captures demand-pull inflationary pressures such as changes in income or insurance status. It also captures supply-push factors such as differential productivity and wage growth and provider-pricing strategies.

*Ua*—This is a factor that reflects the effect of the age-sex composition of the population on use of that good or service. For example, as the proportion of the population 75 years of age or over increases, we can expect to see greater use of nursing home care, even in the absence of any other changes. The construction of this factor, which is exogenous, has been described elsewhere (Arnett et al., 1986).

$\dfrac{\text{Util}}{\text{Pop} \times \text{Ua}}$—This factor captures use per capita other than that generated by demographics. The specific measure varies by type of service. For example, inpatient days are used to project hospital inpatient expenditure, and outpatient visits are used to project hospital outpatient expenditure.

*Ra*—This term captures the effect of the age-sex composition of the population on the intensity of service, that is, on expenditures per unit of use, net of price effects. As with the term "Ua," this factor is exogenous, and its construction is similar to that of the age-sex use factor as well.

$\dfrac{E}{\text{Price} \times \text{Util} \times \text{Ra}}$—This term is a residual. It reflects intensity net of age and sex effects and might be called "real expenditure per unit of service." It incorporates the effects of changes in technology and in the mix of procedures performed during the unit of service. It also reflects changes in regulations or policies that affect the quantity and quality of resources used to produce a unit of service. Like any residual, this term also reflects the accumulation of measurement errors, as well as the effects of all other factors not specifically or implicitly identified elsewhere.

## MACROECONOMIC AND OTHER EXOGENOUS ASSUMPTIONS

### The Economy

The U.S. economic outlook to the year 2000 is characterized by low inflation and modest growth rates in real output (Table 1). The economy is projected to recover from its recession in mid-1991, with real GNP growth increasing from −0.1 percent in 1991 to 3.1 percent in 1992. Real growth rates then eventually stabilize at about 2.2 percent in the second half of the decade. Price inflation (measured by the implicit price deflator for GNP) falls from 4.1 percent in 1990 to 3.5 percent in 1991, before rising gradually to 4.0 percent in 1996 and thereafter. Nominal (current-dollar) GNP therefore reaches a steady 6.2−percent growth rate after the economy recovers from the current business cycle.

The slower growth of real output parallels forecasts of slower civilian labor force growth in the 1990s, as the rate of growth of the working-age population falls and the labor force participation rate (which has increased steadily since the 1960s) levels off. For the 1990s, our projections incorporate average real GNP growth of 2.1 percent, as opposed to 2.7 percent in the 1980s and 2.8 percent in the 1970s. Similarly, inflation in the 1990s will average 3.9 percent, compared with 4.4 percent in the 1980s and 7.4 percent in the 1970s.

### Demographic Change

The total U.S. population is projected to increase about 0.9 percent per year in the 1990s, slowing slightly from the 1.0-percent rate in the 1980s (derived from Table 1). Social Security Administration actuaries project that the population 65 years of age or over will increase 1.1 percent per year and that the population 75 years of age or over will increase 2.3 percent per year in the 1990s (Board of Trustees of the Old Age, Survivors, and Disability Trust Fund, 1991).

## Table 1
### Macroeconomic assumptions used to project national health expenditures: Selected years 1965-2000

| | Gross national product | | | Population in thousands | | |
|---|---|---|---|---|---|---|
| Year | Current dollars in billions | 1982 dollars in billions | Implicit price deflator | Total | 65 years of age or over | 75 years of age or over |
| **Historical** | | | | | | |
| 1965 | $705 | $2,088 | 33.8 | 203,990 | 19,068 | 6,904 |
| 1975 | 1,598 | 2,695 | 59.3 | 224,653 | 23,228 | 9,103 |
| 1980 | 2,732 | 3,187 | 85.7 | 235,252 | 26,125 | 10,413 |
| 1985 | 4,015 | 3,619 | 110.9 | 247,166 | 29,023 | 11,972 |
| 1989 | 5,201 | 4,118 | 126.3 | 256,995 | 31,415 | 13,205 |
| **Projections** | | | | | | |
| 1990 | 5,463 | 4,156 | 131.5 | 259,573 | 31,995 | 13,516 |
| 1991 | 5,650 | 4,152 | 136.1 | 262,102 | 32,527 | 13,827 |
| 1992 | 6,045 | 4,282 | 141.2 | 264,630 | 33,039 | 14,156 |
| 1995 | 7,284 | 4,598 | 158.4 | 271,975 | 34,402 | 15,187 |
| 2000 | 9,865 | 5,118 | 192.7 | 282,889 | 35,682 | 17,035 |

SOURCE: Board of Trustees of the Old Age, Survivors, and Disability trust funds: The 1991 annual report of the board, pursuant to section 201(c)(2) of the Social Security Act as amended. Social Security Administration, May 1991.

The aging of the population is frequently cited as a major factor in the growth of health care expenditures, but such is not yet the case. Although it is true that changes in demographics will have an effect on spending, the impact is relatively small during the projection period. People 65 years of age or over spend an average of four times as much on health care as do those under the age of 65 (Waldo et al., 1989), but the proportion of the population 65 or over is projected to increase only slightly during the 1990s, from 12.3 percent in 1990 to 12.6 percent in 2000. Using age-sex indexes described in . . . Arnett et al., 1986 . . . , we estimate that changes in the age-sex composition of the population will contribute only 4.6 percent to the 147–percent increase in total personal health care expenditures from 1990 to 2000.

## Table 2
### Effects of the age-sex composition of the population on growth in personal health care expenditures, between 1990 and 2000, by selected type of service

| | Percent difference |
|---|---|
| Personal health care | 4.6 |
| Hospital inpatient care | 5.1 |
| Hospital outpatient care | 2.2 |
| Physician services | 2.3 |
| Dentist services | 1.2 |
| Other professional services | 12.6 |
| Home health care | 21.4 |
| Drugs and medical non-durables | 4.8 |
| Nursing home care | 13.4 |

NOTE: Figures reflect how much higher expenditure is projected to be in the year 2000 than it would have been in the absence of demographic change in the population after 1990.

SOURCE: Health Care Financing Administration, Office of the Actuary: Data from the Office of National Health Statistics.

The biggest influence of demographic change will not occur until well into the next century, when the baby boom generation enters the cohorts of 65 years of age and over. After 2015, the aged proportion of the population increases rapidly, reaching 20.4 percent by 2030.

Although the contribution of demographic change to total growth during the next 10 years is small, the impact is not uniform across all services (Table 2). The age-sex factor adds only about one-half of 1 percent per year to the use of inpatient hospital services and actually has a negative effect on the growth in intensity (cost per day is lower for aged patients). The impact on physician expenditures is also small, adding only 0.2 percent a year to its growth. However, an increase in the 1990s of the proportion of the population that is 75 years of age or over has a fairly large effect on the services used by the very old, primarily nursing home and home health services. The age-sex factors add 1.3 percent to the average annual growth of these services during the period.

### Health Professions Manpower

Our model incorporates exogenous estimates of health manpower made by the Public Health Service (Table 3).

The rate of growth in the number of physicians will slow in the 1990s but will remain considerably above the rate of population growth. Thus, the number of physicians per person will continue to increase in the next decade (Table 3).

The rate of growth of the number of practicing dentists fell considerably in the late 1980s, and Public Health Service analysts expect the decline to continue in the 1990s. The number of dentists per capita will begin

## Table 3
### Historical estimates and projections of the number of active physicians and dentists as of December 31: Selected years 1965-2000

| Year | Total | Medical doctors | Doctors of osteopathy | Dentists |
|---|---|---|---|---|
| | | Active physicians | | |
| Historical | | | | |
| 1965 | 288,700 | 277,600 | 11,100 | 95,990 |
| 1975 | 384,400 | 370,400 | 14,000 | 112,450 |
| 1980 | 457,500 | 440,400 | 17,100 | 126,200 |
| 1985 | 534,457 | 512,849 | 21,608 | 140,700 |
| 1989 | 587,454 | 560,937 | 26,517 | 148,300 |
| Projections | | | | |
| 1990 | 601,060 | 573,310 | 27,750 | 149,700 |
| 1991 | 614,300 | 585,400 | 28,900 | 152,000 |
| 1992 | 627,300 | 597,200 | 30,100 | 152,000 |
| 1995 | 664,700 | 631,100 | 33,600 | 154,000 |
| 2000 | 721,600 | 682,120 | 39,480 | 154,600 |

SOURCE: (Bureau of Health Professions, 1990); unpublished data from the Bureau of Health Professions: Data developed by the authors.

falling in the early 1990s, although the absolute number of active dentists will actually peak just before the year 2000 before declining (Bureau of Health Professions, 1990).

## PROJECTION RESULTS: TYPES OF SERVICE

### National Health Expenditures

With the impetus imparted by current laws and practices, NHE will rise to $1.6 trillion in the year 2000, an amount equal to 16.4 percent of that year's GNP (Figure 1). The projected percentage of GNP accounted for by health spending at the end of the century is higher than the 15.0 percent figure reported in the most recent of a series of projections articles produced by the Health Care Financing Administration (Division of National Cost Estimates, 1987). In part, this reflects a higher level of projected health expenditures: The $1.6 trillion is 5.5 percent higher than our projection made 4 years ago. In addition, the projected GNP incorporated in this model is 3 percent lower than our previous projections.

During the 1990s, an increasing share of NHE will be spent for hospital and physician services (Figure 2). Driven by that shift, Medicare and Medicaid will account for an increasing share of total spending as well, because the bulk of Medicare expenditures, and almost one-half of Medicaid's, are devoted to those services.

NHE is projected to increase at an average rate of 9.2 percent from 1990 to 2000, reflecting changes in prices, population, and consumption per capita (Table 4). The overall growth rate is lower than the 12.8–percent average for the 1970s and the 10.4–percent average for the 1980s, mostly because of a projected abatement of price inflation.

In real terms, NHE growth during the last decade of the century is projected to be close to that of the 1980s,

at least in aggregate. "Real NHE" is found by stripping individual service components (hospital care, physician services, etc.) of their own price inflation and summing the resulting figures. Measured thus, it follows that change in real NHE per capita reflects change in "quantity" per capita (an amalgamation of contacts per person and intensity per contact). We project real NHE growth to average 3.8 percent per year from 1990 to 2000, compared with an average rate of 4.8 percent in the 1970s and 3.7 percent in the 1980s. Real growth will vary by type of service, and those variations are discussed later in this article.

We have projected slower health price inflation during the 1990s than had been the case in previous decades. The implicit deflator for health, defined as the ratio of nominal and real NHE, measures price inflation and shifts in use between high-price and low-price services. In our scenario, this deflator increases at an average rate of 5.2 percent between 1990 and 2000; the comparable figures for the 1970s and the 1980s were 7.7 percent and 6.5 percent, respectively. As with real growth, price inflation is projected to vary by type of good or service under consideration.

Using the growth rates just discussed, one may conclude that about one-third of the growth in NHE per capita between now and the end of the century will be attributable to quantity changes and the remainder to price inflation. Population growth will average 0.9 percent per year, a rate very close to that of the 1970s and 1980s. The balance between real growth and price inflation is also similar to that posted for those decades.

In addition to examining growth in nominal and real NHE, it is useful to look at changes in the real opportunity cost of that expenditure. Recall that changes in real NHE reflect changes in the amounts and intensity of health goods and services purchased. The real opportunity cost of expenditure measures the flip side of

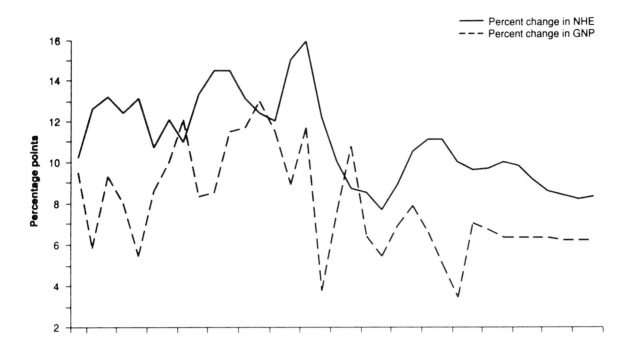

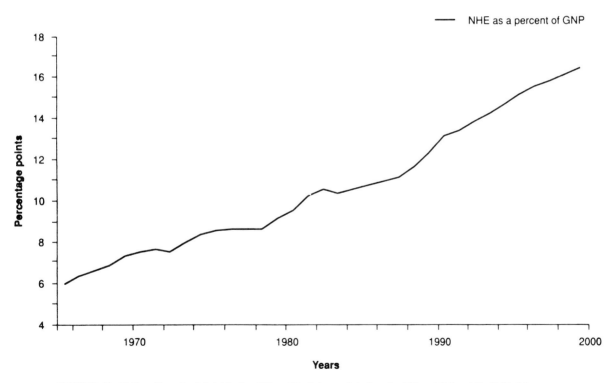

SOURCE: Health Care Financing Administration, Office of the Actuary: Data from the Office of National Health Statistics.

**Figure 1.** Percent change in national health expenditures (NHE) and gross national product (GNP), and NHE as a percent of GNP: 1966–89 and projections 1990–2000

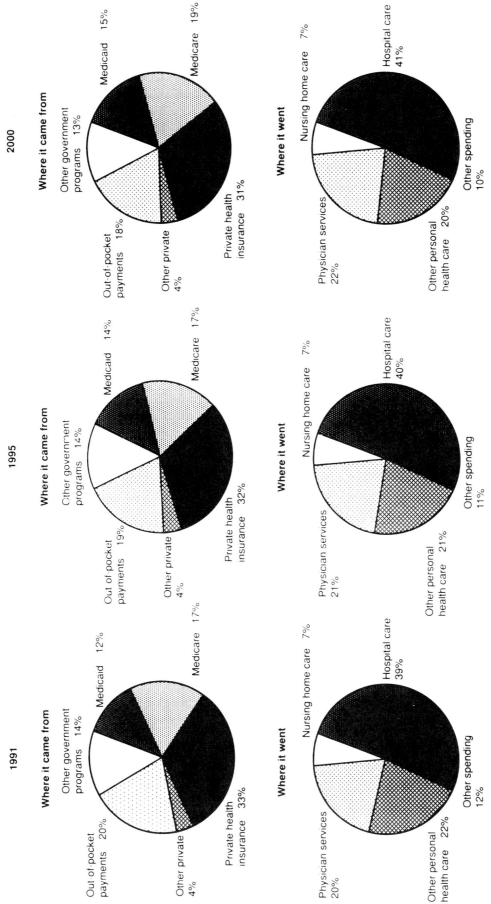

**Figure 2.** The Nation's health dollar—sources and destinations: 1991, 1995, and 2000

1991

**Where it came from**

Other government programs 14%

Medicaid 12%

Medicare 17%

Out-of-pocket payments 20%

Other private 4%

Private health insurance 33%

**Where it went**

Nursing home care 7%

Hospital care 39%

Physician services 20%

Other personal health care 22%

Other spending 12%

1995

**Where it came from**

Other government programs 14%

Medicaid 14%

Medicare 17%

Out-of-pocket payments 19%

Other private 4%

Private health insurance 32%

**Where it went**

Nursing home care 7%

Hospital care 40%

Physician services 21%

Other personal health care 21%

Other spending 11%

2000

**Where it came from**

Other government programs 13%

Medicaid 15%

Medicare 19%

Out-of-pocket payments 18%

Other private 4%

Private health insurance 31%

**Where it went**

Nursing home care 7%

Hospital care 41%

Physician services 22%

Other personal health care 20%

Other spending 10%

NOTES: Other private includes industrial inplant health services, non-patient revenues, and privately financed construction. Other personal health care includes dental, other private professional services, home health care, drugs and other non-durable medical products, and vision products and other durable medical products. Other spending covers program administration and the net cost of private health insurance, government public health, and research and construction.

SOURCE: Health Care Financing Administration, Office of the Actuary: Data from the Office of National Health Statistics.

## Table 4
**Average annual growth of nominal and real national health expenditures (NHE) and gross national product (GNP), of implicit price deflators for NHE and GNP, and of the opportunity cost of NHE: Selected periods, 1965-2000**

| Period | National health expenditures | | | Gross national product | | | Non-health care GNP price deflator | Opportunity cost |
|---|---|---|---|---|---|---|---|---|
| | Nominal | Real | Price | Nominal | Real | Price | | |
| | *Average annual growth* | | | | | | | |
| 1965-70 | 12.3 | 6.7 | 5.3 | 7.6 | 3.0 | 4.5 | 4.4 | 7.5 |
| 1970-75 | 12.3 | 5.3 | 6.7 | 9.5 | 2.2 | 7.1 | 7.2 | 4.8 |
| 1975-80 | 13.4 | 4.3 | 8.7 | 11.3 | 3.4 | 7.6 | 7.5 | 5.4 |
| 1980-85 | 11.0 | 3.3 | 7.5 | 8.0 | 2.6 | 5.3 | 5.1 | 5.7 |
| 1985-90 | 9.8 | 4.0 | 5.5 | 6.4 | 2.8 | 3.4 | 3.2 | 6.5 |
| 1990-95 | 9.8 | 4.3 | 5.3 | 5.9 | 2.0 | 3.8 | 3.5 | 6.1 |
| 1995-00 | 8.5 | 3.4 | 5.0 | 6.3 | 2.2 | 4.0 | 3.8 | 4.6 |
| 1965-75 | 12.3 | 6.0 | 6.0 | 8.5 | 2.6 | 5.8 | 5.8 | 6.2 |
| 1975-85 | 12.2 | 3.8 | 8.1 | 9.6 | 3.0 | 6.5 | 6.3 | 5.5 |
| 1985-95 | 9.8 | 4.2 | 5.4 | 6.1 | 2.4 | 3.6 | 3.3 | 6.3 |
| 1970-80 | 12.8 | 4.8 | 7.7 | 10.4 | 2.8 | 7.4 | 7.4 | 5.1 |
| 1980-90 | 10.4 | 3.7 | 6.5 | 7.2 | 2.7 | 4.4 | 4.1 | 6.1 |
| 1990-00 | 9.2 | 3.8 | 5.1 | 6.1 | 2.1 | 3.9 | 3.6 | 5.4 |
| | *Average annual growth per capita* | | | | | | | |
| 1965-70 | 11.2 | 5.6 | — | 6.5 | 1.9 | — | — | 6.4 |
| 1970-75 | 11.3 | 4.4 | — | 8.5 | 1.3 | — | — | 3.8 |
| 1975-80 | 12.3 | 3.3 | — | 10.3 | 2.5 | — | — | 4.5 |
| 1980-85 | 9.9 | 2.3 | — | 6.9 | 1.6 | — | — | 4.6 |
| 1985-90 | 8.7 | 3.0 | — | 5.3 | 1.8 | — | — | 5.4 |
| 1990-95 | 8.8 | 3.4 | — | 4.9 | 1.1 | — | — | 5.1 |
| 1995-00 | 7.7 | 2.5 | — | 5.4 | 1.4 | — | — | 3.8 |
| 1965-75 | 11.2 | 5.0 | — | 7.5 | 1.6 | — | — | 5.1 |
| 1975-85 | 11.1 | 2.8 | — | 8.6 | 2.0 | — | — | 4.5 |
| 1985-95 | 8.8 | 3.2 | — | 5.1 | 1.4 | — | — | 5.3 |
| 1970-80 | 11.8 | 3.8 | — | 9.4 | 1.9 | — | — | 4.2 |
| 1980-90 | 9.3 | 2.7 | — | 6.1 | 1.7 | — | — | 5.0 |
| 1990-00 | 8.3 | 3.0 | — | 5.2 | 1.2 | — | — | 4.5 |

NOTE: Opportunity cost is defined to be nominal national health expenditures divided by the implicit price deflator for non-health gross national product

SOURCE: Health Care Financing Administration, Office of the Actuary: Data from the Office of National Health Statistics

that coin: the amount of non-health goods and services that the Nation could have purchased with the dollars spent on health care. This measure is found by dividing nominal health care expenditure by the implicit price deflator for non-health GNP, and it is projected to grow 5.3 percent per year between 1990 and 2000. Put in other words, the Nation is projected to spend enough in the 1990s to increase its consumption of health goods and services 3.8 percent per year (real NHE). However, the size of the bundle of non-health goods and services that it could have purchased instead (real opportunity cost) is projected to increase 5.3 percent per year. This rate is similar to the 5.1−percent rate of the 1970s and lower than the 6.1−percent rate of the 1980s.

### Personal Health Care Expenditures

Assuming the continued influence of current laws and practices, expenditures for personal health care are projected to reach $957 billion in 1995 and $1.456 trillion

in 2000. Personal health care expenditures (PHCE) comprise spending for those goods and services used to treat individual patients. PHCE excludes administration expenses, research, construction, and other types of spending that are not directed at patient care. The dollar values mentioned above imply an average annual growth rate of 9.5 percent during the 1990s, compared with 12.9 percent in the 1970s and 10.4 percent in the 1980s.

Our scenario shows a slight shift in the composition of spending for personal health care toward ambulatory services and away from inpatient care (Table 5). In 1990, community hospital outpatient services accounted for 8.7 percent of PHCE, and spending for physician services accounted for another 22.5 percent. By the end of the century, we project that hospital outpatient care will account for 12.8 percent of PHCE, and physician services will account for 24.8 percent. During the same period of time, other hospital revenues (including nonpatient revenues) will decline as a share of total spending, from 35.0 percent in 1990 to 32.1 percent in 2000. Driven by demographic pressures, spending for nursing

## Table 5
## Percent distribution of personal health care expenditures, by type of service: Selected years 1980-2000

| Type of expenditure | 1980 | 1985 | Projected | | |
| --- | --- | --- | --- | --- | --- |
| | | | 1990 | 1995 | 2000 |
| | Percent distribution | | | | |
| Total | 100.0 | 100.0 | 100.0 | 100.0 | 100.0 |
| Hospital care | 46.9 | 45.7 | 43.7 | 44.5 | 44.9 |
| Community inpatient revenue | 31.7 | 30.8 | 28.1 | 26.5 | 26.3 |
| Community outpatient revenue | 4.8 | 6.3 | 8.7 | 11.4 | 12.8 |
| Other hospital care | 10.5 | 8.7 | 7.0 | 6.6 | 5.9 |
| Physician services | 19.2 | 20.1 | 22.5 | 23.6 | 24.8 |
| Dental services | 6.6 | 6.3 | 5.7 | 4.9 | 4.3 |
| Other professional services | 4.0 | 4.5 | 5.2 | 5.4 | 5.2 |
| Home health care | 0.6 | 1.0 | 1.1 | 1.3 | 1.3 |
| Drugs and other medical non-durables | 9.2 | 8.8 | 8.2 | 7.1 | 6.3 |
| Vision products and other medical durables | 2.3 | 2.3 | 2.4 | 2.1 | 2.0 |
| Nursing home care | 9.2 | 9.3 | 9.1 | 9.0 | 9.0 |
| Other personal health care | 2.1 | 1.9 | 2.0 | 2.2 | 2.3 |

NOTES: Columns may not add to totals because of rounding. Non-patient revenues of community hospitals are included in "other hospital care."

SOURCE: Health Care Financing Administration. Office of the Actuary: Data from the Office of National Health Statistics

home care, home health services, and other professional services will maintain their respective shares of the total.

Reflecting the growth of spending for physician services, we also project a strong shift toward government financing of PHCE. Medicaid's share of the total will grow from 12.1 percent in 1990 to 16.1 percent in 2000, a trend that is visible across the spectrum of services. Medicare will also increase in importance, especially in its role of paying for physician services. During the 1990s, the private share of PHCE will shrink from 59.1 percent to 53.6 percent, reflecting the increased share accounted for by government programs.

To understand the trends in consumption and financing of personal health care, it is important to study the individual types of goods and services that comprise the total. The following sections contain a discussion of the major components of expenditures.

### Hospital Care

We project that expenditures for hospital care will reach $425 billion in 1995 and $654 billion at the end of the century. Average annual growth slightly faster than that of the rest of NHE results in hospital care consuming a larger share of the NHE pie in the year 2000: 45 percent of the total compared with 38.5 percent in 1989. During the course of the decade to come, current laws and practices suggest that government programs, especially Medicaid, will finance a larger share of total hospital spending than had been the case in the past. Out-of-pocket expenditures and private health insurance benefits will decline as a percent of the total.

In making our projections of hospital expenditure, we divided that category into five parts. Two parts reflect the inpatient and outpatient revenue of community hospitals—short-term, non-Federal hospitals open to the public, which account for three-quarters of all hospital beds. (The other parts, which reflect activity in non-community hospitals and in Federal hospitals, and community hospital non-patient revenues, are not discussed in detail here.)

*Community Hospital Inpatient Revenue.* Between 1990 and 2000, inpatient revenue of community hospitals is projected to grow at a rate slightly faster than that seen during the previous decade. This roughly similar growth is the result of offsetting changes in the growth of inpatient days and of inpatient intensity, as the relative price of care is projected to grow at rates comparable to those of the past decade (Figure 3).

Medicare's prospective payment system (PPS) and concurrent private and government cost-reduction measures had a profound effect on the growth of community hospital inpatient revenues after 1980. Annual growth of revenues decelerated rapidly between 1980 and 1985, from a high of 18 percent to a low of 4 percent. The average annual rate for the period was 10.3 percent. After 1985, nominal growth rates accelerated, reaching 8.7 percent in 1990, but even that rate was scarcely one-half the average posted prior to 1980. Our projection is that growth will change very little through the end of the century.

A substantial part of the growth in inpatient revenue will continue to be general price inflation, but the decline in inpatient days per capita will reverse itself. Change in the GNP deflator has accounted for about one-half of the growth in inpatient revenue since 1980 and is projected to continue to do so in the future. The differential between hospital prices and prices in general is projected to stay at roughly historical levels as well. However, we project that the 9–year decline in inpatient days per capita will be reversed beginning in 1991. Medicare

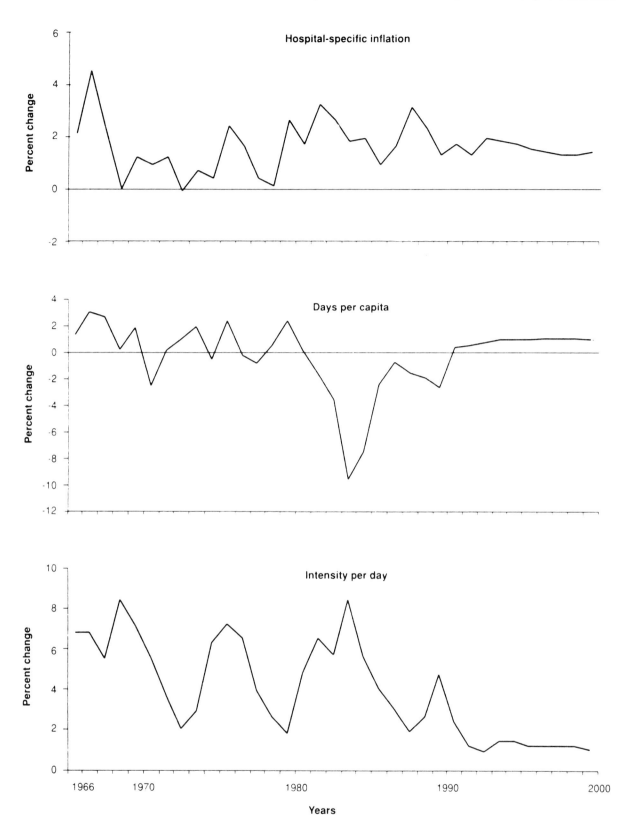

SOURCE: Health Care Financing Administration. Office of the Actuary. Data from the Office of National Health Statistics

**Figure 3.** Annual change in use, intensity, and deflated price of expenditures for community hospital inpatient services: 1966–2000

actuaries predict strong growth in days of care for people 65 years of age or over, as the industry completes its adjustment to PPS. Aging of the elderly population should contribute between one-quarter and one-half of 1 percent per year to growth throughout the decade. The growth of days per capita for the population under the age of 65 is projected to begin midway through the decade. That annual growth will be boosted by an age-sex factor the contribution of which rises from one-quarter of 1 percent per year early in the decade to three-quarters of 1 percent per year by decade end.

At the same time that growth in days per capita accelerates, growth in inpatient intensity decelerates. During the last 25 years, there has been a gradual (if intermittent) deceleration of growth in this factor, and that trend is projected to continue into the next decade.

*Community Hospital Outpatient Revenue.* Growth of community hospital outpatient revenue is projected to continue to subside over the next 10 years. That decline in growth can be traced to both use of outpatient services and the intensity of that use (Figure 4).

Just as PPS and other hospital cost-reduction measures affected use of inpatient services in the mid-1980s, they affected use of outpatient services as well. Throughout the 1970s, the number of outpatient visits per capita had been growing, but the rate of change had dropped steadily, stabilizing at about 1 percent per year in the early 1980s. The introduction of inpatient cost containment resulted in a surge in outpatient visits beginning in 1985, as hospitals responded to changed incentives by shifting much pre-admission testing and many procedures to an outpatient setting. The rate of growth began to decline again after 1986 and is projected to continue to decline through the end of the century, reaching an annual rate of 1 percent by the year 2000.

We also project that outpatient intensity will grow at diminishing rates over the next 10 years. The previous 25 years have been characterized by accelerating growth in intensity, although the rate of acceleration dropped to or below zero in the mid- to late 1980s. We have projected a deceleration in the 1990s, tapering the growth of intensity to just over 2 percent per year by the end of the decade.

In the absence of a good time-series price for outpatient services, we have used the same price measure as for inpatient services. Any differential price changes will be reflected in the outpatient intensity measure already discussed. About one-half of the growth in community hospital outpatient revenues is attributable to price inflation, mostly general inflation. Growth in use and intensity, which is strong relative to growth of inpatient services, accounts for most of the rest of nominal expenditure growth.

Physician Services

National spending for physician services is projected to be $226 billion by 1995 and $360 billion by the year 2000. This growth rate for the 1990s is slightly slower than in the 1970s or 1980s.

General price inflation accounts for slightly more than one-third of the projected increase in physician spending over the next 10 years. The prices that physicians charge in excess of the general inflation rate are expected to comprise less than one-tenth of the growth in the next decade, in part because Medicare is forecasting only slow growth in its allowable fees.

Demographic factors play a fairly small role in our projection of physician expenditures. Population change itself will account for less than one-tenth of the projected growth. The aging of the population does not add much to the use or intensity of physician services, partly because the baby boom does not mature into the higher use ages until the next century and partly because the increase in utilization with age is not as dramatic in the case of physician services as it is for hospitals and nursing homes.

Aside from price inflation, most of the growth in expenditures for physician services has been in intensity. Use of physician services, as measured by office and hospital visits, has changed little in the past two decades, and, in our projections, it grows only slowly in the future. Such is not the case with intensity. Intensity measures the increase in the number and quality of such items as lab tests, radiology for diagnosis and treatment, more complex operative procedures, etc. It has risen steadily in the past and is projected to constitute about one-third of the growth in spending for physician services by 2000.

Nursing Home Care

Nursing homes included in this projection consist of skilled nursing facilities, intermediate care facilities, a large number of homes with both certifications, some homes with neither certification, and some intermediate care facilities for the mentally retarded (ICF/MR). (Certification levels refer to Medicare or Medicaid certification.) Expenditure for this type of care is projected to reach $86 billion in 1995 and $131 billion in 2000.

We project that use of nursing home services will continue to grow less than would be predicted by age-sex-specific use patterns. In part, this is attributable to a bed supply that has grown less rapidly than has the population most at risk. It also is attributable to a trend toward deinstitutionalization of ICF/MR patients. And, in part, it is attributable to a preference on the part of patients and payers for alternative modes of long-term care that are both economical and acceptable to users.

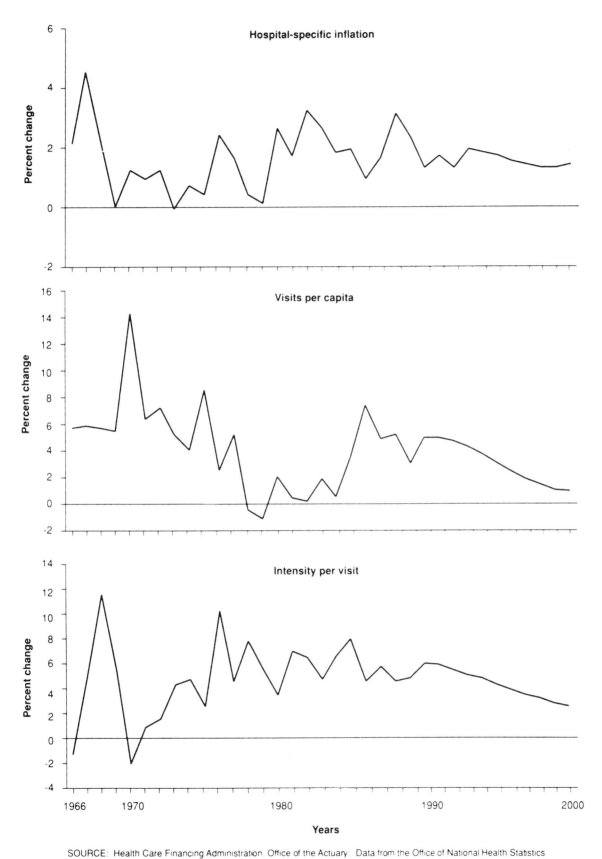

SOURCE: Health Care Financing Administration. Office of the Actuary. Data from the Office of National Health Statistics

**Figure 4.** Annual charge in use, intensity, and deflated price of expenditures for community hospital outpatient services: 1966–2000

Medicaid pays and will continue to pay about 45 percent of the costs of nursing homes. Approximately another 45 percent is paid directly by the patient or the patient's family. The remaining costs are spread among several payers. Of great interest is whether private insurance in either its present form or some modification will meet a significant portion of the cost in the 1990s, helping some private payers budget for these costs and providing relief for the public programs.

### Drugs and Other Non-durable Goods

Total expenditures for drugs and sundries have grown at remarkably stable rates over the last 25 years—average annual growth rates of drug expenditures for 5-year periods from 1965 to 1990 have not been lower than 8.1 percent nor higher than 10 percent. Yet this stability masks some dramatic changes in the composition of that expenditure—price increases as opposed to quantity increases.

Prescription drug prices have followed a different pattern than have prices in general. They fell uniformly from the 1960s through the mid-1970s relative to overall price levels in the economy. From the mid-1970s through 1981, they grew at about the same rate as overall prices, and since then they have grown much more rapidly than have general prices.

The pattern for prescription quantity (expenditures adjusted for price change) is the mirror image of that for price, but less pronounced. During the 1960s and early 1970s, volume increased significantly more rapidly than real GNP. Real spending grew more slowly than did real GNP beginning as early as the late 1970s and especially after 1982.

During the 1990s, we project that relative price inflation will account for less of the growth in expenditure for drugs and non-durable goods than has been the case since the early 1980s. Growth of the relative price of goods in this category will slow during the 1990s from 4 percent in 1990 to 1 percent in 2000. Real spending per capita, although continuing to fall, will do so at diminishing rates and will in fact begin to grow slightly by the end of the decade.

### Other Categories of Personal Health Care

*Dentist Services.* Expenditures for dentist services are expected to be $63 billion in 2000, up from $31 billion in 1989. We project an average annual growth rate for dentist expenditures of 6.4 percent in the 1990s, down from 8.9 percent in the 1980s and 11.9 percent in the 1970s. This reduced rate of growth in the 1990s reflects a forecast of prices increasing 1.8 percent per year faster than the general inflation rate, and slightly negative growth in real (inflation-adjusted) per capita services.

The projected number of practicing dentists will peak in 1999 and actually decline slightly in 2000.

It is widely assumed that past increases in private health insurance coverage of dental services have supported higher dental expenditures despite advances in preventive dental care. We project private health insurance to finance a smaller share of total dental expenditures in the 1990s, reversing the trend toward increasing insurance expenditure shares from 1965 to the present.

*Home Health Care.* In our scenario for the 1990s, recent rapid increases in Medicaid spending for home health care are projected to continue, only slightly abated, through the coming decade. Medicaid spending for home health care was almost $2 billion in 1989 and is projected to reach $5.1 billion in 1995 and $9.7 billion in 2000. State Medicaid programs have been using additional flexibility granted by Congress to attempt to meet the demand for long-term care services that, in the past, have been provided almost exclusively by nursing homes under the Medicaid program. It was intended that the additional flexibility in designing long-term care solutions would result in cost savings and also more satisfactory programs for the aged and disabled who depend on Medicaid for their long-term care needs.

Medicare is anticipating continued growth in its home health outlays at a slower rate than Medicaid. The Medicare benefit is closely circumscribed to be an acute care benefit intended to substitute for more expensive acute institutional care in hospitals and skilled nursing facilities.

Most surveys have noted a very large demand for home health care, some of it met by public or private financial resources, much of it met by volunteers, and some of it not met at all. Most of that care is used by the very elderly, and some pressure on spending is already being exerted by aging cohorts born at the beginning of this century.

*Other Professional Services.* Expenditure growth rates for other professional services are projected to remain moderate in the 1990s. "Other professional services" covers spending for services of licensed health practitioners other than physicians and dentists and expenditures for services rendered in outpatient clinics. Expenditures had increased more than 19 percent per year in the 1970s, a rate of increase that slowed to 13.5 percent per year in the 1980s. We project annual growth rates of 9.4 percent for spending in the 1990s, reflecting price increases of 1.5 percent over the general inflation rate and real expenditure per capita growth of almost 3 percent. Total expenditures for other professional services will reach $75 billion in 2000, up from [$]27 billion in 1989.

Private health insurance coverage for other professional services is expected to moderate in the 1990s. As a result of this and rapid growth in government programs, total spending financed by insurance will peak at about 38 percent early in the decade and fall to less than 35 percent by 2000.

*Eyeglasses and Other Durable Goods.* Expenditures for this class of goods have grown at double-digit rates since the end of the 1982 recession. These high growth rates were driven largely by rapid increases in real spending. In fact, prices seem to have grown slightly less than the GNP deflator in the 1980s. Our projection shows continued strong growth in real spending, but the rates of growth are moderated somewhat from historical rates. Prices are assumed to grow at the rate of general economy prices, so that expenditure grows roughly 1 percent faster than GNP.

Spending for durables has a consistent cyclical pattern, following the economy's business cycles. Thus, spending will be restrained in 1991 and will recover as the economy is predicted to recover in the mid- and late 1900s.

*Other Personal Health Care.* The category labeled "other personal health care" in the tables presented in this article consists of items not definable in the usual categories or not specified by kind by the reporting agency. Much of the spending is financed by government, Medicaid being the largest payer. Total expenditures will reach almost $34 billion in 2000, up from $10.5 billion in 1989. Spending in this category continues to increase more rapidly than GNP, as Medicaid expenditure growth remains very high in the 1990s.

## Research and Construction

Expenditures for biomedical research and research on the delivery of health care will increase at roughly the same rate as GNP in the 1990s, reaching $22.3 billion in 2000. Construction spending will grow more slowly than GNP throughout much of the 1990s, and will reach $17.5 billion in 2000, up from $9.6 billion in 1989. To project construction, we first estimated the capital stock needed to supply our projected hospital and nursing home services; a key variable in the determination was the number of beds in service in the various institutions. We then projected the level of new construction needed to achieve that capital stock.

## PROJECTION RESULTS: SOURCES OF FUNDS

During the 1980s, the proportion of NHE funded by public and private sources stabilized, with the private sector paying just under 60 percent of the total. A gradual shift from private to public sources is projected for the next decade, reducing the private share to 53 percent by the year 2000.

Spending for Medicare and Medicaid, the two major sources of government financing for health, is projected to increase as a percent of the total. The Medicare increase is primarily the result of growth in the proportion of the population 65 years of age or over, especially the cohort 75 or over, which has the highest health care costs. The Medicaid share is projected to rise as a result of several factors, including expanded eligibility.

## Government Financing

Total Federal spending for health care is projected to grow at an average annual rate of 10.4 percent between 1990 and 2000, about the same rate as for the 1980s. We project that Federal expenditures will reach $517.6 billion by 2000 and finance 32 percent of NHE, up from 28.7 percent in 1990. Both the Medicare and Federal Medicaid share of total health spending will increase during the projection period; the share funded by other Federal sources, mainly the Departments of Veterans Affairs and of Defense, is projected to decline slightly.

Although the growth in total Federal spending represents a small increase in the share of total health spending, it represents a sizable increase in the share of total Federal Government spending. In 1980, federally financed health expenditures accounted for 11.7 percent of Federal expenditures; in 1990, the share was 15.1 percent, and it is projected to account for 24.1 percent by the year 2000 (Figure 5).

State and local government expenditures for health care are also projected to rise both as a share of NHE and as a share of total State and local government spending. Driven primarily by projected increases in Medicaid spending. State and local government expenditures are projected to grow from $89.4 billion in 1990 to $238.9 billion in 2000. This results in an increase of 1.6 percent in the State and local share of NHE, and a 6.7 percent increase in health's share of their budget (Figure 5).

*Medicare.* Medicare's HI and SMI programs are projected to account for $182.3 billion of health expenditures in 1995 and for $302.8 billion in 2000. These sums represent an increasing share of total NHE: After remaining relatively stable between 16.5 percent and 17.0 percent of total spending through 1995, Medicare's share of total spending is projected to rise to 18.7 percent by the end of the decade.

Outlays for physician services will consume an increasing amount of Medicare payments. Accounting for 27.6 percent of the Medicare budget in 1990, these payments will rise to 32.6 percent by the year 2000.

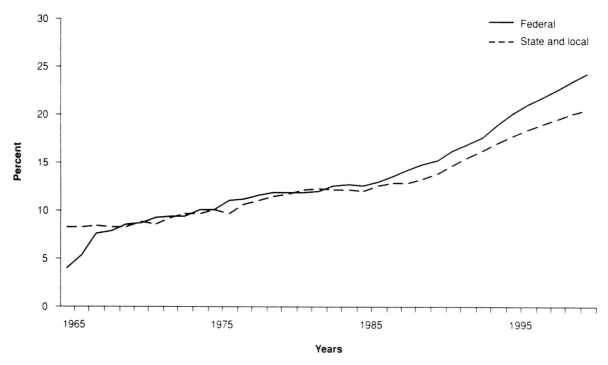

SOURCE: Health Care Financing Administration. Office of the Actuary: Data from the Office of National Health Statistics.

**Figure 5.** Government expenditures for health as a percent of total government expenditures: 1965–97

Effective January 1, 1992, Medicare will begin paying physicians on the basis of a resource-based relative value scale (RBRVS) that is intended to relate payment for any service to the effort, time, and skill required by the physician. The current payment system, based on the lowest of actual, customary, or prevailing fees, has its roots in the traditional charge patterns of physicians in each geographic area, but has been modified substantially by congressional actions over the past several years.

The RBRVS is intended to rationalize Medicare payment levels. To help control increases in utilization and intensity of services, a "volume standard" is promulgated annually. This volume standard is a target growth rate for aggregate Medicare spending on physician services. If physician spending in any year exceeds the target, Medicare will lower a future fee scale increase. If the spending target is exactly met, the fee scale would be increased by the Medicare Economic Index. A bonus fee increase can be paid if spending is less than the volume standard.

There is great interest in how effectively this new payment system will influence future trends in Medicare costs and whether it will affect other payers. During the last half of the 1980s, Medicare payments to physicians rose more than 13 percent per year on average, in spite of fee freezes in some years. In its most recent report, the Board of Trustees of the Federal Supplementary Medical Insurance Trust Fund forecasts physician increases in excess of 10 percent per year through the year 2000 (Alternative II).

Medicare inpatient hospital costs, on the other hand, have increased much more slowly since PPS was instituted in fiscal year 1984. In the 5 years after 1984, Medicare inpatient payments increased less than 6 percent annually. In the 5 years ending with 1984, they increased more than 15 percent annually. The Board of Trustees of the Federal Hospital Insurance Trust Fund projects Medicare hospital inpatient costs to increase about 10 percent annually through the year 2000 (Alternative II). These rates are somewhat higher than in the recent past. In part, this is because Medicare actuaries do not anticipate a continuation of the decreases in hospital use that occurred following PPS. In addition, laws reducing the increase in PPS hospital payment rates will expire in fiscal year 1993.

(For a more detailed discussion of Medicare projections, see the 1991 annual reports by the Board of Trustees of the Hospital Insurance Trust Fund [1991] and Board of Trustees of the Supplementary Medical Insurance Trust Fund [1991].)

*Medicaid.* Preliminary data indicate that Medicaid spending ballooned abruptly in 1990 following several years of much more modest growth rates. Following the 1982 recession, Medicaid grew less than 11 percent per year through 1989. It appears that 1990 costs were about 20 percent above those for 1989. Most spending for acute care services rose much more rapidly than in the recent past and there was sizable growth in home and community-based alternatives to long-term care.

As part of the Federal budget process, State Medicaid programs prepare quarterly estimates of what they expect to be spending in the current and next two fiscal years. These planning estimates indicate that State administrators are forecasting continued high growth through fiscal year 1992.

The reasons for this upturn in spending are not yet well understood, and thus it is difficult to foresee what it implies for the longer term. The current recession probably plays some role. Also, Congress has expanded eligibility somewhat in recent years. Providers in some States have brought successful court cases to increase reimbursement levels. In short, there are many plausible explanations, but so far a shortage of evidence to quantify the effects of most of them.

In light of this uncertainty, our projections follow a middle course. Aggregate Medicaid growth averages 15.5 percent per year through 1995, bringing outlays to $154.1 billion. During the last half of the decade, the average annual growth slows to 9.6 percent, so that spending in the year 2000 is projected to be $243.8 billion.

Private Financing

Private expenditures for health care are projected to reach $859 billion by 2000, financing 53.2 percent of NHE. For the 1990–2000 period, private health expenditures are projected to grow at an average annual rate of 8.2 percent, slower than the 10.5–percent rate of the previous 10–year period, and slower than the projected rate of growth for total NHE.

Private health insurance premiums, which make up about one-third of NHE and 60 percent of total private funding, are projected to more than double in the next 10 years, from $222.5 billion to $507.7 billion. The proportion of personal health care paid for by private health insurance benefits is projected to decline slightly during this period, reversing the trend of the past 10 years, mostly as a result of more rapid relative growth in public payments.

Out-of-pocket payments for health care are projected to increase to $290.9 billion by the turn of the century. The out-of-pocket share of PHCE is projected to continue its decline from 26.8 percent in 1980, through 23.4 percent in 1990, to 20.0 percent by 2000.

Expenditures of other private funds (which include non-patient revenues of hospitals and nursing homes, spending for industrial inplant services, and so on) are projected to reach $61.6 billion by 2000 and account for 3.8 percent of all health spending, including research and construction.

During the past 25 years, there has been a continuous shift from out-of-pocket to private health insurance spending for personal health care. However, this shift is projected to slow during the projection period, resulting in an increase in the insurance share of NHE of only 2 percent, compared with its 5.2-percent share increase during the 1980s.

This projected slowing in the growth of private health insurance is the result of several factors: an increase in the number of uninsured and underinsured people because of the recent recession; the prohibitive cost of purchasing private health insurance by small employers and individuals; and reductions in retiree health care coverage as a result of the implementation of the Financial Accounting Standards Board regulations requiring employers to show future retiree health care costs as a liability on their financial statements.

There also is evidence that employers plan to require employees to pay higher deductibles and copayments and to reduce or eliminate supplemental benefits such as dental and prescription drug coverage in an attempt to control the escalating costs of providing health benefits to employees.

## SUMMARY

Health care expenditures have grown more rapidly than has the rest of the economy during the past 30 years, much of which is attributable to natural factors. Rising income levels, the introduction of new services and new technologies, and changes in the social and demographic composition of the population have all contributed to growth in spending for health. Reimbursement practices, perverse incentives caused by the financing system, and market failures caused by lack of consumer information have played a part as well.

It is clear that at least some of these factors will continue to operate in the future. Real GNP per capita will continue to grow, although more slowly in the long-run than has been the case in the recent past. The aging of America's population will serve to raise the demand for health care, although the effect will be fairly trivial through the next 30 years. Also, there is no reason to doubt that new technologies and new services will continue to be introduced, although when and where is open to debate. Whether perverse incentives to consume care continue into the future is a policy issue to be resolved.

To assist that resolution, we have shown how health care spending would grow in the next 10 years under current law and current practices. Our scenario, however, is only one of an almost infinite number of different scenarios (some more plausible than others) describing the effects of current law and current practice. Each scenario embodies a different set of assumptions about the shape of things to come. For example, extension of our scenario through the year 2030 yields a level of NHE equal to 26.1 percent of the GNP. In testimony before Congress, the director of the Office of Management and Budget suggested that, in the absence of change, health care spending would reach 17 percent of GNP by 2000 and 37 percent by 2030. Even were we to reduce differential price growth to zero immediately and to permit combined use and intensity to grow no more rapidly than real GNP per capita, we would still have a health expenditure figure equal to 15 percent of the 2030 GNP.

[Tables 6 through 10 follow]

Acknowledgments—This article was prepared in the Health Care Financing Administration's Office of National Health Statistics. The authors are grateful for the advice and comments of their colleagues: Ross H. Arnett, III, George Chulis, William Donnelly, Frank Eppig, Charles Fisher, Mark Freedland, Helen Lazenby, Katharine Levit, and John Phelps. Louis Blank and Dawn Li assisted in the preparation of tables and graphs for this article.

## References

Arnett, R. A, III, McKusick, D. R., Sonnefeld, S. T., and Cowell, C. S.: Projections of health care spending to 1990. *Health Care Financing Review* 7(3):1–36. HCFA Pub. No. 03222. Office of Research and Demonstrations. Health Care Financing Administration. Washington, U.S. Government Printing Office, Spring 1986.

Board of Trustees of the Hospital Insurance Trust Fund: *The 1991 annual report of the board, pursuant to section 1817(b) of the Social Security Act as amended.* Baltimore, Md. Health Care Financing Administration, May 1991.

Board of Trustees of the Old Age, Survivors, and Disability Trust Fund: *The 1991 annual report of the board, pursuant to section 201(c)(2) of the Social Security Act as amended.* Baltimore, Md. Social Security Administration, May 1991.

Board of Trustees of the Supplementary Medical Insurance Trust Fund: *The 1991 annual report of the board, pursuant to section 184(b) of the Social Security Act as amended.* Baltimore, Md. Health Care Financing Administration, May 1991.

Bureau of Health Professions: *Seventh report to the President and Congress on the status of health personnel in the United States.* DHHS Pub. No. HRS-P-OD-90-1. Health Resources and Services Administration. U.S. Department of Health and Human Services. Washington, U.S. Government Printing office, March 1990.

Division of National Cost Estimates: National health expenditures, 1986–2000. *Health Care Financing Review* 8(4):1–36. HCFA Pub. No. 03239. Office of Research and Demonstrations, Health Care Financing Administration. Washington, U.S. Government Printing Office, Summer 1987.

Lazenby, H. C., and Letsch, S. W.: National health expenditures, 1989. *Health Care Financing Review* 12(2):1–26. HCFA Pub. No. 03316. Office of Research and Demonstrations, Health Care Financing Administration. Washington, U.S. Government Printing Office, Winter 1990.

Levit, K. R., Lazenby, H. C., Letsch, S. W., and Cowan, C.A.: National health care spending, 1989. *Health Affairs* 10(1):117–130, Spring 1991a.

Levit, K. R., Lazenby, H. C., Cowan, C. A., and Letsch, S. W.: National health expenditures, 1990. *Health Care Financing Review* 13(1):29–54. HCFA Pub. No. 03321. Office of Research and Demonstrations. Health Care Financing Administration. Washington, U.S. Government Printing Office, Fall 1991b.

Waldo, D. R., Sonnefeld, S. T., McKusick, D. R., and Arnett, R. H. III: Health expenditures by age group, 1977 and 1987. *Health Care Financing Review* 10(4):111–120. HCFA Pub No. 03284. Office of Research and Demonstrations. Health Care Financing Administration. Washington, U.S. Government Printing Office, Summer 1989.

## Table 6

## National health expenditures aggregate and per capita amounts, percent distribution, and average annual percent growth, by source of funds: Selected years 1965-2000

| Item | 1965 | 1975 | 1980 | 1985 | 1989 | Projected | | | | |
|---|---|---|---|---|---|---|---|---|---|---|
| | | | | | | 1990 | 1991 | 1992 | 1995 | 2000 |
| | Amount in billions | | | | | | | | | |
| National health expenditures | $41.6 | $132.9 | $249.1 | $420.1 | $604.1 | $670.9 | $738.2 | $809.0 | $1,072.7 | $1,615.9 |
| Private | 31.3 | 77.8 | 143.9 | 245.0 | 350.9 | 389.3 | 421.1 | 457.4 | 592.2 | 859.4 |
| Public | 10.3 | 55.1 | 105.2 | 175.1 | 253.3 | 281.6 | 317.1 | 351.6 | 480.5 | 756.5 |
| Federal | 4.8 | 36.4 | 72.0 | 123.6 | 174.4 | 192.2 | 215.7 | 238.8 | 324.8 | 517.6 |
| State and local | 5.5 | 18.7 | 33.2 | 51.5 | 78.8 | 89.4 | 101.4 | 112.8 | 155.7 | 238.8 |
| | Number in millions | | | | | | | | | |
| U.S. population[1] | 204.0 | 224.7 | 235.3 | 247.2 | 257.0 | 259.6 | 262.1 | 264.6 | 272.0 | 282.9 |
| | Amount in billions | | | | | | | | | |
| Gross national product | 705 | 1,598 | 2,732 | 4,015 | 5,201 | 5,463 | 5,650 | 6,045 | 7,284 | 9,865 |
| | Per capita amount | | | | | | | | | |
| National health expenditures | 204 | 592 | 1,059 | 1,699 | 2,351 | 2,585 | 2,817 | 3,057 | 3,944 | 5,712 |
| Private | 154 | 346 | 612 | 991 | 1,365 | 1,500 | 1,607 | 1,729 | 2,178 | 3,038 |
| Public | 50 | 245 | 447 | 708 | 985 | 1,085 | 1,210 | 1,329 | 1,767 | 2,674 |
| Federal | 24 | 162 | 306 | 500 | 679 | 741 | 823 | 902 | 1,194 | 1,830 |
| State and local | 27 | 83 | 141 | 208 | 307 | 344 | 387 | 426 | 572 | 844 |
| | Percent distribution | | | | | | | | | |
| National health expenditures | 100.0 | 100.0 | 100.0 | 100.0 | 100.0 | 100.0 | 100.0 | 100.0 | 100.0 | 100.0 |
| Private | 75.3 | 58.5 | 57.8 | 58.3 | 58.1 | 58.0 | 57.0 | 56.5 | 55.2 | 53.2 |
| Public | 24.7 | 41.5 | 42.2 | 41.7 | 41.9 | 42.0 | 43.0 | 43.5 | 44.8 | 46.8 |
| Federal | 11.6 | 27.4 | 28.9 | 29.4 | 28.9 | 28.7 | 29.2 | 29.5 | 30.3 | 32.0 |
| State and local | 13.2 | 14.1 | 13.3 | 12.3 | 13.1 | 13.3 | 13.7 | 13.9 | 14.5 | 14.8 |
| | Percent of gross national product | | | | | | | | | |
| National health expenditures | 5.9 | 8.3 | 9.1 | 10.5 | 11.6 | 12.3 | 13.1 | 13.4 | 14.7 | 16.4 |
| | Average annual percent growth from previous year shown | | | | | | | | | |
| National health expenditures | — | 12.3 | 13.4 | 11.0 | 9.5 | 11.1 | 10.0 | 9.6 | 9.9 | 8.5 |
| Private | — | 9.5 | 13.1 | 11.2 | 9.4 | 11.0 | 8.2 | 8.6 | 9.0 | 7.7 |
| Public | — | 18.3 | 13.8 | 10.7 | 9.7 | 11.2 | 12.6 | 10.9 | 11.0 | 9.5 |
| Federal | — | 22.4 | 14.6 | 11.4 | 9.0 | 10.2 | 12.2 | 10.7 | 10.8 | 9.8 |
| State and local | — | 13.1 | 12.1 | 9.2 | 11.3 | 13.3 | 13.4 | 11.3 | 11.3 | 8.9 |
| U.S. population | — | 1.0 | 0.9 | 1.0 | 1.0 | 1.0 | 1.0 | 1.0 | 0.9 | 0.8 |
| Gross national product | — | 8.5 | 11.3 | 8.0 | 6.7 | 5.0 | 3.4 | 7.0 | 6.4 | 6.3 |

[1] July 1 Social Security area population estimates.

NOTE: Columns may not add to totals because of rounding.

SOURCE: Health Care Financing Administration. Office of the Actuary: Data from the Office of National Health Statistics.

## Table 7

## National health expenditures aggregate amounts and average annual percent change, by type of expenditure: Selected years 1965-2000

| Type of expenditure | 1965 | 1975 | 1980 | 1985 | 1989 | 1990 | 1991 | 1992 | 1995 | 2000 |
|---|---|---|---|---|---|---|---|---|---|---|
| | | | | | | Projected | | | | |
| | | | | Amount in billions | | | | | | |
| National health expenditures | $41.6 | $132.9 | $249.1 | $420.1 | $604.1 | $670.9 | $738.2 | $809.0 | $1,072.7 | $1,615.9 |
| Health services and supplies | 38.2 | 124.7 | 237.8 | 404.7 | 583.5 | 648.6 | 714.4 | 783.8 | 1,043.1 | 1,576.1 |
| Personal health care | 35.6 | 116.6 | 218.3 | 367.2 | 530.7 | 589.3 | 651.1 | 716.7 | 956.5 | 1,456.0 |
| Hospital care | 14.0 | 52.4 | 102.4 | 167.9 | 232.8 | 257.7 | 285.4 | 313.9 | 425.4 | 654.2 |
| Physician services | 8.2 | 23.3 | 41.9 | 74.0 | 117.6 | 132.7 | 148.5 | 165.5 | 225.6 | 360.5 |
| Dental services | 2.8 | 8.2 | 14.4 | 23.3 | 31.4 | 33.8 | 36.1 | 38.6 | 47.1 | 63.1 |
| Other professional services | 0.9 | 3.5 | 8.7 | 16.6 | 27.0 | 30.7 | 34.5 | 38.7 | 51.6 | 75.4 |
| Home health care | 0.1 | 0.4 | 1.3 | 3.8 | 5.4 | 6.5 | 7.5 | 8.5 | 12.1 | 18.8 |
| Drugs and other medical non-durables | 5.9 | 13.0 | 20.1 | 32.3 | 44.6 | 48.5 | 51.8 | 55.5 | 67.7 | 91.0 |
| Vision products and other medical durables | 1.2 | 3.1 | 5.0 | 8.4 | 13.5 | 14.3 | 14.9 | 16.1 | 20.0 | 28.4 |
| Nursing home care | 1.7 | 9.9 | 20.0 | 34.1 | 47.9 | 53.6 | 59.1 | 64.9 | 85.8 | 130.8 |
| Other personal health care | 0.8 | 2.7 | 4.6 | 6.8 | 10.5 | 11.5 | 13.3 | 14.9 | 21.3 | 33.9 |
| Program administration and net cost of private health insurance | 1.9 | 5.1 | 12.2 | 25.2 | 35.3 | 40.5 | 43.3 | 45.9 | 60.8 | 85.3 |
| Government public health activities | 0.6 | 3.0 | 7.2 | 12.3 | 17.5 | 18.8 | 20.0 | 21.2 | 25.8 | 34.8 |
| Research and construction | 3.5 | 8.3 | 11.3 | 15.4 | 20.6 | 22.3 | 23.8 | 25.2 | 29.6 | 39.8 |
| Research[1] | 1.5 | 3.3 | 5.4 | 7.8 | 11.0 | 11.7 | 12.5 | 13.3 | 16.1 | 22.3 |
| Construction | 1.9 | 5.0 | 5.8 | 7.6 | 9.6 | 10.6 | 11.3 | 11.9 | 13.5 | 17.5 |
| | | | Average annual percent change from previous year shown | | | | | | | |
| National health expenditures | — | 12.3 | 13.4 | 11.0 | 9.5 | 11.1 | 10.0 | 9.6 | 9.9 | 8.5 |
| Health services and supplies | — | 12.6 | 13.8 | 11.2 | 9.6 | 11.2 | 10.1 | 9.7 | 10.0 | 8.6 |
| Personal health care | — | 12.6 | 13.4 | 11.0 | 9.6 | 11.0 | 10.5 | 10.1 | 10.1 | 8.8 |
| Hospital care | — | 14.1 | 14.3 | 10.4 | 8.5 | 10.7 | 10.7 | 10.0 | 10.7 | 9.0 |
| Physician services | — | 11.0 | 12.5 | 12.1 | 12.3 | 12.8 | 11.9 | 11.5 | 10.9 | 9.8 |
| Dental services | — | 11.4 | 11.7 | 10.1 | 7.8 | 7.6 | 6.8 | 6.9 | 6.8 | 6.0 |
| Other professional services | — | 15.0 | 19.9 | 13.8 | 12.9 | 13.6 | 12.5 | 12.1 | 10.0 | 7.9 |
| Home health care | — | 21.4 | 27.2 | 23.3 | 8.7 | 21.4 | 14.7 | 13.7 | 12.5 | 9.2 |
| Drugs and other medical non-durables | — | 8.3 | 9.1 | 9.9 | 8.4 | 8.6 | 6.8 | 7.2 | 6.8 | 6.1 |
| Vision products and other medical durables | — | 9.4 | 10.1 | 11.0 | 12.7 | 6.0 | 4.2 | 7.9 | 7.5 | 7.3 |
| Nursing home care | — | 19.3 | 15.0 | 11.3 | 8.9 | 11.8 | 10.4 | 9.9 | 9.7 | 8.8 |
| Other personal health care | — | 12.6 | 11.0 | 8.4 | 11.3 | 10.1 | 15.4 | 12.2 | 12.6 | 9.7 |
| Program administration and net cost of private health insurance | — | 10.1 | 19.3 | 15.5 | 8.8 | 14.8 | 6.9 | 5.8 | 9.9 | 7.0 |
| Government public health activities | — | 17.0 | 18.9 | 11.3 | 9.2 | 7.5 | 6.1 | 6.3 | 6.7 | 6.2 |
| Research and construction | — | 9.1 | 6.4 | 6.4 | 7.6 | 8.1 | 6.9 | 5.9 | 5.4 | 6.1 |
| Research[1] | — | 8.1 | 10.4 | 7.4 | 8.9 | 6.4 | 7.3 | 6.4 | 6.4 | 6.8 |
| Construction | — | 9.9 | 3.3 | 5.4 | 6.1 | 10.1 | 6.4 | 5.2 | 4.3 | 5.3 |

[1]Research and development expenditures of drug companies and other manufacturers and providers of medical equipment and supplies are excluded from "research expenditures," but they are included in the expenditure class in which the product falls.

NOTE: Columns may not add to totals because of rounding.

SOURCE: Health Care Financing Administration, Office of the Actuary: Data from the Office of National Health Statistics.

## Table 8

## National health expenditures, by source of funds and type of expenditure: Selected years 1980-2000

| Year and type of expenditure | Total | All private funds | Private Consumer Total | Out-of-Pocket | Private insurance | Other | Government Total | Federal | State and local |
|---|---|---|---|---|---|---|---|---|---|
| **1980** | | | | | Amount in billions | | | | |
| National health expenditures | $249.1 | $143.9 | $131.8 | $58.4 | $73.4 | $12.1 | $105.2 | $72.0 | $33.2 |
| Health services and supplies | 237.8 | 139.7 | 131.8 | 58.4 | 73.4 | 7.8 | 98.1 | 66.8 | 31.4 |
| Personal health care | 218.3 | 131.3 | 123.7 | 58.4 | 65.3 | 7.6 | 87.1 | 63.5 | 23.6 |
| Hospital care | 102.4 | 47.8 | 42.8 | 5.3 | 37.5 | 5.0 | 54.6 | 41.3 | 13.3 |
| Physician services | 41.9 | 29.2 | 29.2 | 11.3 | 18.0 | 0.0 | 12.6 | 9.7 | 3.0 |
| Dental services | 14.4 | 13.7 | 13.7 | 9.4 | 4.4 | — | 0.6 | 0.4 | 0.3 |
| Other professional services | 8.7 | 6.9 | 6.0 | 3.8 | 2.2 | 0.9 | 1.7 | 1.3 | 0.4 |
| Home health care | 1.3 | 0.4 | 0.2 | 0.1 | 0.1 | 0.1 | 1.0 | 0.8 | 0.1 |
| Drugs and other medical non-durables | 20.1 | 18.5 | 18.5 | 16.0 | 2.5 | — | 1.7 | 0.8 | 0.8 |
| Vision products and other medical durables | 5.0 | 4.4 | 4.4 | 3.9 | 0.4 | — | 0.6 | 0.5 | 0.1 |
| Nursing home care | 20.0 | 9.5 | 8.8 | 8.7 | 0.2 | 0.6 | 10.5 | 6.1 | 4.4 |
| Other personal health care | 4.6 | 0.9 | — | — | — | 0.9 | 3.7 | 2.5 | 1.2 |
| Program administration and net cost of private health insurance | 12.2 | 8.4 | 8.1 | — | 8.1 | 0.2 | 3.8 | 2.1 | 1.8 |
| Government public health activities | 7.2 | — | — | — | — | — | 7.2 | 1.2 | 6.0 |
| Research and construction | 11.3 | 4.2 | — | — | — | 4.2 | 7.0 | 5.2 | 1.8 |
| Research | 5.4 | 0.3 | — | — | — | 0.3 | 5.2 | 4.7 | 0.5 |
| Construction | 5.8 | 4.0 | — | — | — | 4.0 | 1.9 | 0.6 | 1.3 |
| | | | | | Percent distribution | | | | |
| National health expenditures | 100.0 | 57.8 | 52.9 | 23.5 | 29.5 | 4.8 | 42.2 | 28.9 | 13.3 |
| Health services and supplies | 100.0 | 58.7 | 55.4 | 24.6 | 30.9 | 3.3 | 41.3 | 28.1 | 13.2 |
| Personal health care | 100.0 | 60.1 | 56.7 | 26.8 | 29.9 | 3.5 | 39.9 | 29.1 | 10.8 |
| Hospital care | 100.0 | 46.7 | 41.8 | 5.2 | 36.6 | 4.9 | 53.3 | 40.4 | 12.9 |
| Physician services | 100.0 | 69.8 | 69.8 | 26.9 | 42.9 | 0.1 | 30.2 | 23.1 | 7.1 |
| Dental services | 100.0 | 95.6 | 95.6 | 65.2 | 30.5 | — | 4.4 | 2.4 | 1.9 |
| Other professional services | 100.0 | 79.9 | 69.3 | 43.5 | 25.8 | 10.6 | 20.1 | 14.9 | 5.2 |
| Home health care | 100.0 | 27.6 | 17.7 | 10.2 | 7.6 | 9.9 | 72.3 | 61.3 | 11.0 |
| Drugs and other medical non-durables | 100.0 | 91.8 | 91.8 | 79.4 | 12.4 | — | 8.2 | 4.1 | 4.2 |
| Vision products and other medical durables | 100.0 | 87.8 | 87.8 | 78.9 | 8.9 | — | 12.2 | 10.3 | 1.9 |
| Nursing home care | 100.0 | 47.3 | 44.2 | 43.3 | 0.9 | 3.1 | 52.7 | 30.7 | 21.9 |
| Other personal health care | 100.0 | 19.1 | — | — | — | 19.1 | 80.9 | 54.7 | 26.2 |
| Program administration and net cost of private health insurance | 100.0 | 68.6 | 66.6 | — | 66.6 | 2.0 | 31.4 | 16.9 | 14.5 |
| Government public health activities | 100.0 | — | — | — | — | — | 100.0 | 17.3 | 82.7 |
| Research and construction | 100.0 | 37.5 | — | — | — | 37.3 | 62.5 | 46.2 | 16.3 |
| Research | 100.0 | 5.0 | — | — | — | 5.5 | 95.0 | 85.4 | 9.6 |
| Construction | 100.0 | 67.8 | — | — | — | 68.6 | 32.2 | 9.6 | 22.6 |

See footnotes at end of table.

## Table 8—Continued

## National health expenditures, by source of funds and type of expenditure: Selected years 1980-2000

| Year and type of expenditure | Total | All private funds | Private Consumer Total | Out-of-Pocket | Private insurance | Other | Government Total | Federal | State and local |
|---|---|---|---|---|---|---|---|---|---|
| **1989** | | | | | Amount in billions | | | | |
| National health expenditures | $604.1 | $350.9 | $324.5 | $124.8 | $199.7 | $26.3 | $253.3 | $174.3 | $78.8 |
| Health services and supplies | 583.5 | 342.7 | 324.5 | 124.8 | 199.7 | 18.2 | 240.8 | 164.8 | 76.1 |
| Personal health care | 530.7 | 315.3 | 297.7 | 124.8 | 172.9 | 17.6 | 215.4 | 158.4 | 57.0 |
| Hospital care | 232.8 | 108.3 | 96.9 | 12.7 | 84.2 | 11.4 | 124.5 | 92.9 | 31.6 |
| Physician services | 117.6 | 78.5 | 78.4 | 22.4 | 56.1 | 0.0 | 39.2 | 31.8 | 7.4 |
| Dental services | 31.4 | 30.7 | 30.7 | 17.2 | 13.4 | — | 0.7 | 0.4 | 0.3 |
| Other professional services | 27.0 | 21.6 | 18.7 | 8.5 | 10.2 | 2.9 | 5.4 | 4.1 | 1.4 |
| Home health care | 5.4 | 1.3 | 1.0 | 0.6 | 0.4 | 0.3 | 4.1 | 3.1 | 0.9 |
| Drugs and other medical non-durables | 44.6 | 39.3 | 39.3 | 32.3 | 7.0 | — | 5.3 | 2.5 | 2.8 |
| Vision products and other medical durables | 13.5 | 11.0 | 11.0 | 9.8 | 1.2 | — | 2.5 | 2.2 | 0.3 |
| Nursing home care | 47.9 | 22.7 | 21.8 | 21.3 | 0.5 | 0.9 | 25.2 | 16.2 | 9.0 |
| Other personal health care | 10.5 | 2.1 | — | — | — | 2.1 | 8.4 | 5.2 | 3.3 |
| Program administration and net cost of private health insurance | 35.3 | 27.4 | 26.8 | — | 26.8 | 0.5 | 8.0 | 4.3 | 3.6 |
| Government public health activities | 17.5 | — | — | — | — | — | 17.5 | 2.1 | 15.4 |
| Research and construction | 20.6 | 8.2 | — | — | — | 8.2 | 12.4 | 9.7 | 2.8 |
| Research | 11.0 | 0.8 | — | — | — | 0.8 | 10.2 | 8.8 | 1.4 |
| Construction | 9.6 | 7.4 | — | — | — | 7.4 | 2.2 | 0.8 | 1.4 |
| | | | | | Percent distribution | | | | |
| National health expenditures | 100.0 | 58.1 | 53.7 | 20.7 | 33.1 | 4.4 | 41.9 | 28.9 | 13.1 |
| Health services and supplies | 100.0 | 58.7 | 55.6 | 21.4 | 34.2 | 3.1 | 41.3 | 28.2 | 13.0 |
| Personal health care | 100.0 | 59.4 | 56.1 | 23.5 | 32.6 | 3.3 | 40.6 | 29.8 | 10.7 |
| Hospital care | 100.0 | 46.5 | 41.6 | 5.5 | 36.2 | 4.9 | 53.5 | 39.9 | 13.6 |
| Physician services | 100.0 | 66.7 | 66.7 | 19.0 | 47.6 | 0.0 | 33.3 | 27.0 | 6.3 |
| Dental services | 100.0 | 97.6 | 97.6 | 54.9 | 42.7 | — | 2.4 | 1.3 | 1.1 |
| Other professional services | 100.0 | 79.8 | 69.2 | 31.5 | 37.7 | 10.6 | 20.2 | 15.2 | 5.0 |
| Home health care | 100.0 | 24.4 | 18.2 | 11.4 | 6.8 | 6.3 | 75.6 | 58.3 | 17.2 |
| Drugs and other medical non-durables | 100.0 | 88.2 | 88.2 | 72.5 | 15.6 | — | 11.8 | 5.6 | 6.3 |
| Vision products and other medical durables | 100.0 | 81.4 | 81.4 | 72.7 | 8.7 | — | 18.6 | 16.6 | 2.1 |
| Nursing home care | 100.0 | 47.4 | 45.4 | 44.4 | 1.1 | 1.9 | 52.6 | 33.8 | 18.8 |
| Other personal health care | 100.0 | 19.6 | — | — | — | 19.6 | 80.4 | 49.3 | 31.1 |
| Program administration and net cost of private health insurance | 100.0 | 77.5 | 76.0 | — | 76.0 | 1.5 | 22.5 | 12.3 | 10.3 |
| Government public health activities | 100.0 | — | — | — | — | — | 100.0 | 11.9 | 88.1 |
| Research and construction | 100.0 | 39.7 | — | — | — | 39.7 | 60.3 | 46.8 | 13.5 |
| Research | 100.0 | 7.1 | — | — | — | 7.1 | 92.9 | 80.3 | 12.6 |
| Construction | 100.0 | 76.7 | — | — | — | 76.7 | 23.2 | 8.7 | 14.5 |

See footnotes at end of table.

**Table 8—Continued**

## National health expenditures, by source of funds and type of expenditure: Selected years 1980-2000

| Year and type of expenditure | Total | All private funds | Private — Consumer — Total | Private — Consumer — Out-of-Pocket | Private — Consumer — Private insurance | Private — Other | Government — Total | Government — Federal | Government — State and local |
|---|---|---|---|---|---|---|---|---|---|
| **1990** | | | | | Amount in billions | | | | |
| National health expenditures | $670.9 | $389.3 | $360.1 | $137.7 | $222.5 | $29.2 | $281.6 | $192.2 | $89.4 |
| Health services and supplies | 648.6 | 380.3 | 360.1 | 137.7 | 222.5 | 20.2 | 268.3 | 182.0 | 86.4 |
| Personal health care | 589.3 | 348.4 | 328.9 | 137.7 | 191.2 | 19.5 | 240.9 | 175.2 | 65.7 |
| Hospital care | 257.7 | 118.6 | 106.1 | 13.6 | 92.5 | 12.5 | 139.1 | 102.5 | 36.6 |
| Physician services | 132.7 | 88.4 | 88.3 | 25.4 | 63.0 | 0.0 | 44.3 | 35.7 | 8.6 |
| Dental services | 33.8 | 32.9 | 32.9 | 18.5 | 14.4 | — | 0.9 | 0.5 | 0.4 |
| Other professional services | 30.7 | 24.4 | 21.1 | 9.5 | 11.6 | 3.2 | 6.3 | 4.7 | 1.6 |
| Home health care | 6.5 | 1.7 | 1.2 | 0.8 | 0.5 | 0.4 | 4.9 | 3.8 | 1.1 |
| Drugs and other medical non-durables | 48.5 | 42.3 | 42.3 | 34.9 | 7.4 | — | 6.2 | 3.0 | 3.1 |
| Vision products and other medical durables | 14.3 | 11.6 | 11.6 | 10.4 | 1.2 | — | 2.7 | 2.4 | 0.3 |
| Nursing home care | 53.6 | 26.3 | 25.2 | 24.6 | 0.6 | 1.1 | 27.3 | 16.9 | 10.3 |
| Other personal health care | 11.5 | 2.2 | — | — | — | 2.2 | 9.3 | 5.7 | 3.6 |
| Program administration and net cost of private health insurance | 40.5 | 31.9 | 31.2 | — | 31.2 | 0.6 | 8.7 | 4.6 | 4.1 |
| Government public health activities | 18.8 | — | — | — | — | — | 18.8 | 2.2 | 16.6 |
| Research and construction | 22.3 | 9.0 | — | — | — | 9.0 | 13.2 | 10.3 | 3.0 |
| Research | 11.7 | 0.8 | — | — | — | 0.8 | 10.9 | 9.4 | 1.5 |
| Construction | 10.6 | 8.2 | — | — | — | 8.2 | 2.4 | 0.9 | 1.5 |
| | | | | | Percent distribution | | | | |
| National health expenditures | 100.0 | 58.0 | 53.7 | 20.5 | 33.2 | 4.4 | 42.0 | 28.7 | 13.3 |
| Health services and supplies | 100.0 | 58.6 | 55.5 | 21.2 | 34.3 | 3.1 | 41.4 | 28.1 | 13.3 |
| Personal health care | 100.0 | 59.1 | 55.8 | 23.4 | 32.5 | 3.3 | 40.9 | 29.7 | 11.1 |
| Hospital care | 100.0 | 46.0 | 41.2 | 5.3 | 35.9 | 4.9 | 54.0 | 39.8 | 14.2 |
| Physician services | 100.0 | 66.6 | 66.6 | 19.1 | 47.5 | 0.0 | 33.4 | 26.9 | 6.5 |
| Dental services | 100.0 | 97.4 | 97.4 | 54.9 | 42.6 | — | 2.6 | 1.4 | 1.2 |
| Other professional services | 100.0 | 79.4 | 68.9 | 30.9 | 37.9 | 10.6 | 20.6 | 15.4 | 5.2 |
| Home health care | 100.0 | 25.3 | 18.9 | 11.7 | 7.1 | 6.5 | 74.7 | 58.1 | 16.5 |
| Drugs and other medical non-durables | 100.0 | 87.3 | 87.3 | 72.0 | 15.3 | — | 12.7 | 6.3 | 6.5 |
| Vision products and other medical durables | 100.0 | 80.9 | 80.9 | 72.3 | 8.6 | — | 19.1 | 17.0 | 2.0 |
| Nursing home care | 100.0 | 49.1 | 47.1 | 45.9 | 1.2 | 2.0 | 50.9 | 31.6 | 19.3 |
| Other personal health care | 100.0 | 19.4 | — | — | — | 19.4 | 80.6 | 49.2 | 31.5 |
| Program administration and net cost of private health insurance | 100.0 | 78.7 | 77.1 | — | 77.1 | 1.6 | 21.3 | 11.2 | 10.1 |
| Government public health activities | 100.0 | — | — | — | — | — | 100.0 | 11.7 | 88.3 |
| Research and construction | 100.0 | 40.6 | — | — | — | 40.6 | 59.4 | 46.1 | 13.3 |
| Research | 100.0 | 7.0 | — | — | — | 7.0 | 93.0 | 80.2 | 12.7 |
| Construction | 100.0 | 77.5 | — | — | — | 77.5 | 22.5 | 8.5 | 14.0 |

See footnotes at end of table.

## Table 8—Continued

## National health expenditures, by source of funds and type of expenditure: Selected years 1980-2000

| Year and type of expenditure | Total | Private All private funds | Private Consumer Total | Out-of-Pocket | Private insurance | Other | Government Total | Federal | State and local |
|---|---|---|---|---|---|---|---|---|---|
| **1991**[1] | | | | | Amount in billions | | | | |
| National health expenditures | $738.2 | $421.1 | $389.4 | $148.0 | $241.5 | $31.7 | $317.1 | $215.7 | $101.4 |
| Health services and supplies | 714.4 | 411.4 | 389.4 | 148.0 | 241.5 | 22.0 | 302.9 | 204.7 | 98.3 |
| Personal health care | 651.1 | 378.4 | 357.1 | 148.0 | 209.1 | 21.3 | 272.6 | 196.9 | 75.8 |
| Hospital care | 285.4 | 128.8 | 115.2 | 14.6 | 100.6 | 13.6 | 156.6 | 114.2 | 42.4 |
| Physician services | 148.5 | 98.4 | 98.4 | 28.4 | 70.0 | 0.1 | 50.0 | 40.1 | 9.9 |
| Dental services | 36.1 | 35.1 | 35.1 | 19.8 | 15.3 | — | 1.0 | 0.6 | 0.5 |
| Other professional services | 34.5 | 27.3 | 23.6 | 10.5 | 13.1 | 3.6 | 7.3 | 5.5 | 1.8 |
| Home health care | 7.5 | 1.8 | 1.4 | 0.8 | 0.5 | 0.5 | 5.7 | 4.4 | 1.3 |
| Drugs and other medical non-durables | 51.8 | 44.5 | 44.5 | 36.8 | 7.7 | — | 7.3 | 3.7 | 3.6 |
| Vision products and other medical durables | 14.9 | 12.0 | 12.0 | 10.7 | 1.3 | — | 3.0 | 2.7 | 0.3 |
| Nursing home care | 59.1 | 28.1 | 27.0 | 26.3 | 0.7 | 1.1 | 31.0 | 19.2 | 11.8 |
| Other personal health care | 13.3 | 2.4 | — | — | — | 2.4 | 10.9 | 6.6 | 4.2 |
| Program administration and net cost of private health insurance | 43.3 | 33.0 | 32.3 | — | 32.3 | 0.7 | 10.3 | 5.5 | 4.9 |
| Government public health activities | 20.0 | — | — | — | — | — | 20.0 | 2.4 | 17.6 |
| Research and construction | 23.8 | 9.7 | — | — | — | 9.7 | 14.2 | 11.1 | 3.1 |
| Research | 12.5 | 0.8 | — | — | — | 0.8 | 11.7 | 10.1 | 1.6 |
| Construction | 11.3 | 8.8 | — | — | — | 8.8 | 2.5 | 1.0 | 1.5 |
| | | | | | Percent distribution | | | | |
| National health expenditures | 100.0 | 57.0 | 52.8 | 20.0 | 32.7 | 4.3 | 43.0 | 29.2 | 13.7 |
| Health services and supplies | 100.0 | 57.6 | 54.5 | 20.7 | 33.8 | 3.1 | 42.4 | 28.7 | 13.8 |
| Personal health care | 100.0 | 58.1 | 54.9 | 22.7 | 32.1 | 3.3 | 41.9 | 30.2 | 11.6 |
| Hospital care | 100.0 | 45.1 | 40.4 | 5.1 | 35.2 | 4.8 | 54.9 | 40.0 | 14.9 |
| Physician services | 100.0 | 66.3 | 66.3 | 19.1 | 47.1 | 0.0 | 33.7 | 27.0 | 6.7 |
| Dental services | 100.0 | 97.2 | 97.2 | 54.9 | 42.3 | — | 2.8 | 1.6 | 1.3 |
| Other professional services | 100.0 | 78.9 | 68.4 | 30.4 | 38.0 | 10.5 | 21.1 | 15.8 | 5.3 |
| Home health care | 100.0 | 24.4 | 18.2 | 11.3 | 6.9 | 6.2 | 75.6 | 58.7 | 16.9 |
| Drugs and other medical non-durables | 100.0 | 85.9 | 85.9 | 71.0 | 14.9 | — | 14.1 | 7.1 | 7.0 |
| Vision products and other medical durables | 100.0 | 80.2 | 80.2 | 71.8 | 8.4 | — | 19.8 | 17.8 | 2.0 |
| Nursing home care | 100.0 | 47.6 | 45.6 | 44.5 | 1.2 | 1.9 | 52.4 | 32.4 | 20.0 |
| Other personal health care | 100.0 | 18.2 | — | — | — | 18.2 | 81.8 | 49.9 | 31.9 |
| Program administration and net cost of private health insurance | 100.0 | 76.2 | 74.6 | — | 74.6 | 1.6 | 23.8 | 12.6 | 11.2 |
| Government public health activities | 100.0 | — | — | — | — | — | 100.0 | 11.9 | 88.1 |
| Research and construction | 100.0 | 40.5 | — | — | — | 40.5 | 59.5 | 46.4 | 13.1 |
| Research | 100.0 | 6.8 | — | — | — | 6.8 | 93.2 | 80.6 | 12.6 |
| Construction | 100.0 | 77.9 | — | — | — | 77.9 | 22.1 | 8.5 | 13.6 |

See footnotes at end of table.

**Table 8—Continued**

## National health expenditures, by source of funds and type of expenditure: Selected years 1980-2000

| Year and type of expenditure | Total | All private funds | Private Consumer Total | Private Consumer Out-of-Pocket | Private Consumer Private insurance | Other | Government Total | Government Federal | Government State and local |
|---|---|---|---|---|---|---|---|---|---|
| **1992**[1] | | | | | Amount in billions | | | | |
| National health expenditures | $809.0 | $457.4 | $423.1 | $160.1 | $263.0 | $34.3 | $351.6 | $238.8 | $112.8 |
| Health services and supplies | 783.8 | 447.2 | 423.1 | 160.1 | 263.0 | 24.1 | 336.6 | 227.1 | 109.5 |
| Personal health care | 716.7 | 412.8 | 389.5 | 160.1 | 229.4 | 23.4 | 303.9 | 218.5 | 85.4 |
| Hospital care | 313.9 | 140.7 | 125.9 | 15.8 | 110.1 | 14.8 | 173.2 | 125.3 | 47.9 |
| Physician services | 165.5 | 109.0 | 108.9 | 31.6 | 77.4 | 0.1 | 56.5 | 45.4 | 11.1 |
| Dental services | 38.6 | 37.5 | 37.5 | 21.2 | 16.3 | — | 1.1 | 0.6 | 0.5 |
| Other professional services | 38.7 | 30.3 | 26.3 | 11.6 | 14.7 | 4.0 | 8.4 | 6.3 | 2.1 |
| Home health care | 8.5 | 2.3 | 1.7 | 1.1 | 0.6 | 0.6 | 6.2 | 4.8 | 1.4 |
| Drugs and other medical non-durables | 55.5 | 47.2 | 47.2 | 39.0 | 8.2 | — | 8.3 | 4.3 | 4.1 |
| Vision products and other medical durables | 16.1 | 12.8 | 12.8 | 11.5 | 1.3 | — | 3.3 | 3.0 | 0.3 |
| Nursing home care | 64.9 | 30.4 | 29.1 | 28.4 | 0.8 | 1.2 | 34.6 | 21.4 | 13.2 |
| Other personal health care | 14.9 | 2.6 | — | — | — | 2.6 | 12.3 | 7.5 | 4.8 |
| Program administration and net cost of private health insurance | 45.9 | 34.4 | 33.7 | — | 33.7 | 0.7 | 11.5 | 6.0 | 5.4 |
| Government public health activities | 21.2 | — | — | — | — | — | 21.2 | 2.5 | 18.7 |
| Research and construction | 25.2 | 10.2 | — | — | — | 10.2 | 15.0 | 11.7 | 3.3 |
| Research | 13.3 | 0.9 | — | — | — | 0.9 | 12.4 | 10.7 | 1.7 |
| Construction | 11.9 | 9.3 | — | — | — | 9.3 | 2.6 | 1.0 | 1.6 |
| | | | | | Percent distribution | | | | |
| National health expenditures | 100.0 | 56.5 | 52.3 | 19.8 | 32.5 | 4.2 | 43.5 | 29.5 | 13.9 |
| Health services and supplies | 100.0 | 57.1 | 54.0 | 20.4 | 33.6 | 3.1 | 42.9 | 29.0 | 14.0 |
| Personal health care | 100.0 | 57.6 | 54.3 | 22.3 | 32.0 | 3.3 | 42.4 | 30.5 | 11.9 |
| Hospital care | 100.0 | 44.8 | 40.1 | 5.0 | 35.1 | 4.7 | 55.2 | 39.9 | 15.3 |
| Physician services | 100.0 | 65.9 | 65.8 | 19.1 | 46.8 | 0.0 | 34.1 | 27.4 | 6.7 |
| Dental services | 100.0 | 97.0 | 97.0 | 54.9 | 42.1 | — | 3.0 | 1.6 | 1.3 |
| Other professional services | 100.0 | 78.4 | 67.9 | 30.0 | 38.0 | 10.4 | 21.6 | 16.3 | 5.4 |
| Home health care | 100.0 | 26.9 | 20.0 | 12.4 | 7.6 | 6.9 | 73.1 | 56.4 | 16.7 |
| Drugs and other medical non-durables | 100.0 | 85.0 | 85.0 | 70.3 | 14.7 | — | 15.0 | 7.7 | 7.3 |
| Vision products and other medical durables | 100.0 | 79.6 | 79.6 | 71.3 | 8.3 | — | 20.4 | 18.3 | 2.0 |
| Nursing home care | 100.0 | 46.8 | 44.9 | 43.7 | 1.2 | 1.9 | 53.2 | 33.0 | 20.3 |
| Other personal health care | 100.0 | 17.6 | — | — | — | 17.6 | 82.4 | 50.1 | 32.3 |
| Program administration and net cost of private health insurance | 100.0 | 75.0 | 73.4 | — | 73.4 | 1.6 | 25.0 | 13.2 | 11.8 |
| Government public health activities | 100.0 | — | — | — | — | — | 100.0 | 11.8 | 88.2 |
| Research and construction | 100.0 | 40.5 | — | — | — | 40.5 | 59.5 | 46.5 | 13.0 |
| Research | 100.0 | 6.8 | — | — | — | 6.8 | 93.2 | 80.4 | 12.8 |
| Construction | 100.0 | 78.2 | — | — | — | 78.2 | 21.8 | 8.5 | 13.3 |

See footnotes at end of table.

## Table 8—Continued

## National health expenditures, by source of funds and type of expenditure: Selected years 1980-2000

| Year and type of expenditure | Total | Private | | | | | Government | | |
|---|---|---|---|---|---|---|---|---|---|
| | | All private funds | Consumer | | | Other | Total | Federal | State and local |
| | | | Total | Out-of-Pocket | Private insurance | | | | |
| **1995**[1] | | | | Amount in billions | | | | | |
| National health expenditures | $1,072.7 | $592.2 | $548.7 | $202.1 | $346.7 | $43.5 | $480.5 | $324.8 | $155.7 |
| Health services and supplies | 1,043.1 | 580.5 | 548.7 | 202.1 | 346.7 | 31.7 | 462.6 | 310.8 | 151.8 |
| Personal health care | 956.5 | 535.4 | 504.7 | 202.1 | 302.6 | 30.8 | 421.1 | 299.7 | 121.4 |
| Hospital care | 425.4 | 188.9 | 169.1 | 20.8 | 148.2 | 19.8 | 236.5 | 167.9 | 68.7 |
| Physician services | 225.6 | 145.2 | 145.1 | 42.5 | 102.7 | 0.1 | 80.4 | 65.1 | 15.3 |
| Dental services | 47.1 | 45.6 | 45.6 | 26.0 | 19.6 | — | 1.5 | 0.8 | 0.7 |
| Other professional services | 51.6 | 38.8 | 33.6 | 14.7 | 18.9 | 5.2 | 12.8 | 9.6 | 3.2 |
| Home health care | 12.1 | 3.0 | 2.2 | 1.4 | 0.9 | 0.8 | 9.1 | 6.7 | 2.4 |
| Drugs and other medical non-durables | 67.7 | 55.6 | 55.6 | 46.0 | 9.5 | — | 12.1 | 6.4 | 5.8 |
| Vision products and other medical durables | 20.0 | 15.5 | 15.5 | 13.9 | 1.6 | — | 4.5 | 4.1 | 0.4 |
| Nursing home care | 85.8 | 39.6 | 38.0 | 36.8 | 1.1 | 1.6 | 46.2 | 28.4 | 17.8 |
| Other personal health care | 21.3 | 3.3 | — | — | — | 3.3 | 18.0 | 10.8 | 7.2 |
| Program administration and net cost of private health insurance | 60.8 | 45.1 | 44.1 | — | 44.1 | 1.0 | 15.7 | 8.1 | 7.7 |
| Government public health activities | 25.8 | — | — | — | — | — | 25.8 | 3.0 | 22.8 |
| Research and construction | 29.6 | 11.7 | — | — | — | 11.7 | 17.8 | 13.9 | 3.9 |
| Research | 16.1 | 1.1 | — | — | — | 1.1 | 15.0 | 12.8 | 2.2 |
| Construction | 13.5 | 10.7 | — | — | — | 10.7 | 2.8 | 1.1 | 1.7 |
| | | | | Percent distribution | | | | | |
| National health expenditures | 100.0 | 55.2 | 51.2 | 18.8 | 32.3 | 4.1 | 44.8 | 30.3 | 14.5 |
| Health services and supplies | 100.0 | 55.6 | 52.6 | 19.4 | 33.2 | 3.0 | 44.4 | 29.8 | 14.6 |
| Personal health care | 100.0 | 56.0 | 52.8 | 21.1 | 31.6 | 3.2 | 44.0 | 31.3 | 12.7 |
| Hospital care | 100.0 | 44.4 | 39.7 | 4.9 | 34.8 | 4.7 | 55.6 | 39.5 | 16.1 |
| Physician services | 100.0 | 64.4 | 64.3 | 18.8 | 45.5 | 0.0 | 35.6 | 28.8 | 6.8 |
| Dental services | 100.0 | 96.8 | 96.8 | 55.1 | 41.7 | — | 3.2 | 1.8 | 1.4 |
| Other professional services | 100.0 | 75.2 | 65.2 | 28.5 | 36.7 | 10.0 | 24.8 | 18.6 | 6.2 |
| Home health care | 100.0 | 24.8 | 18.5 | 11.4 | 7.1 | 6.4 | 75.2 | 55.5 | 19.7 |
| Drugs and other medical non-durables | 100.0 | 82.1 | 82.1 | 68.0 | 14.1 | — | 17.9 | 9.4 | 8.5 |
| Vision products and other medical durables | 100.0 | 77.5 | 77.5 | 69.4 | 8.1 | — | 22.5 | 20.5 | 2.0 |
| Nursing home care | 100.0 | 46.1 | 44.3 | 42.9 | 1.3 | 1.9 | 53.9 | 33.1 | 20.7 |
| Other personal health care | 100.0 | 15.6 | — | — | — | 15.6 | 84.4 | 50.5 | 33.9 |
| Program administration and net cost of private health insurance | 100.0 | 74.1 | 72.5 | — | 72.5 | 1.6 | 25.9 | 13.3 | 12.6 |
| Government public health activities | 100.0 | — | — | — | — | — | 100.0 | 11.6 | 88.4 |
| Research and construction | 100.0 | 39.7 | — | — | — | 39.7 | 60.3 | 47.1 | 13.2 |
| Research | 100.0 | 6.8 | — | — | — | 6.8 | 93.2 | 79.6 | 13.6 |
| Construction | 100.0 | 78.9 | — | — | — | 78.9 | 21.1 | 8.5 | 12.6 |

See footnotes at end of table.

## Table 8—Continued

## National health expenditures, by source of funds and type of expenditure: Selected years 1980-2000

| Year and type of expenditure | Total | Private All private funds | Consumer Total | Out-of-Pocket | Private insurance | Other | Government Total | Federal | State and local |
|---|---|---|---|---|---|---|---|---|---|
| **2000**[1] | | | | Amount in billions | | | | | |
| National health expenditures | $1,615.9 | $859.4 | $797.8 | $290.3 | $507.6 | $61.6 | $756.5 | $517.6 | $238.8 |
| Health services and supplies | 1,576.1 | 844.1 | 797.8 | 290.3 | 507.6 | 46.2 | 732.0 | 498.5 | 233.5 |
| Personal health care | 1,456.0 | 779.6 | 734.8 | 290.3 | 444.6 | 44.8 | 676.4 | 484.2 | 192.1 |
| Hospital care | 654.2 | 279.6 | 250.1 | 30.3 | 219.8 | 29.5 | 374.6 | 263.4 | 111.2 |
| Physician services | 360.5 | 221.1 | 221.0 | 65.8 | 155.2 | 0.1 | 139.3 | 115.7 | 23.6 |
| Dental services | 63.1 | 61.1 | 61.1 | 35.2 | 25.9 | — | 2.0 | 1.1 | 0.9 |
| Other professional services | 75.4 | 52.7 | 45.7 | 20.0 | 25.7 | 7.0 | 22.7 | 17.4 | 5.3 |
| Home health care | 18.8 | 3.3 | 2.5 | 1.6 | 0.9 | 0.8 | 15.5 | 11.0 | 4.5 |
| Drugs and other medical non-durables | 91.0 | 72.5 | 72.5 | 59.9 | 12.6 | — | 18.5 | 9.9 | 8.6 |
| Vision products and other medical durables | 28.4 | 20.9 | 20.9 | 18.7 | 2.2 | — | 7.5 | 7.0 | 0.5 |
| Nursing home care | 130.8 | 63.6 | 61.0 | 58.8 | 2.2 | 2.6 | 67.2 | 41.4 | 25.7 |
| Other personal health care | 33.9 | 4.7 | — | — | — | 4.7 | 29.2 | 17.4 | 11.8 |
| Program administration and net cost of private health insurance | 85.3 | 64.4 | 63.0 | — | 63.0 | 1.4 | 20.9 | 10.1 | 10.8 |
| Government public health activities | 34.8 | — | — | — | — | — | 34.8 | 4.1 | 30.6 |
| Research and construction | 39.8 | 15.4 | — | — | — | 15.4 | 24.5 | 19.1 | 5.3 |
| Research | 22.3 | 1.5 | — | — | — | 1.5 | 20.8 | 17.6 | 3.2 |
| Construction | 17.5 | 13.9 | — | — | — | 13.9 | 3.6 | 1.5 | 2.2 |
| | | | | Percent distribution | | | | | |
| National health expenditures | 100.0 | 53.2 | 49.4 | 18.0 | 31.4 | 3.8 | 46.8 | 32.0 | 14.8 |
| Health services and supplies | 100.0 | 53.6 | 50.6 | 18.4 | 32.2 | 2.9 | 46.4 | 31.6 | 14.8 |
| Personal health care | 100.0 | 53.5 | 50.5 | 19.9 | 30.5 | 3.1 | 46.5 | 33.3 | 13.2 |
| Hospital care | 100.0 | 42.7 | 38.2 | 4.6 | 33.6 | 4.5 | 57.3 | 40.3 | 17.0 |
| Physician services | 100.0 | 61.4 | 61.3 | 18.2 | 43.1 | 0.0 | 38.6 | 32.1 | 6.6 |
| Dental services | 100.0 | 96.9 | 96.9 | 55.8 | 41.1 | — | 3.1 | 1.7 | 1.4 |
| Other professional services | 100.0 | 69.9 | 60.6 | 26.5 | 34.1 | 9.3 | 30.1 | 23.1 | 7.1 |
| Home health care | 100.0 | 17.6 | 13.1 | 8.4 | 4.7 | 4.5 | 82.4 | 58.5 | 23.9 |
| Drugs and other medical non-durables | 100.0 | 79.7 | 79.7 | 65.8 | 13.9 | — | 20.3 | 10.9 | 9.5 |
| Vision products and other medical durables | 100.0 | 73.6 | 73.6 | 65.9 | 7.7 | — | 26.4 | 24.5 | 1.9 |
| Nursing home care | 100.0 | 48.6 | 46.7 | 45.0 | 1.6 | 2.0 | 51.4 | 31.7 | 19.7 |
| Other personal health care | 100.0 | 13.9 | — | — | — | 13.9 | 86.1 | 51.4 | 34.7 |
| Program administration and net cost of private health insurance | 100.0 | 75.5 | 73.8 | — | 73.8 | 1.7 | 24.5 | 11.8 | 12.6 |
| Government public health activities | 100.0 | — | — | — | — | — | 100.0 | 11.9 | 88.1 |
| Research and construction | 100.0 | 38.6 | — | — | — | 38.6 | 61.4 | 48.1 | 13.4 |
| Research | 100.0 | 6.6 | — | — | — | 6.6 | 93.4 | 79.1 | 14.2 |
| Construction | 100.0 | 79.2 | — | — | — | 79.2 | 20.8 | 8.5 | 12.3 |

[1] Projected

NOTES: 0.0 denotes less than $50 million. Research and development expenditures of drug companies and other manufacturers and providers of medical equipment and supplies are excluded from "research expenditures," but are included in the expenditure class in which the product falls. Columns may not add to totals because of rounding

SOURCE: Health Care Financing Administration, Office of the Actuary: Data from the Office of National Health Statistics

# Table 9

## Medicare and Medicaid spending, by type of expenditure: Selected years 1989-2000

| Year and type of expenditure | 1989 Medicare | 1989 Medicaid | 1991 Medicare | 1991 Medicaid | 1992 Medicare | 1992 Medicaid | 1995 Medicare | 1995 Medicaid | 2000 Medicare | 2000 Medicaid |
|---|---|---|---|---|---|---|---|---|---|---|
| | | | | | Amount in billions | | | | | |
| Health services and supplies | $102.1 | $62.5 | $121.2 | $91.1 | $133.4 | $105.0 | $182.3 | $154.1 | $302.8 | $243.8 |
| Personal health care | 99.8 | 59.3 | 118.6 | 86.7 | 130.7 | 99.9 | 179.0 | 146.5 | 298.4 | 234.9 |
| Hospital care | 62.1 | 22.9 | 74.0 | 35.3 | 80.6 | 41.0 | 108.1 | 60.7 | 172.1 | 99.7 |
| Physician services | 27.5 | 4.2 | 33.7 | 7.0 | 37.9 | 8.3 | 54.3 | 12.3 | 98.7 | 19.6 |
| Dental services | — | 0.6 | — | 0.9 | — | 1.0 | — | 1.3 | — | 1.7 |
| Other professional services | 2.5 | 1.7 | 3.3 | 2.4 | 3.8 | 2.9 | 5.7 | 4.9 | 10.7 | 9.0 |
| Home health care | 2.1 | 1.9 | 2.9 | 2.7 | 3.2 | 3.0 | 4.0 | 5.1 | 5.7 | 9.7 |
| Drugs and other medical non-durables | — | 4.1 | — | 6.1 | — | 7.0 | — | 10.6 | — | 16.6 |
| Vision products and other medical durables | 2.1 | — | 2.5 | — | 2.8 | — | 3.9 | — | 6.6 | — |
| Nursing home care | 3.6 | 20.6 | 2.3 | 27.4 | 2.5 | 30.7 | 3.2 | 41.3 | 4.5 | 59.9 |
| Other personal health care | — | 3.2 | — | 4.9 | — | 5.9 | — | 10.4 | — | 18.7 |
| Program administration | 2.3 | 3.1 | 2.6 | 4.4 | 2.8 | 5.1 | 3.3 | 7.6 | 4.4 | 9.0 |
| | | | | | Percent of national expenditure | | | | | |
| Health services and supplies | 17.5 | 10.7 | 17.0 | 12.8 | 17.0 | 13.4 | 17.5 | 14.8 | 19.2 | 15.5 |
| Personal health care | 18.8 | 11.2 | 18.2 | 13.3 | 18.2 | 13.9 | 18.7 | 15.3 | 20.5 | 16.1 |
| Hospital care | 26.7 | 9.8 | 25.9 | 12.4 | 25.7 | 13.1 | 25.4 | 14.3 | 26.3 | 15.2 |
| Physician services | 23.4 | 3.6 | 22.7 | 4.7 | 22.9 | 5.0 | 24.1 | 5.5 | 27.4 | 5.4 |
| Dental services | — | 2.0 | — | 2.4 | — | 2.6 | — | 2.8 | — | 2.7 |
| Other professional services | 9.3 | 6.3 | 9.5 | 7.1 | 9.7 | 7.4 | 11.0 | 9.5 | 14.2 | 12.0 |
| Home health care | 39.1 | 36.0 | 39.4 | 35.8 | 37.2 | 35.5 | 32.7 | 42.0 | 30.5 | 51.6 |
| Drugs and other medical non-durables | — | 9.3 | — | 11.7 | — | 12.7 | — | 15.7 | — | 18.2 |
| Vision products and other medical durables | 15.3 | — | 16.6 | — | 17.1 | — | 19.4 | — | 23.4 | — |
| Nursing home care | 7.5 | 43.1 | 4.0 | 46.4 | 3.9 | 47.3 | 3.7 | 48.2 | 3.4 | 45.8 |
| Other personal health care | — | 30.2 | — | 36.8 | — | 39.8 | — | 48.6 | — | 55.2 |
| Program administration | 6.5 | 8.8 | 6.0 | 10.2 | 6.0 | 11.2 | 5.4 | 12.5 | 5.1 | 10.5 |
| | | | | | Percent of program expenditures | | | | | |
| Health services and supplies | 100.0 | 100.0 | 100.0 | 100.0 | 100.0 | 100.0 | 100.0 | 100.0 | 100.0 | 100.0 |
| Personal health care | 97.8 | 95.0 | 97.9 | 95.1 | 97.9 | 95.1 | 98.2 | 95.1 | 98.6 | 96.3 |
| Hospital care | 60.8 | 36.7 | 61.0 | 38.7 | 60.4 | 39.1 | 59.3 | 39.4 | 56.9 | 40.9 |
| Physician services | 26.9 | 6.8 | 27.8 | 7.7 | 28.4 | 7.9 | 29.8 | 8.0 | 32.6 | 8.0 |
| Dental services | — | 1.0 | — | 1.0 | — | 0.9 | — | 0.8 | — | 0.7 |
| Other professional services | 2.5 | 2.7 | 2.7 | 2.7 | 2.8 | 2.7 | 3.1 | 3.2 | 3.5 | 3.7 |
| Home health care | 2.1 | 3.1 | 2.4 | 2.9 | 2.4 | 2.9 | 2.2 | 3.3 | 1.9 | 4.0 |
| Drugs and other medical non-durables | — | 6.6 | — | 6.7 | — | 6.7 | — | 6.9 | — | 6.8 |
| Vision products and other medical durables | 2.0 | — | 2.0 | — | 2.1 | — | 2.1 | — | 2.2 | — |
| Nursing home care | 3.5 | 33.0 | 1.9 | 30.1 | 1.9 | 29.2 | 1.7 | 26.8 | 1.5 | 24.6 |
| Other personal health care | — | 5.1 | — | 5.4 | — | 5.7 | — | 6.7 | — | 7.7 |
| Program administration | 2.2 | 5.0 | 2.1 | 4.9 | 2.1 | 4.9 | 1.8 | 4.9 | 1.4 | 3.7 |

NOTE: Columns may not add to totals because of rounding

SOURCE: Health Care Financing Administration, Office of the Actuary Data from the Office of National Health Statistics

**Table 10**

**Factors accounting for growth in expenditures for selected categories of national health expenditures, by 5-year periods: 1975-2000**

| Type of expenditure and period | Total | Economywide factors | | Health-sector specific factors | | |
|---|---|---|---|---|---|---|
| | | General inflation[1] | Population | Utilization[2] | Intensity[3] | Sector-specific price inflation |
| **Physician services** | | | Percent distribution | | | |
| 1975-1980 | 100.0 | 63.3 | 7.7 | −5.9 | 20.8 | 14.1 |
| 1980-1985 | 100.0 | 45.7 | 8.6 | 2.0 | 23.3 | 20.4 |
| 1985-1990 | 100.0 | 29.2 | 8.3 | 3.7 | 37.5 | 21.4 |
| 1990-1995 | 100.0 | 35.2 | 8.7 | 7.9 | 37.5 | 10.8 |
| 1995-2000 | 100.0 | 42.0 | 8.3 | 5.2 | 36.5 | 8.0 |
| **Inpatient hospital** | | | | | | |
| 1975-1980 | 100.0 | 50.3 | 6.1 | 5.7 | 28.6 | 9.3 |
| 1980-1985 | 100.0 | 51.4 | 9.7 | −42.8 | 60.1 | 21.6 |
| 1985-1990 | 100.0 | 44.6 | 12.7 | −23.2 | 41.4 | 24.5 |
| 1990-1995 | 100.0 | 44.1 | 10.9 | 8.8 | 16.8 | 19.4 |
| 1995-2000 | 100.0 | 47.8 | 9.5 | 12.5 | 14.0 | 16.1 |
| **Outpatient hospital** | | | | | | |
| 1975-1980 | 100.0 | 43.0 | 5.2 | 8.7 | 35.1 | 8.0 |
| 1980-1985 | 100.0 | 32.7 | 6.1 | 7.7 | 39.9 | 13.7 |
| 1985-1990 | 100.0 | 21.2 | 6.0 | 30.6 | 30.6 | 11.6 |
| 1990-1995 | 100.0 | 24.5 | 6.1 | 26.2 | 32.4 | 10.8 |
| 1995-2000 | 100.0 | 37.2 | 7.4 | 14.0 | 28.9 | 12.6 |
| **Nursing home excluding ICF/MR** | | | | | | |
| 1975-1980 | 100.0 | 56.8 | 6.9 | 14.2 | 16.7 | 5.5 |
| 1980-1985 | 100.0 | 50.6 | 9.5 | 1.1 | 26.8 | 12.0 |
| 1985-1990 | 100.0 | 38.4 | 10.9 | 2.6 | 32.6 | 15.4 |
| 1990-1995 | 100.0 | 40.7 | 10.1 | 8.8 | 31.0 | 9.4 |
| 1995-2000 | 100.0 | 45.9 | 9.1 | 13.6 | 24.4 | 7.1 |
| **Drugs and other medical non-durables** | | | | | | |
| 1975-1980 | 100.0 | 84.9 | 10.3 | 0.0 | 7.8 | −2.9 |
| 1980-1985 | 100.0 | 54.8 | 10.3 | 0.0 | −9.3 | 44.2 |
| 1985-1990 | 100.0 | 41.9 | 11.9 | 0.0 | −0.2 | 46.4 |
| 1990-1995 | 100.0 | 55.7 | 13.8 | 0.0 | −11.3 | 41.8 |
| 1995-2000 | 100.0 | 66.5 | 13.1 | 0.0 | −2.7 | 23.0 |

[1]General inflation is measured by the gross national product implicit price deflator
[2]Per capita days or visits
[3]Real services per day or per visit
NOTE: ICF MR is intermediate care facility for the mentally retarded
SOURCE: Health Care Financing Administration. Office of the Actuary Data from the Office of National Health Statistics

# Chapter 16

## Characteristics of Persons With and Without Health Care Coverage: United States, 1989

Peter Ries, Division of Health Interview Statistics

## PERSONS WITH NO HEALTH CARE COVERAGE

In 1989 an estimated 33.9 million persons in the civilian noninstitutionalized population of the United States (13.9 percent) were reported to lack health care coverage. This point-prevalence estimate represents an average for 52 weeks of household interviews conducted by the U.S. Bureau of the Census for the National Health Interview Survey (NHIS). It is a measure of a person's coverage status at the time of interview, not at any time prior to the interview. Noncoverage was relatively higher for younger persons, males, persons who are not white, those with low incomes, persons 18 years of age and over who were unemployed or had less than 12 years of education, residents of the South and West Regions of the country, and residents of central cities in metropolitan statistical areas (MSA's).

Table 1 shows that more than 20 percent of persons in the following groups lacked coverage: Unemployed workers 18 years of age and over (38.3 percent), persons living below the poverty level (32.5 percent), members of families with low annual incomes (27.7 percent for $5,000–$9,999, 27.1 percent for less than $5,000, and 24.3 for $10,000–$19,999), young adults 18–24 years of age (27.4 percent) and black persons (20.2 percent). In contrast, the lowest proportions of those without health care coverage were among persons 65 years of age and over (1.2 percent) and members of families with an annual income of $50,000 or more (3.6 percent).

Because of Medicare, most persons without any form of health care coverage are under 65 years of age (an estimated 33.6 million persons, or 15.7 percent of those in this age group). In terms of both age and socio-demographic characteristics, more than 40 percent of the persons in some of the resulting subgroups lacked coverage. These included persons 18–44 years of age who were unemployed or were members of families with an annual income of $5,000–$9,999; those 25–44 years of age who had family incomes of less than $5,000 per year or were below the poverty level; and young adults 18–24 years of age with less than 12 years of education.

Figure 1 shows the proportion of persons of all ages and of those under 65 years of age without health care coverage by family income. For all ages combined, the estimates of noncoverage range from 27.7 percent for those in families with an annual family income of $5,000–$9,999 to 3.6 percent for members of families with an annual income of $50,000 or more. The estimates for persons under 65 years of age range from 36.9 to 3.7 percent for the corresponding income groups.

The estimate reported above of the number of persons without health care coverage is similar to the corre-

Reprinted from Advance data from vital and health statistics; No. 201. Hyattsville, Maryland: National Center for Health Statistics. June 1991.

**Table 1. Percent of persons without health care coverage, by age and sociodemographic characteristics: United States, 1989**

| Sociodemographic characteristic | All ages | Under 65 years | | | | | 65 years and over |
| | | Total | Under 18 years | 18–24 years | 25–44 years | 45–64 years | |
|---|---|---|---|---|---|---|---|
| | | | | Percent[1] | | | |
| All persons not covered[2] . . . . . . . . . . . . . . . . . . . . . . | 13.9 | 15.7 | 14.9 | 27.4 | 15.5 | 10.5 | 1.2 |
| **Sex** | | | | | | | |
| Male. . . . . . . . . . . . . . . . . . . . . . . . . . . . . . . . . . . | 15.1 | 16.7 | 15.1 | 31.3 | 17.6 | 9.6 | 1.3 |
| Female . . . . . . . . . . . . . . . . . . . . . . . . . . . . . . . . . | 12.7 | 14.6 | 14.7 | 23.7 | 13.6 | 11.2 | 1.2 |
| **Race** | | | | | | | |
| White . . . . . . . . . . . . . . . . . . . . . . . . . . . . . . . . . . | 12.8 | 14.5 | 14.0 | 26.3 | 14.4 | 9.4 | 1.0 |
| Black . . . . . . . . . . . . . . . . . . . . . . . . . . . . . . . . . . | 20.2 | 21.9 | 18.9 | 34.3 | 22.5 | 17.5 | 2.5 |
| Other . . . . . . . . . . . . . . . . . . . . . . . . . . . . . . . . . . | 19.7 | 20.4 | 18.9 | 27.8 | 20.7 | 17.5 | *8.4 |
| **Family income** | | | | | | | |
| Less than $5,000. . . . . . . . . . . . . . . . . . . . . . . . . . . | 27.1 | 31.3 | 25.5 | 27.3 | 42.4 | 35.5 | *1.5 |
| $5,000–$9,999 . . . . . . . . . . . . . . . . . . . . . . . . . . . . | 27.7 | 36.9 | 31.6 | 43.5 | 43.5 | 32.2 | 1.6 |
| $10,000–$19,999. . . . . . . . . . . . . . . . . . . . . . . . . . | 24.3 | 30.1 | 30.2 | 37.5 | 32.0 | 21.3 | 1.1 |
| $20,000–$34,999. . . . . . . . . . . . . . . . . . . . . . . . . . | 10.6 | 11.6 | 10.9 | 22.1 | 11.8 | 6.8 | 1.0 |
| $35,000–$49,999. . . . . . . . . . . . . . . . . . . . . . . . . . | 5.8 | 6.0 | 4.0 | 18.4 | 5.8 | 3.9 | *0.8 |
| $50,000 or more . . . . . . . . . . . . . . . . . . . . . . . . . . | 3.6 | 3.7 | 2.3 | 12.9 | 3.7 | 1.9 | *1.6 |
| **Poverty status** | | | | | | | |
| In poverty . . . . . . . . . . . . . . . . . . . . . . . . . . . . . . . | 32.5 | 36.0 | 32.5 | 35.9 | 42.2 | 35.9 | 2.3 |
| Not in poverty. . . . . . . . . . . . . . . . . . . . . . . . . . . . . | 10.3 | 11.5 | 9.6 | 23.5 | 11.7 | 7.6 | 1.1 |
| **Employment status[3]** | | | | | | | |
| Currently employed . . . . . . . . . . . . . . . . . . . . . . . . . | 13.9 | 14.3 | . . . | 26.6 | 13.6 | 9.0 | 1.5 |
| Unemployed. . . . . . . . . . . . . . . . . . . . . . . . . . . . . . | 38.3 | 39.2 | . . . | 44.5 | 40.8 | 26.5 | |
| Not in labor force . . . . . . . . . . . . . . . . . . . . . . . . . . | 10.8 | 18.5 | . . . | 26.0 | 21.2 | 12.8 | 1.2 |
| **Education[3]** | | | | | | | |
| Less than 12 years . . . . . . . . . . . . . . . . . . . . . . . . . | 20.8 | 30.1 | . . . | 42.1 | 35.5 | 19.9 | 1.5 |
| 12 years . . . . . . . . . . . . . . . . . . . . . . . . . . . . . . . . | 14.4 | 16.6 | . . . | 29.8 | 16.8 | 8.5 | 0.7 |
| More than 12 years . . . . . . . . . . . . . . . . . . . . . . . . . | 8.4 | 9.2 | . . . | 16.0 | 9.0 | 5.8 | 1.3 |
| **Region** | | | | | | | |
| Northeast . . . . . . . . . . . . . . . . . . . . . . . . . . . . . . . | 9.6 | 11.0 | 9.9 | 22.0 | 10.9 | 6.6 | 1.7 |
| Midwest . . . . . . . . . . . . . . . . . . . . . . . . . . . . . . . . | 9.6 | 10.8 | 8.8 | 22.3 | 10.6 | 7.6 | 0.8 |
| South . . . . . . . . . . . . . . . . . . . . . . . . . . . . . . . . . . | 17.5 | 19.7 | 20.5 | 30.9 | 19.2 | 13.4 | 1.1 |
| West . . . . . . . . . . . . . . . . . . . . . . . . . . . . . . . . . . | 17.1 | 18.9 | 16.7 | 32.7 | 19.7 | 13.1 | 1.6 |
| **Place of residence** | | | | | | | |
| MSA. . . . . . . . . . . . . . . . . . . . . . . . . . . . . . . . . . . | 13.7 | 15.3 | 14.4 | 27.4 | 15.2 | 9.8 | 1.3 |
| Central city . . . . . . . . . . . . . . . . . . . . . . . . . . . . . | 17.2 | 19.4 | 18.2 | 30.0 | 20.1 | 12.9 | 1.6 |
| Not central city . . . . . . . . . . . . . . . . . . . . . . . . . . | 11.4 | 12.7 | 12.1 | 25.4 | 12.1 | 8.0 | 1.1 |
| Not MSA . . . . . . . . . . . . . . . . . . . . . . . . . . . . . . . | 14.7 | 17.1 | 16.5 | 27.6 | 17.0 | 12.6 | 1.1 |

Percent calculated excluding the 9.7 million persons for whom coverage status was not determined.
[1] Includes persons with unknown sociodemographic characteristics.
[3] Excludes persons under 18 years of age.

NOTE: MSA is metropolitan statistical area.

sponding estimate of two recent large-scale U.S. Government surveys. The National Medical Expenditure Survey of 1987 reported point-prevalence estimates for different periods of the year of 34–36 million persons without health care coverage.[1] The preliminary estimate from the March 1990 Current Population Survey indicates that 33.4 million persons had no health care coverage in 1989.[2] The sociodemographic characteristics of persons without health care coverage in those surveys are similar to those shown in table 1 of this report.

Understanding the reasons for the similarities and differences in the results from these three surveys would require a detailed comparison of the procedures and definitions used in each and the possible effect of comparing estimates from different years. . . . Health care coverage as used in this report is defined on the basis of persons' coverage status under four types of plans: Private health insurance, Medicare, public assistance (overwhelmingly Medicaid), and military or Veterans' Administration (military–VA) health benefits. Persons covered by any one of these four plans were classified as

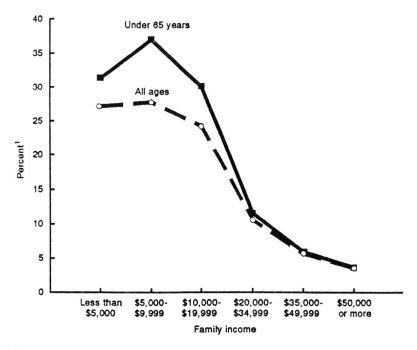

¹Excludes persons with unknown coverage status.

**Figure 1.** Percent of persons without health care coverage, by age and family income: United States, 1989

having health care coverage. In addition, a relatively small number of persons who indicated an unspecified form of coverage were included in this group. Persons classified as not being covered under any of the four plans were classified as not having health care coverage. All other persons were classified as being of unknown coverage status and were excluded in calculating the percents shown in this report. . . . The following four sections highlight the characteristics of persons covered by each of the types of plans.

## PERSON WITH PRIVATE HEALTH INSURANCE COVERAGE

About 76.1 percent (an estimated 185.3 million persons) of the civilian noninstitutionalized population were covered by private health insurance in 1989. Table 2 shows that the estimates do not greatly differ for persons under 65 years of age (75.9 percent) and those 65 years of age and over (77.2 percent). However, in general, these represent different types of plans: For the younger group private plans are the primary form of coverage, whereas for the older group most plans were purchased to supplement Medicare coverage.

Within sociodemographic categories, the proportion of persons covered was relatively high for white persons

(79.3 percent), those not below the poverty line (84.3 percent), currently employed persons (83.6 percent), those with more than 12 years of education (88.2 percent), residents of the Northeast (81.3 percent) and Midwest (81.7 percent) Regions, and persons living outside of central cities in MSA's (82.0 percent).

Figure 2 shows the proportion of persons covered by private health insurance by family income and age. Clearly the percent of persons covered was directly related to the amount of their family incomes, the range for all ages being from 30.5 percent for less than $5,000 to 94.9 percent for $50,000 or more. However, the relationship is not nearly so strong for persons 65 years of age and over (from 42.1 for the lowest to 86.7 percent for the highest income group) as it is for those under 65 years of age (28.7 to 95.2 percent being the corresponding estimates).

Private coverage is determined in the survey by first identifying all plans that pay all or part of hospital or doctor bills for any member of the family and then determining each person's status in relation to each of these plans. Persons are classified as covered if they are covered by one plan or more; they are classified as not covered if they are not covered by any of the plans. Persons not meeting either of these criteria are classified as unknown. Plans covering only one type or condition (such as cancer or injuries) are not included in this definition of private coverage.

**Table 2. Percent of persons with private health insurance coverage, by age and sociodemographic characteristics: United States, 1989**

| Sociodemographic characteristic | All ages | Under 65 years | | | | | 65 years and over |
|---|---|---|---|---|---|---|---|
| | | Total | Under 18 years | 18–24 years | 25–44 years | 45–64 years | |
| | | | | Percent[1] | | | |
| All persons covered[2] . . . . . . . . . . . . . . . . . . . . . . | 76.1 | 75.9 | 71.8 | 64.4 | 79.0 | 82.6 | 77.2 |
| *Sex* | | | | | | | |
| Male. . . . . . . . . . . . . . . . . . . . . . . . . . . . | 76.3 | 76.1 | 71.9 | 65.1 | 78.9 | 83.5 | 78.1 |
| Female . . . . . . . . . . . . . . . . . . . . . . . . . . | 75.8 | 75.7 | 71.7 | 63.9 | 79.1 | 81.8 | 76.6 |
| *Race* | | | | | | | |
| White . . . . . . . . . . . . . . . . . . . . . . . . . . . | 79.3 | 79.1 | 76.3 | 67.4 | 81.4 | 85.0 | 80.8 |
| Black . . . . . . . . . . . . . . . . . . . . . . . . . . . | 56.6 | 57.8 | 51.6 | 48.8 | 64.4 | 64.8 | 43.7 |
| Other . . . . . . . . . . . . . . . . . . . . . . . . . . . | 64.2 | 65.1 | 58.2 | 58.8 | 70.0 | 71.4 | 48.5 |
| *Family income* | | | | | | | |
| Less than $5,000. . . . . . . . . . . . . . . . . . . . . . . | 30.5 | 28.7 | 15.0 | 57.1 | 17.1 | 20.6 | 42.1 |
| $5,000–$9,999 . . . . . . . . . . . . . . . . . . . . . . . | 35.8 | 26.0 | 19.5 | 34.9 | 25.0 | 33.4 | 64.3 |
| $10,000–$19,999. . . . . . . . . . . . . . . . . . . . . . | 62.1 | 57.4 | 51.3 | 52.1 | 59.4 | 67.8 | 81.5 |
| $20,000–$34,999. . . . . . . . . . . . . . . . . . . . . . | 84.4 | 84.2 | 82.9 | 72.6 | 85.7 | 89.3 | 85.9 |
| $35,000–$49,999. . . . . . . . . . . . . . . . . . . . . . | 91.7 | 91.9 | 92.8 | 78.7 | 93.0 | 94.1 | 88.2 |
| $50,000 or more . . . . . . . . . . . . . . . . . . . . . . | 94.9 | 95.2 | 96.5 | 85.6 | 95.7 | 96.8 | 86.7 |
| *Poverty status* | | | | | | | |
| In poverty . . . . . . . . . . . . . . . . . . . . . . . . . | 28.3 | 26.3 | 21.4 | 43.4 | 23.9 | 24.0 | 46.2 |
| Not in poverty. . . . . . . . . . . . . . . . . . . . . . . | 84.3 | 84.6 | 85.0 | 71.6 | 85.8 | 88.1 | 82.3 |
| *Employment status[3]* | | | | | | | |
| Currently employed . . . . . . . . . . . . . . . . . . . . . | 83.6 | 83.5 | . . . | 70.0 | 84.6 | 89.0 | 86.0 |
| Unemployed. . . . . . . . . . . . . . . . . . . . . . . . . | 48.4 | 47.6 | . . . | 42.1 | 44.7 | 64.4 | 81.5 |
| Not in labor force . . . . . . . . . . . . . . . . . . . . . | 67.8 | 61.4 | . . . | 54.1 | 56.4 | 69.2 | 75.9 |
| *Education[3]* | | | | | | | |
| Less than 12 years . . . . . . . . . . . . . . . . . . . . . | 58.4 | 54.3 | . . . | 42.2 | 48.8 | 64.8 | 67.0 |
| 12 years . . . . . . . . . . . . . . . . . . . . . . . . . | 78.5 | 77.5 | . . . | 61.9 | 77.6 | 86.7 | 84.3 |
| More than 12 years . . . . . . . . . . . . . . . . . . . . . | 88.2 | 88.2 | . . . | 80.7 | 88.7 | 91.2 | 88.6 |
| *Region* | | | | | | | |
| Northeast . . . . . . . . . . . . . . . . . . . . . . . . . | 81.3 | 81.9 | 78.9 | 71.7 | 84.1 | 87.2 | 77.5 |
| Midwest . . . . . . . . . . . . . . . . . . . . . . . . . . | 81.7 | 81.5 | 79.1 | 70.0 | 84.1 | 86.8 | 82.7 |
| South. . . . . . . . . . . . . . . . . . . . . . . . . . . | 71.7 | 71.4 | 65.9 | 60.6 | 75.4 | 78.5 | 73.9 |
| West . . . . . . . . . . . . . . . . . . . . . . . . . . . | 71.7 | 71.2 | 67.6 | 57.2 | 74.2 | 79.4 | 75.8 |
| *Place of residence* | | | | | | | |
| MSA. . . . . . . . . . . . . . . . . . . . . . . . . . . . | 76.7 | 76.5 | 72.1 | 64.8 | 79.6 | 83.7 | 78.0 |
| Central city . . . . . . . . . . . . . . . . . . . . . . . . | 68.4 | 67.8 | 60.1 | 59.7 | 71.9 | 76.7 | 72.8 |
| Not central city. . . . . . . . . . . . . . . . . . . . . . . | 82.0 | 82.0 | 79.7 | 68.7 | 84.4 | 87.9 | 81.6 |
| Not MSA. . . . . . . . . . . . . . . . . . . . . . . . . . | 74.0 | 73.8 | 70.8 | 63.1 | 76.8 | 78.8 | 75.2 |

[1] Percent calculated excluding the 8.6 million persons for whom coverage status was not determined.
[2] Includes persons with unknown sociodemographic characteristics.
[3] Excludes persons under 18 years of age.
NOTE: MSA is metropolitan statistical area.

## PERSONS COVERED BY MEDICARE

About 12.6 percent (an estimated 30.7 million persons) of the civilian noninstitutionalized population were covered by Medicare in 1989. Table 3 shows that coverage was 94.3 percent for persons 65 years of age and over and 1.4 percent for those under 65 years of age. Among the older persons, the proportion covered was less than 90 percent for only three of the groups shown in the table: Persons other than white or black (78.1

percent), currently employed persons (87.7 percent), and members of families with an annual income of $50,000 or more (88.3 percent). Among all of the other groups included in the table, coverage was greater than 90 percent, with the lowest percent of coverage among these groups being 90.7 percent for black persons.

Regarding persons under 65 years of age, only four groups had more than 4 percent covered by Medicare: Adults (18 years of age and over) who were not in the labor force (7.4 percent), adults who had less than 12

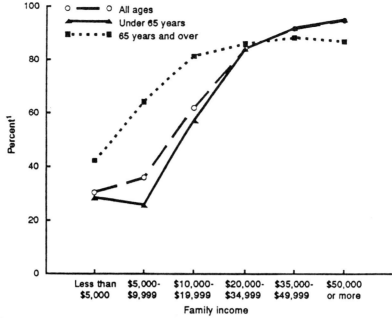

<sup>1</sup>Excludes persons with unknown coverage status.

**Figure 2.** Percent of persons with private health insurance coverage, by age and family income: United States, 1989

years of education (5.0 percent), persons 45–64 years of age (4.3 percent), and members of families with an annual income of $5,000–$9,999 (4.1 percent).

Coverage under Medicare was determined by asking the coverage status of all family members. Respondents were asked to show the Medicare card of persons covered to the interviewer, who determined whether they were covered by Part A, Part B, or both. Persons were classified as covered by Medicare if they were covered by either Part A or B or both.

## PERSONS WITH PUBLIC ASSISTANCE HEALTH CARE COVERAGE

An estimated 15.1 million persons in the civilian non-institutionalized population of the United States (6.2 percent) were covered by public assistance health care programs in 1989. Table 4 shows that proportionately far more persons under 18 years of age (11.1 percent) than adults had this form of coverage. Among persons under 18 years, 60.9 percent of those in families with an annual income of less than $5,000 and 50.3 percent in families in the $5,000–$9,999 income range had public assistance health care coverage. For those living below the poverty level, the corresponding estimate is 46.3 percent. Among the other age groups shown in the table, persons 65 years of age and over had the highest proportion of persons eligible for this form of coverage (6.2 percent).

Disregarding age, the highest proportions of eligible persons were females, persons who are not white, persons with low family income or family income below the poverty level, persons not currently employed, those with less than 12 years of education, and persons living in the central cities of MSA's.

The 1989 NHIS questionnaire included several questions related to eligibility for public assistance health care. Among these were questions on the receipt of Aid to Families with Dependent Children (AFDC) and Supplemental Security Income (SSI), whether the person had a valid Medicaid card, and whether he or she was covered by any public assistance program that paid for medical care. Coverage by public assistance is ascribed to the person if a positive response was obtained to any of these questions. Persons are classified as not covered if a negative response or no response was obtained for all four questions.

Because the eligibility criteria for Medicaid coverage are defined by each of the States and because many people are not aware of the criteria used in their State, it is difficult to obtain point-prevalence estimates of this population based on a household survey using a national rather than a State sampling frame. Thus, extreme caution should be used in comparing the results described in this section with estimates from other sources of the number and characteristics of the Medicaid or public assistance population. Any such comparison should be focused on the criteria used to define this type of cov-

**Table 3. Percent of persons with Medicare coverage, by age and sociodemographic characteristics: United States, 1989**

| Sociodemographic characteristic | All ages | Under 65 years | | | | | 65 years and over |
| --- | --- | --- | --- | --- | --- | --- | --- |
| | | Total | Under 18 years | 18–24 years | 25–44 years | 45–64 years | |
| | | | | Percent[1] | | | |
| All persons covered[2] | 12.6 | 1.4 | 0.2 | 0.4 | 0.9 | 4.3 | 94.3 |
| **Sex** | | | | | | | |
| Male | 11.0 | 1.5 | 0.2 | 0.5 | 1.0 | 4.9 | 93.4 |
| Female | 14.0 | 1.2 | 0.2 | 0.4 | 0.8 | 3.8 | 95.0 |
| **Race** | | | | | | | |
| White | 13.3 | 1.3 | 0.1 | 0.4 | 0.8 | 4.0 | 94.9 |
| Black | 9.4 | 2.1 | 0.5 | *0.5 | 1.7 | 7.5 | 90.7 |
| Other | 5.0 | 0.7 | *0.8 | – | *0.1 | *2.3 | 78.1 |
| **Family income** | | | | | | | |
| Less than $5,000 | 15.7 | 2.9 | *1.0 | *0.3 | 3.1 | 13.3 | 95.0 |
| $5,000–$9,999 | 27.5 | 4.1 | *0.2 | *0.9 | 4.1 | 15.1 | 95.4 |
| $10,000–$19,999 | 20.7 | 2.3 | *0.2 | *0.7 | 1.6 | 8.3 | 96.2 |
| $20,000–$34,999 | 9.7 | 1.1 | *0.2 | *0.5 | 0.6 | 3.7 | 94.4 |
| $35,000–$49,999 | 4.6 | 0.4 | *0.1 | *0.1 | 0.3 | 1.3 | 91.4 |
| $50,000 or more | 4.0 | 0.4 | *0.2 | *0.1 | 0.3 | 0.9 | 88.3 |
| **Poverty status** | | | | | | | |
| In poverty | 11.5 | 2.4 | *0.4 | *0.5 | 2.6 | 13.1 | 94.1 |
| Not in poverty | 11.5 | 1.1 | 0.2 | 0.4 | 0.7 | 3.4 | 94.5 |
| **Employment status[3]** | | | | | | | |
| Currently employed | 3.3 | 0.3 | ... | *0.2 | 0.3 | 0.6 | 87.7 |
| Unemployed | 2.8 | *0.6 | ... | *0.6 | *0.4 | *1.2 | 93.5 |
| Not in labor force | 46.1 | 7.4 | ... | 1.1 | 4.4 | 13.0 | 95.4 |
| **Education[3]** | | | | | | | |
| Less than 12 years | 34.1 | 5.0 | ... | 0.9 | 2.7 | 9.0 | 95.1 |
| 12 years | 14.4 | 1.5 | ... | *0.3 | 0.8 | 3.3 | 94.9 |
| More than 12 years | 9.5 | 0.8 | ... | *0.3 | 0.5 | 2.0 | 92.5 |
| **Region** | | | | | | | |
| Northeast | 14.3 | 1.3 | *0.3 | *0.3 | 0.9 | 3.7 | 93.5 |
| Midwest | 12.3 | 1.2 | *0.1 | *0.4 | 0.8 | 3.9 | 96.0 |
| South | 12.7 | 1.6 | 0.2 | 0.5 | 1.1 | 5.3 | 94.5 |
| West | 10.9 | 1.2 | *0.3 | *0.5 | 0.7 | 3.8 | 92.9 |
| **Place of residence** | | | | | | | |
| MSA | 11.7 | 1.3 | 0.2 | 0.5 | 0.8 | 4.1 | 93.7 |
| Central city | 12.5 | 1.6 | 0.3 | *0.4 | 1.1 | 5.0 | 93.0 |
| Not central city | 11.3 | 1.1 | 0.2 | 0.5 | 0.7 | 3.5 | 94.2 |
| Not MSA | 15.5 | 1.7 | *0.2 | *0.4 | 1.2 | 5.1 | 96.0 |

[1] Percent calculated excluding the 6.9 million persons for whom coverage status was not determined.
[2] Includes persons with unknown sociodemographic characteristics.
[3] Excludes persons under 18 years of age.

NOTE: MSA is metropolitan statistical area.

erage and the procedure used to collect the data that serve as the basis of the estimates.

## PERSONS WITH MILITARY–VETERANS' ADMINISTRATION HEALTH CARE COVERAGE

An estimated 6.3 million persons in the civilian non-institutionalized population (2.6 percent) were covered by military and/or Veterans' Administration health care programs in 1989. Among the sociodemographic cat-

egories included in table 5, the proportion of persons covered was more than 3 percent for the following groups: Persons 45–54 years of age (4.5 percent) and 65 years and over (4.0 percent); males (3.3 percent); persons of other races—that is, not black or white (3.1 percent); members of families with an annual income of $20,000–$34,999 (3.1 percent); persons 18 years of age and over not currently employed (3.1 and 3.9 percent for the unemployed and for those not in the labor force, respectively); and persons living in the South (3.6 percent) and West (3.3 percent) Regions of the country.

**Table 4. Percent of persons with public assistance coverage, by age and sociodemographic characteristics: United States, 1989**

| Sociodemographic characteristic | All ages | Under 65 years | | | | | 65 years and over |
| | | Total | Under 18 years | 18–24 years | 25–44 years | 45–64 years | |
|---|---|---|---|---|---|---|---|
| | | | | Percent[1] | | | |
| All persons covered[2] . . . . . . . . . . . . . . . . . . . . . . . . | 6.2 | 6.2 | 11.1 | 5.6 | 3.9 | 3.7 | 6.2 |
| **Sex** | | | | | | | |
| Male. . . . . . . . . . . . . . . . . . . . . . . . . . . . . . . . . . | 4.8 | 4.9 | 10.8 | 2.2 | 2.0 | 2.7 | 4.4 |
| Female . . . . . . . . . . . . . . . . . . . . . . . . . . . . . . . . | 7.5 | 7.5 | 11.3 | 8.8 | 5.8 | 4.6 | 7.6 |
| **Race** | | | | | | | |
| White . . . . . . . . . . . . . . . . . . . . . . . . . . . . . . . . . | 4.4 | 4.4 | 7.6 | 4.2 | 2.9 | 2.7 | 4.8 |
| Black . . . . . . . . . . . . . . . . . . . . . . . . . . . . . . . . . | 16.8 | 16.6 | 26.9 | 12.5 | 10.1 | 10.8 | 18.4 |
| Other . . . . . . . . . . . . . . . . . . . . . . . . . . . . . . . . . | 12.7 | 12.1 | 19.9 | 10.7 | 7.3 | 9.5 | 22.8 |
| **Family income** | | | | | | | |
| Less than $5,000. . . . . . . . . . . . . . . . . . . . . . . . . . | 37.8 | 38.4 | 60.9 | 13.0 | 39.7 | 37.7 | 34.2 |
| $5,000–$9,999 . . . . . . . . . . . . . . . . . . . . . . . . . . | 28.5 | 34.3 | 50.3 | 18.7 | 29.4 | 22.8 | 12.0 |
| $10,000–$19,999. . . . . . . . . . . . . . . . . . . . . . . . . | 7.9 | 8.9 | 15.1 | 6.6 | 6.0 | 5.6 | 3.6 |
| $20,000–$34,999. . . . . . . . . . . . . . . . . . . . . . . . . | 2.2 | 2.2 | 3.6 | 3.3 | 1.2 | 1.3 | 2.8 |
| $35,000–$49,999. . . . . . . . . . . . . . . . . . . . . . . . . | 1.0 | 0.9 | 1.7 | *1.0 | 0.5 | 0.8 | *2.1 |
| $50,000 or more . . . . . . . . . . . . . . . . . . . . . . . . . | 0.5 | 0.4 | 0.6 | *0.8 | 0.3 | *0.2 | *1.5 |
| **Poverty status** | | | | | | | |
| In poverty . . . . . . . . . . . . . . . . . . . . . . . . . . . . . . | 35.1 | 35.8 | 46.3 | 17.6 | 32.3 | 32.0 | 28.3 |
| Not in poverty. . . . . . . . . . . . . . . . . . . . . . . . . . . . | 2.3 | 2.1 | 3.3 | 2.7 | 1.3 | 1.8 | 3.5 |
| **Employment status[3]** | | | | | | | |
| Currently employed . . . . . . . . . . . . . . . . . . . . . . . . | 1.1 | 1.0 | . . . | 1.5 | 1.1 | 0.7 | 2.3 |
| Unemployed. . . . . . . . . . . . . . . . . . . . . . . . . . . . . | 9.7 | 9.8 | . . . | 11.1 | 10.8 | 5.1 | *1.8 |
| Not in labor force . . . . . . . . . . . . . . . . . . . . . . . . . | 11.1 | 14.4 | . . . | 15.9 | 17.9 | 10.6 | 6.9 |
| **Education[3]** | | | | | | | |
| Less than 12 years . . . . . . . . . . . . . . . . . . . . . . . . | 11.5 | 12.0 | . . . | 13.0 | 13.7 | 10.0 | 10.4 |
| 12 years . . . . . . . . . . . . . . . . . . . . . . . . . . . . . . . | 3.6 | 3.6 | . . . | 5.5 | 3.9 | 2.1 | 3.2 |
| More than 12 years . . . . . . . . . . . . . . . . . . . . . . . . | 1.3 | 1.2 | . . . | 1.3 | 1.2 | 1.1 | 2.4 |
| **Region** | | | | | | | |
| Northeast . . . . . . . . . . . . . . . . . . . . . . . . . . . . . . | 5.1 | 5.2 | 9.2 | 4.2 | 3.8 | 3.6 | 4.4 |
| Midwest . . . . . . . . . . . . . . . . . . . . . . . . . . . . . . . | 6.4 | 6.8 | 12.2 | 6.6 | 4.4 | 3.3 | 3.2 |
| South. . . . . . . . . . . . . . . . . . . . . . . . . . . . . . . . . | 6.0 | 5.7 | 10.1 | 4.8 | 3.4 | 3.8 | 8.5 |
| West . . . . . . . . . . . . . . . . . . . . . . . . . . . . . . . . . | 7.3 | 7.2 | 12.9 | 6.9 | 4.3 | 4.1 | 8.3 |
| **Place of residence** | | | | | | | |
| MSA. . . . . . . . . . . . . . . . . . . . . . . . . . . . . . . . . . | 6.0 | 6.0 | 11.2 | 5.2 | 3.7 | 3.5 | 5.6 |
| Central city . . . . . . . . . . . . . . . . . . . . . . . . . . . | 9.6 | 9.9 | 18.7 | 7.2 | 6.0 | 6.2 | 7.6 |
| Not central city. . . . . . . . . . . . . . . . . . . . . . . . . | 3.6 | 3.6 | 6.4 | 3.7 | 2.3 | 1.8 | 4.2 |
| Not MSA . . . . . . . . . . . . . . . . . . . . . . . . . . . . . . . | 7.0 | 6.8 | 10.8 | 7.1 | 4.7 | 4.5 | 7.9 |

[1]Persons not administered the supplement were classified as not covered. About 2.0 million persons for whom unknown responses were obtained were excluded in calculating the percents.
[2]Includes persons with unknown sociodemographic characteristics.
[3]Excludes persons under 18 years of age.

NOTE: MSA is metropolitan statistical area.

As was the case with public assistance health care plans, coverage for civilians under military or VA health benefits is much more difficult to define than coverage under private health insurance or Medicare. This is especially so in the case of VA health benefits, which operate for most veterans and their eligible dependents under a system of priority eligibility.

In this report persons are classified as covered by military–VA health benefits if it was determined that (a) they received a military or VA pension; (b) they were covered by CHAMPUS (Civilian Health and Medical Program of the Uniformed Services), CHAMPVA (Civilian Health and Medical Program of the Veterans' Administration), or any other program that provides health care for military dependents or survivors of military persons; or (c) they received compensation for a disability from the VA. Other circumstantial criteria by which a person might qualify for military–VA health care benefits (such as advanced age or low income) were not used.

**Table 5. Percent of persons with military–Veterans' Administration coverage, by age and sociodemographic characteristics: United States, 1989**

| Sociodemographic characteristic | All ages | Under 65 years | | | | | 65 years and over |
|---|---|---|---|---|---|---|---|
| | | Total | Under 18 years | 18–24 years | 25–44 years | 45–64 years | |
| | | | Percent[1] | | | | |
| All persons covered[2] . . . . . . . . . . . . . . . . . . . . . | 2.6 | 2.4 | 2.1 | 1.9 | 1.5 | 4.5 | 4.0 |
| *Sex* | | | | | | | |
| Male. . . . . . . . . . . . . . . . . . . . . . . . . . . . . . . | 3.3 | 2.6 | 2.2 | 1.0 | 1.5 | 6.3 | 8.7 |
| Female . . . . . . . . . . . . . . . . . . . . . . . . . . . . . | 1.9 | 2.1 | 2.0 | 2.8 | 1.5 | 2.9 | 0.7 |
| *Race* | | | | | | | |
| White . . . . . . . . . . . . . . . . . . . . . . . . . . . . . . | 2.5 | 2.3 | 2.0 | 1.8 | 1.4 | 4.5 | 4.1 |
| Black . . . . . . . . . . . . . . . . . . . . . . . . . . . . . . | 2.5 | 2.4 | 2.2 | 2.1 | 2.0 | 4.0 | 3.5 |
| Other . . . . . . . . . . . . . . . . . . . . . . . . . . . . . . | 3.1 | 3.2 | 2.7 | *3.8 | 2.2 | 5.7 | *2.0 |
| *Family income* | | | | | | | |
| Less than $5,000. . . . . . . . . . . . . . . . . . . . . . . . | 1.5 | 1.4 | *0.6 | 2.1 | *1.0 | *3.2 | *1.6 |
| $5,000–$9,999 . . . . . . . . . . . . . . . . . . . . . . . . | 1.6 | 1.4 | *0.8 | *0.9 | *1.0 | 3.9 | 2.2 |
| $10,000–$19,999. . . . . . . . . . . . . . . . . . . . . . . | 2.7 | 2.6 | 3.0 | 2.6 | 1.7 | 3.5 | 3.4 |
| $20,000–$34,999. . . . . . . . . . . . . . . . . . . . . . . | 3.1 | 2.9 | 2.7 | 2.2 | 1.9 | 5.6 | 5.8 |
| $35,000–$49,999. . . . . . . . . . . . . . . . . . . . . . . | 3.0 | 2.7 | 2.5 | 1.9 | 1.7 | 5.5 | 8.4 |
| $50,000 or more . . . . . . . . . . . . . . . . . . . . . . . | 2.3 | 2.1 | 1.2 | 1.5 | 1.1 | 4.8 | 5.5 |
| *Poverty status* | | | | | | | |
| In poverty . . . . . . . . . . . . . . . . . . . . . . . . . . . | 1.2 | 1.2 | 0.9 | 1.5 | 0.9 | 2.5 | *1.3 |
| Not in poverty. . . . . . . . . . . . . . . . . . . . . . . . . | 2.8 | 2.6 | 2.4 | 2.1 | 1.6 | 4.8 | 4.5 |
| *Employment status[3]* | | | | | | | |
| Currently employed . . . . . . . . . . . . . . . . . . . . . . | 2.1 | 2.0 | . . . | 1.6 | 1.3 | 3.8 | 5.5 |
| Unemployed. . . . . . . . . . . . . . . . . . . . . . . . . . | 3.1 | 3.0 | . . . | *1.5 | 2.6 | 6.3 | *6.2 |
| Not in labor force . . . . . . . . . . . . . . . . . . . . . . | 3.9 | 4.0 | . . . | 2.8 | 2.5 | 5.8 | 3.8 |
| *Education[3]* | | | | | | | |
| Less than 12 years . . . . . . . . . . . . . . . . . . . . . . | 2.3 | 2.0 | . . . | 1.3 | 1.0 | 3.2 | 3.1 |
| 12 years . . . . . . . . . . . . . . . . . . . . . . . . . . . . | 2.8 | 2.7 | . . . | 2.2 | 1.6 | 4.7 | 4.0 |
| More than 12 years . . . . . . . . . . . . . . . . . . . . . . | 2.9 | 2.6 | . . . | 2.0 | 1.6 | 5.2 | 5.9 |
| *Region* | | | | | | | |
| Northeast . . . . . . . . . . . . . . . . . . . . . . . . . . . | 1.4 | 1.1 | 0.5 | *0.7 | 0.7 | 2.9 | 2.9 |
| Midwest . . . . . . . . . . . . . . . . . . . . . . . . . . . . | 1.4 | 1.2 | 0.9 | *0.6 | 1.0 | 2.2 | 2.6 |
| South . . . . . . . . . . . . . . . . . . . . . . . . . . . . . . | 3.6 | 3.5 | 3.4 | 3.2 | 2.1 | 6.2 | 4.6 |
| West . . . . . . . . . . . . . . . . . . . . . . . . . . . . . . | 3.3 | 3.0 | 2.7 | 2.6 | 1.9 | 5.9 | 5.9 |
| *Place of residence* | | | | | | | |
| MSA. . . . . . . . . . . . . . . . . . . . . . . . . . . . . . . | 2.5 | 2.3 | 2.1 | 1.9 | 1.5 | 4.4 | 4.1 |
| Central city . . . . . . . . . . . . . . . . . . . . . . . . . | 2.5 | 2.4 | 2.3 | 1.7 | 1.6 | 4.4 | 3.8 |
| Not central city. . . . . . . . . . . . . . . . . . . . . . . | 2.5 | 2.3 | 2.0 | 2.0 | 1.4 | 4.5 | 4.2 |
| Not MSA . . . . . . . . . . . . . . . . . . . . . . . . . . . . | 2.6 | 2.4 | 2.0 | 2.0 | 1.6 | 4.6 | 3.8 |

Persons not administered the supplement were classified as not covered. About 2.0 million persons for whom unknown responses were obtained were excluded in calculating the percents.
[1] Includes persons with unknown sociodemographic characteristics.
[3] Excludes persons under 18 years of age.

NOTE: MSA is metropolitan statistical area.

## TRENDS

Although data on health care coverage have been collected by means of NHIS since the 1960's, the questions related to public assistance and military–VA coverage were periodically changed until 1984. Because these types of coverage are included in the more general category of health care coverage it is not possible to show trends in coverage for the earlier periods. However, since 1984 the questions used to determine coverage have undergone only minimal changes. Thus, comparisons between the levels of coverage and noncoverage from 1984 to 1989 are possible.

The percent of persons with no health care coverage increased from 13.0 percent in 1984 to 13.9 percent in 1989 (table 6). For persons under 65 years of age the increase was from 14.6 to 15.7 percent. Of all of the sociodemographic characteristics shown in table 1, the largest differential change occurred for family income groups. Figure 3 shows the ratio of the 1989 to the

**Table 6. Percent of persons without health care coverage, by family income: United States, 1984 and 1989**

| Family income | 1984 | 1989 |
|---|---|---|
| | Percent[1] | |
| All incomes[2] | 13.0 | 13.9 |
| Less than $5,000 | 25.8 | 27.1 |
| $5,000–$9,999 | 28.0 | 27.7 |
| $10,000–$19,999 | 17.4 | 24.3 |
| $20,000–$34,999 | 6.7 | 10.6 |
| $35,000–$49,999 | 3.5 | 5.8 |
| $50,000 or more | 3.1 | 3.6 |

[1]Excludes persons with unknown coverage status.
[2]Includes unknown income.

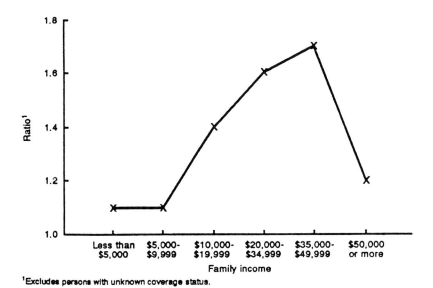

'Excludes persons with unknown coverage status.

**Figure 3.** Ratio of 1989 to 1984 percents of persons without health care coverage, by family income: United States

1984 estimates of noncoverage by income category. The largest increases were in the income range $10,000–$49,999, the ratio of increase being 1.7 for persons in families with an annual income of $35,000–$49,999. Some of this increase is only apparent, though, because inflation tends to move families to higher income categories over time without necessarily improving their health care coverage. Thus, higher income groups appear to be losing coverage. However, inflation is taken into account in the definition of poverty status, and the increase in noncoverage during this period was greater for those above the poverty level (10.8 percent) than it was for those below the poverty level (5.2 percent). This indicates that the increases noted above are not solely a function of inflation.

The NHIS questions related to private health insurance coverage have changed little since 1974. Table 7 shows the proportions of persons covered by private health insurance for each of the survey years from 1974 to 1989. There has been a slow decline in this type of coverage from 79.9 percent in 1974 to 75.9 percent in 1989.

Two previously published reports (3,4) include more extensive information on NHIS estimates of health care coverage prior to 1989.

**Table 7. Percent of persons with private health care coverage: United States, 1974–89**

| Year | Percent[1] |
|---|---|
| 1974 | 79.9 |
| 1976 | 78.9 |
| 1978 | 79.3 |
| 1980 | 79.4 |
| 1982 | 78.1 |
| 1984 | 76.7 |
| 1986 | 76.6 |
| 1989 | 75.9 |

[1]Excludes persons with unknown coverage status.

## References

1. Short PF. Estimates of the uninsured population, calendar year 1987. Data Summary no 2. Rockville, Maryland: Agency for Health Care Policy and Research. 1990.
2. U.S. Bureau of the Census: Preliminary unpublished estimates from the Current Population Survey. Washington. 1990.
3. Ries PW. Health care coverage by sociodemographic and health characteristics: United States, 1984. National Center for Health Statistics. *Vital Health Stat* 10(162). 1987.
4. Ries PW. Health care coverage by age, sex, race, and family income: United States, 1986. Advance data from vital and health statistics; no 139. Hyattsville, Maryland: National Center for Health Statistics. 1987.
5. Adams PF, Benson V. Current estimates from the National Health Interview Survey, 1989. National Center for Health Statistics. *Vital Health Stat* 10(176). 1990.

# Chapter 17
# Conventional Health Insurance: A Decade Later

Steven DiCarlo and Jon Gabel

*In this article, the 1987 conventional health plans are examined and 1987 group health insurance is compared with that of 1977. The source of information for 1987 is the national survey of 771 private and public employers conducted by the Health Insurance Association of America. Data for 1977 are from the National Medical Care Expenditures Survey. Findings show that conventional health plans' share of the group market declined from 95 to 73 percent during the decade; the majority of Americans covered by conventional group insurance are now enrolled in a plan that self-insures; prospective utilization review grew dramatically after 1984; and patient cost sharing increased, but not as significantly as conventional wisdom holds.*

## INTRODUCTION

In 1977, the National Center for Health Services Research conducted the most comprehensive survey of health insurance and use of health care services in this Nation's history. From this survey emerged a vivid picture of the American health care system in the 1970's—a system almost entirely financed by conventional insurance (defined as non-health maintenance and non-preferred provider organization health plans). It is from this survey that much of our understanding of the economics of health care has been derived.

In this article, after a decade of extraordinary change in American health care, we examine the 1987 conventional health plans. Where there are comparable data, we compare private health insurance of 1987 with that of 1977. The focus is on conventional health insurance, the source of protection for approximately 96 percent of Americans in 1977 and 73 percent in 1987 who secured health insurance through their employers.

Conventional fee-for-service insurance has been the traditional form of health coverage for Americans. This type of arrangement has few incentives for the provider or the patient to minimize the cost of treatment. Historically, insurers reimbursed providers' charges with few questions asked. The insurer's role was simply to forecast expenditures, determine risk, collect premiums, and pay the bills.

As health care costs escalated, employers and insurers turned increasingly to health maintenance organizations (HMO's) and preferred provider organizations (PPO's) as the means of controlling costs (Gabel et al., 1988; Rice et al., 1989). Patients in these plans no longer have unrestricted access to physicians and hospitals, and they almost always have to secure approval for admission to a hospital. HMO's and PPO's may review other steps in

Reprinted from *Health Care Financing Review,* Spring 1989, Vol 10, No. 3.

the medical treatment to make sure the treatment is necessary. If a patient does not follow guidelines, the HMO or PPO may deny payment (totally or partially), and the patient may face larger out-of-pocket costs.

This article is organized as follows:

- We review the health insurance data available in the past decade.
- We review the methodology for the Health Insurance Association of America (HIAA) health benefit survey.
- We compare characteristics of conventional health insurance plans of 1987 with those of 1977.
- We take a closer look at conventional plans of 1987 according to their sponsorship and employer size.

Our conclusion assesses the future of conventional insurance.

## NEED FOR NEW INFORMATION

To examine 1977 conventional health insurance, we turn to the landmark National Medical Care Expenditures Survey (NMCES)—a household interview survey during which family health insurance coverage and use and costs of services were investigated (Farley, 1986). NMCES supplemental surveys explored in detail additional aspects of each person's health coverage. During a smaller survey, the Employer Health Insurance Cost Survey (EHICS), employment-related health insurance plans were investigated by interviewing the employer of the individuals in the household survey (Taylor and Lawson, 1981). EHICS includes information about the availability of health coverage for employees, the cost of premiums, and how these were distributed between the employer and employee. For our analysis of health insurance in 1977, we used only the employer-based results from the EHICS. Data are on a national and a regional basis.

In recent years, health care analysts have relied on three sources of information for trends in health benefit coverage—consulting firm studies, coalition studies, and the Bureau of Labor Statistics (BLS) annual survey of mid-sized and large employers (Jensen et al., 1987). All of these studies have serious limitations, however, when one extrapolates the results to the U.S. population.

Consulting firms generally select their samples from their client base. They often fail to report their response rate or assess the representativeness of their sample. Thus, samples tend to be subject to selection bias and lack the ability to extrapolate findings to the entire U.S. population.

Several local employer communities have formed coalitions. These coalitions have, at times, commissioned studies of employer-sponsored health insurance. Coalition studies are usually better statistically designed than consulting firm studies but tend to focus on small regions of the country, thereby hampering the ability to extrapolate the findings to national figures.

The BLS annual survey is the best available source of national data. However, its major flaw is that the sample includes only medium- and large-sized private firms. Thus, employers that have fewer than 100 employees are not represented in the study. There is ample evidence to suggest that small employer premiums and benefit packages differ from those of larger employers and that public employers offer richer benefit packages than do private ones (Small Business Administration, 1987). Moreover, small employers make up the majority of the employers in the country (U.S. Bureau of the Census, 1987). Thus, a substantial portion of the group insurance marketplace is omitted from the BLS survey, thereby biasing any extrapolations to the population as a whole.

## HEALTH BENEFIT SURVEY

The source of information for 1987 is the national health benefit survey of 771 private and public employers conducted by the Health Insurance Association of America (HIAA) in conjunction with the Johns Hopkins University and the University of North Carolina in the spring of 1987.

Attempting to remedy many of the flaws of the post-NMCES surveys, we designed the HIAA survey with the objective of deriving a representative sample from which to draw conclusions about the Nation's employment-related health insurance population. We stratified the sample according to region, the firm's total number of employees, and private-public status. Because we are interested primarily in firms that offered health benefits to their employees, we undersampled small employers (those with fewer than 100 employees) and disproportionately selected large employers (those with 100 or more employees). Many small employers do not offer health coverage to their employees, and large employers, though fewer in number, cover a plurality of employees with group coverage (Employee Benefits Research Institute, 1988).

The survey questionnaire asked about the firm's largest conventional, HMO, and PPO plans (according to the number of subscribers). Questions examined eligibility, plan design, cost, and employer satisfaction.

Using a sample frame originally designed by the Health Care Financing Administration (HCFA) to adjust the accuracy of its national health care expenditure estimates, National Research Inc., a Maryland-based research firm, conducted telephone interviews with employee benefit managers from 771 firms in the spring of 1987. The sample frame includes an estimated 84 percent of Americans who receive health insurance through an employer. The sample frame included few employers that do not offer health insurance to their employees. Two major employer groups that provide health insurance to their employees are missing from our sample frame: Federal employees and workers who receive health insurance directly through a union. Another limitation of our data is that we did not gather information regarding the specific benefits offered in each plan. Therefore, the richness of the benefit plan is not a variable in our analysis.

Our response rate was 45 percent. With the exception of the BLS survey, this response rate exceeds that achieved in most surveys of employer-based health plans. Using the information in the sample frame collected by HCFA, we compared characteristics of responding and nonresponding employers. We found no difference between the two groups for all variables including industry, region, firm size, self-insurance status, and availability of an HMO plan.

We were able to compare the data from the HIAA survey of employers with those of the NMCEs and the EHICS. The figures are comparable, with the exception that the 1977 NMCES included HMO's. In 1977, the private health insurance market was almost entirely conventional fee for service. Employers were predominantly covered by the Blue Cross and Blue Shield plans and commercial insurance carrier plans. HMO's represented only 4.3 percent of the private health insurance market for persons under 65 years of age (Farley, 1985), PPO's did not emerge as a significant force until the early

eighties (Gabel et al., 1986). In our analysis of the 1977 conventional market, it was not possible to segregate HMO enrollment. Because of the small share of the HMO business, however, its impact on the results should be minimal.

In this article, we have applied a series of weights to the survey findings to derive employee-based national estimates for the U.S. population that secures its health insurance through employers. Where appropriate in the tables, we have reported the number of firms in each category analyzed as well as the standard error associated with the given statistics. However, we could not determine the sample size or the standard errors for the 1977 NMCES data and could not compare these statistics with the 1987 data in Tables 1 and 2.

## CONVENTIONAL HEALTH INSURANCE: 1977 VERSUS 1987

Changes in eligibility and premium costs for 1987 and 1977 are given in Table 1. The number of employees eligible for employer-sponsored conventional health insurance has remained high in the past 10 years. Among firms that offered health benefits to their employees, 95 percent of the employees were eligible for benefits in 1987. This compares with 93 percent of employees

## Table 1

### Employer and employee contributions in conventional plans, by region and selected variables: 1977 and 1987

| Selected variable | United States | Region | | | |
|---|---|---|---|---|---|
| | | Northeast | North Central | South | West |
| **1977** | | | | | |
| Percent of eligible employees | 93 | 93 | 91 | 96 | 94 |
| Total annual premium: | | | | | |
| In 1987 dollars[1] | $1,111 | $1,192 | $1,215 | $943 | $1,131 |
| In 1977 dollars | 609 | 653 | 666 | 517 | 620 |
| Employer contribution: | | | | | |
| In 1987 dollars | $943 | $1,053 | $1,051 | $741 | $992 |
| In 1977 dollars | 517 | 577 | 576 | 406 | 544 |
| Employee contribution: | | | | | |
| In 1987 dollars | $168 | $139 | $164 | $202 | $139 |
| In 1977 dollars | 92 | 76 | 90 | 111 | 76 |
| Percent of premium contributed by employer | 85 | 88 | 87 | 79 | 88 |
| **1987** | | | | | |
| Percent of eligible employees | 95 | 99 | 97 | 95 | 95 |
| Total annual premium[2] | $1,656 | $1,602 | $1,698 | $1,614 | $1,794 |
| Employer contribution | $1,374 | $1,512 | $1,524 | $1,236 | $1,404 |
| Employee contribution | $282 | $90 | $174 | $378 | $390 |
| Percent of premium contributed by employer | 83 | 94 | 90 | 77 | 78 |

[1]Dollars are in constant 1987 dollars; adjustments made using the Consumer Price Index, all items.
[2]Total annual premium was calculated with a weighted adjustment for single and for family plans.

SOURCE: Health Insurance Association of America, 1987; National Center for Health Services Research, 1977.

eligible for employee benefits in 1977. Eligibility increased in all regions except in the South, where it showed a slight decrease of less than 1 percent.

Premiums per eligible employee for conventional insurance in 1987 amounted to $1,656 nationwide and ranged from $1,602 in the Northeast to $1,794 in the West (Figure 1). Compared with the national average cost of $609 per eligible employee in 1977, premiums increased 171.9 percent during the last 10 years. This is an average annual increase of 10.5 percent. In constant 1987 dollars, premiums increased from $1,111 in 1977 to $1,656 in 1987. To illustrate how premiums have escalated, during the same period, general prices increased 82.4 percent (an average of 6.2 percent per year); and medical prices went up 120.8 percent (a rate of 8.3 percent per year). The difference between the rate of increase in medical care prices and insurance premiums largely reflects increases in the number of covered services, utilization, and intensity of services. Insurer administrative expenses and profits as a percent of premiums fluctuated greatly during the 10–year period but showed no clear upward movement and, thus, are not a major factor in explaining the difference in premium increases and medical care prices (Musco, 1988).

Employees who share in the cost of health insurance premiums have greater incentives for choosing cost-effective plans than employees who receive their health insurance free from their employers. Contrary to conventional wisdom, as a percent of the overall premium cost, employees are contributing only slightly more than they were 10 years ago. On the average, employers paid 83 percent of the premium in 1987 as compared with 85 percent in 1977 (Figure 2). In regional comparisons, however, our survey data show that employers are actually paying a greater percent of the premium in two of the four regions of the country. The greatest change occurred in the West Region, which showed a significant decrease in the proportion of premiums paid by employers, from 88 percent of premiums in 1977 to 78 percent in 1987.

Overall, employers in the Northeast continue to pay the largest portion of the premium cost. Those in the South pay the lowest portion, as was true a decade ago. During the 1977 NMCES, there was a strong correlation between the cost of the insurance and the percent the employer paid—the higher the proportion paid by the employer, the higher the overall premium cost. In 1987, this pattern was no longer true. In fact, the Northeast had the lowest conventional premium cost and the second highest employer contribution, and the West had the highest premium cost and the second lowest employer contribution of the four regions.

In terms of dollar outlays, employers paid the most money in the North Central Region, $1,524 per employee; and employers in the South contributed the least, $1,236 per employee annually. There was a decided

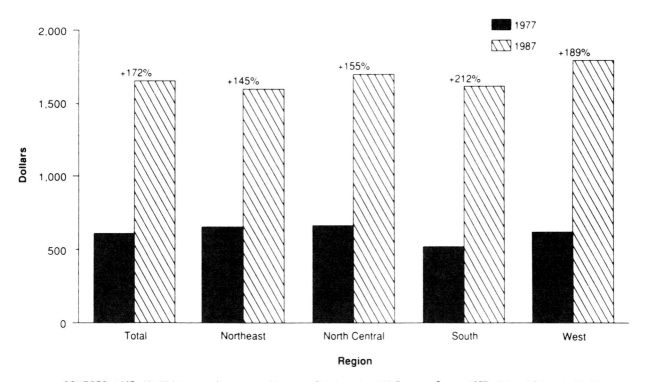

Figure 1. Premium increases for conventional plans, by region: 1977 and 1987

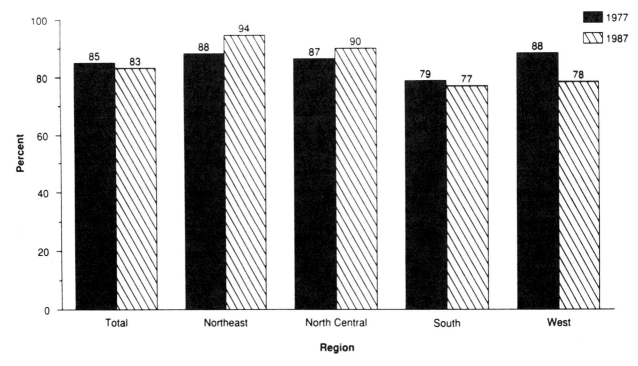

SOURCES: 1987—Health Insurance Association of America: Data from the 1987 Employer Survey; 1977—National Center for Health Services Research: Data from the National Medical Care Expenditure Survey.

**Figure 2.** Percent of conventional premium paid by employers, by region: 1977 and 1987

contrast on the employee side, where employees paid $390 annually in the West, as compared with only $90 a year in the Northeast. Increases in the employer contribution did not vary significantly from the national average. However, growth in employee contributions varied widely from a low of 18 percent in the Northeast to a high of 413 percent in the West. In fact, after adjusting for general inflation, employees in the Northeast actually contributed less toward the premium than they did a decade ago.

We also collected data on the contribution levels for both employer-based individual and family coverage. Employers pay a greater share of the individual plan than they do of the family plan. Employers pay 95 percent of the individual premium, as compared with 77 percent of the family plan. In the Northeast and West, the employer paid 100 percent of the cost for the majority of the employees with individual coverage. For family coverage, the percent of total contributions picked up by the employer varied greatly by region, with employers in the Northeast Region paying the most—92 percent of the family cost for their employees. The West showed the lowest contribution by employers, who paid only 68 percent of the premium.

Changes in patient cost sharing between 1977 and 1987 are shown in Table 2 (Wilensky et al., 1984). Figures for deductibles and coinsurance are for physician services. Figures for lifetime maximum benefits and out-of-pocket maximums apply to all services. The num-

ber of employees with first-dollar coverage for physician services declined from 15 percent to 5 percent (Table 2). The number of workers having to pay less than 20 percent coinsurance has declined from 21 percent to 9 percent.

## Table 2

### Percent distribution of employment-related cost-sharing features: United States, 1977 and 1987

| Feature | 1977 | 1987 |
|---|---|---|
| No deductible, less than 20 percent coinsurance | 7.8 | 1.7 |
| No deductible, 20 percent or more coinsurance | 6.9 | 3.3 |
| Deductible, less than 20 percent coinsurance | 13.2 | 7.5 |
| Deductible, 20 percent or more coinsurance | 60.1 | 75.4 |
| No coverage or don't know | 12.0 | 12.1 |
| Lifetime maximum benefits: | | |
| Limited dollars | 77.0 | 72.7 |
| Unlimited dollars | 10.1 | 17.2 |
| No coverage or don't know | 12.9 | 10.1 |
| Out-of-pocket maximum: | | |
| Limited liability | 45.6 | 88.0 |
| Unlimited liability | 41.5 | 6.1 |
| No coverage or don't know | 12.9 | 5.9 |

SOURCE: Health Insurance Association of America, 1987; National Center for Health Services Research, 1977.

These increases in cost sharing, however, have been somewhat offset by a dramatic increase in the number of workers with catastrophic protection. In an area of high-tech medicine, catastrophic cases assumed increasing importance in cost-control efforts. For example, one study of 1.2 million insured persons found that individuals incurring more than $1,000 in claims accounted for nearly 90 percent of insurer payments (Medstat, 1988). In 1987, nearly 90 percent of employees have out-of-pocket maximums; only 46 percent had these in 1977. The number of workers with unlimited maximum benefits increased from 10 to 17 percent.

## COMPARING CONVENTIONAL PLANS BY SPONSOR

One major change in the conventional insurance market during the past decade has been the decline of traditional insurers—Blue Cross and Blue Shield and commercial insurers—and the rise of third-party administrators and self-administered plans. The dramatic growth of self-insurance is largely responsible for this shift.

Traditionally, Blue Cross and Blue Shield and commercial insurer policies completely insured a plan's expenses and provided all administered duties—insurer and administrator were synonymous. This meant that insurers would calculate their risk to provide health insurance protection as well as the added expense of administrative duties and would charge a premium to cover this cost. The insurer was then responsible for all of the expenses that arose.

The growth of self-insurance, spurred by the passage of the Employee Retirement and Income Security Act in 1974, led to a debundling of the risk and administrative functions of insurers. By exempting self-insured plans from State regulation of health insurance, the act bestowed strong financial rewards to self-insured employers. Self-insured plans were not subject to State laws requiring health plans to provide specified benefits mandated by State legislation, such as chiropractic services. Self-insured plans also were not subject to State premium taxes. Self-insurance also allowed firms to pay claims as they were submitted, rather than paying an insurance premium each month. Thus, employers were able to earn interest on their working capital.

Because self-insured firms did not require the services of Blue Cross and Blue Shield and commercial insurance companies to insure financial risk, companies quickly came into the business under a generic term called "third-party administrators" (TPA's). These companies specialize in providing administrative services (i.e., paying claims, keeping track of eligibility) without the additional expenses that are incurred with underwriting costs. Several employers also felt their needs would be best served if they administered their own plan. Not to be

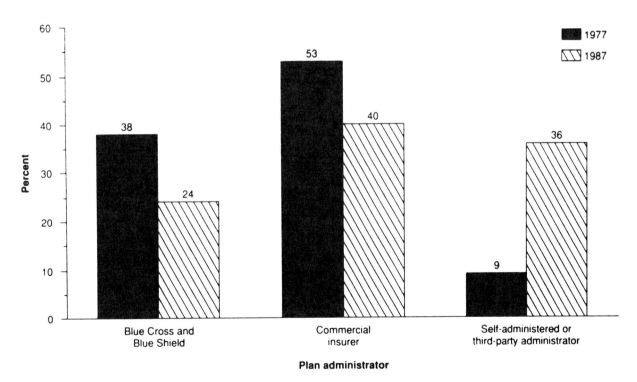

SOURCES: 1987—Health Insurance Association of America: Data from the 1987 Employer Survey; 1977—(Carroll and Arnett, 1979).

**Figure 3.** Market shares of conventional plan administrators: United States, 1977 and 1987

outdone, the Blue Cross and Blue Shield and commercial carriers also marketed products that provided administrative services only or partial insurance protection plans called minimum premium or stop-loss plans. These latter plans allow employers to self-insure their plan up to a certain dollar amount (and gain the savings afforded by self-insuring a plan). When this dollar figure is reached, the insurer pays the rest of the claims. Thus, these plans protect the employer from an unusual or catastrophic experience in any given year.

Hence, in 1977, commercial insurers held approximately 53 percent of the market, Blue Cross and Blue Shield retained 38 percent, and self-administered, TPA, and independent plans held 9 percent of the group market (Carroll and Arnett, 1979). One decade later, data from the 1987 HIAA survey show commercial insurance companies now administer 40 percent of the conventional insurance market, Blue Cross and Blue Shield plans administer 24 percent, and self-administered and TPA plans administer the remaining 36 percent (Figure 3). Blue Cross and Blue Shield sponsored plans have their greatest share of the market in the East Region of the United States, as they did a decade ago. Plans sponsored by commercial insurance companies are strongest in the East and North Central Regions, as was the case in 1977. The self-administered and TPA plans are strongest in the South and the West.

When employers provide health insurance for their employees, very often they give employees an opportunity to choose from more than one plan. For example, employers may offer two conventional plans—one administered by Blue Cross and Blue Shield and one administered by a commercial carrier—or they may make available one conventional plan and one or more HMO or PPO plans.

Firms that self-administered or had TPA-administered conventional plans faced more competition from HMO and PPO plans than the other administrators (Table 3). Seventy percent of these employers gave their employees the opportunity to choose an HMO, and 2 percent, the opportunity to join a PPO. Only 38 percent of the employees administered by Blue Cross and Blue Shield had the opportunity to choose an HMO, and 7 percent had the opportunity to select a PPO plan. Commercially administered plans were between these groups on both accounts. Regardless of their opportunities of choice, when an employer offered a conventional plan, an overwhelming majority of employees made it their choice (roughly 9 out of 10).

Self-insurance status varies greatly according to the plan administrator (Table 3). For the Blue Cross and Blue Shield and commercial insurers, fully insured business was the dominant mode of funding at 69 and 51 percent, respectively. A partly insured plan (presumably where an employer would be self-insuring a plan and

### Table 3
### Conventional plan administrators, by selected variables: United States, 1987

| Selected variable | Plan administrator | | |
| --- | --- | --- | --- |
| | Blue Cross and Blue Shield | Commercial insurance companies | Other plans |
| Percent of market | 24 | 40 | 36 |
| Percent of employees choosing conventional plan when also given choice of HMO and/or PPO | 91 (1.8) | 91 (1.2) | 90 (1.5) |
| Percent of employees in a conventional plan given choice of PPO | 7 (8.8) | 6 (6.7) | 2 (4.8) |
| Percent of employees in a conventional plan given choice of HMO | 38 (6.0) | 40 (3.7) | 70 (5.2) |
| Percent of employees in first year of plan contract with current insurer | 11 (2.3) | 18 (2.3) | 7 (1.8) |
| Retiree per active employees | 1-13 (2.0) | 1-11 (1.9) | 1-7 (2.9) |
| Percent of plans with specified insured status: | | | |
| Fully insured | 69 (3.4) | 51 (3.0) | 2 (1.8) |
| Self-insured | 11 (2.2) | 8 (1.7) | 72 (3.7) |
| Partly insured | 19 (2.7) | 38 (2.8) | 26 (3.5) |
| Percent of plans with preadmission certification: | | | |
| Always required | 24 (3.1) | 37 (3.0) | 37 (4.0) |
| Sometimes required | 14 (2.4) | 7 (1.8) | 4 (2.2) |
| Never required | 57 (3.7) | 52 (3.1) | 59 (4.1) |
| Percent of plans with second surgical opinion: | | | |
| Always required | 23 (3.0) | 55 (3.1) | 39 (4.0) |
| Sometimes required | 11 (2.2) | 9 (1.8) | 10 (2.5) |
| Never required | 58 (3.7) | 33 (2.9) | 50 (4.1) |

NOTES: Standard errors are in parentheses. Percents may not add to 100 because of "Don't know" responses. HMO is health maintenance organization; PPO is preferred provider organization.

SOURCE: Health Insurance Association of America, 1987.

have a stop-loss arrangement with an insurer) made up the next greatest portion of the Blue Cross and Blue Shield and commercial insurer business. Plans administered by employers and TPA's were predominantly self-insured (72 percent), with an additional 26 percent of these plans having a stop-loss arrangement.

Almost as striking as the growth of self-insurance during the decade has been the emergence of prospective utilization review among conventional plans. Earlier studies have established that there was little prospective utilization review prior to 1984 (Gabel et al., 1987). Since then, it has grown at a rapid pace, with commercial insurers instituting more prospective review than Blue Cross and Blue Shield and the other plans. A mandatory second surgical opinion was always or sometimes required for 64 percent of the employees covered by commercial insurer plans. Blue Cross and Blue Shield had this provision for only 34 percent of the employees in plans administered by them, and self-administered and TPA plans had this provision for 49 percent of those covered (Figure 4). Preadmission certification was always or sometimes required for 44 percent of the commercial insurer covered employees, 38 percent of the Blue Cross and Blue Shield employees, and 41 percent of the self-administered and TPA employees (Figure 5).

Blue Cross and Blue Shield administered plans placed smaller cost-sharing burdens on employees than the commercials or self-administered and TPA plans (Table 4). An employee covered by Blue Cross and Blue Shield typically faced a modest $100 individual deductible and a low $200 family deductible. The self-administered and TPA plans had the highest deductibles ($150 for an individual and $400 for a family), and the commercial insurers had a $150 individual deductible and a $300 family deductible. Lifetime family maximums were the least generous under the Blue Cross and Blue Shield

plans, where almost one-quarter of the employees had less than $1 million of coverage. However, lifetime maximums for the most part were very generous. Across all plans, the most common maximum out-of-pocket expenditure was between $501 and $1,000. The most common coinsurance rate was 80–20, where the employer paid 80 percent and the employee paid 20 percent.

Premium costs did not vary significantly among plan sponsors. Individual coverage costs ranged by only $6 dollars a month, from a high of $97 for commercial insurers to a low of $91 for self-administered and TPA plans (Table 4). Family coverage ranged from a high of $220 a month for commercial insurers to a low of $191 for self-administered and TPA plans.

Overall cost increases from 1986 to 1987 were very modest. Among the different plan sponsors, Blue Cross and Blue Shield had the greatest increase from 1986 of 7.4 percent. The commercial insurers had the lowest increase, with only a 5.7 percent increase in premiums. Employers are passing on a greater share of the premium cost to their employees in the commercially sponsored benefit plans. In these plans, employees saw a 7.8–percent increase in their premium contributions. Self-administered and TPA plans increased their employee contributions the lowest amount—only 1.1 percent from the previous year.

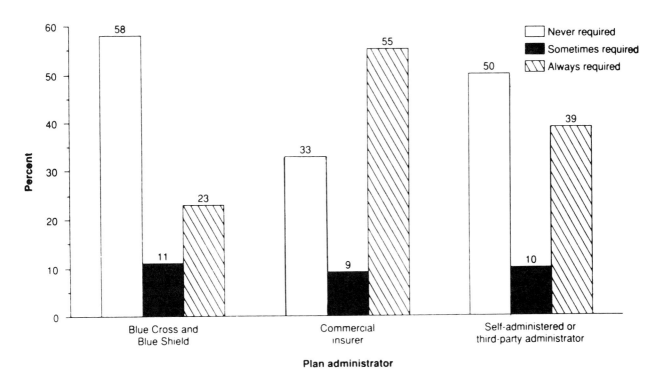

SOURCE  Health Insurance Association of America  Data from the 1987 Employer Survey

**Figure 4.** Mandatory second surgical opinion, by plan administrator: United States, 1987

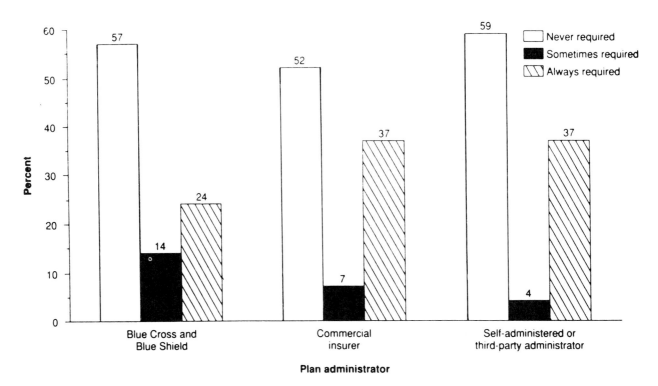

SOURCE: Health Insurance Association of America: Data from the 1987 Employer Survey.

**Figure 5.** Preadmission certification, by plan administrator: United States, 1987

## COMPARING CONVENTIONAL PLANS BY SIZE

Conventional wisdom holds that small employers pay more for health insurance coverage than large or mid-sized employers and that the characteristics of their plans differ too. The HIAA survey of employers allows an examination of insurance coverage among small employers and a comparison with coverage of other employers.

Characteristics of conventional health plans of small employers (25 employees or fewer), small to medium employers (26 to 99 employees), medium to large employers (100 to 999 employees), and large employers (1,000 employees or more) are shown in Table 5. Three facets seem to distinguish small (1 to 25 workers) employers' conventional plans from the plans of other employers. First, employees within the small-employer sector rarely are free to choose between a conventional plan and an HMO or PPO. In no case did a conventional plan compete with a PPO plan, and in only 7 percent of the firms did it compete with an HMO plan. Second, nearly 90 percent of the conventional plans among small firms are fully insured plans. In contrast, more than 85 percent of the large firms self-insure in some capacity, either through an administrative-services only arrangement, or through a minimum-premium (stop-loss) plan. Third, insurers have moved more slowly to have small employers adopt prospective utilization review than they have with mid-sized and large employers. For example,

nearly one-half of the large firms had a preadmission certification program, whereas only 29 percent of small firms did. Large employers tend to be better informed about the health insurance marketplace and, thus, are more likely to adopt innovations before small employers do.

Cost-sharing arrangements in conventional plans are compared according to the size of the employer in Table 6. Employees in small firms face a $100 individual deductible and a $300 family deductible, the same as their peers in mid-sized firms. The 80–20 coinsurance rate is the predominate method for conventional plans, regardless of the size of the employer. Small employers are more likely than either mid-sized or large firms to offer a coinsurance-free plan, however. Employees in small firms contribute a slightly lower percent of the health insurance premium for their conventional plan than their peers in large or mid-sized firms, particularly for individual coverage. More employees in small firms are without catastrophic out-of-pocket protection; nonetheless, when present, these thresholds tend to be lower than those in mid-sized and large firms.

To protect themselves against poor risks, many insurers individually underwrite employees in small firms. Because small firms must spread these costs and other administrative expenses across a smaller base and at greater risk because of the smaller base, conventional wisdom holds that these employers must pay substantially more for a given amount of financial protection.

## Table 4

### Cost sharing in conventional plans, by plan administrator and selected variables: United States, 1987

| Selected variable | Plan administrator | | |
| --- | --- | --- | --- |
| | Blue Cross and Blue Shield | Commercial insurance companies | Other plans |
| Premium cost: | | | |
| Individual coverage | $ 93 | $ 97 | $ 91 |
| | (3.6) | (3.2) | (3.3) |
| Family coverage | 203 | 220 | 191 |
| | (6.0) | (4.5) | (5.7) |
| Percent of premium contributed by firm: | | | |
| Individual coverage | 88.8 | 82.0 | 81.0 |
| | (1.6) | (1.5) | (1.9) |
| Family coverage | 75.9 | 78.2 | 76.2 |
| | (4.9) | (4.5) | (5.7) |
| Percent change in employee contribution from previous year | +4.7 | +7.8 | +1.1 |
| | (1.4) | (3.4) | (0.8) |
| Percent change in family premium from previous year | +7.4 | +5.7 | +6.4 |
| | (1.1) | (0.8) | (0.8) |
| Plan deductible: | | | |
| Individual coverage | $100 | $150 | $150 |
| | (12.5) | (5.6) | (6.8) |
| Family coverage | 200 | 300 | 450 |
| | (26.1) | (13.4) | (13.4) |
| Percent of plans with specified coinsurance rate: | | | |
| 100-0 | 12 | 4 | 4 |
| | (2.8) | (1.4) | (1.2) |
| 90-10 | 9 | 4 | 1 |
| | (1.9) | (1.4) | (0.8) |
| 80-20 | 64 | 75 | 86 |
| | (3.9) | (2.6) | (3.0) |
| 70-30 | 2 | 1 | 1 |
| | (1.1) | (0.6) | (0.8) |
| Other | 13 | 16 | 8 |
| | (2.8) | (2.2) | (2.2) |
| Percent of plans with specified maximum out-of-pocket expense: | | | |
| $500 or less | 27 | 23 | 13 |
| | (3.7) | (2.6) | (2.9) |
| $501-1,000 | 30 | 28 | 55 |
| | (3.8) | (2.9) | (4.1) |
| $1,001-2,000 | 14 | 27 | 22 |
| | (3.0) | (2.9) | (3.5) |
| $2,001 or more | 6 | 10 | 6 |
| | (1.7) | (2.0) | (2.3) |
| No limit | 7 | 5 | 4 |
| | (1.7) | (1.4) | (1.8) |
| Percent of plans with specified lifetime family maximum benefit: | | | |
| Less than $1,000,000 | 22 | 17 | 3 |
| | (3.4) | (2.6) | (1.4) |
| $1,000,000 or more | 46 | 43 | 74 |
| | (4.0) | (3.2) | (3.7) |
| Unlimited | 15 | 28 | 8 |
| | (3.1) | (2.7) | (2.3) |

NOTES: Standard errors are in parentheses. Percents may not add to 100 because of "Don't know" responses.

SOURCE: Health Insurance Association of America, 1987.

Some individuals have estimated that the difference in cost between small and large firms is 40 percent for similar policies (U.S. Senate, 1988).

Table 6 suggests that the differences between large and small employers in fact are modest. Single coverage costs approximately 10 percent more for small employers. Family coverage costs less, on the average, than for large and mid-sized employers. There are a number of serious limitations to these comparisons, however. Our analysis does not control for the richness of the benefit package nor for the geographic location of the employer. Presumably, small employers are disproportionately located in low-cost rural areas; in addition, large employers offer richer benefits (Farley, 1986). One other possible explanation is that insurers may screen many of the high-risk small groups as uninsurable.

In a year of modest increases in the price of health insurance (1986 to 1987), small employers experienced significantly smaller increases (2.6 percent) than did large and mid-sized firms. In fact, employers with 1,000 employees or more experienced the highest rate of change (up 6.9 percent). One possible contributing factor to this pattern of increases is adverse selection— where conventional plans attract a disproportionate share of the poor health risks. Many health analysts contend that individuals with closer ties to their doctors are less willing to joint an HMO—and heavy users of health care are more likely to have close ties (Wilensky and Rossiter, 1986). HMO's and PPO's held approximately 15 percent of the market among large employers that offered conventional coverage and less than 2 percent among small employers.

## ASSESSING CONVENTIONAL HEALTH PLANS

In 1977, conventional health plans reigned as the unchallenged monarch of the private health insurance world. In the following decade, insurance premiums increased at an average annual rate of 10.5 percent, almost double the rate of increase of the Consumer Price Index. As purchasers searched for ways to contain the rising cost of health care, the conventional plan's market share declined from 95 percent to 73 percent of the group insurance marketplace, with most of the decrease experienced in the latter part of the 10-year span.

As insurers of conventional plans fought to retain their market share, the conventional plan underwent significant change. Most obvious was the growth of self-insurance. There was little self-insurance in 1977. One decade later, nearly 60 percent of the Nation's employees with conventional coverage were enrolled in a plan with some aspect of self-insurance.

As self-insurance grew, employers took responsibilities formerly held by insurers, including the assumption of risk. New organizations entered the marketplace, and enrollment with the traditional insurers—Blue Cross and

## Table 5
### Number of conventional plans, by size of employer and selected variables: United States, 1987

| Selected variable | Size of employer | | | |
| --- | --- | --- | --- | --- |
| | Large (1,000+) | Medium-large (100-999) | Medium-small (26-99) | Small (1-25) |
| Percent of employees choosing conventional plan when also given choice of HMO and/or PPO | 86 (1.4) | 93 (1.6) | 96 (2.0) | 98 (0.6) |
| Percent of employees in a conventional plan given choice of PPO | 6 (6.3) | 4 (7.5) | 2 (9.9) | 0 (0.0) |
| Percent of employees in a conventional plan given choice of HMO | 80 (5.4) | 26 (6.3) | 16 (7.7) | 7 (14.9) |
| Percent of employees in first year of plan | 6 (1.5) | 9 (2.5) | 25 (4.1) | 26 (5.3) |
| **Percent of plans with specified insured status:** | | | | |
| Fully insured | 13 (2.6) | 42 (3.7) | 74 (4.0) | 89 (3.7) |
| Self-insured | 56 (3.4) | 21 (3.0) | 5 (2.1) | 3 (1.7) |
| Partly insured | 31 (2.9) | 36 (3.5) | 19 (3.5) | 5 (2.9) |
| **Percent of plans with preadmission certification:** | | | | |
| Always required | 43 (3.3) | 30 (3.4) | 24 (4.1) | 19 (3.8) |
| Sometimes required | 4 (1.6) | 10 (2.2) | 13 (3.1) | 10 (3.7) |
| Never required | 53 (3.4) | 56 (3.7) | 60 (4.7) | 58 (6.5) |
| **Percent of plans with second surgical opinion:** | | | | |
| Always required | 50 (3.2) | 42 (3.6) | 23 (4.0) | 31 (5.6) |
| Sometimes required | 9 (1.5) | 7 (2.0) | 16 (3.6) | 2 (2.4) |
| Never required | 41 (3.0) | 45 (3.7) | 54 (4.8) | 63 (5.7) |

NOTES: Standard errors are in parentheses. Percents may not add to 100 because of "Don't know" responses. HMO is health maintenance organization; PPO is preferred provider organization.

SOURCE: Health Insurance Association of America, 1987.

Blue Shield plans and commercial insurers—declined. In 1977, the traditional insurers held 95 percent of the market. One decade later, TPAs's and self-administered plans had more than one-third of the market, surpassing Blue Cross and Blue Shield plans in market share.

Prospective utilization review illustrates another dramatic development affecting conventional plans. A majority of employees in 1987 were covered by a mandatory surgical second opinion program, and 45 percent were covered by preadmission certification review. As recently as 1984, only about 5 percent of conventional plan had preadmission review programs. Utilization review should continue this growth, particularly among small employers, in the immediate future.

Meeting the challenge of rising health care costs requires sacrifice, and one of the most unpleasant of these sacrifices is patient cost sharing. Yet, as long as it costs employees very little each time they seek care, there will be little reward for employees for choosing cost-effective

health plans and for seeking efficient care. One surprising finding from the 1987 HIAA survey was that, after adjusting for inflation, employees today bear only modestly increased cost-sharing burdens over those of a decade ago. Employers pay for 83 percent of the cost of health insurance, down from 85 percent in 1977. For physician services, there was a modest decline in first-dollar coverage, and fewer workers today face coinsurance rates of less than 20 percent. These increases in cost sharing, however, were somewhat offset by a dramatic increase in the number of workers with limits on out-of-pocket costs.

What does the HIAA survey suggest about the future of conventional insurance? With the rapid growth of HMO's and PPO's in this decade, many health experts are predicting a quick demise for the conventional insurance market. Our survey suggests that this dire forecast may be a bit premature. Conventional plans are still the largest form of private health insurance coverage in

## Table 6
## Cost sharing in conventional plans, by size of employer: United States, 1987

| Selected variable | Size of employer | | | |
| --- | --- | --- | --- | --- |
| | Large (1,000 + ) | Medium-large (100-999) | Medium-small (26-99) | Small (1-25) |
| Premium cost: | | | | |
| Individual coverage | $ 94 | $ 90 | $ 98 | $107 |
| | (2.7) | (3.9) | (5.3) | (6.7) |
| Family coverage | 205 | 191 | 210 | 189 |
| | (4.3) | (5.0) | (10.1) | (7.2) |
| Percent of premium contributed by firm: | | | | |
| Individual coverage | 82.2 | 86.5 | 82.4 | 87.8 |
| | (1.5) | (1.5) | (2.7) | (2.6) |
| Family coverage | 80.0 | 72.3 | 73.3 | 78.8 |
| | (4.1) | (5.1) | (8.8) | (6.6) |
| Percent change in employee contribution from previous year | + 1.8 | + 2.9 | + 12.0 | – 1.0 |
| | (1.4) | (1.0) | (7.8) | (1.6) |
| Percent change in family premium from previous year | + 6.9 | + 6.7 | + 5.4 | + 2.6 |
| | (0.7) | (1.0) | (1.4) | (1.3) |
| Plan deductible: | | | | |
| Individual coverage | $150 | $100 | $100 | $100 |
| | (5.3) | (7.8) | (17.3) | (12.5) |
| Family coverage | 400 | 300 | 300 | 300 |
| | (11.7) | (21.0) | (30.1) | (31.5) |
| Percent of plans with specified coinsurance rate: | | | | |
| 100-0 | 3 | 9 | 7 | 15 |
| | (1.3) | (2.4) | (2.6) | (4.9) |
| 90-10 | 3 | 6 | 3 | 0 |
| | (1.3) | (1.7) | (1.6) | (0.0) |
| 80-20 | 85 | 66 | 73 | 73 |
| | (2.6) | (3.7) | (4.1) | (6.1) |
| 70-30 | 0 | 0 | 4 | 0 |
| | (0.0) | (0.0) | (1.8) | (0.0) |
| Other | 8 | 9 | 14 | 1 |
| | (1.8) | (1.7) | (2.8) | (1.3) |
| Percent of plans with specified maximum out-of-pocket expense: | | | | |
| $500 or less | 15 | 19 | 29 | 28 |
| | (2.4) | (3.0) | (4.5) | (6.0) |
| $501-$1,000 | 46 | 37 | 30 | 16 |
| | (3.1) | (3.6) | (4.7) | (5.1) |
| $1,001-$2,000 | 27 | 14 | 16 | 23 |
| | (2.9) | (2.6) | (3.4) | (5.7) |
| $2,001 or more | 6 | 14 | 5 | 13 |
| | (1.7) | (2.6) | (2.4) | (4.5) |
| No limit | 5 | 9 | 5 | 13 |
| | (1.5) | (1.9) | (2.4) | (4.5) |
| Percent of plans with specified lifetime family maximum benefit: | | | | |
| Less than $1,000,000 | 16 | 25 | 12 | 8 |
| | (2.6) | (3.2) | (3.6) | (3.8) |
| $1,000,000 or more | 63 | 45 | 52 | 37 |
| | (3.1) | (4.0) | (5.4) | (6.9) |
| Unlimited | 16 | 19 | 17 | 26 |
| | (2.6) | (3.2) | (3.7) | (6.2) |

NOTES: Standard errors are in parentheses. Percents may not add to 100 because of "Don't know" responses.

SOURCE: Health Insurance Association of America, 1987.

this country. When employees have their choice of plans, they still choose the conventional plans in large numbers; meanwhile, employers express high levels of overall satisfaction with these plans.

There are, to be sure, some forces working against conventional plans. For example, it appears that Medi-

care will continue to tighten its prospective payments to hospitals during the next few years. As Medicare payments fail to increase as rapidly as hospital expenses, hospitals are likely to attempt to recoup their lost revenues from insurers who reimburse on the basis of billed charges. HMO's and PPO's that negotiate prices with hospitals are in a stronger position to fend off so-called "hospital cost-shifting" than conventional plans (Frech and Ginsburg, 1988). Thus, a major weakness of conventional insurance is its inability to negotiate prices with hospitals and doctors, unlike their competitors, the HMO's and PPO's.

A major strength of conventional plans is their flexibility. This has allowed conventional plans to look increasingly similar to PPO and HMO plans with prospective-utilization review, without relinquishing patients' freedom to choose their doctors and hospitals.

Ultimately, the conventional market's fate will be determined by its ability to control costs. Cost control, after all, is the reason for the existence of HMO's and PPO's in the first place. In a year of modest premium increases, 1986 to 1987, conventional plans to compete with alternative delivery systems shall be revealed in the not-too-distant future.

Acknowledgments—The authors thank Tony Wang for his excellent support as a statistical and research assistant. We also wish to thank Cindy Jajich-Toth, Tom Rice, Greg de Lissovoy, Gail Jensen, Tom Musco, Pam Farley, and Marsha Preble for comments on earlier drafts.

## References

Carroll, M., and Arnett, R.: Private health insurance plans in 1977: Coverage, enrollment, and financial experience. *Health Care Financing Review*, Vol. 1, No. 2. Office of Research, Demonstrations, and Statistics, Health Care Financing Administration. Washington. U.S. Government Printing Office, Fall 1979.

Employee Benefit Research Institute: Personal communication on Current Population Survey. Washington. 1988.

Farley, P.: Private health insurance in the United States. *National Health Care Expenditures Study*. Data Preview 23. DHHS Publication No. (PHS) 86–3406. National Center for Health Services Research, Public Health Service. Washington. U.S. Government Printing Office, Sept. 1986.

Farley, P.: Private insurance and public programs: Coverage of health services. *National Health Care Expenditures Study*. Data Preview 20. DHHS Publication No. (PHS) 85–3374. National Center for Health Services Research, Public Health

Service. Washington. U.S. Government Printing Office, Mar. 1985.

Frech, H., III and Ginsburg, P.: Competition among health insurers, revisited. *Journal of Health Politics, Policy and Law* 13(2):279–291, Summer 1988.

Gabel, J., Ermann, D., Rice, T., and de Lissovoy, G.: The emergence and future of PPOs. *Journal of Health Politics, Policy and Law* 11(2):305–322, Summer 1986.

Gabel, J., Jajich-Toth, C., de Lissovoy, G., et al.: The changing world of group health insurance. *Health Affairs* 7(3):48–66, Summer 1988.

Gabel, J., Jajich-Toth, D., Williams, K., et al.: The commercial health insurance industry in transition. *Health Affairs* 6(3):46–60, Fall 1987.

Jensen, G., Morrisey, M., and Marcus, J.: Cost-sharing and the changing pattern of employer-sponsored health benefits. *Milbank Memorial Fund Quarterly* 65(4):521–550, 1987.

Medstat Systems Incorporated: *Sample Insured Population Study*. Prepared for the Health Insurance Association of America. Washington, D.C., 1988.

Musco, T.: Operating results from the leading writers of group and individual health insurance. *Research and Statistics Bulletin*. Health Insurance Association of America. Washington, D.C., 1988.

Rice, T., Gabel, J., and de Lissovoy, G.: PPOs: The employer perspective. *Journal of Health Politics, Policy and Law*, 1989.

Small Business Administration: *Health Care Coverage and Costs in Small and Large Business*. Washington. Apr. 1987.

Taylor, A. K., and Lawson, W. R. Jr.: Employer and employee expenditures for private health insurance. *National Health Care Expenditures Study*. Data Preview 7. DHHS Publication No. (PHS) 81–397. National Center for Health Services Research, Public Health Service. Washington. U.S. Government Printing Office, June 1981.

U.S. Bureau of the Census: *Statistical Abstract of the United States, 1988*. 108th Edition. Washington. U.S. Government Printing Office, 1987.

U.S. Senate, Committee on Labor and Human Resources: *Minimum Health Benefits For All Workers Act of 1988*. Washington, 1988.

Wilensky, G., Farley, P., and Taylor, A.: Variations in health insurance coverage: Benefits vs. premiums. *Milbank Memorial Fund Quarterly* 62(1):53–81, 1984.

Wilensky, G., and Rossiter, L.: Patient self-selection in HMOs. *Health Affairs* 5(1):66–80, 1986.

# Chapter 18

# The Effect of Prospective Payment on Medicare Expenditures

Louise B. Russell, Ph.D., and Carrie Lynn Manning, B.A.

**Abstract:** Medicare's prospective payment system was introduced in 1983 to show the growth of expenditures for hospital care, which form the bulk of Medicare costs. Instead of reimbursing hospitals for the actual costs of patient care, the system pays them at fixed rates for each admission.

In this study, we estimated the savings to Medicare from the use of prospective payment. We analyzed the expenditure projections published in 10 successive annual reports (1979 to 1988) by the trustees of the federal Hospital Insurance Trust Fund, which pays hospital bills for Medicare beneficiaries. To show the effect of prospective payment, these projections were adjusted to correct for the different assumptions about inflation and admissions made in each report. We also examined trends in expenditures from the Supplementary Medical Insurance Trust Fund, which pays for outpatient services, to see whether the savings in hospital expenses were offset by higher spending for out-of-hospital services.

We found that prospective payment has reduced Medicare's hospital costs substantially. Expenditures from the Hospital Insurance Trust Fund for 1990 are expected to be $12 billion less in 1980 dollars, and $18 billion less in 1990 dollars, than was expected shortly before prospective payment went into effect—the equivalent of a savings of approximately 20 percent. By contrast, the effect of prospective payment on the supplementary fund has not been great. We conclude that the prospective payment system is having a major impact on Medicare's hospital expenditures and that the savings is not offset by an increase in outpatient expenditures. (*N Engl J Med* 1989; 320:439–44.)

On October 1, 1983, Medicare replaced its cost-based system of reimbursement for hospitals with prospective payment. Instead of receiving payment for the costs actually incurred in caring for Medicare patients, hospitals now receive a rate fixed in advance for each admission. The rate depends on the patient's diagnosis-related group (DRG) and on certain characteristics of the hospital. The primary purpose of the new payment system was to slow the rapid growth of Medicare expenditures, the bulk of which are for hospital care. Indeed, when prospective payment was under consideration in 1982 and early 1983, the Hospital Insurance Trust Fund, which pays hospital bills for Medicare beneficiaries, faced imminent bankruptcy.[1]

A critical test of the success of prospective payment, though not the only important one, is its effect on Medicare expenditures: How much money has it saved?

From the Institute for Health, Health Care Policy, and Aging Research and the Department of Economics, Rutgers University, New Brunswick, N.J.

This article is drawn from a larger study of prospective payment that will be published as a book by the Brookings Institution. The opinions expressed are those of the authors and should not be attributed to the Brookings Institution, the Colorado Trust, or Rutgers University.

This study addresses that issue by analyzing the annual expenditure projections made by the trustees of the federal Hospital Insurance Trust Fund. The estimates of expenditures made shortly before prospective payment was introduced can be compared with those made subsequently, in order to show the effect of the new system.

We examined the projections published in the annual reports for the years 1979 through 1988.[1-10] These projections are based on the trustees' best estimates of probable trends in the demographic, economic, and policy variables that influence expenditures. The effect of one such variable, payment policy, was the focus of interest in our study. In order to see its effect clearly, it is important to adjust for two other variables that have changed substantially over the period in question—inflation and admissions. During the late 1970s and early 1980s, the rate of inflation was high, and the trustees assumed that it would remain so in the future. As inflation wound down during the mid-1980s, the trustees lowered their estimates of future inflation accordingly. The projections made in various reports differ substantially because different inflation rates were assumed. The projections must therefore be adjusted for the effect of these rates before the effect of prospective payment can be seen.

Similarly, the projections must be adjusted to reflect the rate of change in the number of hospital admissions assumed in each report. Before prospective payment went into effect, admissions under Medicare rose every year. The fixed rates paid under prospective payment gave hospitals an incentive to continue increasing the number of admissions, in order to bring in more revenue. Despite this incentive, however, admissions declined for several years after the introduction of prospective payment,[11] probably because of the admission-monitoring system instituted by the Health Care Financing Administration (HFCA). The assumptions made in each report reflect the recent experience at the time. In the early 1980s, the trustees assumed admissions would continue to rise, but after a year or two of prospective payment, they showed the number falling and continuing to fall for a few years. The projected expenditures must therefore be adjusted to show how much of any change should be attributed to prospective payment, and how much to the change in the number of admissions.

We report here on the expenditures of the Hospital Insurance Trust Fund, adjusted and unadjusted. To test the possibility that any savings in hospital expenses may have been offset by an increase in spending for outpatient services, which are covered by the Supplementary Medical Insurance Trust Fund, we also report on trends in the expenditures projected for that fund.

## METHODS

The expenditure projections for the Hospital Insurance Trust Fund were taken from the annual reports of the fund's trustees for the years 1979 through 1988,[1-10] along with the assumptions about hospital admissions that accompanied each set of projections. Projections about inflation were taken from the corresponding annual reports of the Social Security trust fund.[12-21]

To make their projections, the trustees establish the levels of actual expenditures in the most recent year as accurately as possible for each type of care, given lags in payment and reporting (see, for example, Appendix A of the 1988 report[10]). They then project these expenditures to future years, using assumptions about future growth that seem reasonable in the light of past experience; the assumptions are published with each year's report. In the case of inpatient hospital expenditures, which account for 93 percent of the expenditures of the Hospital Insurance Trust Fund, the projections are based on expected increases in admissions and in the cost per admission. Changes in Medicare enrollment and in the hospital admission rate determine the expected number of admissions. Growth in the cost per admission depends on increases of two kinds—those stemming from the rising costs of labor and nonlabor inputs, as projected on the basis of general inflation plus differentials that reflect experience in the hospital industry, and those arising from "intensity," or payments over and above the amounts needed to keep pace with price increases, which allow the hospital to use more real resources per admission. Presented as a single number before the start of prospective payment, intensity is now reflected in the trustees' assumptions as the official allowance made for intensity in the prospective rates, plus growth from other sources; changes in the coding of cases ("DRG creep") have accounted for much of the recent growth from other sources. This sum averaged 3.4 percent during the years from 1979 to 1983—somewhat less than in the previous decade—and 6.6 percent annually during the first three years of prospective payment, from 1984 to 1986 (see Table A1 of the 1988 report[10]).

The trustees project expenditures for 75 years into the future, but they do not publish their estimates beyond the year in which they expect the trust fund's revenues to be exhausted. Since the state of the trust fund in the early 1980s was such that it was expected to be exhausted by the late 1980s or soon thereafter, the number of years for which projections were actually published is much smaller than 75. In every report but one, however, projections were published at least through 1990—long enough to show the effect of prospective payment. We collected all available projections through the year 2000.

In each report, the trustees make three sets of projections, which they label Series I, II, and III. Series II is based on the economic and demographic circumstances considered to be most likely in the future. Series I is a more optimistic set of forecasts, incorporating demographic and economic assumptions more favorable to the trust fund (for example, a lower rate of inflation). Series III is a more pessimistic set of forecasts, incorporating less favorable assumptions. Starting in 1981, the trustees published two sets of short-term projections for Series II, assuming a more favorable and a less favorable economic outlook, respectively, for the near term; after a few years, the two converge to the same projection. In this study we present the Series II projections, although we also analyzed the Series I and III projections. After completing our computations, we averaged the two Series II projections (for years in which two projections were made) and show the average projection (adjusted and unadjusted) for each year in this article.

We chose 1980 as the base year. Using the trustees' assumptions about inflation that appear in each report, we developed a separate price index for each year's set of projections and deflated all expenditures to 1980 dollars. Similarly, we adjusted for the trustees' assumptions about hospital admissions by creating an admissions index for each set of projections and using it to produce numbers showing what the expenditures would have been if admissions had remained at the 1980 level. We present here the original expenditure projections, the expenditures as adjusted for inflation, and the expenditures as adjusted for inflation and changes in the number of admissions.

## RESULTS

Table 1 shows expenditures in 1980 dollars (i.e., adjusted for inflation) for the years 1980, 1985, 1990, 1995, and 2000. When the projections in the different reports are adjusted to the price level of a particular year, it becomes possible to see how expenditures projected for a given year changed as prospective payment took effect. The year 1990 provides a useful focus. The projections for this year show the effects of seven years of prospective payment—a period long enough for those effects to show up clearly. At the same time, the actual expenditures for the years in question are now either already known or so few years away that the estimates are likely to be quite accurate.

In the reports for 1979 through 1984, the trustees consistently projected expenditures for 1990 of $54 to $56 billion (in 1980 dollars). Thus, the average projection for 1990 was about $55 billion in the period just before prospective payment went into effect. The only exception was the estimate made in 1980. In that report, the trustees noted that the growth of resources per hospital admission had slowed sharply in 1979, a marked

Table 1. Projected Expenditures of the Hospital Insurance Trust Fund, Adjusted for Inflation, 1980 to 2000.*

| YEAR OF REPORT | 1980 | 1985 | 1990 | 1995 | 2000 |
|---|---|---|---|---|---|
| | *billions of 1980 dollars* | | | | |
| 1979 | 24.80 | 38.15 | 55.87 | — | — |
| 1980 | 24.80 | 34.33 | 50.94 | — | — |
| 1981 | 25.60 | 35.65 | 55.19 | — | — |
| 1982 | 25.60 | 38.56 | — | — | — |
| 1983 | 25.60 | 39.79 | 54.20 | — | — |
| 1984 | 25.60 | 39.88 | 54.33 | — | — |
| 1985 | 25.60 | 37.78 | 46.62 | 60.38† | 76.56† |
| 1986 | 25.60 | 37.55 | 47.49 | 62.68 | — |
| 1987 | 25.60 | 37.55 | 44.92 | 57.69 | 70.09 |
| 1988 | 25.60 | 37.55 | 42.71 | 55.30 | 68.37 |

*Figures shown are Series II projections. Starting with the year 1981, two variants of Series II projections were published; numbers shown are the average of the two projections. Numbers in italics represent actual expenditures for the year shown. Expenditures are adjusted for inflation according to the price levels assumed in the reports. Dashes indicate years in which the trust fund would be depleted, according to estimates. Data were taken from Tables 11 and A1 of the annual reports for the years 1979 to 1988 of the Board of Trustees of the United States Federal Hospital Insurance Trust Fund[1-10] and from Table 10 of the annual reports of the Board of Trustees of the United States Federal Old-Age and Survivors Insurance and Disability Insurance Trust Funds for the same years.[12-21]

†Projection II-A only; according to projection II-B, the trust fund would be depleted in 2000.

departure from the steady increases of the preceding decades.[3] In making their projections, they assumed that the amount of resources per admission would decline in 1980 and stay below the long-term trend until 1982. Subsequent events did not support their assumption, and the rates of increase reported for 1979 and 1980, as well as those assumed for later years, were raised again in the next year's report.

In the 1985 report, which came out midway through the second year of prospective payment, the trustees lowered their estimate for 1990 to $47 billion (in 1980 dollars). The 1986 report presented a similar estimate. In the next two reports the projection for 1990 dropped again—to $43 billion in the 1988 report. The difference (in 1980 dollars) between the projections made before prospective payment and that made in 1988 was thus approximately $12 billion. Expressed in terms of the price level for 1990 assumed in the 1988 report, this figure means that expenditures in 1990 will be approximately $18 billion less than was estimated before prospective payment was initiated.

Part of the savings must be attributed to the decline in admissions that occurred with prospective payment. To identify the effect of this decline, Table 2 shows the projections for each year in three forms: without adjustment, in 1980 dollars (as in Table 1), and in 1980 dollars adjusted for the changes in the number of admissions assumed by the trustees. As noted in the Methods section, the third of these numbers shows what the level of expenditures would have been if both the number of admissions and the price level had remained at the 1980 levels. Comparing these numbers with the figures for expenditures adjusted only for inflation shows the effect of lower admissions on total savings.

Table 2. Projected Expenditures of the Hospital Insurance Trust Fund, 1980 to 2000, in Current Dollars, Adjusted for Inflation, and Adjusted for Both Inflation and Changes in the Admission Rate.*

| YEAR OF REPORT | 1980 | 1985 | 1990 | 1995 | 2000 |
|---|---|---|---|---|---|
| | | | *billions of dollars* | | |
| **1979** | | | | | |
| Current dollars | 24.80 | 48.50 | 86.40 | — | — |
| 1980 Dollars | 24.80 | 38.15 | 55.87 | — | — |
| 1980 Dollars adjusted | 24.80 | 37.22 | 53.41 | — | — |
| **1980** | | | | | |
| Current dollars | 24.80 | 52.00 | 105.70 | — | — |
| 1980 Dollars | 24.80 | 34.33 | 50.94 | — | — |
| 1980 Dollars adjusted | 24.80 | 33.15 | 48.22 | — | — |
| **1981** | | | | | |
| Current dollars | 25.60 | 52.55 | 96.65 | — | — |
| 1980 Dollars | 25.60 | 35.65 | 55.19 | — | — |
| 1980 Dollars adjusted | 25.60 | 34.43 | 52.25 | — | — |
| **1982** | | | | | |
| Current dollars | 25.60 | 54.45 | — | — | — |
| 1980 Dollars | 25.60 | 38.56 | — | — | — |
| 1980 Dollars adjusted | 25.60 | 36.87 | — | — | — |
| **1983** | | | | | |
| Current dollars | 25.60 | 52.05 | 85.05 | — | — |
| 1980 Dollars | 25.60 | 39.79 | 54.20 | — | — |
| 1980 Dollars adjusted | 25.60 | 36.54 | 47.08 | — | — |
| **1984** | | | | | |
| Current dollars | 25.60 | 52.65 | 88.60 | — | — |
| 1980 Dollars | 25.60 | 39.88 | 54.33 | — | — |
| 1980 Dollars adjusted | 25.60 | 35.85 | 45.10 | — | — |
| **1985** | | | | | |
| Current dollars | 25.60 | 48.80 | 74.30 | 114.35† | 160.10† |
| 1980 Dollars | 25.60 | 37.78 | 46.62 | 60.38 | 76.56 |
| 1980 Dollars adjusted | 25.60 | 36.99 | 42.67 | 51.82 | 62.51 |
| **1986** | | | | | |
| Current dollars | 25.60 | 48.40 | 73.85 | 115.85 | — |
| 1980 Dollars | 25.60 | 37.55 | 47.49 | 62.68 | — |
| 1980 Dollars adjusted | 25.60 | 40.04 | 50.13 | 62.02 | — |
| **1987** | | | | | |
| Current dollars | 25.60 | 48.40 | 68.10 | 104.05 | 150.20 |
| 1980 Dollars | 25.60 | 37.55 | 44.92 | 57.69 | 70.00 |
| 1980 Dollars adjusted | 25.60 | 40.65 | 48.08 | 57.89 | 66.92 |
| **1988** | | | | | |
| Current dollars | 25.60 | 48.40 | 65.10 | 100.30 | 147.35 |
| 1980 Dollars | 25.60 | 37.55 | 42.71 | 55.29 | 68.37 |
| 1980 Dollars adjusted | 25.60 | 40.65 | 47.10 | 57.17 | 67.60 |

*Figures shown are Series II projections. Starting with the year 1981, two variants of Series II projections were published; numbers shown are the average of the two projections. Numbers in italics represent actual expenditures for the year shown. Expenditures are adjusted according to the price levels and the growth in the admissions rate assumed in the reports. Dashes indicate years for which the trust fund would be depleted, according to estimates. Data were taken from Tables 11 and A1 of the annual reports for the years 1979 to 1988 of the Board of Trustees of the United States Federal Hospital Insurance Trust Fund [1-10] and from Table 10 of the annual reports of the Board of Trustees of the United States Federal Old-Age and Survivors Insurance and Disability Insurance Trust Funds for the same years. [12-21]

†Projection II-A only; according to projection II-B, the trust fund would be depleted in 2000.

The decline in admissions was clearly established by 1986. In the report for that year, the projection for 1990 is, after adjustment for inflation and admissions, higher than that adjusted for inflation alone: $2.6 billion of the savings for 1990 (the difference between $50.13 billion and $47.49 billion) was due to lower admissions. In the 1988 report, more than $4 billion of the savings projected for 1990 was due to lower admissions ($47.10 billion minus $42.71 billion). Thus, about one third of the savings projected for 1990 comes not from the

prospective rates themselves, but from the decline in admissions that accompanied them.

Some of the savings in the Hospital Insurance Trust Fund may be offset by higher spending from Medicare's other fund, the Supplementary Medical Insurance Trust Fund, which pays for doctors' services and outpatient care. Expenditures from this fund have grown rapidly, and some have attributed the growth to the substitution of outpatient services for inpatient services—a possible consequence of prospective payment.

Table 3 shows expenditures through 1990 from the 1988 report of the Supplementary Medical Insurance Trust Fund, actual and projected, and adjusted for inflation; again, the base year is 1980.[22] Because expenditures from this trust fund are financed by a combination of enrollee premiums, which are adjusted every year, and general federal revenues, the trustees project expenditures only for the current year and the two subsequent years. Thus, 1990 is the last year for which projections appear in the 1988 report. If the unusually high growth in real expenditures between 1982 and 1983 is omitted, the average growth rate was 9.4 percent in the period before prospective payment (1979 to 1982) and 10.3 percent in the period from 1983 to 1987—the years for which the experience with prospective payment was complete at the time of the 1988 report. If the 1982–1983 growth rate is included in the first period, the rates of growth are nearly identical for the two periods—10.4 percent as compared with 10.3 percent.

In these calculations, we used the rates most favorable to the possibility that prospective payment has contributed to higher expenditures from the Supplementary Medical Insurance Trust Fund. We thus omitted the

Table 3. Expenditures of the Supplementary Medical Insurance Trust Fund, 1978 to 1990, in Current Dollars and Adjusted for Inflation.*

| YEAR | CURRENT DOLLARS | 1980 DOLLARS | PERCENT CHANGE, IN 1980 DOLLARS |
|---|---|---|---|
| | | *billions of dollars* | |
| 1978 | 7.80 | 9.69 | — |
| 1979 | 9.30 | 10.57 | 9.1 |
| 1980 | 11.20 | 11.20 | 6.0 |
| 1981 | 14.00 | 12.73 | 13.7 |
| 1982 | 16.20 | 13.85 | 8.8 |
| 1983 | 19.00 | 15.82 | 14.2 |
| 1984 | 20.60 | 16.48 | 4.2 |
| 1985 | 23.90 | 18.53 | 12.4 |
| 1986 | 27.30 | 20.84 | 12.5 |
| 1987 | 31.70 | 23.31 | 11.9 |
| 1988 | 36.10† | 25.60† | 9.8 |
| 1989 | 40.70† | 27.79† | 8.6 |
| 1990 | 46.30† | 30.33† | 9.1 |

*Sources: Table 6, 1988 annual report of the Board of Trustees of the Federal Supplementary Medical Insurance Trust Fund.[22]

†Figures shown are Series II projections. Numbers shown are the average of Series II-A and II-B. Expenditures are adjusted for inflation according to the price levels given in the report.

1982–1983 growth rate and reestimated the projections for 1990 as if the average rate found in the early 1980s had applied during the entire period. Applying the 9.4 percent growth rate to project expenditures for 1984 and subsequent years yields an estimate of $29.7 billion for 1990—$0.6 billion less than the trustees' estimate. Thus, the effect, if any, of prospective payment on this fund has not been great.

## DISCUSSION

According to our results, prospective payment has reduced Medicare expenditures from the Hospital Insurance Trust Fund to a level substantially below the levels projected shortly before the introduction of prospective payment. In 1980 dollars, the savings in 1990 are estimated to be about $12 billion. At the price level now expected for 1990, these savings amount to about $18 billion. Whether they are expressed in inflation-adjusted dollars or in 1990 dollars, prospective payment has reduced the expenditures projected for 1990 by more than 20 percent. Our analysis shows that this reduction has not been offset by higher expenses for out-of-hospital services; at most, prospective payment may increase the expenditures from the Supplementary Medical Insurance Trust Fund in 1990 by about $0.6 billion (in 1980 dollars).

About one third of the savings can be attributed to the decline in Medicare admissions during the first few years of the new payment system. Rates that are fixed in advance give hospitals an incentive to increase admissions, in order to bring in more revenues. The HCFA was well aware of this incentive and acted forcefully to counter it. During the early years of prospective payment, the Peer Review Organizations and their predecessors, the Professional Standards Review Organizations, were directed to focus on reducing admissions, not simply on holding the line.[23,24] The reviewers questioned the necessity of many admissions and encouraged the use of outpatient care whenever possible. The HCFA even warned that if admissions did rise, the prospective payment rates would be adjusted downward to compensate.[24] Thus, the decline in admissions appears to have been a result of the review system that accompanied prospective payment, and not of the prospective rates.

The state of the Medicare trust funds is a politically sensitive issue, and some may ask whether the projections are a credible base for the estimation of savings. It was partly for this reason that we analyzed projections from 10 reports, rather than the 2 that would have been minimally necessary (1 just before prospective payment and the most recent report). The reports for the period before prospective payment began span two administrations. The 1980 projections, which were substantially lower than any others in this period, were released during an election year and suggest that the projections may sometimes be subject to political pressures, although the lower estimate was based on an actual event—the sharply lower growth in intensity in 1979. The consistency found in the remaining estimates indicates that the 1980 projections were the exception, not the rule. Since the beginning of prospective payment, the projections have also demonstrated a consistent pattern and those for 1990 are further constrained by the fact that that year is rapidly approaching.

Possibly some Medicare costs have been shifted to other payers. If so, the true savings would not be as large as our estimates indicate. We could not test this possibility comprehensively among different groups of payers. We did examine the growth in out-of-pocket payments by Medicare beneficiaries, which has been rapid in recent years. Even so, data published by the Prospective Payment Assessment Commission show that beneficiary payments have not increased as a share of total payments (payments by Medicare plus payments by beneficiaries) for Medicare-covered services.[25] Beneficiaries paid 23 percent of the total in 1980 and the same percentage in 1987.

Furthermore, in its June 1988 report, the Prospective Payment Assessment Commission noted that Medicare's prospective payment system appeared to have contributed to slower growth in medical expenditures for the nation as a whole, indicating that any cost shifting that has taken place has not been large enough to offset the savings produced by the system.[25] Prospective payment cannot be expected to have a major effect on national health expenditures, since Medicare accounts for only a portion of the national total. In 1986, Medicare expenses made up slightly under 17 percent of the national total for health expenditures and 19 percent of expenditures for personal health care (as compared with just over 14 percent and 16 percent, respectively, in 1980).[26] Nonetheless, our results support the conclusion of the Prospective Payment Assessment Commission— that the new system may have helped slow the growth in national expenditures, which are expected to approach $650 billion in 1990.[26] The $18 billion Medicare savings we estimate for that year amounts to a reduction of almost 3 percent in the national total.

The trustees of the Hospital Insurance Trust Fund now estimate that the fund will remain financially sound until about the year 2005. Although this is a considerable improvement over the prospects of only a few years ago, the trustees warn against complacency. Instead, they see the improvement as providing time for further gradual changes and they urge Congress to begin making these changes as soon as possible.[10]

Savings are the first test of prospective payment's success, but not the only one. As has been widely recognized, it is important to determine whether, in the course of saving money, prospective payment has also changed the quality of medical care, and if so, in what ways.[11] A full assessment must consider the effects of prospective payment on quality and access, as well as the financial consequences for Medicare. We do not address the issue of quality here, but raise it to emphasize that our results should not be interpreted to mean that prospective payment is an unqualified success. We have provided only a part, although an important part, of the information needed to make that assessment.

## References

1. Board of Trustees of the United States Federal Hospital Insurance Trust Fund. 1982 Annual report of the board of trustees of the federal hospital insurance trust fund. House document 97–166, 97th Congress, 2nd session. Washington, D.C.: Government Printing Office, 1982.
2. Board of Trustees of the United States Federal Hospital Insurance Trust Fund. 1979 Annual report of the board of trustees of the federal hospital insurance trust fund. House document 96–102, 96th Congress, 1st session. Washington, D.C.: Government Printing Office, 1979.
3. Board of Trustees of the United States Federal Hospital Insurance Trust Fund. 1980 Annual report of the board of trustees of the federal hospital insurance trust fund. House document 96–333, 96th Congress, 2nd session. Washington, D.C.: Government Printing Office, 1980.
4. Board of Trustees of the United States Federal Hospital Insurance Trust Fund. 1981 Annual report of the board of trustees of the federal hospital insurance trust fund. House document 97–67, 97th Congress, 1st session. Washington, D.C.: Government Printing Office, 1981.
5. Board of Trustees of the United States Federal Hospital Insurance Trust Fund. 1983 Annual report of the board of trustees of the federal hospital insurance trust fund. House document 98–75, 98th Congress, 1st session. Washington, D.C.: Government Printing Office, 1983.
6. Board of Trustees of the United States Federal Hospital Insurance Trust Fund. 1984 Annual report of the board of trustees of the federal hospital insurance trust fund. House document 98–199, 98th Congress, 2nd session. Washington, D.C.: Government Printing Office, 1984.
7. Board of Trustees of the United States Federal Hospital Insurance Trust Fund. 1985 Annual report of the board of trustees of the federal hospital insurance trust fund. House document 99–47, 99th Congress, 1st session. Washington, D.C.: Government Printing Office, 1985.
8. Board of Trustees of the United States Federal Hospital Insurance Trust Fund. 1986 Annual report of the board of trustees of the federal hospital insurance trust fund. House document 99–190, 99th Congress, 2nd session. Washington, D.C.: Government Printing Office, 1986.
9. Board of Trustees of the United States Federal Hospital Insurance Trust Fund. 1987 Annual report of the board of trustees of the federal hospital insurance trust fund. House document 100–56, 100th Congress, 1st session. Washington, D.C.: Government Printing Office, 1987.
10. Board of Trustees of the United States Federal Hospital Insurance Trust Fund. 1988 Annual report of the board of trustees of the federal hospital insurance trust fund. House document 100–193, 100th Congress, 2nd session. Washington, D.C.: Government Printing Office, 1988.
11. Impact of the Medicare hospital prospective payment system. Baltimore, Md.: Department of Health and Human Services, Health Care Financing Administration, Office of Research and Demonstrations, 1986.
12. Board of Trustees of the United States Federal Old-Age and Survivors Insurance and Disability Insurance Trust Funds. 1979 Annual report of the board of trustees of the federal old-age and survivors insurance and disability insurance trust funds. House document 96–101, 96th Congress, 1st session. Washington, D.C.: Government Printing Office, 1979.
13. Board of Trustees of the United States Federal Old-Age and Survivors Insurance and Disability Insurance Trust Funds. 1980 Annual report of the board of trustees of the federal old-age and survivors insurance and disability insurance trust funds. House document 96–332, 96th Congress, 2nd session. Washington, D.C.: Government Printing Office, 1980.
14. Board of Trustees of the United States Federal Old-Age and Survivors Insurance and Disability Insurance Trust Funds. 1981 Annual report of the board of trustees of the federal old-age and survivors insurance and disability insurance trust funds. House document 97–66, 97th Congress, 1st session. Washington, D.C.: Government Printing Office, 1981.
15. Board of Trustees of the United States Federal Old-Age and Survivors Insurance and Disability Insurance Trust Funds. 1982 Annual report of the board of trustees of the federal old-age and survivors insurance and disability insurance trust funds. House document 97–163, 97th Congress, 2nd session. Washington, D.C.: Government Printing Office, 1982.
16. Board of Trustees of the United States Federal Old-Age and Survivors Insurance and Disability Insurance Trust Funds. 1983 Annual report of the board of trustees of the federal old-age and survivors insurance and disability insurance trust funds. House document 98–74, 98th Congress, 1st session. Washington, D.C.: Government Printing Office, 1983.
17. Board of Trustees of the United States Federal Old-Age and Survivors Insurance and Disability Insurance Trust Funds. 1984 Annual report of the board of trustees of the federal old-age and survivors insurance and disability insurance trust funds. House document 98–200, 98th Congress, 2nd session. Washington, D.C.: Government Printing Office, 1984.
18. Board of Trustees of the United States Federal Old-Age and Survivors Insurance and Disability Insurance Trust Funds. 1985 Annual report of the board of trustees of the federal old-age and survivors insurance and disability insurance trust funds. House document 99–46, 99th Congress, 1st session. Washington, D.C.: Government Printing Office, 1985.
19. Board of Trustees of the United States Federal Old-Age and Survivors Insurance and Disability Insurance Trust Funds. 1986 Annual report of the board of trustees of the

federal old-age and survivors insurance and disability insurance trust funds. House document 99–189, 99th Congress, 2nd session. Washington, D.C.: Government Printing Office, 1986.

20. Board of Trustees of the United States Federal Old-Age and Survivors Insurance and Disability Insurance Trust Funds. 1987 Annual report of the board of trustees of the federal old-age and survivors insurance and disability insurance trust funds. House document 100–55, 100th Congress, 1st session. Washington, D.C.: Government Printing Office, 1987.

21. Board of Trustees of the United States Federal Old-Age and Survivors Insurance and Disability Insurance Trust Funds. 1988 Annual report of the board of trustees of the federal old-age and survivors insurance and disability insurance trust funds. House document 100–192, 100th Congress, 2nd session. Washington, D.C.: Government Printing Office, 1988.

22. Board of Trustees of the United States Federal Supplementary Medical Insurance Trust Fund. 1988 Annual report of the board of trustees of the federal supplementary medical insurance trust fund. House document 100–194, 100th Congress, 2nd session. Washington, D.C.: Government Printing Office, 1988.

23. Admissions increase will cost money. *McGraw-Hill's Med Health* 1984; 38(5):1.

24. PRO goals, realistic or risky? *McGraw-Hill's Med Health* 1984; 38:31.

25. Medicare prospective payment and the American health care system. Washington, D.C.: Prospective Payment Assessment Commission, 1988.

26. Division of National Cost Estimates, Office of the Actuary, Health Care Financing Administration. National health expenditures, 1986–2000. *Health Care Financ Rev* 1987; 8(4):1–36.

# Chapter 19

# Estimating Physicians' Work for a Resource-Based Relative-Value Scale

William C. Hsiao, Ph.D., Peter Braun, M.D., Douwe Yntema, Ph.D., and Edmund R. Becker, Ph.D.

**Abstract:** We have developed a resource-based relative-value scale as an alternative to the system of payment based on charges for physicians' services. Resource inputs by physicians include (1) total work input performed by the physician for each service; (2) practice costs, including malpractice premiums; and (3) the cost of specialty training. These factors were combined to produce a relative-value scale denominated in nonmonetary units.

We describe here the process by which the physician's work was defined and estimated. The study asked two questions: What is the physician's work for each service performed? and Can work be estimated reliably and validly? We concluded that a physician's work has four major dimensions: time, mental effort and judgment, technical skill and physical effort, and psychological stress.

We found that physicians can rate the relative amount of work of the services within their specialty directly, taking into account all the dimensions of work. Moreover, these ratings are highly reproducible, consistent, and therefore probably valid. (*N Engl J Med* 1988; 319:835–41).

There is a growing consensus that the prevailing method of paying for physicians' services should be fundamentally reformed. Increasingly, physicians, patients, and insurers find the current system based on usual, customary, and reasonable charges to be cumbersome and administratively complex.[1] The current method of payment has also been faulted for "creating patterns of allowed charges that embody inappropriate incentives for the use of medical services, as well as for physicians' decisions on where to locate and what to specialize in."[2] Yet another criticism is that the system "encourages physicians to specialize, to practice in urban and suburban areas, and to perform services in hospital settings—all in the face of stated national policies of encouraging primary care, rural practice, and out-of-hospital services."[3] The current method of payment produces these perverse effects, it is argued, because physicians' charges are distorted by serious imperfections in the marketplace.

The market for physicians' services does not satisfy the conditions that define a reasonably competitive market. First, widespread health insurance coverage reduces patients' sensitivity to fees. Patients generally choose physicians and services with little concern for price.

Reprinted with permission from William C. Hsiao, Ph.D., Peter Braun, M.D., Douwe Yntema, Ph.D., and Edmund R. Becker, Ph.D., Estimating Physicians' Work for a Resource-Based Relative-Value Scale. *The New England Journal of Medicine*, Vol. 319 No. 13, pp. 835–841, 1988.

From the Department of Health Policy and Management, Harvard School of Public Health (W.C.H., P.B., E.R.B.), and the Department of Psychology (D.Y.), Harvard University.

Supported in part by the Office of Research and Demonstrations, Health Care Financing Administration, under a cooperative agreement (17-C-98795/1–03). The opinions expressed are those of the authors and not necessarily those of the Health Care Financing Administration.

Second, patients often lack adequate knowledge on which to base their choices of medical services and judgments about technical quality; they typically rely on their physicians for advice in making medical decisions. Physicians are often not subject to the checks and balances generated by traditional competitive forces. Finally, legal restrictions specify who can provide medical services, admit patients to hospitals, and prescribe drugs. Although such restrictions protect patients from unqualified providers, they also tend to grant monopoly power to the medical profession.

Because of these failures of the medical marketplace, charges (prices) are distorted. Policy makers, third-party payers, and many physicians are exploring alternative methods of payment that are not based solely on physicians' charges. One such approach is to base reimbursement on the resource-input cost. That is the approach we have taken.

Three major resource inputs are required to produce medical services or procedures: (1) the total work input by the physician; (2) practice costs, including malpractice premiums; and (3) the opportunity costs of postgraduate training to become a qualified specialist.

These three factors combine to produce the resource-based relative value (RBRV) of a given medical service. One way to merge these factors into a relative value is as follows:

$$RBRV = (TW) (1 + RPC) (1 + AST),$$

where TW denotes total work input by the physician, RPC an index of relative specialty-practice costs, and AST an index of amortized value for the opportunity cost of specialized training.

We have further divided total work into pre-, intra-, and postservice work. The intraservice period is the time when a physician sees the patient or performs a procedure, and preservice and postservice periods are the times spent on the patient before and after the intraservice period.

There already exists a detailed classification of physicians' services, designed by physicians, for use in billing patients and insurers. The *Physician's Current Procedural Terminology*, fourth edition, known as the CPT-4,[4] identifies more than 7000 distinct services and procedures (henceforth jointly denoted here by the word "services"), taking into account variations in the level of service provided to patients with conditions of differing complexity and severity. In seeking to measure relative physician work input, we used the CRT-4's classification of services. We dealt with the issue of variation in the complexity of patients' conditions within CPT-4 codes by describing, with the assistance of the technical consulting physicians, average patients for each service.

Information about practice costs can be obtained from physicians' tax returns or from national surveys, and the opportunity costs of specialty training can be estimated in a conventional manner. We then distributed these costs among all the services performed in each specialty, in proportion to the physicians' total work input for each service.

The principal research questions remaining were these: What is the physician's work input for each service performed? and Can work be measured in a reliable and valid manner?

Our primary objective here has been to understand and define the work input of physicians' services and to measure such work in a reliable and valid manner. In this paper we examine the definition and dimensions of work, and explore a method of measuring the work of given services. We will present quantitative estimates of work, derived from surveys of physicians, and we will examine the reliability and validity of these results. We will be concerned here only with estimates of intraservice work, which generally constitutes roughly 60 percent of the total work input. In a companion report,[5] we include data on preservice and postservice work, as well as on the two other components of the relative value estimate (i.e., RPC and AST).

## FINDINGS OF PREVIOUS STUDIES

The present study is constructed on the foundation of two previous studies of resource-based relative values.[6,7] In an initial exploratory study in 1979,[6] we posited four inputs for quantitative assessment: time, complexity per unit of time, investment in professional training, and overhead expenses of practice. We assumed that time and complexity could be assessed independently.

Our approach to quantifying the physician's work was to measure the duration and the complexity per unit of time of each service. We obtained measures of time from published data on the total duration of surgical procedures. We obtained measures of complexity by asking surgeons for their subjective estimates of the relative complexity per unit of time of various procedures. The work for each procedure was then calculated as the product of the values for time and complexity obtained separately.

Examination of the data revealed a high degree of correlation between the duration of a procedure and physicians' estimates of its complexity per unit of time. As a result, we questioned whether physicians could hold time constant when providing estimates of complexity. Overlap between time and complexity, we hypothesized, led to an exaggeration of their product.

In a second study,[7] we tried to avoid the confounding of time and complexity estimates by obtaining direct global estimates of work, incorporating both dimensions. The estimates were elicited with use of a closed numeric scale, from 1 to 100, with the most difficult procedure assigned a value of 100. The results appeared to be unrealistically low in the case of lengthy procedures. Moreover, the longer the procedure, the more the work appeared to be underestimated. The physicians interviewed seemed to have given inadequate weight to the duration of the procedures.

In both previous studies, the physicians' estimates were strikingly consistent, particularly with respect to the rank-ordering of procedures. However, both studies produced primary data that we and the physicians who served as technical consultants considered to be unreasonable as estimates of the work required. Our measure of reasonableness was the degree to which the estimates of work conformed to the "reality" of work input as physicians experience it.

## METHODS

A general discussion of our methodologic strategy has already been published.[8]

### Defining Work and Its Dimensions

The present investigation began with a systematic reexamination of work and its dimensions, resulting in a major revision of our methods. Instead of assuming that work consists of two independent factors, time and complexity, we asked a total of 20 Boston clinicians in six specialties to participate in hour-long face-to-face interviews with a psychologist and to identify the important dimensions of their work.

The physicians typically described the important variables in their work as time; mental effort; knowledge, judgment, and diagnostic acumen; technical skill; physical effort; and psychological stress. These six dimensions initially seemed to encompass the varied aspects of work.

In addition, asked what factors determined the level of work input for an individual patient, the physicians commonly cited the complexity of the patient's problem, the seriousness of the patient's condition, uncertainty about the diagnosis or treatment, and the possibility of iatrogenic harm to the patient.

In analyzing the six dimensions of work identified by physicians, we suspected that some might overlap greatly and thus be highly correlated. We collected preliminary data and performed some exploratory data analysis, including multidimensional scaling analysis[9] to identify the major independent dimensions. This exploratory analysis led us to combine mental effort and judgment into a single dimension and technical skill and physical effort into another. Thus, we ultimately postulated the dimension of work as (1) time, (2) mental effort and

judgment, (3) technical skill and physical effort, and (4) psychological stress.

Mental effort, technical skill, and stress, of course, are almost impossible to measure objectively. We have had to rely on the subjective judgments of the physicians who perform particular procedures. Reliable and valid measurement of subjective judgments is difficult to obtain, however, and the method of measurement is crucial.

Our central approach in the present study was to obtain global ratings of the relative work of selected services, embracing all the important dimensions of work. We then examined these ratings in terms of separate ratings of the individual dimensions to determine whether our direct measures of work were valid measures of all its important parts.

### Magnitude Estimation

After consultation with psychologists, statisticians, economists, and sociologists, we selected the method magnitude estimation[10] as the best means of obtaining subjective assessments of work and its dimensions. Magnitude estimation is a means of measuring subjective perceptions and judgments; its usefulness in obtaining reliable, reproducible, and valid results has been demonstrated.[11-13] For example, it can yield a close correspondence between objective physical measures of sensation and subjective ratings of perceptions, such as the correspondence between the intensity of light and a subjective rating of brightness. Moreover, it has been found to be reliable in the replication of results among many groups of people.

Using this method, we asked respondents to rate services in relation to a reference service, using a ratio scale rather than a cardinal or ordinal scale. Respondents could rate a service as high or low as they thought necessary to reflect reality. In general surgery, for example, we chose uncomplicated inguinal hernia repair as the reference service and assigned a value of 100 to the work it required. A surgeon who judged the work of a lower anterior resection for rectal carcinoma to be $4\frac{1}{2}$ times that of an uncomplicated inguinal hernia repair responded with a rating of 450.

### Survey Design

To gather ratings of work and its dimensions from a large sample of physicians, we designed a straightforward questionnaire that could be administered over the telephone. The questionnaire was carefully tested to minimize any potential misunderstanding that could result in survey bias. We surveyed a stratified random sample of physicians from the American Medical Association's (AMA's) 1986 Physician Masterfile, which lists every known physician in the United States, including nonmembers of the AMA. We stratified the sample according to 10 geographic regions,[14] the national percentage of board-certified physicians in each specialty, and the specialty-specific proportions in each region. We excluded physicians who worked in patient care fewer than 20 hours a week, were in residency training or over 65, or lacked a current address in the AMA Physician Masterfile. Approximately 250 names were drawn in each specialty, in case there was a large number of physicians who did not meet the criteria. The first 185 names drawn constituted the initial sample.

Pilot Survey

As a pilot test of the questionnaire and the magnitude estimation method, we chose four representative specialties—general surgery, internal medicine, radiology, and anesthesiology. We then selected from the Physician Masterfile a random sample of about 90 specialists in each of the four specialties, drawn from among physicians practicing in the New England states and New York who were not employed by the federal government.

A professional survey firm (the Center for Survey Research of the University of Massachusetts) sent each physician a letter from the principal investigators explaining the survey's purpose, a letter of endorsement from the AMA, an instruction sheet describing the magnitude estimation method with illustrative examples, and a list of selected services and procedures in the physician's specialty, along with definitions of the four dimensions on which to rate them. Several days after the mailing, the survey firm contacted each physician's office to arrange a telephone interview. The physician had to respond personally; no substitute was acceptable. The overall response rate for the pilot study was 73.1 percent, ranging from 85.4 percent for radiologists to 59.3 percent for internists.

National Survey

Before starting the national survey, we tested the questionnaire again with physicians from each of the four specialties, using telephone interviews that were recorded and reviewed by members of the project staff and professionals from the Center for Survey Research. At the end of the interview, the interviewers also asked the respondents about problems or shortcomings in the questionnaire. Ninety such interviews were conducted, and the questionnaire or interview process was revised where appropriate.

In the national survey, we set a response-rate goal of 60 percent in each specialty. To protect confidentiality, each physician in the sample was assigned a random number by the survey firm. After an initial telephone call to verify specialty and address, the survey firm administered the questionnaire in the same manner as in the pilot study.

We surveyed 3164 physicians, with whom 1977 interviews were completed, for an overall response rate of 62.5 percent. Response rates ranged from 69 percent for radiologists to 56 percent for practitioners of obstetrics and gynecology. The survey firm worked assiduously to obtain high response rates. For instance, an average of 36 calls were made per nonresponding obstetrician/gynecologist.

To ascertain whether the quantitative measurement of work obtained from the survey was reliable and valid, we performed statistical analyses on the data collected from the pilot study and the national survey. First, the data were edited to remove extremely high and low outlines (those that differed by more than 3 SD from the mean of those remaining). Fewer than 1.0 percent of the ratings were eliminated for this reason. After editing, we used the Estimation and Maximization algorithm[15] to calculate the means and standard deviations of the ratings, taking missing values into account. For the vast majority of services, 2 to 5 percent of the physicians gave no rating. Summary statistics were computed for each service according to specialty.

## RESULTS

We found that physicians were able to give reliable and valid ratings of the work entailed in performing services within their specialties. For purposes of brevity, we report here the summary data on intraservice work of 33 services selected from four specialists—internal medicine, general surgery, radiology, and anesthesiology. Additional information, including the complete survey data and detailed statistical analyses of this study, may be found in the final report to the Health Care Financing Administration, September 1988.[16]

Table 1 shows the mean value of ratings of work and time for both the pilot and the national survey. Analysis of the survey data showed that the ratings of work and its dimensions followed a logarithmic normal distribution. Thus, we transformed the data into a logarithmic scale, as is commonly done in analyzing data obtained with the magnitude estimation method, and calculated the means, standard deviations, and other statistics on the basis of the log-normal distribution.

The ratings show that work input for different services can vary more than 30-fold in surgery and 8-fold in internal medicine. The standard errors for the ratings of work and time were higher in the pilot survey than in the national survey, because the standard errors are a function of sample size; the pilot survey had a much smaller sample. Table 1 shows that the standard errors

Table 1. Physicians' Estimates of Intraservice Work and Time for Selected Services, According to Specialty.*

| | WORK† | | TIME† | |
|---|---|---|---|---|
| | PILOT SURVEY | NATIONAL SURVEY | PILOT SURVEY | NATIONAL SURVEY |
| | | | | *minutes* |
| **Internal medicine‡** | | | | |
| Electrocardiogram, with interpretation, in a 50-year-old man | 96 (9.4) | 80  (6.9) | 9.4 (9.0) | 7.7§ (7.7) |
| Office visit, sore throat, fever, and fatigue in a 19-year-old college student, established patient | 100 — | 100  (5.7) | 13.6 (4.7) | 13.8  (4.1) |
| Office phone consultation regarding possible adverse drug reaction in established patient | 107 (12.5) | 80  (6.3) | 9.4 (8.3) | 7.9§ (4.9) |
| Follow-up visit of a 55-year-old man for management of hypertension, mild fatigue, on beta-blocker and thiazide regimen¶ | 153 (12.5) | 123  — | 15.4 (4.0) | 15.6  (2.7) |
| Aspiration of synovial fluid from knee | 180 (9.1) | 166  (6.6) | 15.1 (6.8) | 14.6  (6.1) |
| Office evaluation of new-onset right-lower-quadrant pain in a 32-year-old woman, established patient | 272 (6.7) | 253  (3.6) | 26.1 (4.8) | 29.0  (3.8) |
| Hospital consultation for diagnosis and management of fever after abdominal surgery | 374 (7.2) | 411  (4.6) | 48.1 (4.3) | 48.4  (3.2) |
| Management of patient with acute pulmonary edema in emergency room, who is subsequently admitted to hospital | 518 (7.3) | 650  (4.6) | 56.6 (5.1) | 66.1§ (4.5) |
| **General surgery** | | | | |
| Hospital visit, three days after uncomplicated cholecystectomy with exploration of common bile duct | 17 (14.7) | 13 (10.7) | 10.4 (6.7) | 11.0  (4.5) |
| Rigid sigmoidoscopy, without biopsy, in office | 23 (7.8) | 23  (6.8) | 10.7 (8.3) | 12.0  (5.3) |
| Office evaluation of new-onset right-lower-quadrant pain in a 32-year-old woman, established patient | 40 (14.4) | 31  (9.9) | 24.2 (5.5) | 26.0  (3.9) |
| Insertion of Swan–Ganz catheter | 72 (11.3) | 58  (9.0) | 29.5 (6.6) | 31.7  (7.1) |
| Uncomplicated indirect inguinal hernia repair, 45-year-old man¶ | 100 — | 100 — | 46.0 (4.6) | 41.4  (3.2) |
| Cholecystectomy for cholelithiasis | 235 (4.5) | 231  (4.0) | 73.3 (5.1) | 61.0§ (3.3) |
| Abdominal hysterectomy for cancer in situ of cervix in a 50-year-old woman | 247 (5.5) | 255  (4.9) | 95.5 (4.2) | 84.9  (3.4) |
| Modified radical mastectomy | 263 (5.1) | 293  (4.4) | 107.2 (4.3) | 102.9  (3.3) |
| Low anterior resection for rectal carcinoma | 445 (5.2) | 447  (4.1) | 163.7 (3.5) | 151.9  (2.5) |
| **Radiology** | | | | |
| Interpretation of lumbar spine x-ray films, complete radiographic exam, adult patient with low back pain | 47 (7.0) | 45  (5.1) | 6.7 (12.6) | 5.4  (6.9) |
| Upper gastrointestinal series, air-contrast technique with KUB, for abdominal pain after meals and heme-positive stools, performance and interpretation¶ | 100 — | 100 — | 15.1 (10.7) | 17.1  (5.2) |
| Intravenous urography, pyelography, including kidneys, ureters, and bladder, patient with hematuria and flank pain, performance and interpretation | 124 (4.7) | 115  (4.2) | 21.8 (9.8) | 22.6  (6.0) |
| Hysterosalpingography, complete procedure, in a 26-year-old woman with infertility | 124 (9.6) | 153  (6.0) | 21.6 (8.6) | 23.6  (6.2) |
| Barium enema, double contrast, complete procedure, for occult gastrointestinal bleeding in a 55-year-old man, performance and interpretation | 167 (4.5) | 153  (3.0) | 23.8 (6.4) | 23.6  (4.6) |
| Ethography of the pregnant uterus, B-scan, real time, or both, image documentation, complete for questionable fetal abnormality, performance and interpretation | 167 (8.8) | 197  (5.6) | 21.3 (8.7) | 22.6  (5.5) |
| Venography, unilateral, complete procedure, for possible deep-vein thrombosis of lower extremity, performance and interpretation | 186 (6.1) | 181  (5.5) | 28.4 (6.3) | 27.7  (4.2) |
| Anesthesiology‖ | | | | |
| Anesthesia for dilation and curettage of uterus | 67 (4.2) | 68  (4.2) | | |
| Anesthesia for cystoscopy | 79 (4.6) | 76  (5.0) | | |
| Anesthesia for inguinal hernia repair¶ | 100 — | 100 — | | |
| Anesthesia for knee arthroscopy | 106 (4.0) | 110  (2.8) | | |
| Anesthesia for modified radical mastectomy | 175 (3.6) | 185  (3.4) | | |
| Anesthesia for transurethral resection of prostate | 186 (4.2) | 181  (3.5) | | |
| Anesthesia for colectomy | 236 (4.0) | 268§ (3.7) | | |
| Anesthesia for total hip replacement | 321 (4.5) | 306  (3.9) | | |
| Anesthesia for repair of abdominal aortic aneurysm | 518 (5.1) | 533  (4.3) | | |

*Relative values assigned to a physician's work are specific to the specialty in question and cannot be compared across specialties.

†Values shown are means with the standard error of the mean expressed as a percentage of the mean.

‡Different reference services and procedures were used in the pilot and national surveys for internal medicine. KUB denotes kidney and upper bladder.

§Mean values for this service from the pilot and national surveys differ significantly (P<0.05).

¶Used as a reference service in the national survey.

‖No comparison of time is shown for anesthesiology, because of a different specification between the two surveys for time during a service.

for the ratings of most services ranged between 4.0 and 8.0 percent in the national survey.

## Reliability and Reproducibility

A fundamental question in our study concerns the degree to which physicians in a given specialty agree in their ratings of work. We first compared the ratings from the pilot survey with those from the national survey. For only 5 of 33 services were the t-statistics for differences in estimates of work or time between the pilot and the national study significant beyond the 0.05 level. This finding implies that the ratings are reproducible and that they were obtained by a reliable method.

In general, the ratings of work obtained independently in the two studies were within 10 percent of each other. Only in a few instances did they differ by more than 15 percent. When all services were classified as evaluation-and-management, invasive, imaging, or laboratory, the category of service with the greatest difference was evaluation-and-management. The estimates of time were also in agreement.

In the specialty of internal medicine, we used different reference services in the two surveys. Until the reference services were standardized, ratings for the same service were not comparable. To align the two scales, we used the office visit of a 19-year-old established patient with a sore throat, fever, and fatigue. As Table 1 shows, the ratings for work for most services in internal medicine differed by less than 10 percent across studies. Significant differences appeared, however, in the ratings of work for services performed in the emergency room and by telephone consultation. The mean estimates of time required for most services were, again, surprisingly similar between the two surveys.

In general surgery, the mean ratings of work for all surgical procedures were similar between the two surveys; two thirds of the values are nearly identical. There is also close agreement in the two sets of time estimates. The same is true of the comparative results for anesthesiology and radiology. Estimated times are not shown for anesthesiology because we changed the definition of anesthesia intraservice time between the pilot and national surveys.

To evaluate the reliability of the ratings of work, we used the intraclass correlation method,[17] which indicates the degree to which two physicians in the same specialty agree in their ratings of various services. The results appear in Table 2, in the column headed "Individual Physician." All correlations are above 0.5, and most are above 0.7. These values apply to all the services studied, not just those shown in Table 1. Although there is no universal standard by which to judge what value of intraclass correlation reflects reliable subjective judg-

### Table 2. Reliability of Ratings of Intraservice Work.*

| SPECIALTY | PILOT SURVEY | | NATIONAL SURVEY | |
|---|---|---|---|---|
| | INDIVIDUAL PHYSICIAN | MEAN OF SAMPLE | INDIVIDUAL PHYSICIAN | MEAN OF SAMPLE |
| Anesthesiology | 0.647 | 0.992 | 0.720 | 0.997 |
| General surgery | 0.709 | 0.993 | 0.717 | 0.996 |
| Internal medicine | 0.614 | 0.988 | 0.713 | 0.996 |
| Radiology | 0.740 | 0.994 | 0.784 | 0.998 |

*The reliability of the ratings for an individual physician is the intraclass correlation. The reliability of the mean ratings is calculated from the intraclass correlation with use of the Spearman–Brown prediction formula.

ments, it is commonly agreed that values above 0.6 are very good and that values over 0.75 are excellent.

Although the intraclass correlation is customarily reported for reliability tests, it is less meaningful for our present purpose than the reliability measure provided in Table 2 in the column headed "Mean of Sample." This measurement, obtained from the intraclass correlation by the Spearman-Brown predictor formula,[17] predicts that the coefficient of correlation would be between two sets of means of the ratings of work if we had drawn from the population of all specialists two samples of the size we actually obtained in our national survey. These coefficients, which range from 0.988 to 0.998, predict that the mean values for each service would be very close to each other. When different groups of experts agree this closely, it is likely that their judgments reflect reality.

## Consistency and Validity

It is possible, however, for two groups of experts to agree and for both to be wrong. We therefore evaluated whether the ratings of work can be predicted from the ratings of the dimensions of work—a test of the consistency between the whole and its parts. These predictions were made separately for each specialty, with use of the mean value of work for each service and the mean values of their respective dimensions. The regression results appear in Table 3. The multiple correlation coefficients ($R^2$) are surprisingly close to unity. That is, the estimates of the means of ratings for work can be predicted from, and are therefore consistent with, the estimates of the means of ratings of the dimensions.

### Table 3. Prediction of the Mean Ratings of Intraservice Work from the Mean Ratings of Its Dimensions.*

| SPECIALTY | PILOT SURVEY | NATIONAL SURVEY |
|---|---|---|
| Anesthesiology | 0.994 | 0.993 |
| General surgery | 0.999 | 0.996 |
| Internal medicine | 0.990 | 0.988 |
| Radiology | 0.996 | 0.991 |

*Values shown are the squares of the multiple correlation coefficients

Table 4. Prediction of Individual Ratings of Intra-service Work from Individual Ratings of Its Dimensions.*

| SPECIALTY | PILOT SURVEY | NATIONAL SURVEY |
|---|---|---|
| Anesthesiology | 0.845 | 0.872 |
| General surgery | 0.909 | 0.887 |
| Internal medicine | 0.860 | 0.836 |
| Radiology | 0.876 | 0.903 |

*Values shown are the squares of the multiple correlation coefficients.

This high degree of consistency constitutes statistical evidence that the ratings of work are probably valid.

A similar analysis was performed for each specialty at the level of the individual physician. Each physician's rating of the work entailed in performing a given service was predicted from that physician's ratings of its dimensions. Since it does not use group means, this analysis allows for differences among physicians in experience and judgment. The results are shown in Table 4. Ratings by individual physicians are, of course, more variable than group means, but the multiple correlation coefficients are very high, all exceeding 0.83. In other words, individual ratings of work are consistent with individual ratings of the dimensions of work. Once again, these results provide evidence that the ratings of work are reproducible and valid.

We validated a major dimension of work on the basis of external objective information, comparing the durations of surgical procedures obtained from the national survey, which are based on physicians' recall, with the times logged in 1986 in the operating rooms of eight hospitals in two regions of the United States. Table 5 shows a comparison of the durations, from the operating room logs and in our survey, of several procedures that were defined and coded identically. The survey times

are very similar to the operating room times, providing external validation for physicians' judgments of time.

## DISCUSSION

The relative values of work presented in this chapter are expressed in scales specific to different specialties, we developed a method of aligning the scales for different specialties onto a common scale. The method and results are reported in detail elsewhere.[16]

Our results show that the relative work input for physicians' services can be defined and estimated reliably. We developed a topography of work, consisting of four dimensions. The means of the ratings of work obtained from a group of about 100 specialists proved reproducible and highly reliable in every specialty. Moreover, the data display validity and a high degree of consistency.

There is no objective standard against which to compare our results in order to ascertain how well the measured work represents reality. Thus, we had to rely on the next best choice—to subject the results to review for reasonableness by practicing physicians. For this purpose, we organized technical consulting groups, consisting of 100 physicians in private practice and academic medicine from across the United States. The panelists reviewed the ratings of work and its dimensions obtained in the survey. In general, they found the ratings to be reasonable and to conform to the reality they had experienced in clinical practice.

Some secondary questions remain about the results of this study. First, it can be argued that nonrespondents to the survey may differ systematically from the respondents. If so, and if we could obtain ratings from the nonrespondents, their ratings of work might be significantly different. This possibility, however slight, cannot be completely ruled out. Our further analyses have shown

Table 5. Comparison of Estimates from the National Survey of the Time Required for Selected Services with Actual Hospital Operating Room Times.*

| SERVICE | NATIONAL SURVEY ESTIMATES | OPERATING ROOM TIME |
|---|---|---|
| | *mean minutes* | |
| Decompression of carpal tunnel in a 48-year-old woman, unilateral, ambulatory surgery unit | 30.5 | 25.2 |
| Carotid endarterectomy, unilateral, in a 58-year-old woman with a history of transient ischemic attacks | 99.4 | 91.0 |
| Transurethral resection of prostate, medium-sized gland for benign prostatic hypertrophy in a 70-year-old man | 64.6 | 56.4 |
| Abdominal hysterectomy for cancer in situ of cervix in a 50-year-old woman | 91.9 | 96.6 |
| Diagnostic dilation and curettage for menometrorrhagia in a 50-year-old woman | 13.9 | 8.8 |
| Primary total hip replacement for osteoarthritis | 135.1 | 145.6 |
| Modified radical mastectomy | 109.4 | 106.8 |
| Primary triple-vessel coronary-artery bypass graft, in a 65-year-old man, ejection fraction = 50 percent, with no complicating associated disease | 202.1 | 194.7 |

*Extremely high and low outliers were deleted. Outliers were defined as time values that differed by more than three standard deviations from the mean of the remaining values.

no significant differences between respondents and non-respondents in specialty-board-certification status or in geographic distribution. Other analyses failed to show differences between ratings by physicians who responded only after many calls and those by physicians who responded after fewer calls.[16]

Second, some of the specialists we surveyed may have offered ratings for services that they are not well trained to perform, or perform infrequently. The responses from these less-qualified specialists could have biased our data, though in what direction we cannot be sure. Nevertheless, the possibility that ratings may vary systematically with professional qualifications cannot be ruled out. Another study, however, offers evidence that ratings do not vary according to the frequency with which a physician performs a particular service.[18]

This study has demonstrated that physicians' work input into services within each specialty can be defined. We assumed work input to consist of time, mental effort and judgment, technical skill and physical effort, and stress. Relative work input can be measured by magnitude estimation, with results that are reproducible, reliable, and consistent, and therefore probably valid. Because ratings of work do not vary greatly among physicians, it is feasible to quantify systematically the relative resource-input costs of physicians' services in each specialty. This study indicates that resource-based relative values could serve as a rational foundation for compensating physicians according to the work and effort they exert in performing services.

We are indebted to Robert Rosenthal, Ph.D., and to Jack Langenbrunner, M.P.P., our project officer at the Health Care Financing Administration, for their helpful comments and suggestions; to the many physicians on our technical consulting panels who took time from their busy schedules to attend our meetings and provide their expertise; and to the many physicians whose participation in our surveys made this work possible.

## References

1. Roe BB: The UCR boondoggle; a death knell for private practice? *N Engl J Med* 1981; 305:41–5.
2. Physician Payment Review Commission. Medicare physician payment: an agenda for reform. Annual report to Congress. Washington, D.C.: Government Printing Office, 1982:27.
3. Jencks SF, Dobson A. Strategies for reforming Medicare's physician payments: physician diagnosis-related groups and other approaches. *N Engl J Med* 1985; 312:1492–9.
4. Fanta CM, Finkel AJ, Kirshner CG, Perlman JM. Physician's current procedural terminology. 4th ed. Chicago: American Medical Association, 1986.
5. Hsiao WC, Braun P, Dunn D, Becker ER, DeNicola M, Ketcham TR. Results and policy implications of the resource-based relative-value scale. *N Engl J Med* 1988; 319:881–8.
6. Hsiao WC, Stason W. Toward developing a relative value scale for medical and surgical societies. *Health Care Financ Rev* 1979; 1:23–8.
7. Hsiao WC, Braun P, Goldman P, et al. Resource-based relative values of selected medical and surgical procedures in Massachusetts: final report on research contract for Rate Setting Commission, Commonwealth of Massachusetts. Boston: Harvard School of Public Health, 1985.
8. Hsiao WC, Braun P, Becker ER, Thomas SR. The resource-based relative value scale: toward the development of an alternative physician payment system. *JAMA* 1987; 258:799–802.
9. Kruskal WB, Wish M. Multi-dimensional scaling. Beverly Hills, Calif.: Sage, 1978.
10. Stevens SS. Psychophysics. New York: John Wiley, 1975.
11. Sellin T, Wolfgang ME: The measurement of delinquency. New York: John Wiley, 1964.
12. Bohrnstedt GW. A quick method for determining the reliability and validity of multiple-item scales. *Am Sociol Rev* 1969; 34:542–8.
13. Cronbach LJ. Coefficient alpha and the internal structure of texts. *Psychometrika* 1951; 16:297–334.
14. American Medical Association Center for Health Policy Research. Socioeconomic characteristics of medical practice, 1987. Chicago: American Medical Association, 1987:137.
15. Dempster AP, Laird NM, Rubin DB. Maximum likelihood estimation via the EM algorithm. *J Am Stat Assoc* 1966; 61:595–604.
16. Hsiao WC, Braun P, Becker ER, et al. A national study of resource-based relative value scale for physician services: final report to the Health Care Financing Administration. Boston: Harvard School of Public Health, 1988. (Publication no. 18–C-98795/1–03.)
17. Winer BJ. Statistical principles in experimental design. 2nd ed. New York: McGraw-Hill, 1971:28–7.
18. Mitchell JB, Cromwell J, Rosenbach ML, et al. Using relative physician effort to identify mispriced procedures: final report to U.S. Department of Health and Human Services under HHS research contract 100–86–0023. Needham, Mass.: Health Economics Research, 1988.

# Chapter 20

## Managed Mental Health Care: Myths and Realities in the 1990s

Robert A. Dorwart, M.D., M.P.H.

*Managed care may be viewed as the most recent attempt to control the rate of increase of health and mental health care costs in the United States. The majority of people who receive insured mental health services do so through some form of managed care program. Now increasing concerns are being raised about whether managed care really reduces costs, whether it adversely affects the quality of care, and whether it restricts access to care. The author discusses the origins, actors, and major issues involved in managed health care in terms of prevailing myths and future realities. He calls for more and better research to answer important clinical and policy questions about managed care and for improved communication between mental health professionals and managed care organizations.*

It is a fact that over the past decade health care costs have rapidly increased due to inflation, increased demand for and volume of services and providers, new technology and treatments, and the growing corporatization of health care. Additional factors have contributed to the growth of mental health care costs, including increased availability of insurance coverage for psychiatric disorders; increased demand from the baby boom population for help with family problems, drug abuse, and serious psychiatric disorders; continued proliferation of psychiatric medications and effective therapies; and growth in the number of mental health professionals as well as psychiatric units in general hospitals. Moreover, during this time the number of psychiatric (specialty) hospitals, often owned by large multihospital, investor-owned corporations, has roughly tripled.[1]

It is a myth that utilization management alone will control the rising costs of health and mental health care. Numerous strategies have been used in efforts to reduce the rate of increase of costs, including insurance benefit limitations and exclusions, prepaid health plans, prospective payment systems, fee schedules, and utilization management or "managed care" approaches. However, current evidence suggests that despite managed care efforts, the costs of care will continue to rise rapidly and that, in response, managed care activities and arrangements will continue to increase dramatically. It has already been estimated that within a few years three out of four psychiatric patients will have their care overseen by some type of managed care program.[2]

The hypothesis that managed care will not halt the rise in health care costs presents two major dilemmas

Robert A. Dorwart, M.D., M.P.H., *Managed Mental Health Care: Myths and Realities in the 1990s,* Vol. 41 No. 10, pp. 1087–1091, 1990. Copyright 1991, the American Psychiatric Association. Reprinted by permission.

for psychiatric clinicians. First, the use of managed care to control costs may adversely affect the quality of mental health care as well as patients' access to it. Second, clinicians must nonetheless decide how to react to, or participate in, managed care efforts. This paper briefly reviews the background of managed mental health care and identifies some of the myths and realities associated with it.

## FORMS OF MANAGED CARE

The specter of managed care has hovered over mental health care for more than a decade. In its various guises—health maintenance organizations (HMOs), preferred provider organizations, and utilization review—managed care claims to offer solutions to the pressing concerns of insurers, employers, and policymakers about rising costs and overuse of services.[3] Managed care now has so many different forms that it is difficult to know exactly what is meant by the term. In looking carefully at managed care, however, we discover shifting practice patterns among providers of mental health services.

The trend of rising health care cost is multidetermined, and there is often synergy among the forces driving the increases. The upward trend, like inflation itself, seems inevitable. Perhaps it is not surprising, then, that according to the recent review by the Institute of Medicine (IOM), utilization management results in one-time savings after implementation but does not continue to control costs.[3] This review also suggested that the HMO, which controls both supply and demand, is no longer the most widespread form of managed care. The concept of managed care refers increasingly to the more common external review by third parties using utilization management companies; managed care is defined as "a set of techniques used by or on behalf of purchasers of health care benefits to manage health care costs by influencing patient care decision-making through case-by-case assessments of the appropriateness of care prior to its provision."[3]

Over the last decade there has been a monumental debate in health policy about whether the direction of health and mental health care services should be shaped by the invisible hand of the market, the guiding hand of professional planning and peer review, or the controlling hand of governmental regulation and utilization review.[3] In near desperation over rising costs, health care professionals and policymakers have tried using all three approaches, resulting at times in confusion, inconsistency, and overmanagement.

So-called first and second parties (patients and health care providers) often differ from third, fourth, and fifth parties (insurers or government, employers, and utilization management organizations) on what the outcome of the policy debate over managed care should be.

Gradually, the theme of the debate has shifted from clinical concerns about management of patient care to an emphasis on combining reduction of cost with effectiveness and efficiency. As mental health professionals, we must be concerned about the methods and goals of proposed cost-containment measures; we must shift the balance of concern from cost to quality of care.[4]

Only recently have individual and institutional providers begun to realize the stakes involved in the changes in the patterns of practice resulting from managed care approaches and to confront such questions as, Who benefits and who pays under managed care? What are the options and trade-offs? Beyond the arguably effective cost-control strategies of today loom issues such as, Who will control clinical decision making and standard setting? Will providers be financially stable? And who will be responsible for preserving the rights of patients? In other words, we have begun to question the why, how, and who of managed care. . . .

### The Why of Managed Care

The Commerce Department estimates that expenditures in 1990 for health care services in the United States will exceed $660 billion, or roughly 12 percent of the gross national product.[5] Furthermore, it predicts that despite efforts to slow the rate of growth, spending for health care and physicians' services will continue to increase at an annual rate of between 12 and 15 percent for the next five years.

Although estimates vary, it appears the overall funds allocated for mental health care (including drug and alcohol abuse services and all state mental health funding) represent between 12 and 14 percent of total health care expenditures. Spending has been at this level for many years; whether these amounts are viewed as too much, the right amount, or not enough clearly depends on one's perspective and values. By any measure, however, an increasing proportion of resources is being used to pay for health care in our society, and costs for psychiatric and substance abuse services are often said to be growing much more rapidly than are costs for other types of medical care.[6]

### The How of Managed Care

Health maintenance organizations and preferred (or exclusive) provider organizations were the economic crucible of mental health managed care approaches in the 1980s.[7,8] Originally, HMOs were intended to increase access and comprehensiveness of health care by reducing the fee-for-service disincentives to seeking medical care. When HMOs were seen as cost-effective, they were asked to care for more patients who were more costly to treat.

Today HMOs are seen as one means of balancing the demand for health care services with a fixed supply of primary medical care and specialty providers in a controlled organizational and fiscal environment.[9] However, according to Bennett,[10] "Over the past 15 years the health maintenance organization (HMO) movement has abandoned its social objectives in favor of economic ones."

Actually, the picture is not so clear cut. Because HMOs have evolved into many different models, they represent not only a shift in thinking about practice but an evolutionary organization form as well. The emphasis in HMOs is on limiting the supply of services and, at times, managing providers and their behavior. As Bennett notes, both HMO and utilization review strategies use financing mechanisms as a critical tool to limit use to that below ostensibly allowed covered benefits. HMOs rely on prospective or prepayment financing and selective contracting at discounts with hospitals, whereas utilization review relies on precertification of admissions, concurrent review of treatment, and discharge planning.[3] Given that nearly 40 million Americans are enrolled in some kind of HMO and probably twice that many subscribe to other forms of health insurance involving utilization management, the question of whether to support or oppose managed care may be less salient than the issue of how best to shape and participate in the processes of managed care.

Economists and providers alike believe there are special threats to mental health from managed care, including the longstanding problem of apparent discriminatory insurance coverage for alcohol, drug abuse, and mental disorders. Demand for mental health and substance abuse services may be more sensitive to a variety of constraints than are other medical services, suggesting the need to pay particular attention to how mental health care is monitored and controlled.[11-14] If demand varies according to subgroups of patients or among insured populations, restricting services could result in trade-offs that reduce needed care as well as unnecessary care. In the context of HMOs, such restrictions pose special difficulties for patients who have major chronic disorders, such as schizophrenia or Alzheimer's disease.[9,12]

Because policymakers have turned their attention from altering demand to altering the supply of services, denial or rationing of care does occur. Services are either excluded entirely, as happens when a hospital closes its emergency room, or they are severely limited, as happens when an HMO provides little or no psychiatric hospital or specialty care.[15] This latter tactic has been adopted by HMOs in several states that do not have mandated minimum inpatient mental health benefits.

Another approach to restricting the supply of care—utilization review—is designed to assess the medical necessity for care, the appropriateness of specific services, or even the particular treatment modalities employed. For indemnity insurers, this function may be performed by a separate utilization review firm. For self-insured groups, the employer's personnel department may carry out this review. HMOs may do their own internal utilization review or use an outside contractor.

## The Who of Managed Care

In an early era, before public and private insurance coverage was available for psychiatric disorders, two parties were involved in managing patient care—the physician and the patient. The psychiatrist managed the patient's care according to his or her best professional judgment, and physician autonomy was the hallmark of the medical profession. The situation we face today is dramatically different.

Patients and providers are now accustomed to many more key actors in the drama of patient care, including hospital administrators, non-physician mental health professionals, and ancillary support and technical staff. Provider autonomy is highly constricted. The unfolding scenario of the 1990s includes the direct involvement of new actors, such as government regulators, insurance medical departments, and employee assistance and utilization review staff, not to mention legislators and judges who may try to appropriate minimal coverage policies. Ginzberg[16] describes this situation as today's medical triangle, involving physicians, the government, and the public.

This rapid multiplication of managers in response to concern over cost and appropriateness of care is creating much of the concern about managed care. Among the familiar and worrisome issues are the monitoring of care by anonymous reviewers, interprofessional or non-physician "peer review," and inconsistent or nonexistent review criteria. As the IOM report states, "Utilization management brings patient-based and system-based concerns together and represents a new nexus of relations among payers, practitioners, hospitals, and patients."[3] Given these trends, what can we expect in the 1990s?

## POLICY ISSUES OF THE 1990S

It is not easy to predict with much specificity the future of managed mental health care, but issues of costs, access to care, and appropriateness of care are likely to increase in importance. The challenge will be to continue to find acceptable and responsible approaches to balance, as Goldman[17] recently put it, "the tension between access [to services] and excess [utilization]."

This systems-level focus has a counterpart concern at the patient cost-cutting and quality assurance. From a policy perspective, these issues of equity versus efficiency and cost versus quality of care are ones that will engage clinicians, policymakers, and researchers in the 1990s. At present, however, there appear to be many myths about managed care.

## Myths About Managed Care

One myth is that utilization management is a new phenomenon or a transitional state. It is not. Rather, it represents part of a much larger set of strategies designed to stem the rising cost of health care. As such, the drama of managed care often involves not new and unknown actors but the same actors in different makeup and in new, more active (some would say intrusive) roles. The reality is that utilization management is growing and will soon involve outpatient as well as inpatient practice.

A second myth is that utilization management alone will reduce costs in the long run. It will not. In fact, nobody knows what will work. Beyond one-time savings when new approaches, such as utilization review, are instituted, there is no evidence that costs are under control. Perhaps more cost-effective treatments would help. Excellent treatment-specific clinical research has been done,[18] but much more research is needed before we have credible and useful data about treatment effectiveness and cost-effectiveness in mental health for a full range of services.

A third myth is that managed care will of itself resolve our policy dilemma concerning who is treated or how care is allocated. It will not. These broader issues of priorities and equity require much more attention, and managed care is only one short-term response to the current cost crisis. Systemic approaches that link financial incentives and quality of care remain an elusive goal. Other policy tools, such as prospective payment with capitation, spending caps, and fee schedules, are more likely to contain costs but are also likely to raise equally distressing professional, ethical, and procedural concerns. In an era of cost containment and accountability, we must acknowledge that our policy devices involve explicit trade-offs, such as those faced earlier by the early form of staff model HMOs, which found they had to limit the quantity of care to stay within budgets.[19,20]

A fourth myth is that managed care is entirely about costs. It is not. Providers should not think that if we could magically reduce costs for mental health care, all would be well and there would be no pressure for utilization review. Actually, many employers would willingly spend the same or even more money if they were confident their employees were receiving competent, effective, high-quality care.

A fifth myth is that managed care does not affect quality of care. It does. Sometimes it affects quality for the better, but often it is for the worse. Admittedly, this is a generalization that needs further investigation, but the trade-off of lesser quantity or lower quality in exchange for lower costs is implicit in many managed care plans.[21]

A sixth myth is that managed care alone is the cause of current problems of mental health care. It is not. No single factor is responsible for raising costs or lowering the quality of care. Managed care does challenge our assumptions about who should determine what care is provided, how much autonomy we should have, and what are the rules of engagement in case of disagreements among the many parties.[22]

## Changing Roles and Realities

Like it or not, clinicians must advocate for patients as well as for themselves. Most managed care activities occur out of sight of patients and families, but they often have a major impact on the amount and cost of treatment that families receive.

Clinicians must participate in the development of treatment guidelines. Most managed care companies have developed, or are developing, specific criteria for judging the appropriateness of treatment according to diagnosis, facility type, and cost, and even to preferred modalities of treatment. These criteria are being developed outside the view of most mental health professionals, resulting in widely disparate rather than uniform professional standards of care. Each state agency, insurance company, utilization management firm, and HMO is seemingly eager to develop its own standards. The clinicians' role in all this, especially through their professional associations, is to develop clinically oriented treatment guidelines or "parameters of care." Models for such collaborative processes, such as that used by the American Psychiatric Association to develop its forthcoming diagnostic and statistical manual (DSM-IV), are not being widely used to improve quality of care.

Another role for clinicians may be as providers of service or consultants to managed care organizations. Such involvement sometimes requires careful attention to issues of potential conflict of interest; practitioners must avoid pressures to deny needed treatment. Researchers have a special obligation to see that members of the profession participate in services research, such as studies of access to care and quality and costs of care, and that they do not leave this important work entirely to nonclinicians.

The major issue facing government is to what extent should managed care, both in HMOs and utilization management companies, be monitored, certified, or otherwise regulated.[23] There is currently very little regulation, and little is known about the activities of the more than 50 companies involved in providing psychiatric utilization review services across the country. At a minimum, policymakers could create advisory committees, regulatory agencies, or research centers that permit ample and open professional input to their deliberations about managed care. Other proposals to regulate utilization review activities, such as licensure and certification of staff and disclosure of criteria, are also being considered by individual states.

## WHAT LIES AHEAD?

The growing body of information about HMOs and managed care suggests the need for concern. A national survey of psychiatric hospitals, for example, indicated that in 1988 psychiatric units in general hospitals and private psychiatric hospitals received an average of less than 5 percent of their revenues from HMOs and preferred provider organizations, but that private hospitals received nearly 60 percent of their revenue from private insurance.[24] This difference suggests that managed care for private insurance should be of much greater concern than the already tightly managed utilization of most HMOs. In the survey, administrators were asked what strategies they used to contend with increasing competition for patients: out of more than 900 respondent hospitals, none reported placing great emphasis on lowering their prices, but more than 40 percent said they strongly encouraged the use of shorter lengths of treatment.

It is important to recognize that shortening lengths of stay does not necessarily reduce the cost of care. More intensive diagnostic and treatment services may, for example, be provided in slightly fewer days and result in care that is just as good and costs just as much; however, an increase in cost for the utilization management service itself may offset savings from an increase in efficiency.

In a national survey of psychiatrists conducted by the American Psychiatric Association, 60 percent of the respondents reported pressure from outside influences, such as utilization review firms, to shorten the length of stay or even to discourage the treatment of some patients. The extent and impact of this pressure has not been widely studied. Research needs to continue to document the effects of managed care. To the extent that well-designed research suggests that some forms of managed care do not result in differences in outcome, we can expect continued pressure for more managed care.[25]

## CONCLUSIONS

Many excellent reviews of general social and economic trends in health care affecting mental health today have described emerging conflicts in more detail.[26–28] In her historical analysis of hospital care in the United States in the 20th century, Stevens[29] concluded that the root causes of rising health care costs are an ingrained part of the character of American health policy. Consequently, conflicts (sometimes latent) revolving around costs of care versus access to care lead to episodic reactions to stem the rise in the costs of health care. This dynamic tension over costs may explain the stringent and harsh—some say harassing—reactions of some utilization management efforts. It also may make a well-designed HMO seem a more rational approach by comparison. However, the main lesson from this perspective is clear: both increasing costs of care and efforts to manage services will continue to characterize health policy in the 1990s.[30]

It is a myth prevalent among health care providers that we can ignore the problem of rising costs as a necessary, if not desirable, burden, but the reality of political economics is that we do so at the peril of relinquishing our social role in preserving access to, and quality of, mental health care.

Acknowledgments—This work was supported in part by National Institute of Mental Health grant K20-MH-00848-01. The author thanks Sherrie Epstein for research assistance.

## References

1. Redick RW, Stroup A, Witkin M, et al: Private Psychiatric Hospitals, United States: 1983–84 and 1986 Statistical Note 191. Rockville, Md. National Institute of Mental Health, Oct 1989
2. Preliminary Report of the Resource Symposium on Psychiatry and Managed Care. Washington, DC, American Psychiatric Association, Sept 1989
3. Institute of Medicine Committee on Utilization Management by Third Parties: Controlling Costs and Changing Patient Care? The Role of Utilization Management. Edited by Gray BH, Field MJ. Washington, DC, National Academy Press, 1989
4. Langman N, Wahl R, Singer C, et al: Mental health managed care: from cost containment to quality assurance. Administration and Policy in Mental Health, in press
5. Health and medical services, in US Industrial Outlook. Washington, DC, US Department of Commerce, 1990
6. Issues in Mental Health Care. Issue Brief no 98. Washington, DC, Employee Benefit Research Institute, 1990
7. Dorwart RA, Epstein S: Economics and mental health care: the HMO as a crucible for cost-effective care, in Mental Health and Managed Care. Edited by Fitzpatrick R, Feldman J. Washington, DC, American Psychiatric Press, in press
8. Sederer LI, St Clair LURE: Managed health care and the Massachusetts experience. *American Journal of Psychiatry* 146:1142–1148, 1989

9. Schlesinger M: On the limits of expanding health care reform: chronic care in prepaid settings. *Milbank Quarterly* 64:189–215, 1986

10. Bennett MJ: The greening of the HMO: implications for prepaid psychiatry. *American Journal of Psychiatry* 145:1544–1549, 1988

11. McGuire TG: Financing and reimbursement for mental health services, in The Future of Mental Health Services Research. Edited by Taube CA, Mechanic D, Hohmann A. DHHS Pub no (ADM) 86–1600. Rockville, Md, National Institute of Mental Health, 1989

12. Schlesinger M: Striking a balance: capitation, the mentally ill, and public policy, in Integrating Mental Health Services Through Capitation. Edited by Mechanic D, Aiken L. San Francisco, Jossey-Bass, 1989

13. Keeler EB, Wells KB, Manning WG, et al: The Demand for Episodes of Mental Health Services. Santa Monica, Calif, Rand Corp, 1986

14. Manning WG, Wells KB, Benjamin B: Use of Outpatient Mental Health Care: Trial of a Prepaid Group Practice Versus Fee-for-Service. Santa Monica, Calif, Rand Corp, 1986

15. Levinson DF: Toward full disclosure of referral restrictions and financial incentives by prepaid health plans. *New England Journal of Medicine* 317:1729–1731, 1987

16. Ginzberg E: The Medical Triangle: Physicians, Politicians, and the Public. Cambridge, Mass, Harvard University Press, 1990

17. News Analysis. *Mental Health Report* 13:201, 1990

18. Agency for Health Care Policy and Research: Research Activities. No 125, Rockville, Md, Public Health Service, Jan 1990

19. Shadle M, Christianson JB: The impact of HMO development on mental health and chemical dependency services. *Hospital and Community Psychiatry* 40:1145–1151, 1989

20. Lehman AF: Capitation payment and mental health care: a review of the opportunities and risks. *Hospital and Community Psychiatry* 38:31–38, 1987

21. Sharfstein SS, Dunn L, Kent J: The clinical consequences of payment limitations: the experience of a private psychiatric hospital. *Psychiatric Hospital* 19:63–66, 1988

22. Veatch RM: The HMO physician's duty to cut costs. *Hastings Center Report* 15(4):13–15, 1985

23. Field MJ, Gray BH: Should we regulate "utilization management?" *Health Affairs* 8(4):103–112, 1989

24. Dorwart RA, Schlesinger M, Davidson H, et al: Changing Psychiatric Hospital Care: A National Study. Cambridge, Mass, Malcolm Wiener Center for Social Policy, John F Kennedy School of Government, Harvard University, 1990

25. Wells KB, Manning WG, Valdez RB: The Effects of a Prepaid Group Practice on Mental Health Outcomes in a General Population: Results of a Randomized Trial. Santa Monica, Calif, Rand Corp, 1989

26. Sharfstein S, Beigel A: The New Economics of Managed Care. Washington, DC, American Psychiatric Press, 1985

27. Starr P: The Social Transformation of American Medicine. New York, Basic Books, 1982

28. Dorwart RA, Schlesinger M: Privatization of psychiatric services. *American Journal of Psychiatry* 145:543–553, 1988

29. Stevens R: In Sickness and in Wealth: American Hospitals in the 20th Century. New York, Basic Books, 1989

30. Tischler GL: Utilization management of mental health services by private third parties. *American Journal of Psychiatry* 147:967–973, 1990

# PART SIX

## Assessing and Regulating System Performance

This section is designed to examine critically the ways in which the health care system itself is evaluated and assessed. The first article is a look at the efficiency of our current approach to administering services. This relatively critical article by Steffie Woolhandler and David U. Himmelstein raises very interesting and challenging questions about the structure of the system itself and its administration.

This article is followed by an equally challenging examination of the way the system, particularly third-party payers, utilizes inconvenience as a means to ration services. The author, Gerald W. Grumet, raises fundamental questions about the underlying nature of the system and its efficiency and approaches.

The next three articles in this section address the evaluation of the quality of care provided in health care systems. The first two articles, by Avedis Donabedian, provide a comprehensive overview of the measurement and evaluation of the quality of care and associated issues, such as reliability, validity, and efficiency. The first of these articles examines twenty years of research on the quality of medical care, and the second discusses the epidemiology of quality, particularly looking at variations in quality among different groups within the population and at systems characteristics associated with differences in quality of care.

The third quality-of-care-related article, by Arnold M. Epstein, critically discusses the topic of outcome evaluation, a current emphasis in national policy making and health services research.

The final article in this section, by Curtis P. McLaughlin and Arnold D. Kaluzny, is an excellent discussion of total quality management and its application to the health care system. Total quality management has been of great interest in the United States, particularly in the industrial sector, and is currently gaining adherents in the health care industry as well. This article is especially timely and relevant to examining the role of total quality management in health care.

# Chapter 21

# The Deteriorating Administrative Efficiency of the U.S. Health Care System

Steffie Woolhandler, M.D., M.P.H., and
David U. Himmelstein, M.D.

**Abstract:** *Background and Methods.* In 1983 the proportion of health care expenditures consumed by administration in the United States was 60 percent higher than in Canada and 97 percent higher than in Britain. To assess the effects of recent health policy initiatives on the administrative efficiency of health care, we examined four components of administrative costs in the United States and Canada for 1987: insurance overhead, hospital administration, nursing home administration, and physicians' billing and overhead expenses. Most data were provided by the two nations; federal health and statistics agencies, supplemented by state and provincial data and published sources. Because data on physicians' billing costs were limited, we estimated a range for these costs by two methods that rely on different sources of data. All figures are reported in 1987 U.S. dollars.

*Results.* In 1987 health care administration cost between $96.8 billion and $120.4 billion in the United States, amounting to 19.3 to 24.1 percent of total spending on health care, or $400 to $497 per capita. In Canada, between 8.4 and 11.1 percent of health care spending ($117 to $156 per capita) was devoted to administration. Administrative costs in the United States increased 37 percent in real dollars between 1983 and 1987, whereas in Canada they declined. The proportion of health care spending consumed by administration is now at least 117 percent higher in the United States than in Canada and accounts for about half the total difference in health care spending between the two nations. If health care administration in the United States had been as efficient as in Canada, $69.0 billion to $83.2 billion would have been saved in 1987.

*Conclusions.* The administrative structure of the U.S. health care system is increasingly inefficient as compared with that of Canada's national health program. Recent health policies with the avowed goal of improving the efficiency of care have imposed substantial new bureaucratic costs and burdens. *(N Engl J Med* 1991; 324:1253–8.)

Medicine is increasingly a spectator sport. Doctors, patients, and nurses perform before an enlarging audience of utilization reviewers, efficiency experts, and cost managers (Fig.1). A cynic viewing the uninflected curve of rising health care spending might wonder whether the cost-containment experts cost more than they contain; one is reminded of the Chinese proverb "There is no use going to bed early to save candles if the result is twins."

In 1983 the proportion of health care spending consumed by administrative costs in the United States was 60 percent higher than in Canada and 97 percent higher than in Britain.[2] Recent U.S. health policies have increased bureaucratic burdens and curtailed access to care. Yet they have failed to contain overall costs. This study updates and expands estimates of the costs of

Reprinted with permission from Steffie Woolhandler, M.D., M.P.H., and David U. Himmelstein, M.D., The Deteriorating Administrative Efficiency of the U.S. Health Care System, *The New England Journal of Medicine,* Vol. 324 No. 18, pp. 1253–1258, 1991.

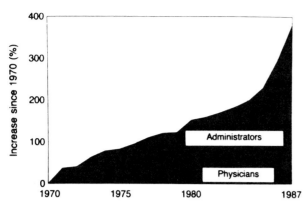

**Figure 1.** Growth in the Numbers of Physicians and Health Care Administrators from 1970 to 1987.
The data are from *Statistical Abstract of the United States* for these years (Table 64–2, 109th edition).[1] Because of a modification in the Bureau of the Census' definition of "health administrators," the change between 1982 and 1983 is interpolated rather than actual.

health administration in North America through 1987.[2] The results demonstrate that the bureaucratic profligacy of the U.S. health care system has increased sharply, while in Canada the proportion of spending on health care consumed by administration has declined.

## METHODS

We examined four components of administrative costs in the United States and Canada: insurance overhead, hospital administration, nursing home administration, and physicians' overhead and billing expenses. All estimates are for fiscal year 1987, the most recent year for which complete data were available. Costs are reported in 1987 U.S. dollars, based on the 1987 exchange rate of $1.33 (Canadian) = $1 (U.S.); calculations of per capita spending were based on populations of 243,934,000 in the United States and 25,652,000 in Canada.

Figures on insurance overhead in the United States were obtained from the Health Care Financing Administration.[3] Although nationwide data on the costs of hospital and nursing home administration were not available, the California Health Facilities Commission regularly compiles detailed cost data, based on Medicare cost reports, on that state's hospitals and nursing homes. Four years ago we confirmed that administrative costs in California's health facilities were similar to those in at least two other states.[2] Since then, trends in hospital and nursing home financing and organization in California have paralleled developments in the nation as a whole.[4,5] We computed total hospital administrative costs by summing costs in the following categories: general accounting, patient accounting, credit and collection, admitting, other fiscal services, hospital administration, public re-

lations, personnel department, auxiliary groups, data processing, communications, purchasing, medical library, medical records, medical-staff administration, nursing administration, in-service education, and other administrative services. We excluded costs attributed to research administration, administration of educational programs, printing and duplicating, depreciation, amortization, leases and rentals, insurance, licenses, taxes, central services and supply, other ancillary services, and unassigned costs. We assumed that administration represented the same proportion of total hospital costs in California as nationwide. We derived estimates of nationwide administrative costs for nursing homes from the California data in a similar manner.

Although Canada's 10 provincial health programs differ in some details, they share common structural features that tend to streamline bureaucracy. Each program provides comprehensive coverage for virtually all provincial residents under a single publicly administered plan. Private insurance may cover additional services, but duplication of the public coverage is proscribed; hospitals are paid a lump-sum (global) amount to cover operating expenses, and physicians bill the program directly for all fees.

The Health Statistics Branch of Health and Welfare Canada and Statistics Canada's Canadian Center for Health Information provided unpublished data on nationwide spending for insurance, hospitals, and nursing homes. These data were derived from the provincial governments' reports of their expenditures for insurance administration and from detailed cost reports submitted by hospitals and nursing homes. We computed total hospital administrative costs by summing costs in the following categories: hospital administration ("other"), advertising, association-membership fees, business machines, collection fees, postage, auditing and accounting fees, other professional fees (such as legal fees but excluding medical fees), service-bureau fees, telephone and telegraph, indemnity to board members, travel and convention expenses, medical records and hospital library, and nursing administration. We excluded administrative and support services for educational and research programs, insurance, interest, printing, stationery and office supplies, material management, and central supply. Statistics Canada tabulates administrative costs for nursing homes as a single category. These data are less reliable than the hospital figures, since cost reporting by nursing homes is voluntary, and the number of facilities reporting varies substantially from year to year.

We confirmed the accuracy of the Canadian federal data, using more detailed but incomplete data from British Columbia, the Maritimes, Ontario, Quebec, and Saskatchewan[6–10] (and personal communications: Cunningham D, British Columbia Ministry of Health; Lim P,

Continuing Care Employee Relations Association of British Columbia; and Davis J, Ontario Ministry of Health). Because these data generally matched the national figures, we have not reported them separately.

Only indirect or incomplete information is available on the billing costs of Canadian and U.S. physicians. We therefore used two different methods to estimate these costs, one based on physicians' reports of their professional expenses and the other on the numbers of employees in physicians' offices. The expense-based method (Method 1) probably overestimates the actual difference in billing costs between the two nations, whereas the personnel-based approach (Method 2) may underestimate the difference.

Our first approach, Method 1, rests on the assumption that the entire difference in physicians' billing and overhead expenses (excluding malpractice premiums[11,12]) between the United States and Canada is attributable to the excess administrative costs borne by American doctors. The American Medical Association (AMA) estimates U.S. physicians' incomes and practice expenses on the basis of the results of a survey of a representative sample of nonfederal, practicing physicians (excluding interns and residents).[12] Revenue Canada tabulates physicians' professional expenses on the basis of tax returns (Rehmer L, Health Information Division, Health and Welfare Canada: personal communication). Because these figures are "distorted, primarily because of the way group practice physicians tend to report expenses" (Rehmer L, Health Information Division, Health and Welfare Canada: personal communication), we used Revenue Canada's corrected tabulation, which included only the 91 percent of physicians who reported professional expenses amounting to between 5 percent and 300 percent of their net incomes. We added to both the U.S. and Canadian figures an estimate of the value of the physicians' time devoted to billing[13] (and Peachey D: personal communication); we assumed that this time was valued at the same rate as other professional activity.

Using Method 2, we also estimated physicians' billing costs on the basis of data on the number of clerical and managerial personnel employed in their offices, as well as the costs of outside billing services. For the United States, we obtained information on physicians' office personnel from data tapes from the Census Bureau's March 1988 Current Population Survey (CPS).[14] Since comparable survey data were unavailable for Canada, we used information from a detailed study of office staffing patterns in the province of Quebec in 1977.[15] These earlier figures were slightly higher than informal current estimates provided by the Ontario Medical Association (Peachey D: personal communication). For both the United States and Canada, we assumed that the total annual cost per employee averaged $35,000

(including wages, benefits, taxes, work space, equipment, telephone, supplies, and other costs attributable to the employee) and that the ratio of clerical workers to physicians (excluding residents) was identical in offices and other settings. We added to both the U.S. and Canadian figures estimates of the value of physicians' personal time spent on billing, calculated as described above. For the United States we added the cost of outside billing services as determined by a recent survey by the AMA.[13]

Finally, to evaluate trends over time, we recalculated the 1987 figures to maintain strict comparability with the less detailed and less complete data for 1983.[2] As in our earlier paper,[2] we estimated physicians' billing and overhead costs by the expense-based method (Method 1). However, we excluded the cost of physicians' time spent on billing because comparable data were unavailable for 1983. In keeping with our earlier method, we included malpractice costs in physicians' overhead expenses but corrected for increases over time in these costs.[11,12,16] For each country we took average total professional expenses in 1987, subtracted the average 1987 malpractice premium, then added the average 1983 malpractice premium (all expressed as a percentage of gross income). The 1983 figures were converted to 1987 dollars with use of the gross-domestic-product price index for each country.[17]

## RESULTS

Insurance Overhead

In 1986 private insurance firms in the United States retained $18.7 billion for administration and profits out of total premium revenues of $157.8 billion.[3] Their average overhead costs (11.9 percent of premiums) were considerably higher than the 3.2 percent administrative costs of government health programs such as Medicare and Medicaid ($6.6 billion out of total expenditures of $207.3 billion).[3] Together, administration of private and public insurance programs consumed 5.1 percent of the $500.3 billion spent for health care, or $106 per capita.

The overhead costs for Canada's provincial insurance plans amounted to $235 million (0.9 percent) of the $26.57 billion spent by the plans[17] (and Health Information Division, Health and Welfare Canada; personal communication). The administrative costs of Canadian private insurers averaged 10.9 percent of premiums ($200 million of the $1.83 billion spent for such coverage) (Health Information Division, Health and Welfare Canada: personal communication). Total administrative costs for Canadian health insurance consumed 1.2 percent of health care spending, or $17 per capita.

## Hospital Administration

Hospital administration represented 20.2 percent of hospital costs in California in 1987–1988.[18] Extrapolating this figure to the total U.S. hospital expenditures of $194.7 billion in 1987[2] yielded an estimate of $39.3 billion, or $162 per capita, consumed by hospital administration. In Canada, hospital administration cost $1.27 billion, amounting to 9.0 percent of total hospital expenditures of $14.14 billion (Health Information Division, Health and Welfare Canada: personal communication), or $50 per capita.

## Nursing Home Administration

The administrative costs in California's nursing homes accounted for 15.8 percent of total revenues in 1987–1988.[19] On the basis of this figure, we estimate that administration cost $6.4 billion of the $40.6 billion spent nationally for nursing home care,[3] or $26 per capita. Canadian nursing homes spent $231 million on administration in 1987–1988, amounting to 13.7 percent of the total expenditures of $1.69 billion (Statistics Canada, Canadian Center for Health Information: personal communication), or $9 per capita.

## Physicians' Billing Expense

*Method 1.* When calculated according to Method 1, U.S. physicians' overhead and billing expenses, excluding malpractice premiums, made up 43.7 percent of their gross professional income[12]—$44.9 billion of the $102.7 billion spent for physicians' services.[3] In addition, physicians spent an average of six minutes on each Medicare and Blue Shield claim.[13] Assuming that the time required to bill other insurers was similar, the average physician spent about 134.4 hours per year (4.4 percent of his or her total professional activity) on billing; this time had a total value of $4.5 billion. Thus, the total value of U.S. physicians' billing and overhead was $49.4 billion, or $203 per capita.

Canadian physicians' professional expenses, excluding malpractice premiums, amounted to $1.99 billion, or 34.4 percent of their gross income (Rehmer L: personal communication). According to the director of professional affairs of the Ontario Medical Association, "The commitment of time to billing . . . is trivial and can be measured in seconds [per claim]" (Peachey D: personal communication). Assuming that the average physician spends 1 percent of his or her professional time on billing, with a total value of $58 million annually, the total cost of physicians' billing and overhead was $2.04 billion, or $80 per capita.

*Method 2.* The average office-based physician in the United States employed 1.47 clerical and managerial workers (Himmelstein DU, Woolhandler S: unpublished data), at an annual cost of $51,564 per physician, for a total of $20.0 billion. As calculated above (Method 1), the time physicians spent on billing was valued at $4.5 billion. In addition, 13.9 percent of physicians contracted with outside billing firms, at an average annual cost of $23,196 each,[13] for a total of $1.3 billion. Physicians' total billing and clerical expenses amounted to $25.8 billion, or $106 per capita.

The average office-based general practitioner in Quebec employed 0.733 receptionists and secretaries[15] at an annual cost of $25,655 per physician, for a total of $1.0 billion for Canadian physicians. In addition, the time physicians spent on billing was valued at $58 million. Physicians' total billing and clerical expenses were thus $1.06 billion, or $41 per capita.

## Total Costs of Administration

Table 1 summarizes the per capita costs of health care administration in the United States and Canada, including physicians' billing and overhead costs as calculated by the two different methods. Overall expenditures for health care administration in the United States totaled $96.8 billion to $120.4 billion ($400 to $497 per capita), accounting for 19.3 to 24.1 percent of the $500.3 billion spent for health care. Canadians spent $3.00 billion to $3.98 billion for health care administration ($117 to $156 per capita), amounting to 8.4 to 11.1 percent of the $35.9 billion spent for health care. The difference of $283 to $341 in the per capita cost of health care administration and billing accounted for 43.5 and 52.5 percent of the total difference in health spending between the two nations. If U.S. health care administration had been as efficient as Canada's, $69.0 to $83.2 billion (13.8 to 16.6 percent of total spending on health care) would have been saved in 1987.

**Table 1. Cost of Health Care Administration in the United States and Canada, 1987.**

| COST CATEGORY | SPENDING PER CAPITA* | |
|---|---|---|
| | U.S. | CANADA |
| Insurance administration | 106 | 17 |
| Hospital administration | 162 | 50 |
| Nursing home administration | 26 | 9 |
| Physicians' overhead and billing expenses | | |
|   Expense-based estimate | 203 | 80 |
|   Personnel-based estimate | 106 | 41 |
| Total costs of health care administration† | | |
|   High estimate | 497 | 156 |
|   Low estimate | 400 | 117 |

*All costs are expressed in U.S. dollars.

†The high estimate incorporates physicians' administrative costs derived by the expense-based method, and the low estimate costs derived by the personnel-based method.

The difference between the United States and Canada in billing and administrative costs has markedly increased since 1983.[2] Insurance overhead in the United States has risen from 4.4 percent to 5.1 percent of total health care spending, whereas insurance overhead in Canada has declined from 2.5 percent to 1.2 percent.[2] Hospital administrative costs have risen from 18.3 percent to 20.2 percent of total hospital spending in the United States, whereas in Canada these costs have climbed slightly from 8.0 percent to 9.0 percent.[2] Administrative expenses in U.S. nursing homes rose from 14.4 percent to 15.8 percent of costs, whereas administration's share of total costs rose from 10.5 to 13.7 percent in Canada.[2] Physicians' professional expenses (excluding malpractice premiums) have increased from 41.4 percent to 43.8 percent of gross income in the United States, whereas the Canadian figure declined from 35.5 percent to 34.4 percent.[2]

When we recalculated the 1987 figures to maintain comparability with the less complete 1983 data, we found that U.S. administrative costs rose from 21.9 percent to 23.9 percent of health care spending between 1983 and 1987, whereas in Canada administrative costs declined from 13.7 percent to 11.0 percent.[2] After adjustment for inflation, the divergence was even more striking. The costs of the health care bureaucracy in the United States rose by $32.2 billion (37 percent) between 1983 and 1987, an increase of $118 per capita. Administrative costs in the Canadian health care system fell by $161 million during this period, a decrease of $6 per capita.

## DISCUSSION

Most of our analysis is based on well-substantiated data, although in some areas reliable figures are sparse. The comparability of the data on hospital administrative costs in Canada and the United States is uncertain. However, we relied on detailed budgetary categories that appeared closely matched in the two nations. Although data on the administrative costs of health maintenance organizations are limited, they do not appear to differ substantially from those in the U.S. fee-for-service sector.[20–22]

Both of our methods for estimating physicians' billing costs are imprecise. The expense-based method (Method 1) may overstate the difference between the United States and Canada, since it assumes that the entire discrepancy in the proportion of income devoted to professional expenses was accounted for by malpractice premiums, billing, and administration. The personnel-based method (Method 2) may understate the difference because it assumes that aides and other clinical personnel employed in physicians' offices performed no activ-

ities related to billing, that the total annual cost per clerical worker was no less in Canada than in the United States, and that Canadian billing operations have not been streamlined since 1977 despite computerization. An official of the Ontario Medical Association estimates that electronic claims submission and reconciliation takes about one sixth as much staff time as paper-based billing (Peachey D: personal communication).

In the United States, clerical and managerial staff accounted for 59.5 percent of the nonphysician employees in doctors' offices in 1988, and 74,700 more were added over the ensuing two years (Himmelstein DU, Woolhandler S: unpublished data). In contrast, technicians and technologists accounted for only 7.3 percent of nonphysician office workers in 1988 and for only 5.7 percent in 1990 (Himmelstein DU, Woolhandler S: unpublished data). In 1988, the staff in a typical U.S. physician's office spent about one hour on each Blue Shield or Medicare claim,[13] at least 20 times more than in Ontario (Peachey D: personal communication; Weinkauf D: personal communication). In a typical practice in Canada, "One person does all the billing, bookkeeping and typing . . . for 8 physicians."[23]

Our estimates omit the administrative costs of union and employer health-benefit programs and the administrative work done by hospital nurses and other nonphysician clinical personnel—all probably greater in the United States than in Canada. Moreover, patients in the United States spend far more time (and anguish) on insurance paperwork than do Canadians; these costs are not reflected in our figures. On the other hand, some argue that funding health services through taxes, as in Canada, erodes productivity throughout the economy by discouraging work and investment—the so-called dead-weight loss.[24] Within the range of tax rates in North America, however, the magnitude, and even existence of this dead-weight loss is controversial.[25]

The United States spent 37 percent more in real dollars on health administration in 1987 than in 1983.[2] The recent quest for efficiency has apparently amplified inefficiency. Cost-containment programs predicated on stringent scrutiny of the clinical encounter have required an army of bureaucrats to eliminate modest amounts of unnecessary care. Each piece of medical terrain is meticulously inspected except that beneath the inspectors' feet. Paradoxically, the cost-management industry is among the fastest-growing segments of the health care economy and is expected to generate $7 billion in revenues by 1993.[26] The focus on micromanagement has obscured the fundamentally inefficient structure required to implement such policies. In contrast, Canada has evolved simple mechanisms to enforce an overall budget, but it allows doctors and patients wide latitude in deciding how the funds are spent. Reducing our administrative costs to Canadian levels would save enough money to fund coverage for all uninsured and underinsured Americans.[27] Universal comprehensive coverage under a single, publicly administered insurance program is the sine qua non of such administrative simplification.

The fragmented and complex payment structure of the U.S. health care system is inherently less efficient than the Canadian single-payer system. The existence of numerous insurers necessitates determinations of eligibility that would be superfluous if everyone were covered under a single, comprehensive program. Rather than a single claims-processing apparatus in each region, there are hundreds. Fragmentation also reduces the size of the insured group, limiting savings from economies of scale. Insurance overhead for U.S. employee groups with fewer than 5 members is 40 percent of premiums but falls to 5.5 percent for groups of more than 10,000.[28] Competition among insurers leads to marketing and cost shifting, which benefit the individual insurance firm but raise systemwide costs.

A lack of comprehensiveness in coverage also drives up administrative costs. Copayments, deductibles, and exclusions are expensive to enforce and lead many enrollees to purchase secondary "Medigap" policies. The secondary insurers maintain redundant and expensive burcaucracies.[29]

The efficiency of U.S. health care is further compromised by the extensive participation of private insurance firms whose overhead consumes 11.9 percent of premiums, as compared with 3.2 percent in U.S. public programs.[3] Even the "public" figure reflects the inefficiency of the private firms that process claims for Medicare for an average of $2.74 per claim,[30] whereas Ontario's Ministry of Health processes claims for $0.41 each (Davis J: personal communication). Moreover, the inefficiency of private insurers is not unique to the United States. The small private-insurance sectors of Canada, the United Kingdom, and Germany have overheads of 10.9 percent, 16 percent, and 15.7 percent, respectively.[31,32] A major advantage of public programs in terms of efficiency is their use of existing tax-collection structures, obviating the need for a redundant bureaucracy to collect money for health services. Thus, the overhead in Germany's premium-based, quasi-public sickness funds is between 4.6 percent[33] and 4.8 percent (Kuhn H: personal communication)—considerably higher than the overhead in tax-funded systems.

The scale of waste among private carriers is illustrated by Blue Cross/Blue Shield of Massachusetts, which covers 2.7 million subscribers and employs 6682 workers[34]— more than work for all of Canada's provincial health plans, which together cover more than 25 million people[7–10] (and Davis J: personal communication; Cunningham D: personal communication); 435 provincial employees administer the coverage for more than 3 million people

in British Columbia (Cunningham D: personal communication).

The existence of multiple payers in the United States also imposes bureaucratic costs on health care providers. Hospitals must bill several insurance programs with varying and voluminous regulations on coverage, eligibility, and documentation. Moreover, billing on a per-patient basis requires an extensive internal accounting apparatus for attributing costs and charges to individual patients and insurers. In contrast, Canada's single-payer system funds hospitals through global budgets, eliminating almost all hospital billing. The striking administrative efficiency of the Shriners' hospitals in the United States, which bill neither patients nor third parties and devote only 2 percent of their revenues to administration,[35] suggests that payment mechanisms rather than cultural or political milieus determine administrative costs. Here, too, the European experience parallels North America's. British hospitals that are assigned global budgets devote 6.9 percent of spending to administration,[36] but those paid on a per-patient basis (such as Humana's Wellington Hospital in London) spend 18 percent.[37]

The synchronous growth of bureaucratic profligacy and unmet health needs is reminiscent of Dickens' somber take of six poor travelers who were relegated to outbuildings when the hostel built for them was fully occupied by its charitable administrators.

> I found, too, that about a thirtieth part of the annual revenue was now expended on the purposes commemorated in the inscription over the door; the rest being handsomely laid out in Chancery, law expenses, collectorship, receivership, poundage, and other appendages of management, highly complimentary to the importance of the six Poor Travellers.[38]

The house of medicine is host to a growing array of specialists in fields unconnected to healing. At its present rate of growth, administration will consume a third of spending on health care 12 years hence, and half of the health care budget in the year 2020.

We are indebted to Mr. Lothar Rehmer, Ms. Judith Dowler, Dr. Jane Fulton, and Mr. Gilles Fortin for providing much of the raw data on Canadian health spending and to Dr. David H. Bor for his invaluable advice.

## References

1. Bureau of the Census. Statistical abstract of the United States. 102nd–109th eds. Washington, D.C.: Government Printing Office, 1981–1989.
2. Himmelstein DU, Woolhandler S. Cost without benefit: administrative waste in U.S. health care. N Engl J Med 1986; 314:441–5.

3. Letsch SW, Levit KR, Waldo DR. National health expenditures, 1987. *Health Care Financ Rev* 1988; 10(2):109–22.

4. American Hospital Association. Hospital statistics: 1984 ed. Chicago: American Hospital Association, 1984.

5. *Idem.* Hospital statistics: 1988 ed. Chicago: American Hospital Association, 1988.

6. Hospital statistics 1986–1987. Toronto: Queen's Printer, 1987.

7. Ontario Ministry of Health. Annual report 1988–1989. Kingston: Ontario Ministry of Health, 1989.

8. Regie de L'assurance-maladie du Quebec. Rapport Annuel 1986–1987. Quebec: Government of Quebec, 1987:30.

9. Saskatchewan Medical Care Insurance Commission. Annual report 1985–86. Regina: Government of Saskatchewan, 1986.

10. Nova Scotia Medical Services Insurance. Annual statistical tables: fiscal year 1985–86. Halifax: Government of Nova Scotia, 1986:3.

11. Canadian Medical Protective Association (CMPA) membership fees, 1971–1990. Toronto: Canadian Medical Association, 1989.

12. Gonzalez ML, Emmons DW, eds. Socioeconomic characteristics of medical practice 1989. Chicago: American Medical Association, 1989.

13. AMA Center for Health Policy Research. The administrative burden of health insurance on physicians. *SMS Report* 1989; 3(2):2–4.

14. Bureau of the Census. Current population survey, March 1988: technical documentation. Washington, D.C.: Department of Commerce, 1988.

15. Berry C, Brewster JA, Held PJ, Kehrer BH, Manheim LM, Reinhardt U. A study of the responses of Canadian physicians to the introduction of universal medical care insurance: the first five years in Quebec. Princeton, N.J.: Mathematica Policy Research, 1978.

16. Reynolds RA, Abram JB, eds. Socioeconomic characteristics of medical practice 1983. Chicago: American Medical Association, 1983.

17. Poullier J-P. Compendium: health care expenditure and other data. *Health Care Financ Rev* 1989; 11:Suppl:111–94.

18. Aggregate hospital financial data for California: report periods ending June 30, 1987–June 29, 1988. Sacramento: California Health Facilities Commission, 1989.

19. Aggregate long-term care facility financial data: report periods ending December 31, 1987–December 30, 1988. Sacramento: California Health Facilities Commission, 1989.

20. PHS will be challenged to maintain unbroken streak of profitability. *Mod Healthcare* 1989; 19(31):32–4.

21. Kenkel PJ. Improving managed care's management. *Mod Healthcare* 1990; 20(19):27–34.

22. *Idem.* Medicaid HMOs struggle for viability: federal plan aims to ease the burden. *Mod Healthcare* 1990; 20(16):32.

23. Gerber PC. What your life would be like under a Canadian-type NHI. *Physician's Manage* 1990; 30(5):32–9.

24. Ballad CA, Shoven JB, Wholley J. The total welfare costs of the U.S. tax system: a general equilibrium approach. *Natl Tax J* 1985; 38:125–40.

25. MacEwan A, Campen J. Crisis, contradiction, and conservative controversies in contemporary U.S. capitalism. *Rev Radical Polit Econ* 1982; 14(3):1–22.

26. Cost-management industry grew in 1988. *Mod Healthcare* 1989; 19(33):64.

27. Woolhandler S, Himmelstein DU. Free care: a quantitative analysis of health and cost effects of a national health program for the United States. *Int J Health Serv* 1988; 18:393–9.

28. Congressional Research Service. Library of Congress. Cost and effects of extending health insurance coverage. Washington, D.C.: Government Printing Office, 1988. (Education and Labor serial number 100–EE.)

29. Statement of Janet L. Shikles, Director, Health Finance and Policy Issues, Human Resources Division, General Accounting Office, before the Subcommittee of Health, Committee on Ways and Means, U.S. House of Representatives, March 13, 1990. Washington, D.C.: Government Printing Office, 1990. (SUDOC no. GAO/T-HRD-90–16.)

30. Statement of Janet L. Shikles, Director, Health Financing and Policy Issues, Human Resources Division, General Accounting Office, before the Subcommittee of Health, Committee on Ways and Means, U.S. House of Representatives, June 14, 1990. Washington, D.C.: Government Printing Office, 1990. (SUDOC no. GAO/T-HRD-90-42.)

31. Vayda E. Private practice in the United Kingdom: a growing concern. *J Public Health Policy* 1989; 10:359–76.

32. Verband der privaten Krankenversicherung e.V. Die private Krankenversicherung, Zahlenbericht 1988/1989.

33. Die gesetzliche Krankenversicherung in der Bundersrepublik Deutschland im Jahre 1988. Bonn, Germany: Bundesministerium für Arbeit und Sozialordnung, 1989.

34. Blue Cross/Blue Shield corporate report. Boston: Blue Cross/Blue Shield of Massachusetts, May 1990.

35. Guest DB. Health care policies in the United States: can the "American Way" succeed? *Lancet* 1985; 2:997–1000.

36. Compendium of health statistics. London: Office of Health Economics, 1984.

37. Parker P. A free market in health care. Lancet 1988, 1:1210–4.

38. Dickens C. Seven poor travellers. In: Dickens the Younger C, ed. Stories from the Christmas numbers of "Household Words" and "All the Year Round" 1852–1867. New York: Macmillan, 1896.

# Chapter 22

# Health Care Rationing Through Inconvenience

## The Third Party's Secret Weapon

**Gerald W. Grumet, M.D.**

Many strategies for the containment of medical costs have emerged from systems of managed care—gatekeeping by a primary care physician, prior authorization and utilization review, assumption of financial risk through capitation payments to the provider with financial disincentives for hospitalization or referral to specialists, and so forth. But another feature has crept into the managed care formula and has been largely overlooked: that of slowing and controlling the use of services and payment for services by impeding, inconveniencing, and confusing providers and consumers alike. In managed care's arsenal of cost-control weaponry, probably none is more potent—except for restricting hospital admission—than superseding the physician's autonomy by a managerial-review process in which armies of claims clerks, administrators, auditors, form processors, peer reviewers, functionaries, and technocrats of every description insinuate themselves into a complex system that authorizes, delivers, and pays for medical service.

Paradoxically, the savings that ordinarily accrue to an efficiently managed business are reversed in the case of insurance carriers, whose bungling, confusion, and delay impede the outflow of funds. For carriers, inefficiency is profitable. The result is a mounting number of dysfunctional bureaucracies with eye-catching logos and slick marketing techniques that contrast sharply with the difficulties encountered each time medical services are used. Such problems are not the exclusive province of managed care systems but are found as well in other third-party carriers, especially those that are governmentally based and use public funds. Some of the mechanisms used by carriers to impede the delivery process are examined here.

## PROCEDURAL COMPLEXITY

The university elaboration of simple procedures may explain in part why each visit to a physician's office is estimated to generate 10 pieces of paper.[1] Take, for example, the procedure required to obtain a nebulizer through the New York State Medicaid program:

> When physicians or clinics write a fiscal order for this appliance, they are required to complete their portion of a prior authorization form #3706, for the item ordered, along with the requested recipient information. The ordering provider will retain one copy of the form and the recipient will present the remaining three copies to the dispensing provider of their choice. The dispensing provider will retain one copy of the order and forward the remaining two parts of the form to the New York State

Reprinted with permission from Gerald W. Grumet, M.D., Health Care Rationing Through Inconvenience: The Third Party's Secret Weapon, *The New England Journal of Medicine,* Vol. 321 No. 9, pp. 607–611, 1989.

Department of Social Services. . . . The Bureau of MMIS [Medical Management Information System] will review the request and return to the dispensing provider a copy of the document with an assigned prior authorization number. That prior authorization number must be entered on the MMIS claim form. . . .[2]

The complexity of this particular Medicaid system is reflected in the huge procedure manuals sent to physicians: the instructions for filing a one-page billing form run for 135 pages, followed by 260 pages of procedural codes.[3] But New York is not alone. Former Governor Richard Riley of South Carolina has reported that his state once required pregnant women to fill out a 43–page questionnaire to gain eligibility for Medicaid.[4] Nor can the word "simplicity" be found in the Medicare lexicon. The tendency of the federal Medicare program to complicate the simple is evident in this excerpt from a "general information" message accompanying a benefit statement:

> Where the hospital collects the charges in full and the intermediary later finds the deductibles were fully or partially met, you will receive payment, along with this notice, for 80% of the paid hospital charges in excess of the cash deductible and any charges for the Part B blood deductible.

The marriage of the federal military and medical bureaucracies is seen in the "CHAMPUS/CHAMPVA [Civilian Health and Medical Program of the Uniformed Services/Civilian Health and Medical Program of the Veterans Administration] UB-82/HCT-A-1450" claim form for hospital services, which manages to include 96 "form locator" items on a single billing sheet.

The hindering effects of procedural complexity are reflected in the statistics of those denied Medicaid or welfare: 59.7 percent of the denials occurred because of problems with paperwork or documentation, whereas only 21.4 percent occurred because of excess income.[5]

## EXOTIC TERMS

Some carriers create a unique or exotic system of procedures, terms, codes, or acronyms, fostering a sense of alienation and unfamiliarity with the insurance plan and its benefits. Sociologist Max Weber, who popularized the concept of bureaucracy, noted that professional bureaucrats attempt to maintain their power and superiority over the general public by keeping secret their motives and technical expertise. This tendency can be seen in the rarefied terminology of insurance planners— "corridor deductibles," "disbursed self-funded plans," "cost-office effects," "per cause plans," and so forth— as well as in the alphabet soup of acronyms and buzzwords confected by managed care insurers. Besides the familiar HMOs (health maintenance organizations), there

are many hybrid and derivative terms, such as "swing PPOs," "HMO leaks," "HPOs" (hospital provider organizations), and "CPUs" (combined provider units). These are paralleled by an unending proliferation of acronyms that often puzzle the uninitiated. Awkwardness poses no barrier to such proliferation, as reflected in the CHAMPUS Program for the Handicapped (PFTH), New York Medicaid's Child-Teen Health Program (C/THP), or its Early Periodic Screening, Diagnosis, and Treatment Program (EPSDT). These acronyms join other jargon— "retrobilling," "claims processing edits," "multisource drugs," "magnetic media,"—to become standard idiom in the health care system. Thus, Medicare's "DME patrol" describes the effort to prevent duplicate billing for durable medical equipment, and "MAAC monitoring" indicates an effort to ensure that providers do not exceed the maximal actual allowable charges. The "final outcome" is an abstruse and enigmatic bit of jargon that frequently puzzles all but the most thoroughly initiated. An item from the *Champus News* exemplifies this tendency: "When the Nonavailability Statement is on file in the patient record at the hospital, a rubber stamp indicating 'DD1251 IS ON FILE' may be stamped on the claim form (HCFA 1500/CHAMPUS 501 or FORM 500) since, unlike the UB-82, there is no item number to indicate a code. . . ." To counter the obscure and convoluted billing procedures of Medicare and other insurers, private companies have sprung up with workshops and seminars to assist providers in coping with "carrier intimidation" and to explain esoteric terms like "no pay," "desperation," or "junk" codes, "carrier screens," "unbundling," and "blended rates."

## SLOWDOWNS

There are assorted techniques of slowing down the operations that lead to the outflow of funds, including authorizations for care, processing of claims, and responses to telephoned or written inquiries or appeals. In Great Britain and to some extent Canada, slowdowns in care delivery are the result of limitations in facilities, whereas in the United States they are operational. By one recent count, 848,246 people were awaiting treatment in Britain's National Health Service, where delays of three or four years for elective surgery are commonplace.[6] Similarly, as recently as 1986 there was a wait of 8 to 12 weeks for a CT scan in New Brunswick, and elective surgery often involved a one- or two-year delay.[7] In the United States, slowdowns focus on bureaucratic processes that restrain access to information, delaying the communications required to authorize care or disburse funds. Sometimes exchanges of information that could take a fraction of a second take weeks.

The average U.S. hospital waited 67.9 days to receive Medicare payments in 1986, and 73.2 days in 1987.[8] By early 1988, the average hospital had to wait 81 days for Medicare and other bills to be paid.[9] Such delays have been used in the fiscal cosmetology of budget-deficit reduction: in July 1988, Medicare adopted a 10-day delay in sending out its checks (extended to 14 days in October), deferring an estimated $815 million of liability for 1988 into fiscal 1989. A slowdown is seen likewise in the strenuous litigating, appealing, and delaying tactics of the Department of Health and Human Services and the Health Care Financing Administration as they attempt to thwart the efforts of hospitals to collect contested Medicare fees; such tactics sometimes hold up cases in court for as long as nine years.[10] Medicare providers encounter shorter delays: one otolaryngologist reported that half of his claims appeals were never answered, and those that were answered were delayed an average of 93 days.[11] Similarly, in early 1987 the state of Oklahoma was reported to have 400,000 unprocessed Medicaid claims,[12] whereas in Illinois delay in Medicaid payments led to the closing of two Chicago hospitals and the bankruptcy of a third.[13]

Among the 36 percent of 460 HMO enrollees who responded unfavorably to a survey, many indicated that delays and impediments were a major source of dissatisfaction. The complaints included being placed on hold on the telephone for as long as 50 minutes and waiting as long as four or five months for a physical examination under nonemergency conditions.[14] Among private carriers, the delaying techniques may include the dubious practice of shifting a claims review into a clinical review. A newsletter from Group Health Incorporated notes:

> When submitting claims for a complete Pulmonary Function Study. . .please attach a copy of the test results to the claim form and a statement describing why this particular method was medically indicated. This will facilitate handling and assure prompt and accurate settlement of your claim.[15]

A potentially lethal form of delay is observed among some HMOs who warn their patients that they must obtain authorization before using an emergency department or ambulance, unless the situation is life-threatening or the bill will not be paid. This places patients in the predicament of having to decide whether or not they are dying. Three critically ill patients in Milwaukee nearly lost their lives because of the delays of HMO triage, which circumvented the highly effective emergency medical system of that city.[16]

## SHIFTING OF PROCEDURES

Some third-party agencies shift their procedures, codes, forms, or policies frequently, leaving providers unable to systematize their operations for maximal efficiency. In sharp contrast to the rigid procedures typical of older,

entrenched bureaucracies, modern health carriers typically maintain a state of kinetic chaos by frequent mailings of directories, brochures, newsletters, memos, bulletins, benefit updates, and fee schedules. The situation is often compounded by rapid turnover and efforts to resolve difficulties by adding new layers of bureaucracy or shifting organizational responsibility. When Preferred Care, an independent practice association–model HMO in Rochester, New York, had problems with providers' claims, a newsletter announced that a new Provider Services Unit, formerly part of the Provider Relations Department, had been created within the Claims Administration Department, headed by the Policy and Project Administrator, and staffed by Provider Service Representatives, to deal with these issues.

On a national scale, widespread chaos can result when changes are imposed with inadequate time to adapt. When the Health Care Financing Administration approved a new Medicare coding system for U.S. hospitals on September 1, 1987, even the most sophisticated hospital systems were left scrambling to minimize the economic damage. According to one estimate, the new system called for 375,000 changes to be made within one month in codes for diagnosis-related groups.[17] The difficulties encountered by providers in coping with changes by carriers were exemplified by the need for CHAMPUS Transition Workshops throughout the northeastern United States when the CHAMPUS program was shifted from a carrier in Rhode Island to one in Indiana.

## FAIL-SAFE PAYMENT SYSTEMS

The computer programs and protocols of third-party payers have a strong tilt toward inhibition when approving claims. As with the fail-safe system for launching nuclear weapons, any one of a large number of negative conditions can restrain the system, but a long and unbroken sequence of positive conditions is required for its operation. Within the insurance organization's claims-processing mechanism, one envisions multiple subsystem circuit loops able to inhibit the claim for any of a myriad of minor errors, such as a one-letter misspelling of a name. Simple human events—a change in address, employment, or marital status, or the substitution for a vacationing physician by a colleague—will trip the system to a halt. Usually no one takes personal responsibility for an "adverse determination," which is typically ascribed to "fixed policy," a "committee decision," or "computer error."

## OVERLAPPING COVERAGE

Warring between carriers may occur in cases of overlapping coverage. An obvious example is the client who is covered for mental illness by carrier A and for substance abuse by carrier B. If such a client were admitted to a hospital in a depressed or drunken state, carrier A might refuse payment because "alcoholism was involved," whereas carrier B might note that "the primary diagnosis was depression." An example of boundary blurring in the obligations acknowledged by carriers is seen in the CHAMPUS program: the surgical care of a temporomandibular-joint problem is handled by one carrier, whereas the application of an occlusal splint to stabilize the joint is considered dental care and directed to a second carrier. Efforts by CHAMPUS to clarify this boundary lead to a pirouette of confusion:

> Adjunctive dental care is that dental care which is medically necessary in the treatment of an otherwise covered medical (not dental) condition, is an integral part of the treatment of such medical condition and is essential to the control of the primary medical condition; or which is the result of dental trauma caused by medically necessary treatment of an injury or disease. Adjunctive dental care requires prior approval and written preauthorization from the Dental Fiscal Intermediary. . . . Where adjunctive dental care involves a medical (not dental) *emergency*, preauthorization is waived. . . .[18]

## FRAGMENTATION OF TRANSACTIONS

Many health care transactions are divided or disassembled into multiple parts, complicating and slowing operations. An example familiar to Medicaid providers in New York State is the submission of a claim for perhaps seven charges on a single billing form, of which three charges are paid, two are "pended," one is submitted for "manual review," and one is lost. Another example of such fragmentation, often observed within the collective evasiveness and anonymity of bureaucracy, is the predicament of the provider who must scurry around for answers within a multipartite insurance organization, calling the Claims Department, the Member Services Department, the Provider Relations Department, the Continuing Care Department, and so forth. Fragmentation is also exemplified by the tendency of many carriers to subdivide levels of service into "minimal," "brief," "limited," "intermediate," "extended," "comprehensive," provided to a "new" as compared with an "established" patient in the setting of "hospital," "office," or "nursing home"—even though all these services rest on the single variable of professional time.

## UNCERTAINTY OF COVERAGE

Many carriers have a tendency to keep the care giver and the care recipient on tenterhooks with regard to authorization and payment for care. This is seen commonly in the delivery of psychiatric services, an area in which behavioral and emotional factors exert a powerful influence on one's willingness to treat or be treated. If a patient is highly apprehensive about a carrier's willingness to pay a medical bill or if the patient's physician harbors a high level of similar uncertainty, the provision of inpatient or outpatient care may become tentative. The problem is exacerbated by concurrent reviewers, who sometimes parcel out a series of 72–hour approvals for hospital psychiatric care, inconveniencing the physician and maintaining an unsettled climate. This may happen regardless of the clinical situation—even at the start of a course of electroconvulsive therapy that requires two to three weeks of inpatient care.

The same phenomenon is seen with regard to telephone authorization for care in which written confirmations are promised but slow in arriving. When the written approval does arrive, it too may be tentative and accompanied by disclaimers, such as these included in the Equicor-Equitable "Part Services" authorizations:

"PAR authorization does not guarantee payment."

"Benefits are subject to eligibility and coverage at the time of service and must be verified separately."

"The proposed treatment/surgery may *not* by covered by the patient's benefit plan. The PAR authorization only verifies that a hospital stay is medically necessary. You *must* contact the benefit office/claims payer to discuss what benefits will be paid. . . ."

Similar phenomena are apparent in the rise in Medicare denials of payment for home care services—up from 1.2 percent in 1983 to 6.0 percent in 1986. The ambiguity of definitions of crucial words such as "homebound" and the unpredictability of Medicare payments are given as reasons for the growing hesitancy of many agencies to accept Medicare patients.[19] The same is true for the retrospective denials of payment to hospitalized Medicare and Medicaid patients who do not fulfill review criteria.

A new, special form of uncertainty arises from the investigations of billing errors by physicians or alleged fraud in the treatment of Medicare and Medicaid patients. The Committee on Government Health Programs of the New York State Psychiatric Association has learned that Medicaid investigators posing as patients are furnished with hidden recording devices to tape psychotherapy sessions, in order to compare the actual length of the session with the length of treatment reported on the bill. A former fraud investigator for the Department of Health and Human Services has said that to the "Medicops" there is no such thing as "an honest mistake."[20]

## EMERGING TRENDS AND DANGERS

Although there are few statistics to document the numbers of patients deterred from seeking care or the numbers of physicians discouraged from offering it, a discernible pattern of restraint is emerging in various sectors of the health care system. There is a frequent impression that HMO patients sometimes believe their physicians to be less interested and less responsive than fee-for-service doctors.[21] During an 18–month period, a survey of 245 California patients found that those who subscribed to a prepaid insurance plan became disenchanted with the level of access to care, as compared with fee-for-service patients who saw the same doctors.[22] Reduced access to care because of financial barriers or the unavailability of medical resources within the community has a disproportionate effect on poor people, who may lack the sophistication, mobility, or assertiveness to secure the care they require. Such persons make fewer uninsured visits to hospitals or public health clinics if Medicaid-insured visits to local doctors are unavailable.[23] In California, physicians fought strenuously against "punitive" audits and claims reviews of their Medicaid (Medi-Cal) patients; the ultimate outcome was often a reduced willingness to continue treating indigent patients. One family practitioner who located his office in a Los Angeles ghetto and established a practice in which 98 percent of the patients were indigent reduced his Medi-Cal caseload to 30 percent after audits forced him to mortgage his home to pay legal fees.[24]

The inspector general of the Department of Health and Human Services imposed 466 sanctions for abuse of the Medicare and Medicaid programs in the fiscal year 1988—a 1200 percent increase over the 39 sanctions levied in 1981.[25] But a curious contrast is seen when these statistics are compared with those on the activities of the Provider Reimbursement Review Board, which makes the initial review for large Medicare providers who appeal decisions about reimbursement. In fiscal 1984 this board adjudicated 683 cases. By 1988 the number of decisions dwindled to 48, and by early 1989 its director estimated that he had a backlog of 3000 unheard cases.[26] Even before Medicare cost-containment initiatives reached Congress, a report of the American Medical Association indicated that 22 percent of American physicians had already cut their Medicare patient loads, stopped taking new patients, performed fewer procedures, and discontinued certain types of care.

Physicians are oriented toward advocacy of patients' interests and are trained for clinical rather than economic decision making. Admittedly, they have not been in the forefront of cost-control efforts, but now they must face a "second generation" of impediments to managed care that promises further challenges to physicians' autonomy in medical decision making. Carl Schramm, president of the Health Insurance Association of America, which represents about 350 commercial insurers, sees an expanded role for nurses in challenging the judgments of physicians—raising the spector of internecine conflict between fellow professionals. Schramm says,

"Many nurses have saved people from death by second-guessing physicians."[27]

American health care is now controlled haphazardly and is financed by multiple cumbersome, poorly integrated bureaucracies in desperate need of coordination, simplification, and streamlining. Perhaps the emerging Joint Commission on Accreditation of Healthcare Organizations can play a part by rewarding insurers who simplify and streamline operations, and by penalizing obstructive carriers. The methods of medical cost containment that we choose to invoke must be rational, explicit, equitable, and free of ambiguity, deception, or harassment.

## References

1. Wohl S. The medical industrial complex. New York: Harmony Books, 1984.
2. Noonan BJ. Letter no. 880781 to N.Y. State Medicaid providers, Albany, N.Y., 1988.
3. Medical management information system provider manual—physicians. Albany, N.Y.: Computer Science Corporation, 1988.
4. Richmond J. Comments made on the MacNeil/Lehrer Newshour, September 21, 1988. New York: WNET, 1988.
5. Tolchin M. Many rejected for welfare aid over paperwork. New York Times. October 29, 1988:1.
6. Harper T. Is Britain scrapping the National Health Service? Med Econ 1988; 65(July 18):23–6.
7. Robertson D. Is Canadian health care really such a great bargain? Med Econ 1988; 65(January 18):171–8.
8. Hospitals report slower Medicare reimbursement. Mod Healthcare 1988; 18(25):60.
9. Hospitals report modest rise in uncollectible bills. Mod Healthcare 1988; 18(37):104.
10. Burda D. HHS antics trying courts' patience. Mod Healthcare 1988; 18(36):65–6.
11. Watts JD. Mandatory assignment would kill our practice. Med Econ 1988; 65(July 18):70–80.
12. Lutz S. 'Automated Medicaid claims processing system creating a backlog of hospital bills.' Mod Healthcare 1987; 17(10):93.
13. Bell CW. Stop the shenanigans. Mod Healthcare. 1988; 18(24):16.
14. Cohn V. HMO members share their feelings. Washington Post (Health Supplement). November 10, 1987:9–11.
15. Group Health Incorporated. Professional News and Notes. Dec. 1987:4.
16. Kerr HD. Prehospital emergency services and health maintenance organizations. Ann Emerg Med 1986; 15:727–9.
17. Gardner E. Coding changes delay reimbursement. Mod Healthcare 1987; 17(25):11.
18. Blue Cross & Blue Shield of Rhode Island. Champus News. January 1988.
19. Lutz S. Home health denials prompting mergers, reductions in services to Medicare patients. Mod Healthcare 1987; 17(23):119, 122.

20. Starks S. To the Medicops, there are no honest mistakes. *Med Econ* 1988; 65(July 4):52–7.
21. Mechanic D. Cost containment and the quality of medical care: rationing strategies in an era of constrained resources. *Milbank Mem Fund Q* 1985; 63:453–75.
22. Murray JP. A follow-up comparison of patient satisfaction among prepaid and fee-for-service patients. *J Fam Pract* 1988; 26:576–81.
23. Blendon RJ, Aiken LH, Freeman HE, Kirkman-Liff BL, Murphy JW. Uncompensated care by hospitals or public insurance for the poor: does it make a difference? *N Engl J Med* 1986; 314:1160–3.
24. Holoweiko M. These doctors turned the tables on Medicaid auditors. *Med Econ* 1987; 64(June 27):62–8, 732–80.
25. Record number of sanctions levied in Medicare program. *Medical World News.* February 27, 1989:24.
26. Holthaus D. First step in Medicare appeal can be a long one. *Hospitals* 1989; 63(May 5):40–2.
27. Schramm CJ. Insurance companies to intensify claims review. *Hospitals* 1988; 63(December 5):58–9.

# Chapter 23

# Twenty Years of Research on the Quality of Medical Care 1964–1984

## Avedis Donabedian, M.D., M.P.H.

*Since 1964 we have built on earlier work, with some refinements, particularly in the formulation of explicit criteria of process and outcome; the detailed standardization of case mix when outcomes signify quality; the prespecification of outcomes for follow-up, when adverse outcomes are only the occasion for later assessment of process; a greater emphasis on more subtle organizational characteristics in the study of structure; and the identification of the separate effects of structural attributes by multivariate analysis. We have also paid more systematic attention to questions of measurement, including the veracity and completeness of the record; the procedures of criteria formulation; and the reliability, validity, and screening efficiency of the criteria. A notable advance is the use of decision analysis to identify optimal strategies of care, including the introduction of patient preferences and monetary cost in the specification of such strategies, and the use of decisional algorithms to portray the criteria of quality.*

AUTHOR'S NOTE: This article is based on a presentation for "Twenty Years of Research, Two Days of Celebration," Kaiser Permanente Health Services Research Center, Portland, Oregon, September 29–30, 1984. It is one product of work supported by the Commonwealth Fund, the W.K. Kellogg Foundation, and the National Center for Health Services Research. The opinions expressed in it are mine alone.

When I was first asked to consider this subject, my immediate reaction was that the last 20 years were a time of momentous advances in quality assessment. But a rapid scanning of several bibliographies led me to an additional discovery. I must now conclude that (1) by 1964 the foundations of almost all the major approaches to quality assessment had been laid down; (2) between 1964 and 1984, despite the astounding proliferation of quality studies, we achieved mainly refinements in what we already knew how to do; and (3) regrettably, some of the more fundamental questions pertinent to quality assessment are still not asked, or are misspecified, let alone systematically addressed.

## DEVELOPMENTS PRIOR TO 1964

Let me give some examples of accomplishments prior to 1964, using date of publication as the criterion of dating.

Reprinted with permission from Sage Publications, Inc. From *Evaluation and the Health Professions,* vol. 8(3) pp. 243–265, September 1985.

## Studies of "Outcomes"

The stream of studies that use health status as a means of measuring quality can begin, most properly, with the work of Ernest Amory Codman, a great, yet tragic, figure. By 1916 Codman fully understood the place of what he called the "end result" of care in the evaluation of clinical practice, not only as a professional activity, but also as an organizational, administrative, and economic enterprise; and he had proposed and tested a method for monitoring "end results." His published work, though rather confused and flawed by excessive dogmatism, is arresting for its creativity and insightfulness, and also deeply moving for the clear evidence we see in it of both his courage and personal anguish. He is a man whose memory we should forever cherish.

In the same tradition was the later study on preventable maternal mortality conducted under the aegis of the New York Academy of Medicine. The monograph (published in 1933) in which Hooker described this study is so elegant in style, searching in its analysis, and uncompromising in its commitment to human welfare, that it must be recognized as one of the treasures of a literature not overly rich in such accomplishments.

Quite a bit later—1955, to be precise—we find a parallel piece of work sponsored by the same organization, but this time on preventable perinatal deaths (Kohl, 1955). We also see, at about this time, notable examples of comparative mortality in the work of Shapiro and his associates (1958, 1960) at the Health Insurance Plan of Greater New York (HIP), and later of Lipworth et al. (1963) in Britain, the former concerned with prematurity and perinatal mortality, and the latter with case fatality in teaching and nonteaching hospitals.

## Studies of "Process"

Let us now visit the second major stream of quality studies, that which includes the assessments of the process of care.

Here again, we encounter an early, awe-inspiring landmark in the monumental work of Lee and Jones (1933) on the "Fundamental of Good Medical Care." This work offers a concept of quality rarely equaled in profundity or comprehensiveness, an uncompromising declaration of socially responsible professional norms as the standards of assessment, and an explicit enunciation of these standards. By a remarkable coincidence, this work was published in 1933, the same year the work on preventable maternal mortality appeared. Equally interesting, the next major advances occurred in the 1950s, but with some separation into several recognizably different offshoots, all similar in using professional norms as a foundation for assessment, but differing in the degree to which the criteria are specified in advance, the method of obtaining information on practice, the locus of care

subject to assessment, and the extent of interest in the relationship between structural attributes and the process of care.

*"Implicit" criteria.* Let me first follow the offshoot made up of the studies that adopted implicit criteria, with varying degrees of superimposed guidance, to assess the quality of care. We find, in this group, the landmark study of general practice in rural North Carolina by Peterson et al. (1956): an assessment of office practice, based on direct observation of the practitioner-client transaction, by a trained visitor who used his own implicit criteria to arrive at a judgment of the quality of care.

At about the same time, a series of studies unfolded at the Health Insurance Plan of Greater New York, led at first by Makover and then by Morehead, assessing the quality of care, mainly based on information obtained by a review of records and conversations with physicians, and basing the judgments of quality primarily on the implicit criteria of expert clinicians (Makover, 1951; Daily and Morehead, 1945; Morehead, 1958, 1967). The apotheosis of the implicit criteria approach, however, is to be found in the assessment of the quality of hospital care received by members of the Teamsters Union and their families, as reported by Morehead and her associates (1964).

It is important to note that in all these studies there were explorations of the relationships between performance and structural characteristics that set the pattern for much that was to come. For example, in their study of hospital care, Morehead et al. (1964) paid much attention to the organizational characteristics of hospitals (such as ownership and medical school affiliation), the professional characteristics of physicians (such as specialty certification and hospital privileges), and the interaction of the two sets of characteristics. Peterson et al. (1956), who measured the quality of care only because they wished to find out what attributes and experiences were conducive to good general practice, included in their exhaustive inquiry factors such as the type of medical school, performance as a medical student, the nature and duration of postgraduate training, continuing education through refresher courses and subscription to medical journals, medical society membership, hospital affiliation, practice alone or in a group, access to laboratory services, the presence of specific pieces of technical equipment in the doctor's office, seeing patients by appointment, and duration of the workday. Attributes such as education, training, hospital affiliation, and seeing patients by appointment were also included in the studies conducted at HIP, but there were added questions of special interest, such as length of association with the Plan, percentage of time devoted to HIP enrollees, and percentage of work done at a group-practice facility.

*"Explicit" criteria.* Let us now follow developments along another branch, that on which cluster the studies using explicit criteria. The premise that the norms of practice must be expressed in explicit criteria was the rock on which Lembcke (1956) built what he hoped to be a "science" of assessment. We find in his work the fundamental precepts that have guided the formulation of such criteria ever since.

A little later, quite independently, a group of workers at the University of Michigan—a group that included Fitzpatrick, Riedel, and Payne (1962)—adopted the use of explicit criteria to assess what they called "hospital effectiveness."

There are a few other offshoots that, although smaller, foreshadow later developments. We find, for example, in another work by Lembcke (1952), an epidemiological approach to quality assessment based on comparisons among hospital service areas. This is the prototype of, and a fully equal companion to, the spate of small-area studies that we have recently experienced. Similarly, the statistical indexes of outpatient care developed by Ciocco et al. (1950) and the indexes of hospital activities by Eisele et al. (1956) are the prototypes of what later came to be recognized as "professional activities studies" and "profiles." In fact, Lembcke (1967) has traced the origins of the statistical indexes of hospital performance even further back, first to measures used by the staff of the Commonwealth Fund to assess the members of its rural hospital program (Southmayd and Smith, 1944) and then to Lembcke's own elaboration of these measures in assessing the performance of participants in the Council of Rochester Regional Hospitals, also under the aegis of the Commonwealth Fund (Lembcke, 1947:27–29).

### Studies of "Structure"

I have one final major stream I must mention, even if briefly. It is the stream of studies that are concerned with the assessment of structural attributes.

Here, again, the foundations are rather old. For example, we find in the work of Goldmann and Graham (1954) a detailed model for assessing an ambulatory care program by means of a variety of structural characteristics. The work of Georgopoulos and Mann (1962) on "The Community General Hospital" also introduced a new set of more subtle organizational attributes that either appear to influence, or can, with good reason be expected to influence, the quality of care.

### Use and Abuse of the Past

I ask you to forgive me for this overly length retrospective. Perhaps it is merely a failing of old age that prompts me to be so backward looking. But it seems to me that no field of intellectual endeavor can afford to

remain as unmindful of its roots and indifferent to its indebtedness to its past as ours appears to be. Without a more widely shared knowledge of our antecedents, some of us remain condemned to reinventing what we already know, often in less successful forms; some less scrupulous others are tempted to plunder the past by failing to reveal their sources. We should, instead, do homage to our past by building upon it.

## MORE RECENT DEVELOPMENTS

### Lines of Continuity

Let me now survey the work published during 1964 and since. To begin with, I shall mention briefly some lines of continuity that one observes when old methods are used, with variable degrees of improvement, to obtain new information in new settings.

Perhaps the most notably derivative of all recent efforts was the near duplication of the Lee-Jones study (1933) by a group of investigators at Yale, led first by I.S. Falk (Falk et al., 1967) and then by Schonfeld (Schonfeld et al., 1975). In this reincarnation, the original work was in many ways improved upon, but in some ways the new failed to measure up to its majestic predecessor.

The comparisons of small geographic areas with respect to a large variety of attributes has continued—without striking improvements in method—in the work of many investigators, including that of Lewis (1969) in Kansas, Wennberg and Gittlesohn (1973) in New England, Griffith and his colleagues (1981) in Michigan, and Stockwell and Vayda (1979) in Ontario. A succession of international comparisons could also be placed in this category. (See, for example, Bunker, 1970; Vayda, 1973; McPherson et al., 1982).

During the period under examination, Morehead and her associates used the method developed originally at HIP, with relatively small refinements, to study the quality of care in neighborhood health centers and some other ambulatory care settings (Morehead, 1970; Morehead et al., 1971, Morehead and Donaldson, 1974). Similarly, Payne extended the scope of his activities by using the method originally devised to study hospital effectiveness in Michigan to assess the quality of care in Hawaii—an admittedly more pleasant locale! There were some refinements of method as well. These included the joint consideration of in-hospital and out-of-hospital care in each episode of hospitalization, the differential weighting of the criteria, attention to the reliability of abstracting records, and the development of explicit criteria for ambulatory care (Payne et al., 1976).

### Advances in Studies of "Process"

The extension of explicit criteria to assessing the process of ambulatory care appears to usher in a new stage in the assessment of process in general, a stage characterized by much greater interest in some basic questions of method. I shall mention only some of these.

*The medical record.* Because the study of process depends so heavily on what appears in the medical records, there has been a fair amount of attention to the completeness and accuracy of the record, and to the implications of this to quality assessment, as well as clinical management. The work of Starfield and her associates at Johns Hopkins is a good example (Zuckerman et al., 1975; Starfield et al., 1979). At the same time, there has been a great deal of interest, notably represented by the work of Weed (1969, 1971), in redesigning the medical record to make it a better tool in clinical management. By stretching our category a little, we might include here the introduction and testing of computerized record systems as well. (See, for example, McDonald, 1976; Barnett et al., 1978; Barnett, 1984). I believe that in these kinds of developments there is a growing realization that the nature of recording influences what is possible in quality assessment, and that the requirements of quality assessment can and should influence the design of the record system, although a thorough, systematic exploration of this interrelationship is yet to come.

*Criteria formulation.* A more important development in studying the assessment of process, and also of outcome, has been the exploration of criteria formulation itself. One sees here several strands that cannot be—indeed should not be—separated, as they are so intimately intertwined.

One strand represents the interest in criteria formulation as a consensus-achieving process; another comprises work on the choice of criteria and the design of criteria lists so as to achieve greater correspondence between assessments of process and of outcome; still another strand consists of explorations of the relation between criteria design and the ability of the criteria to screen cases so as to achieve the most accurate separation between acceptable and unacceptable care at lowest cost in effort and money. Briefly, these are studies of consensus or reliability, causal validity, and screening efficiency.

*Consensus.* The study of criteria formulation as a social process leading to consensus is represented by the deliberate application of techniques such as the Delphi method or the Nominal Group Process (Delbecq and Van de Ven, 1971; Dalkey et al., 1972). Many investigators borrowed elements from these and other methods of arriving at consensus, and have described the consequences with variable degrees of attention to reliability and validity.

Notable among the many studies of process that have looked into these matters are, in rough chronological order, the early work of Brook (1973) in Baltimore, Hare and Barnoon (1973) for the American Society of Internal Medicine in several regions of the United States, Osborne, and Thompson (1975) under the leadership of the American Academy of Pediatrics, Hulka et al. (1979) in North Carolina, Riedel and Riedel (1979) in New Haven and Hartford, and Palmer et al. (1984) in Boston.

Among other things, these studies have described the changes that occur in the inclusion or exclusion of criteria when these are selected according to degree of "importance" based on perceived contributions to making the right diagnosis or achieving the best outcomes, and according to the information called for by the criteria being subject to recording. The degree of agreement on the criteria has been studied among members of a group of physicians, as well as among groups of physicians differentiated by specialty or other attributes. There are only fragments of information about the stability of such choices over time (Wagner et al., 1976, 1978). There is also some information, again not enough, about the relation between the perceived importance of the criteria and the likelihood of finding that they have been complied with in practice. We also do not know on what basis the criteria that have been chosen might be differentially weighted and whether the weighting materially alters the judgments on quality. Nor do we know whether one method of arriving at consensus is better than another, and in what ways (Donabedian, 1982).

*Screening efficiency and validity.* The more elaborate methods of achieving and testing consensus on the explicit criteria of process are, of course, only a means of obtaining criteria that are efficient and valid. To test validity it is necessary to examine the correspondence among judgments based on explicit criteria of process, implicit criteria of process, and either implicit or explicit criteria of outcome. If one of any pair of methods can be taken as more valid, the efficiency of the less valid method is judged by a comparison of the proportion of "positives" that it detects and the proportion of "negatives" that it mistakenly identifies as "positive." McClain and Riedel (1973) and Greenfield et al. (1982) offer examples of such comparisons in the screening of cases for utilization review and for appropriateness of admission, respectively. Judgments resulting from the use of explicit and implicit criteria have been compared, among others, by Brook (1973), Novick et al. (1976), Hulka et al. (1979), and Kane et al. (1981). Comparisons of judgments based on explicit criteria or process with those based on either implicit or explicit criteria of outcome include those reported by Brook (1973), Hulka et al. (1979), Mushlin and Appel (1980), and Mates and Sidel (1981).

Though much more remains to be done, the findings of these comparisons suggest, on the whole, coherence and rationality rather than—as some have claimed—failure and disarray. We have, moreover, yet another refinement in the criteria of process—one that, by more directly linking criteria formulation to decision analysis, promises to yield progressively more valid conceptions and measures of quality.

*Decision analysis and the criteria of care.* As early as 1964, the year I arbitrarily chose to usher in the new age, Peterson and Barsamian described an approach to quality assessment based on the then burgeoning science of decision analysis as applied to clinical practice (Peterson and Barsamian 1964, Peterson et al., 1966). This approach was soon forgotten, but only to reemerge later, based on different antecedents, and in different hands, as the "criteria mapping" approach described by Greenfield et al. (1975, 1981).

In their original forms, the decision maps can be seen as more true-to-life representations of the sequences by which physicians arrive at clinical decisions. But they are similar to the more traditional lists of criteria in being merely current embodiments of the conventional wisdom. They do, however, offer opportunities for more formal testing, based on subjective probabilities of the relationship between successive branchings of the stepwise progression that they represent. Besides defining more precisely which of several possible alternative strategies is to be preferred, this testing can lead to an assigning of differential penalties to different kinds of failures to pursue the optimal path. At the same time, the empirical testing of such decisional algorithms through epidemiological observations, or by means of more rigorous clinical trials, can be directly translated to revised criteria maps. If one goes on to include monetary cost as well as patient preferences as important criteria for judging the success of alternative strategies of care, one arrives at a fundamental reformulation of the meaning of quality itself.

The various currents and crosscurrents of research that have brought about this last development are too diverse, widely dispersed, and complex to permit a ready review. But illustrative stages may be observed in the work of a single group of investigators led by McNeil (McNeil et al., 1976). We see (1) how the choice of strategies depends on the specificity and sensitivity of each step in a stepwise progression of diagnostic tests; (2) an example of how the choice of a therapeutic regimen depends not only on the benefits and risks associated with alternative regimens when these are implemented, but also, as one would expect, on the propensity of patients to adhere to each of the contending regimens (McNeil and Adelstein, 1975); (3) the importance of monetary cost as a factor in determining how far successively more exhaustive testing is to continue, and which regimen of therapy is preferable (McNeil et al., 1975); (4) how different patients make different choices when offered a treatment with higher immediate mortality but greater subsequent longevity for the survivors, as compared to a lower immediate mortality attained at the price of shorter subsequent longevity

(McNeil et al., 1978); and finally (5) we are also shown analogous differences in preferences when there is a prospect of a shorter life with less disability contrasted with a longer life, but with greater disability (McNeil et al., 1981).

It is easy to see even from these sketchy examples why these developments promise to reform clinical practice by redefining the meaning of quality and its standards, and why I believe that they are the single most important advance pertinent to quality assessment in recent years. Needless to say, the advance I refer to rests on an expansion of the meaning of outcomes and a reexamination of the relationship between outcomes and process. Thus, we are brought back to a category of methods that use outcomes to assess the quality of care.

### Advances in Studies of Outcome

You will have noticed that the earlier studies of outcome that I described are divisible into two classes. In the first of these classes are studies in which favorable adverse outcomes, such as mortality and case fatality, serve to indicate—or at least suggest—a judgment on quality, in and of themselves.

The stream of such studies continues, stimulated primarily by the observation of remarkable differences in postsurgical morbidity and fatality among hospitals, particularly in the national Halothane study (Bunker et al., 1969). The chief refinement of method in such studies has been a greater sophistication in making adjustments for differences in case mix that might influence outcome independently of the quality of care. The earliest adjustments, as in the work of Lipworth et al. (1963) to which I have referred, were simply for diagnosis, age, and sex. Later Roemer et al. (1968) proposed an ingenious adjustment for length of stay and hospital occupancy. More recent studies have supplemented information about age and sex by information gleaned from hospital discharge abstracts. Perhaps the most elaborate system of adjustments, using information on the relative risk of postsurgical fatality collected expressly for the purpose, is to be found in one part of the study of "institutional differences" conducted by a group of investigators at Stanford University (Staff of the Stanford Center for Health Care Research, 1976). The system devised by Gonnella for staging the progression of illness can also be considered to serve a similar purpose, among others, and to be a more recent, more highly elaborated form of an approach with rather ancient beginnings (Gonnella and Gorban, 1975; Gonnella et al., 1976).

In a second class of outcome studies are those in which the identification of adverse outcomes is merely a trigger to the assessment of antecedent process. These studies derive their parentage, at least in part, from the "end result" system of Codman (1916), and the studies of preventable maternal and perinatal mortality that I mentioned earlier (Hooker, 1933; Kohl, 1955).

Most important among these more recent developments is the work of John Williamson (1971, 1978a) at Johns Hopkins University. In essence, the method consists of the specification of outcomes that one expects to achieve, the verification of whether or not the expectations have been met, and an assessment of antecedent process, as well as of structure, if the expectations have not been met. With regard to method, the more notable features of this procedure include:

(1) an order of priority for selecting conditions for study based on the principle of "maximum achievable benefit";
(2) a carefully specified procedure, based on the Nominal Group Process, for selecting conditions and specifying goals;
(3) an insistence that these conditions and these goals be specific to any given institution and to the population they serve, and that representatives of all members of the institution participate in their selection;
(4) a recognition that outcomes may include a wider range of phenomena, beyond the conventional measures of morbidity and mortality;
(5) a recognition that randomness introduces a specifiable degree of variability in the outcomes experienced by samples of patients, and that action is not indicated unless the observed frequency of such events is not easily explained by chance; and
(6) the development of a standardized scale of functional states that can be used to measure outcomes in all conditions instead of, or in addition to, more discrete measures of outcomes more specific to each condition.

Besides contributing to methodological improvements of its own, Williamson's method has produced offspring, the most important of which is the "Problem Status Index" developed by Mushlin and Appel (1980) based on earlier work by Barr (1974)—all the work being based at Johns Hopkins. The method is adaptable to setting goals either for individual patients or categories of patients in groups, and it is designed to identify individual patients whose care is suspected of having been substandard. Mushlin and Appel have supplied a fair amount of information on the sensitivity and specificity of the method, and on the reasons for the failure to achieve expected outcomes.

As might have been expected, studies of outcome have shared in the more systematic attention to the process by which criteria are selected and specified. The work of Williamson is particularly notable for its early adoption of a carefully specified procedure for selecting conditions that could be accorded high priority in the assessment of outcomes, and for checking the reliability and, to some extent, the validity of such choices (Williamson, 1978b; Williamson et al., 1978, 1979). Another scheme for selecting conditions for assessment is the "tracer method" proposed by Kessner et al. (1973) with a view to obtaining a representative or illustrative view of a health-care system.

As to the studies of how outcome criteria can be and perhaps should be formulated, the work of the group of investigators at the Rand Corporation stands as the supreme example (Brook et al., 1977). Notable in this work, in addition to careful description of the method by which the criteria were arrived at, is the emphasis on carefully specifying the categories of patients to be assessed, the method for measuring outcomes, the precise time at which outcome measurement should occur, and the sources of information concerning patient characteristics and outcomes. We still need to see, however, how the method performs in full-scale field tests.

Another line of development promises to contribute to quality assessment by providing measures of outcome that represent more accurately and comprehensively several aspects of the quantity and quality of life. Notable in this regard is the series of studies that began with the seminal work of Fanshel and Bush (Fanshel and Bush, 1970); the progressive refinements of the Sickness Impact Profile (Gilson et al., 1975; Bergner et al., 1981), and the measures of functional status developed at the Rand Corporation (Brook et al., 1979).

Advances in Studies of "Structure"

As I move closer to my conclusions, allow me to review very briefly some developments in the assessment of structure as it influences either the process of care or its outcomes.

Perhaps the first significant improvement over the early studies of this relationship occurred when methods of multivariate analysis allowed an assessment of the independent effects of several coexisting variables, and of the extent of variation in quality that they are able to explain. An excellent example is the more thorough analysis of the findings of Payne et al. in Hawaii, conducted by Rhee, under the guidance of Darsky in our own department at the University of Michigan (Rhee, 1976).

A second development of major importance is a growing interest in the more intimate structures and processes of formal organizations and of their influence on quality. Continuing in a tradition already clearly established in the early work of Georgopoulos and Mann (1962), more recent investigators such as Scott et al. (1976, 1979) and Shortell et al. (1976) have studied the influence of variables such as "differentiation," "coordination," "power," "specification of work procedures," "visibility of consequences," and so on. The operational measurement of these variables in health-care organizations is, itself, a matter of great interest and considerable difficulty. Unfortunately, in many studies of such organizational characteristics, the measures of the dependent variable, which is quality, tend to be rather crude, being primarily measures of case fatality, postoperative complications, or reputations for good performance. Therefore, the findings, which are often rather unexpected as well, are difficult to interpret or accept. We urgently need to supplement the mere observation of adverse outcomes with investigations of how these outcomes were brought about.

Let me also point out that the studies of the relationship between structural attributes and quality are now and always have been primarily concerned with the attributes of the individual or institutional providers of care. Study of variations in the quality of care received by consumers with different characteristics is a much neglected field, though this is a matter of utmost importance to social policy (Wyszewianski and Donabedian, 1981). Perhaps we are unwilling to face the possibility that even if near equality in access is achieved, subsequent differences in the quality of care might persist.

## CONCLUSIONS

Although during the last twenty years of research on the quality of health care we have seen a consolidation of some previous gains, as well as a number of notable advances, we still face, as I have detailed elsewhere, a formidable array of challenging problems (Donabedian, 1978). Among these are two that I believe demand our most dedicated attention.

First, and at a most fundamental level, we need to look into the nature of quality itself, so that the conceptions we have of it are socially more relevant and scientifically more valid. This requires that all presumed relationships between process and outcome be rigorously tested while our technical concerns are supplemented by attention to the interpersonal, social, even moral dimensions of quality. It follows that individual and social valuations must enter the assessment of both the means and the results of health care. As for the means, we cannot continue as if monetary cost were still of no concern. We are obligated, it seems to me, to devise and test strategies of care that achieve the greatest improvements in health at lowest cost. Having such strategies at hand, we would be better able to resist the pressure to accept lower levels of quality because we cannot afford the cost. And if not, we would at least be able to show a truer picture of the losses and gains.

Second, we must pay much more attention than we have done in the past to the determinants of clinically relevant behaviors in the health-care system, and to the means of bringing about desired changes in behavior. The truest concepts of quality and the most elegant methods of assessment will mean little unless we are able to bring about the changes that make our realities correspond to our aspirations much more closely than they now do.

## References

Barnett, G.O. (1984) "The application of computer-based medical-record systems in ambulatory practice." New England J. of Medicine 310 (June 21): 1643–1650.

—— R. Winickoff, J.L. Dorsey, M. Morgan, and R.S. Lurie (1978) "Quality assurance through automated monitoring and feedback using a computer-based medical information system." Medical Care 16 (November): 962–970.

Barr, D.M. (1974) "The patient's problem: concept, method, and use in health services research." Unpublished master's thesis, Johns Hopkins University.

Bergner, M. and R.A. Bobbitt with W.B. Carter and B.S. Gilson (1981) "The Sickness Impact Profile: development and final revision of a health status measure." Medical Care 19 (August): 787–805.

Brook, R.H. (1973) Quality of Care Assessment: A Comparison of Five Methods of Peer Review. Washington, DC: Department of Health, Education, and Welfare, Bureau of Health Services Research.

—— A. Davies-Avery, S. Greenfield, L.J. Harris, T. Lelah, N.E. Solomon, and J.E. Ware, Jr. (1977) "Assessing the quality of medical care using outcome measures: an overview of the method." Medical Care 15 (September Supplement): 1–165.

Brook, R.K., J.E. Ware, A. Davies-Avery, A.L. Stewart, C.A. Donald, W.H. Rogers, K.N. Williams, and S.A. Johnston (1979) "Overview of adult health status measures fielded in Rand's Health Insurance Study." Medical Care 17 (July Supplement): 1–131.

Bunker, J. (1970) "Surgical manpower: a comparison of operations and surgeons in the United States and in England and Wales." New England J. of Medicine 282 (January 15): 135–144.

Bunker, J.P., W.H. Forrest, Jr., F. Mosteller, and L.D. Vandam [eds.] (1969) The National Halothane Study: A Study of the Possible Association between Halothane Anesthesia and Postoperative Hepatic Necrosis. Bethesda, MD: National Institutes of Health.

Ciocco, A., G.H. Hunt, and I. Altman (1950) "Statistics on clinical services to new patients in medical groups." Public Health Reports 65 (January): 99–115.

Codman, E.A. (1916) A Study in Hospital Efficiency. Boston: Thomas Todd.

Daily, E.F. and M.A. Morehead (1956) "A method of evaluating and improving the quality of medical care." Amer. J. of Public Health 46 (July): 848–854.

Dalkey, N.C., D.L. Rourke, R. Lewis, and D. Snyder (1972) The Qualify of Life: Delphi Decision-Making, Lexington, MA: D. C. Heath.

Delbecq, A.L. and A.H. Van de Ven (1971) "A group process model for problem identification and program planning." J. of Applied Behavioral Sci. 7 (July-August): 466–492.

Donabedian, A. (1982) Explorations in Quality Assessment and Monitoring, Volume 2. The Criteria and Standards of

Quality. Ann Arbor, MI: Health Administration Press. [See Methods of Deriving the Criteria, pp. 149–199; Stringency of the Standards and Importance of the Criteria, pp. 203–292; Consensus, Replicability, Stability, and Relevance, pp. 297–347.]

—— (1978) Needed Research in the Assessment and Monitoring of the Quality of Medical Care. Hyattsville, MD: National Center for Health Services Research, Office of Scientific and Technical Information.

Eisele, C.W., V.N. Slee, and R.G. Hoffman (1956) "Can the practice of internal medicine be evaluated?" *Annals of Internal Medicine* 44 (January): 144–161.

Fanshel, S. and J.W. Bush (1970) "A health status index and its application to health services outcomes." *Operations Research* 18 (November-December): 1021–1060.

Falk, I.S., H.K. Schonfeld, B.R. Harris, S. Landau, and S.S. Mills (1967) "The development of standards for the audit and planning of medical care. I. concepts, research design and the content of primary care." *Amer. J. of Public Health* 57 (July): 1118–1136.

Fitzpatrick, T.B., D.C. Riedel, and B.C. Payne (1962) "The effectiveness of hospital use," "Criteria and data collection," "Appropriateness of admission and length of stay," "The physician interview," "Summary and conclusions," and "Criteria of effectiveness of hospital use," chapters 24–28 and Appendix 2-B, pages 449–526 and 545–559 in W.J. McNerney and study staff, Hospital Economics: Services, Costs, Methods of Payment, and Controls, Volume 1. Chicago: Hospital Research and Educational Trust.

Georgopoulos, B.S. and F.C. Mann (1962) The Community General Hospital. New York: Macmillan.

Gilson, B.S., J.S. Gilson, and M. Bergner (1975) "The sickness impact profile: development of an outcome measure of health care." *Amer. J. of Public Health* 65 (December): 1304–1310.

Goldman, F. and E.A. Graham (1954) The Quality of Medical Care Provided at the Labor Health Institute, St. Louis, Missouri. St. Louis: The Labor Health Institute.

Gonnella, J.S. and M.J. Goran (1975) "Quality of patient care—a measurement of change: the staging concept." *Medical Care* 14 (June): 467–473.

Gonnella, J.S., D.Z. Louis, and J. J. McCord (1976) "The staging concept-an approach to the assessment of outcome of ambulatory care." *Medical Care* 14 (January): 13–21.

Greenfield, S., C.E. Lewis, S.H. Kaplan, and M.B. Davidson (1975) "Peer review by criteria mapping: criteria for diabetes mellitus, the use of decision-making in chart audit." *Annals of Internal Medicine* 83 (December): 761–770.

Greenfield, S., S. Cretin, L.G. Worthman, F.J. Dorey, N.E. Solomon, and G.A. Goldberg (1981) "Comparison of a criteria map to a criteria list in quality-of-care assessment for patients with chest pain: the relation each to outcome." *Medical Care* 19 (March): 255–272.

Greenfield, S., S. Cretin, L.G. Worthman, and F. Dorey (1982) "The use of an ROC curve to express quality of care results." *Medical Decision Making* 2 (Spring): 23–31.

Griffith, J.R., J.D. Restuccia, P.J. Tedeschi, P.A. Wilson, and H. S. Zuckerman (1981) "Measuring community hospital services in Michigan." *Health Services Research* 16 (Summer): 135–160.

Hare, R.L. and S. Barnoon (1973) Medical Care Appraisal and Quality Assurance in the Office Practice of Internal Medicine. San Francisco: American Society of Internal Medicine.

Hooker, R.S. (1933) Maternal Morality in New York City: A Study of All Puerperal Deaths 1930–1932. New York: Oxford Univ. Press.

Hulka, B.S., F.J. Romm, G.R. Parkerson, Jr., I.T. Russell, N.E. Clapp, and F.S. Johnson (1979) "Peer review in ambulatory care: use of explicit criteria and implicit judgments." *Medical Care* (March Supplement): 1–73.

Kane, R.E., L.Z. Rubinstein, R.H. Brook, J. Van Ryzin, P. Masthay, E. Schoenrich, and B. Harrell (1981) "Utilization review in nursing homes: making implicit level-of-care judgments explicit." *Medical Care* 19 (January): 3–13.

Kessner, D.M., G.E. Kalk, and J. Singer (1973) "Assessing health quality—the case for tracers." *New England J. of Medicine* 288 (January 25): 189–194.

Kohl, S.G. (1955) Perinatal Mortality in New York City: Responsible Factors. Cambridge, MA: Harvard Univ. Press.

Lee, R.I. and L.W. Jones (1933) The Fundamentals of Good Medical Care. Chicago: Univ. of Chicago Press.

Lembcke, P.A. (1967) "Evolution of the medical audit." *J. of the Amer. Medical Assn.* 199 (February 20):543–550.

——(1956) "Medical auditing by scientific methods: illustrated by major female pelvic surgery." *J. of the Amer. Medical Assn.* 162 (October 13):646–655.

——(1952) "Measuring the quality of medical care through vital statistics based on hospital service areas: 1. Comparative study of appendectomy rates." *Amer. J. of Public Health* (March): 276–286.

——[ed.] (1947) The Regional Hospital Plan—The Second Year's Experience. Rochester, NY: Council of Rochester Regional Hospitals, pp. 27–29.

Lewis, C.E. (1969) "Variations in the incidence of surgery." *New England J. of Medicine* 281 (October 16): 880–884.

Lipworth, L., J.A.H. Lee, and J.N. Morris (1963) "Case fatality in teaching and non-teaching hospitals 1956–159." *Medical Care* 1 (April-June): 71–76.

Makover, H.B. (1951) "The quality of medical care." *Amer. J. of Public Health* 41 (July): 824–832.

Mates, S. and V.W. Sidel (1981) "Quality assessment by process and outcome methods: evaluation of emergency room care of asthmatic adults." *Amer. J. of Public Health* 71 (July): 687–693.

McClain, J.O. and D.C. Riedel (1973) "Screening for utilization review: on the use of explicit criteria and non-physicians in case selection." *Amer. J. of Public Health* 63 (March): 247–251.

McDonald, C.T. (1976) "Protocol-based computer reminders, the quality of care and the non-perfectibility of man." *New England J. of Medicine* 295 (December 9): 1351–1355.

McNeil, B.J. and S.J. Adelstein (1975) "Measures of clinical efficacy: the values of case finding in hypertensive renovascular disease." *New England J. of Medicine* 293 (July 31): 221–226.

McNeil, B.J., S.J. Hessel, W.T. Branch, L. Bjork, and S.J. Adelstein (1976) "Measures of clinical efficacy. III. The value of the lung scan in the evaluation of young patients with pleuritic chest pain." *J. of Nuclear Medicine* 17 (March): 163–169.

McNeil, B.J., P.D. Varady, B.A. Burrows, and S.J. Adelstein (1975) "Measures of clinical efficacy: cost-effectiveness calculations in the diagnosis and treatment of hypertensive renovascular disease." *New England J. of Medicine* 293 (July 31):216–221.

McNeil, B.J., R. Weichselbaum, and S.G. Pauker (1981) "Speech and Survival: tradeoffs between quality and quantity of life in laryngeal cancer." *New England J. of Medicine* 305 (October 22): 982–987.

——(1978) "Fallacy of the five year survival in lung cancer." *New England J. of Medicine* 299 (December 21): 1397–1401.

McPherson, K., J.E. Wennberg, O.B. Hovind, and P. Clifford (1982) "Small-area variations in the use of common surgical procedures: an international comparison of New England, England, and Norway." *New England J. of Medicine* 307 (November 18): 1310–1314.

Morehead, M.A. (1970) "Evaluating the quality of medical care in the neighborhood center program of the Office of Economic Opportunity." *Medical Care* 8 (March-April): 118–1131.

——(1967) "The medical audit as an operational tool." *Amer. J. of Public Health* 57 (September): 1643–1656.

——(1958) Quality of Medical Care Provided by Family Physicians as Related to Their Education, Training and Methods of Practice. New York: Health Insurance Plan of Greater New York.

——and R. Donaldson (1974) "Quality of clinical management of disease in comprehensive neighborhood health centers." *Medical Care* 12 (April): 301–315.

——and others (1964) A Study of the Quality of Hospital Care Secured by a Sample of Teamster Family Members in New York City. New York: School of Public Health and Administrative Medicine, Columbia University.

Morehead, M.A., R.S. Donaldson, and M.R. Seravelli (1971) "Comparisons between DEO Neighborhood Health Centers and other health care providers of ratings of the quality of health care." *Amer. J. of Public Health* 61 (July): 1294–1306.

Mushlin, A.I. and F.A. Appel (1980) "Testing and outcome-based quality assurance strategy in primary care." *Medical Care* 18 (May Supplement): 1–100.

Novick, L.F., K. Dickinson, R. Asnes, S-P.M. Lan, and R. Lowenstein (1976) "Assessment of ambulatory care: applications of the tracer methodology." *Medical Care* 19 (January): 1–12.

Osborne, C.E. and H.C. Thompson (1975) "Criteria for evaluation of ambulatory child health care by chart audit: development and testing of a methodology." *Pediatrics* 56 (October, Part 2): 625–692.

Palmer, R.H., R. Strain, J.V.W. Maurer, J.K. Rothrock, and M.S. Thompson (1984) "Quality assurance in eight adult medicine group practices." *Medical Care* 22 (July): 632–643.

Payne, B.C., T.F. Lyons, L. Dwarshius, M. Kolton, and W. Morris (1976) The Quality of Medical Care: Evaluation and Improvement. Chicago: Hospital Research and Educational Trust.

Peterson, O.L. and E. Barsamian (1964) "Diagnostic performance," pp. 347–362 in J.A. Jacquez (ed.) The Diagnostic Process. Ann Arbor: University of Michigan School of Medicine.

——and E. Murray (1966) "A study of diagnostic performance: preliminary report." *J. of Medical Education* 41 (August): 797–803.

Peterson, O.L., L.P. Andrews, R.S. Spain, and B.G. Greenberg (1956) "An analytical study of North Carolina general practice, 1953–54." *J. of Medical Education* 31 (December, part 2): 1–165.

Rhee, S.-O. (1976) "Factors determining the quality of physician performance in patient care." *Medical Care* 14 (September): 733–750.

Riedel, R.L. and D.C. Riedel (1979) Practice and Performance: An Assessment of Ambulatory Care. Ann Arbor, MI: Health Administration Press.

Roemer, M.I., A.T. Moustafa, and C.E. Hopkins (1968) "A proposed hospital quality index: hospital death rates adjusted for case severity." *Health Services Research* 3 (Summer): 96–118.

Schonfeld, H.K., J.F. Henston, and I.S. Falk (1975) Standards for Good Medical Care, Vols. 1–4. Washington, DC: Government Printing Office.

Scott, W.R., W.H. Forrest, Jr., and B.W. Brown (1976) "Hospital structure and postoperative mortality and morbidity," pp. 72–89 in S.M. Shortell and M. Brown (eds.) Organizational Research in Hospitals. Chicago: Blue Cross Association.

Scott, W.R., A.B. Flood, and W. Ewy (1979) "Organizational determinants of services, quality and cost of care in hospitals." *Milbank Memorial Fund. Q./Health and Society* 57 (Spring): 234–264.

Shapiro, S., L. Weiner, and P.M. Densen (1958) "Comparison of prematurity and perinatal mortality in a general population and in the population of a prepaid group practice, medical care plan." *Amer. J. of Public Health* 48 (February): 170–187.

Shapiro, S., H. Jacobziner, P.M. Densen, and L. Weiner (1960) "Further observations on prematurity and perinatal mortality in a general population and in the population of a prepaid group practice medical care plan." *Amer. J. of Public Health* 50 (September): 1304–1317.

Shortell, S.M., S.W. Becker, and D. Neuhauser (1976) "The effects of managerial practices on hospital efficiency and quality of care," pp. 90–107 in S.M. Shortell and M. Brown (eds.) Organizational Research in Hospitals: Blue Cross Association.

Southmayd, H.J. and G. Smith (1944) Small Community Hospitals. Cambridge, MA: Harvard Univ. Press.

Staff of the Stanford Center for Health Care Research (1976) "Comparison of hospitals with regard to outcomes of surgery." *Health Services Research* (Summer): 112–127.

Starfield. B., D. Steinwachs, I. Morris, G. Bause, S. Siebert, and C. Westin (1979) "Concordance between medical records and observations regarding information on coordination of care." *Medical Care* 17 (July): 758–766.

Stockwell, H. and E. Vayda (1979) "Variations in surgery in Ontario." *Medical Care* 17 (April): 390–396.

Vayda, E. (1973) "A comparison of surgical rates in Canada and in England and Wales." *New England J. of Medicine* 289 (December 6): 1224–1229.

Wagner, E.H., R.A. Greenberg, P.B. Imprey, C.A. Williams, S.H. Wolf, and M.A. Ibrahim (1976) "Influence of training and experience on selecting criteria to evaluate medical care." *New England J. of Medicine* 294 (April 16): 871–876.

Wagner, E.H., C.A. Williams, R. Greenberg, D. Kleinbaum, S. Wolf, and M.A. Ibrahim (1978 "A method for selecting criteria to evaluate medical care." *Amer. J. of Public Health* 68 (May): 464–470.

Weed, L.L. (1971) "Quality control and the medical record." *Archives of Internal Medicine* 127 (January): 101–105.

Weed, L.L. (1969) Medical Records, Medical Education, and Patient Care. Chicago: Year Book Medical.

Wennberg, J. and A. Gittelsohn (1973) "Small area variations in health care delivery." *Science* 182 (December 14): 1102–1108.

Williamson, J.W. (1978a) Assessing and Improving Health Care Outcomes: The Health Accounting Approach to Quality Assurance. Cambridge, MA: Ballinger.

——(1978b) "Formulating priorities for quality assurance: de-scription of a method and its application." *J. of the Amer. Medical Assn.* 239 (February 13): 631–637.

——(1971) "Evaluating quality of patient care: a strategy relating outcome and process assessment." *J. of the Amer. Medical Assn.* 218 (October 25): 564–569.

——H.R. Braswell, and S.D. Horn (1979) "Validity of medical staff judgments in establishing quality assurance priorities." *Medical Care* 17 (April): 331–346.

——and S. Lohmeyer (1978) "Priority setting in quality assurance: reliability of staff judgments in medical institutions." *Medical Care* 16 (November): 931–940.

Wyszewianski, L. and A. Donabedian (1981) "Equity in the distribution of quality of care." *Medical Care* 19 (December Supplement): 28–56.

Zuckerman, A.E., B. Starfield, C. Hochreiter, and B. Kovaszmay (1975) "Validating the content of pediatric outpatient medical records by means of tape recording doctor-patient encounters." *Pediatrics* 56 (September): 407–411.

# Chapter 24

# The Epidemiology
# of Quality

## Avedis Donabedian, M.D., M.P.H.

*The quality of care can be perceived to have an "epidemiology" in that it is distributed in each of two populations, one of providers and another of clients. In this review of the pertinent literature, I found, overall, that the quality of technical care is better when practitioners have better or more training, are more specialized, and are more experienced though not too old; when they provide ambulatory care by appointment to a not overly large caseload in well-equipped premises and possibly in association with colleagues; and when they provide hospital care in larger institutions with significant teaching functions. I fund no consistent correlation between quality and age, sex, rurality, occupation, income, and ethnicity of patients, but there were enough intimations of a relation between socioeconomic disadvantage and poorer technical care to prompt careful study.*

The epidemiology of quality is the study of the distribution of quality at any given time and of changes in its distribution through time. Time, place, and person, the traditional triad of descriptive epidemiology, apply to the study of the quality of medical care as well. But the epidemiology of quality seems to be distinctive in having, simultaneously, two sets of populations to which it pertains: one of providers and another of clients. This duality, if nothing else, should invest the epidemiology of quality with a peculiar appeal.

Knowledge of the distribution of quality among the providers of health care services (whether these providers are individual practitioners, teams, organizational units, or entire institutions) is the product of the more usual studies of quality that throw light on the relation between structure, on the one hand, and either process or outcome on the other.[1] Often, the more immediate purpose of these studies is to demonstrate that certain attributes of providers can be used to indicate a greater or lesser likelihood that good quality will be delivered. In this way, structural attributes become indirect measures of the quality of care as well as indicators of where the quality of care is likely to be deficient and, therefore, worthy of more assiduous supervision. But more fundamentally, elucidation of the relation between structure and performance is central to the science of health care organization, insofar as such a science can be said to exist. We must understand the determinants of performance, for example, if we are to design a more effective system of health care.

The distribution of specified levels of quality among various groupings of the consumers of care is, of course, the ultimate measure of success or failure in achieving

Reprinted with permission from *Inquiry*, 22: 282–292 (Fall 1985). Copyright 1985 Blue Cross and Blue Shield Association.

the social objectives of a health care system. It is necessary, therefore, to know who receives better care and who worse, and what the reasons for the inequality are.

We see that the epidemiology of quality has functions analogous to those of the more familiar epidemiology of health states: It is both a method of scientific inquiry and a tool for action. To the extent that health states are used in studies of quality as a measure of outcome, the two epidemiologies do, in fact, overlap, except that in order to serve the epidemiology of quality, observed disparities in health states must be attributable to corresponding differences in antecedent care.

It is not the purpose of this paper to deal with the epidemiology of quality as a method of scientific inquiry. The paper will merely offer a review of what we know about the relation between attributes of providers and clients and the quality of care that they, respectively, provide and receive. The reader can look elsewhere for a general discussion of the definition and measurement of quality[2] and for a detailed assessment of the methods used in the studies from which most of the information in this paper is culled.[3]

Even as a vehicle for the empirical findings, this paper, though reasonably detailed, is incomplete. First, studies that do not offer, or lead to, reasonably direct judgments on the quantitative or qualitative adequacy of care have been omitted. The vast literature on patterns of differential utilization was, therefore, excluded. Quality was then defined quite narrowly so that attention focused on the technical care provided mainly by physicians. The consequent omission of client satisfaction is a particularly limiting exclusion. Finally, even within the narrower field delineated above, the information gathered in this paper is meant only to be illustrative rather than exhaustive.

It is also important to realize that there are no national studies of quality from which we could obtain an undistorted picture of the level and distribution of quality, either here or abroad. For that purpose, and also to obtain a picture of temporal trends in quality, we must depend on reports of mortality, morbidity, longevity, and use of service—reports that are, insofar as their implications for the quality of care are concerned, extremely difficult to interpret. What we do have is a rather large assemblage of studies, using methods that vary in accuracy and stringency, to assess diverse aspects of the quality of care provided by selected practitioners to circumscribed populations at different periods. As a result, there is little we can say about the levels of quality in the United States as a whole, besides noting that almost invariably performance seems to fall far short of the criteria and standards used to judge the quality of care. And because one expects that as medical science progresses these criteria and standards will become correspondingly more stringent, there is little to be learned

about secular trends from comparisons of current studies with those in the past, even if on other grounds the comparison might seem appropriate. For the same reasons, what is said concerning the factors that influence quality should also be treated with caution, even though in this case we can be somewhat more assured of the general applicability of the observed associations, particularly when they are repeatedly encountered and seem to be reasonable in the light of what we know about the health care system in general.

## VARIABILITY AND LOCALIZATION

The distribution of behaviors that directly or indirectly connote quality reveals an astounding degree of variability among geographic areas, practitioners, and institutions. Particular attention has been paid in recent years to the poorly understood variations in the incidence of surgical procedures among small areas within the United States,[4] within other countries,[5] and among countries.[6] There is also considerable variation among practitioners and institutions in any given, rather circumscribed geographic area, and even among practitioners within a given institution. Adherence to the implicit or explicit criteria of good care has been observed to vary among general practitioners[7] and internists[8] practicing in an area. The same is true for physicians in a set of associated group practices.[9] There are wide variations in the cost of care provided by physicians in a group practice[10] and by physicians and other practitioners in a university-affiliated clinic.[11] The number and cost of diagnostic procedures vary considerably among physicians who practice in a geographic locale,[12] a hospital,[13] or a group practice.[14] The propensity to remove normal tissue in primary appendectomies is astoundingly variable among physicians in a hospital and also among the staffs of different hospitals, each taken as a whole.[15]

Hospitals and ambulatory care institutions are known to vary with regard to other aspects of quality as well. For example, hospitals have been observed to differ greatly in the proportion of unjustified hysterectomies performed in them,[16] in the incidence of postoperative fatality and complications,[17] in the occurrence of preventable maternal mortality,[18] and in the adherence of their staffs to the implicit or explicit criteria of appropriate use and quality.[19] The quality of care provided by organized ambulatory care settings has been observed to be similarly variable.[20]

Greatly variable though the practice of health care may be, the variability is far from random. Questionable practices, on the contrary, are known to be highly concentrated or localized. It has been observed, for example, that relatively small proportions of physicians account for a relatively large share of questionable drugs[21] and injections.[22] The concentration of tonsillectomies[23] and of other surgery[24] in relatively few hands raises the suspicion that those who are responsible for most of the operations may be doing too many, whereas those who are doing too few are not able to maintain their surgical skills.

Variability and localization are the twin necessities of epidemiology. What remains is to identify the attributes with which appropriate use and quality are associated.

## TRAINING, EXPERIENCE, SPECIALIZATION, AND AGE OF PRACTITIONERS

The key attributes that influence physician performance (beyond the possible influence of personality traits, a subject concerning which I have no information) are apparently training, experience, and specialization.

The effect of training is illustrated repeatedly in the literature. General practice has been observed to be of higher quality among physicians who were better students,[25] who were educated in certain categories of medical schools,[26] and who had longer periods of certain kinds of training,[27] there being a mutually reinforcing effect when two or more of these attributes coexist.[28] Generalists taken as a group, however, are usually found to maintain a lower standard of practice compared with their more highly specialized colleagues, at least when judged by criteria that usually correspond more closely to the opinions of specialists.

Specialists appear to perform better than generalists in many aspects of ambulatory and inpatient care. Specialists use x-ray examinations more appropriately,[29] give fewer questionable injections,[30] use the hospital more appropriately,[31] more often comply with the implicit or explicit criteria of hospital care[32] and of ambulatory care,[33] and are responsible for fewer "preventable" perinatal deaths.[34] There is evidence, moreover, that the effect of specialization is contingent on a specialist's restricting his or her domain of practice to the cases that fall strictly within the corresponding area of specialization.[35] Furthermore, organizations that as a whole are more specialized in their functions appear to provide better care.[36]

Training and specialization are, of course, intimately related to experience. There are two additional components to experience: 1) years in practice and 2) volume of similar cases treated or of nearly identical procedures performed each year. As concerns the second of these two (the volume of care), there is evidence that larger hospitals provide better technical care,[37] though not necessarily care with which patients are satisfied.[38] But institutional size is an attribute with several connotations; experience with larger volumes of similar cases, either by individual practitioners or by the hospital's staff as a whole, is only one of these. It is interesting to find,

therefore, that fatality following certain surgical procedures is lower in hospitals where more of these procedures are performed[39] and that preventable maternal deaths are judged to occur less often in hospitals where a large number of deliveries take place.[40] A contrary observation, perhaps attributable to adverse factors associated with hospital size, is a positive association of the annual number of births with neonatal and maternal mortality in a national sample of hospitals.[41]

The effect of the experience that accrues with longer duration of practice seems to be obscured by the obsolescence of medical knowledge that apparently occurs at the same time. As a result, advanced age seems almost always to be associated with lower levels of performance. Although it is not clear whether it is good or bad to do so, older physicians use fewer laboratory tests and x-rays.[42] Other observations, more clearly indicative of quality, have shown that older physicians with more years in practice use x-ray procedures less appropriately;[43] more often use questionable injections;[44] perform less appropriately as general practitioners in a community,[45] as family physicians in group practice,[46] and as physicians in a variety of ambulatory care settings;[47] and provide hospital care that is less likely to conform to preformulated explicit criteria than that provided by physicians in their intermediate years of practice.[48] In a study that found a bimodal pattern that is the opposite of this last one, the best pediatricians in one community were found to have been in practice for either less than 12 years or more than 40; but on the whole, the longer general practitioners were in practice, the lower their adherence to the criteria of ambulatory care.[49]

Because these studies of the relation between age and performance are all cross-sectional in design, having observed only contemporaneous differences among physicians, we cannot tell how much of the difference between the young and the old is due to a failure of the latter to acquire new knowledge or skill and how much is the result of a loss of knowledge or skill originally possessed. It is also likely, as the foregoing comparisons between pediatricians and general practitioners imply, that under certain circumstances that now can only be surmised, the balance of these two tendencies (the acquisition and loss of competence) will remain favorable, at least until extreme old age inevitably takes its toll.

## CONDITIONS OF OFFICE PRACTICE

The performance of physicians is also influenced by the conditions in their own practices and in the organizations or institutions where they work. For example, general practitioners in rural North Carolina in the early 1950s seemed to do better work when they had a larger variety of certain kinds of equipment (a microscope, a clinical centrifuge, an electrocardiograph, an apparatus for determining basal metabolic rate, and a photoelectric calorimeter) in their offices.[50] Seeing patients by appointment was found to be correlated with higher levels of performance by general practitioners in rural North Carolina,[51] by general practitioners in the Canadian provinces of Ontario and Nova Scotia,[52] and by family physicians in an association of group practices in New York City and vicinity.[53] Family physicians in this last setting were also observed to provide better care if they had a full-time office assistant or if they used a medical record with a larger format.[54]

Physicians who are very busy may begin to provide less complete care (as judged by the records they keep) when the number of patients seen each hour becomes too large.[55] As physicians become busier, their office records have been found to show evidence of less compliance with criteria for history taking and physical examination while there is greater compliance with criteria for laboratory test.[56] This suggests that the latter could be a substitute for the former.

## FINANCING AND ORGANIZATION OF CARE

There is also evidence, not always fully convincing, that financial incentives may influence practice. It appears that physicians who own x-ray equipment are more likely to use it, and to do so less appropriately;[57] that more surgery is performed when surgeons are less able or willing to make charges beyond those approved by an insurer;[58] that appendectomies are probably less often justified when the hospital stay is financed by a Blue Cross Plan;[59] and that patients who have help in paying for their hospital stays experience overstays more often and understays less often than do patients who pay the entire bill themselves.[60] These observations can be supplemented by a wealth of evidence showing that when prepayment is combined with group practice, there is a more parsimonious, and perhaps more appropriate, use of services.[61]

Participation in an organized group, clinic, or similar institution can be expected to alter radically the terms and conditions of practice, bringing about corresponding changes in the quality of technical care. It has been observed, for example, that the quality of ambulatory care for children is better in hospital outpatient departments than in office practice, at least as judged by entries in the medical record.[62] In rural North Carolina, general practitioners who worked in associations of two or more were observed to provide better care, perhaps because they were on the average better qualified by education and training, were younger, and had organized and equipped their practices in a manner more favorable to good performance.[63] No such relationship between quality

and working in an association of two or more was observed for general practitioners in the Canadian provinces of Ontario and Nova Scotia.[64]

In the same vein, a more recent study in Hawaii suggests that physicians in multispecialty groups did not provide ambulatory care that was indisputably better than that provided by solo practitioners.[65] The physicians in such groups did, however, clearly use the hospital more appropriately, and provided better hospital care, than did physicians in solo practice.[66] But this association between belonging to a group practice and the nature of hospital care was explained by the fact that the groups employed specialists who restricted their practice to the domains of their respective specialties.[67]

It would be interesting and important to know whether group practice exerts an effect on quality through mechanisms in addition to the mere selection of the physicians who participate in the group, important though that is. Evidence for more subtle forms of influence may be inferred from observations that the quality of care provided by family physicians in a set of associated group practices was better when the physicians had a longer affiliation with the group, gave more of their time to the group, and spent more time in the facility owned by the group.[68] The importance of an active hospital affiliation is confirmed by the observation that the quality of ambulatory care was better when the physicians had such an appointment, when the appointment was at a higher rank, and when more hospital visits were made.[69] But, as if to highlight the complexity of the physician-hospital relationship, there was no association in rural North Carolina between the quality of office care and the degree to which the physician was "active" in the use of the hospital, though the better doctors were more selective and skillful in their use of hospital services.[70]

There is some evidence about the association between access by patients to an organized practice and the outcome of care. The incidence of first attacks of rheumatic fever has been observed to be lower after the establishment of a comprehensive care center in a low-income area.[71] Enrollees in one prepaid group practice plan received more prenatal care and experienced a lower rate of neonatal mortality than a sample of the general population, the advantage being greater for blacks than whites.[72] But a more recent study in another community shows that the enrollees of a prepaid group practice received less prenatal care but had an equal level of neonatal mortality, leading the investigators to suggest a higher degree of efficiency in the attainment of a given outcome.[73]

## HOSPITAL CHARACTERISTICS

Of all the organizations that provide health care, hospitals are perhaps the most likely to control the quality of care provided in them. The attributes of hospitals, alone or in association with the characteristics of the physicians who work in them therefore, can be expected to have a large influence on the quality of care. I have already alluded to the possible effects of hospital size. More important by far appears to be the teaching function of the hospital, particularly when that function is reinforced by a close affiliation with a medical school.

Teaching hospitals are more often appropriately used.[74] Appendectomies in teaching hospitals more often appear to be justified.[75] The care provided in teaching hospitals more often conforms to implicit and explicit criteria of quality, at least as shown by the medical record.[76] Case fatality was found to be lower in teaching hospitals in England and Wales,[77] and preventable perinatal deaths were lower in teaching hospitals in New York City compared with their voluntary or municipal counterparts that had no teaching functions.[78]

There are some disquieting exceptions to this general harmony of praise. In one national study of obstetrical care, maternal mortality, neonatal mortality, and the stillbirth ratio were all higher in hospitals affiliated with medical schools, conceivably because differences in case mix were not adjusted for.[79] The same possible explanation does not hold for some other studies that, having made extensive corrections for differences among patients, still found that adverse postoperative events and teaching status—when the latter was indicated by measures such as medical school affiliation, the presence of residency training, or the number of house staff per hospital bed—were either unrelated[80] or were perhaps positively related.[81]

Information about the quality of care in proprietary hospitals is fragmentary; it is also difficult to interpret, since these hospitals differ so much from one another and are so influenced by the circumstances of time and place. After an adjustment for differences in length of stay were made, the case fatality for patients hospitalized in proprietary hospitals was reported to be higher than that for patients in voluntary hospitals in Los Angeles County in 1964,[82] but not unequivocally so in New York City in 1971.[83] By contrast, during 1950–51, preventable perinatal deaths occurred less frequently in the proprietary hospitals of New York City than in any other category of institutions except voluntary teaching hospitals.[84] But again in New York City, care in proprietary hospitals, at least for a certain segment of the population during 1961 or 1962, was much more often inappropriate and of "less than optimal" quality, particularly in the hands of physicians to whom only the proprietary hospitals would grant privileges.[85]

Seeing how much importance is given to hospital accreditation, it is remarkable how little is known about its relationship to the demonstrated quality of care. This may be because all the better hospitals are already

accredited, so that the contribution that might be specifically attributed to accreditation is difficult to tease out. In one study of national scope, no significant association was found between accreditation status and postoperative fatality for three conditions after differences in case mix had been corrected for.[86] Among other fragments of information on the subject, hospital case fatality adjusted for length of stay is lower in accredited hospitals[87] and accreditation seems to be associated with somewhat higher quality when otherwise similar voluntary hospitals are compared but not when similar accredited and unaccredited proprietary hospitals are compared.[88] A study of 30 hospitals in the Chicago area, all accredited, showed that the more detailed ratings of medical departments by the surveyors of the Joint Commission on Accreditation of Hospitals were associated, when favorable, with lower case fatality rates, after adjustment for differences in length of stay, and with better reputations for the hospitals among knowledgeable informants.[89]

Hospitals no doubt influence quality partly through the facilities and equipment they provide and partly through selecting the physicians and other personnel who are permitted to work in them. There appears to be, however, yet another effect, one mediated through organizational controls. In any event, there is an interaction between the characteristics of hospitals and the attributes of the physicians who practice in them. The formal qualifications of individual physicians seem less important indicators of quality in a hospital affiliated with a university than in one that is not. By contrast, the less able the hospital and its medical staff are to control the practice of medicine in the hospital, the more likely is the care received by patients to depend on the qualifications of individual physicians.[90] Irrespective of university affiliation, the quality of technical care seems to be best in the hands of highly trained physicians in tightly organized hospitals and worst in the hands of less highly trained physicians in hospitals with looser forms of organization.[91]

A growing number of studies draw on the theory of organizations to explore the relation between quality and the details of organizational structure and behavior. These studies offer possible explanations for some of the more obvious correlations we have known about, but they also reveal new associations we had not suspected and occasionally find difficult to understand or believe.[92] We find, for example, that although hospital size, teaching status, or a higher proportion of more qualified personnel is sometimes not associated with better outcomes (either surgical or both medical and surgical), such outcomes seem to be better when there are higher levels of coordination in the hospital as a whole, in patient care wards, or in operating rooms,[93] and when there is greater control over the privileges and activities of the surgical staff.[94] By contrast, one study unexpectedly revealed that when nursing administrators had a greater degree of power in their own "domain," postoperative mortality was worse rather than better.[95] Although we hesitate to accept this finding, unless it signifies less communication between doctors and nurses, we think we gain a new perspective on the relation between age and performance when we are told that hospitals that employ a higher proportion of doctors who have been in practice for many years are also hospitals characterized by a greater laxity in coordination and control.[96]

## CHARACTERISTICS OF CLIENTS

So far, we have been concerned with the distribution of technical quality among providers. Much less is known about its distribution among clients, although this should be a matter of the greatest importance to public policy.[97]

Differences in the quality of care provided to different categories of persons may arise in one of two ways. Different people may have different degrees of access to different kinds of practitioners and institutions. This is a form of social differentiation that we seem willing to tolerate, even when we regard it as unfortunate. We are less able to contemplate the second possibility: that patients with similar needs for technical care will be treated differently when seen by the same practitioner, or cared for in the same institution, unless the difference is only in the amenities of care. This reluctance may partly explain our unwillingness or inability even to study the subject, with the result that there is very little known about it. More is known about a third factor that influences the quality of care, namely, the ability or willingness of clients to participate in influencing the recommendations of the physician and in carrying them out. This paper, however, does not include studies of patient participation and compliance.

The variability in the quantity and quality of provider care already noted must have its counterpart among the people who use these providers. We can expect to see, therefore, corresponding differences among those who reside in different geographic areas or who are clients of different hospitals and practitioners. The clients of any given set of practitioners can also be expected to vary a great deal in the quality of care they receive.[98]

As to the association between client attributes and the quality of care received, there are snippets of information about the effects of place of residence, age, sex, race, occupation, having insurance, and indexes of socioeconomic status.

It is reasonable to expect that rural residents experience the adverse consequences of reduced access to care, particularly to care by more highly specialized physicians and those in the larger, university-affiliated hospitals. For example, the improper use of an antibiotic has been shown to be more frequent in rural areas, even

when physician specialty status has been taken into account.[99] Surgical procedures are less often performed for residents of less highly urbanized areas.[100] But if the possibility of unnecessary intervention is considered, being less subject to surgery may not necessarily be a bad thing. At least one study has noted an association of urban residence with more frequent appendectomies and higher fatality from appendicitis.[101]

The evidence concerning the possible effect of age and sex is fragmentary and inconclusive. On the one hand, there appears to be no consistent association between the age of the patient and the quality of either hospital care or office care in Hawaii.[102] On the other hand, the quality of nursing services in a selected group of urban hospitals has been observed to be somewhat better for younger males than for younger females, and better for older females than for older males.[103] In one study abroad, females were found to be more subject to appendectomy, and the surgery more often yielded normal tissue, but this could possibly be explained by the greater difficulty of diagnosing appendicitis in females.[104]

Comparisons based on differences in race are equally sparse and inconclusive. There was no association between ethnic origin and the quality of hospital care in Hawaii, nor was the quality of hospital care, at least in its conformity to technical standards, influenced in a consistent manner by whether the patient received care from a physician of similar or disparate ethnic origin.[105] Hawaii could be atypical in this regard. Other studies have found that surgical operations are fewer among nonwhites,[106] that nonwhites may be receiving nursing care of lower quality,[107] and that when surgery is done, it is more often performed by resident staff than by surgeons with more experience or higher qualifications.[108] One cannot conclude, of course, that the care provided by resident staff is necessarily inferior. In one study, house staff were found to perform quite well,[109] whereas in another study their performance was reported to be rather poor.[110]

Occupational differences are interesting partly because occupation is an important indicator of socioeconomic status (as is, unfortunately, ethnic origin) and partly because the use of services by physicians and members of their families may be used as a standard of care.[111] It has been noted, for example, that the wives of physicians are much more likely to have had a hysterectomy than are women in general.[112] This may also mean, however, that the wives of physicians are more exposed to unnecessary surgery. Hysterectomies are known to be frequently proposed and performed when not completely justified.[113] A study in the German city of Hannover shows that white-collar workers have more appendectomies but that the tissue removed is less often acutely inflamed.[114] Much more to the point is the observation that persons connected with medicine or nursing may experience higher risk because of the much greater readiness to subject them to appendectomies that prove not to have been justified.[115]

These observations suggest that greater access to care may have adverse as well as beneficial consequences. This principle appears to apply when coverage by private health insurance or by a governmental program improves the ability to pay for care. It has been observed that such coverage decreases underuse of the hospital but at the same time increases overuse.[116] Appendectomies for patients whose hospital stays were financed by Blue Cross Plans appeared to yield normal or questionable tissue in a higher proportion of cases.[117]

In some studies, the outcomes of care have been used to tell us something about the influence of social and economic factors on the quality of care and its consequences. It has been reported, for example, that patients with higher incomes are less likely to suffer post-operative morbidity or death, even when many extraneous factors that might account for the finding are corrected for.[118] Mothers assigned to lower socioeconomic categories on the basis of average house rents have been shown to experience higher rates of preventable maternal mortality, the difference being largely attributable to failure of the expectant mother to obtain suitable care.[119] The proportion of perinatal deaths considered preventable is larger when the birth takes place in a municipal hospital rather than a voluntary one, or when the mother and child are cared for in a ward rather than the private service of a hospital.[120] When the organization of care is improved, there may be an associated improvement in prenatal care and a reduction in neonatal mortality, the relative improvements being greater for those who are ordinarily disadvantaged. But the disadvantage is not completely remedied.[121] Even approximately equal access to reasonably equal care does not necessarily result in equal enjoyment of health.

That does not mean, of course, that we must abandon hope; it only means that we must try harder, and on a wider front.

**Notes:** *This paper is based on the epilogue to the author's book* The Methods and Findings of Quality Assessment and Monitoring: An Illustrated Analysis, *published by the Health Administration Press. Copyright to the book is held by the Regents of the University of Michigan. The work was supported by the Commonwealth Fund, the Carnegie Corporation of New York, the Milbank Memorial Fund, the W. K. Kellogg Foundation, and the National Center for Health Services Research. The views expressed are those of the author; they do not in any way represent his sponsors.*

# References

1. A. Donabedian. *Explorations in Quality Assessment and Monitoring,* vol. 1: *The Definition of Quality and Approaches to Its Assessment* (Ann Arbor, MI: Health Administration Press, 1980).

2. Ibid.; A. Donabedian, *Explorations in Quality Assessment and Monitoring,* vol. 2: *The Criteria and Standards of Quality* (Ann Arbor, MI: Health Administration Press, 1982).

3. A. Donabedian, *Explorations in Quality Assessment and Monitoring,* vol. 3: *The Methods and Findings of Quality Assessment and Monitoring: An Illustrated Analysis* (Ann Arbor, MI: Health Administration Press, 1985).

4. P. A. Lembcke, "Measuring the Quality of Medical Care Through Vital Statistics Based on Hospital Service Areas, 1: Comparative Study of Appendectomy Rates," *American Journal of Public Health* 42 (1952): 276–286; C. E. Lewis, "Variations in the Incidence of Surgery," *New England Journal of Medicine* 281 (1969): 880–884; J. Wennberg and A. Gittelsohn, "Small Area Variations in Health Care Delivery," *Science* 182 (1973): 1102–1108; A. M. Gittelsohn and J. E. Wennberg, "On the Incidence of Tonsillectomy and Other Common Surgical Procedures," in *Costs, Risks, and Benefits of Surgery,* ed. J. P. Bunker, B. A. Barnes, and F. Mosteller (New York: Oxford University Press, 1977); J. R. Griffith, J. D. Restuccia, P. J. Tedeschi, P. A. Wilson, and H. S. Zuckerman, "Measuring Community Hospital Services in Michigan," *Health Services Research* 16 (1981):135–160.

5. H. Stockwell and E. Vayda, "Variations in Surgery in Ontario," *Medical Care* 17 (1979): 390–396.

6. J.P. Bunker, "Surgical Manpower: A Comparison of Operations and Surgeons in the United States and in England and Wales," *New England Journal of Medicine* 282 (1970): 135–144; E. Vayda, "A Comparison of Surgical Rates in Canada and in England and Wales," *New England Journal of Medicine* 289 (1973): 1224–1229; K. McPherson, J. E. Wennberg, O. B. Hovind, and P. Clifford, "Small-Area Variations in the Use of Common Surgical Procedures: An International Comparison of New England, England, and Norway," *New England Journal of Medicine* 307 (1982): 1310–1314.

7. O. L. Peterson, L. P. Andrews, R. S. Spain, and B. G. Greenberg, "An Analytical Study of North Carolina General Practice, 1953–1954, " *Journal of Medical Education* 31, pt. 2 (December 1956): 1–165; K. F. Clute, *The General Practitioner: A Study of Medical Education and Practice in Ontario and Nova Scotia* (Toronto: University of Toronto Press, 1963).

8. B. S. Hulka, F. J. Romm, G. R. Parkerson, Jr., I. T. Russell, N. E. Clapp, and F. S. Johnson, "Peer Review in Ambulaory Care: Use of Explicit Criteria and Implicit Judgments," *Medical Care* 17, suppl. (March 1979): 1–73.

9. M. A. Morehead, *Quality of Medical Care Provided by Family Physicians as Related to Their Education, Training and Methods of Practice* (New York: Health Insurance Plan of Greater New York, 1958).

10. C. B. Lyle, D. S. Citron, W. C. Sugg, and O. D. Williams, "Cost of Medical Care in a Practice of Internal Medicine: A Study in a Group of Seven Internists," *Annals of Internal Medicine* 81 (1974): 1–6.

11. D. D. Wright, R. L. Kane, G. F. Snell, and F. R. Wolley, "Costs and Outcomes for Different Primary Care Providers," *Journal of the American Medical Association* 238 (1977): 46–50.

12. J. M. Eisenberg and D. Nicklin, "Use of Diagnostic Services by Physicians in Community Practice," *Medical Care* 19 (1981): 297–309.

13. S. A. Schroeder, A. Schliftman, and T. E. Piemme, "Variation Among Physicians in the Use of Laboratory Tests: Relation to Quality of Care," *Medical Care* 12 (1974): 709–713.

14. D. K. Freeborn, D. Baer, M. R. Greenlick, and J. W. Bailey, "Determinants of Medical Care Utilization: Physicians' Use of Laboratory Services," *American Journal of Public Health* 62 (1972): 846–853.

15. H. A. Weeks, *Tightness of Organization Related to Patterns of Patient Care* (Ann Arbor: University of Michigan, School of Public Health, Bureau of Public Health Economics, n.d.); J. F. Sparling, "Measuring Medical Care Quality: A Comparative Study," *Hospitals* 36 (Mar. 16, 1962): 62–68; 36 (Apr. 1, 1962): 56–57, 60–61.

16. J. C. Doyle, "Unnecessary Hysterectomies: Study of 6,248 Operations in Thirty-Five Hospitals During 1948," *Journal of the American Medical Association* 51 (1953): 360–365.

17. J. P. Bunker, W. H. Forrest, Jr., F. Mosteller, and L. D. Vandam (eds.), *The National Halothane Study: A Study of the Possible Association Between Halothane Anesthesia and Postoperative Hepatic Necrosis* (Bethesda, MD: National Institutes of Health, National Institute of General Medical Sciences, 1969); Stanford Center for Health Care Research, "Comparison of Hospitals With Regard to Outcomes of Surgery," *Health Services Research* 11 (1976): 112–127; W. R. Scott, W. H. Forrest, Jr., and B. W. Brown, "Hospital Structure and Postoperative Mortality and Morbidity," in *Organizational Research in Hospitals,* ed. S. M. Shortell and M. Brown (Chicago: Blue Cross Association, 1976); W. R. Scott, A. B. Flood, and W. Ewy, "Organizational Determinants of Services, Quality and Cost of Care in Hospitals," *Milbank Memorial Fund Quarterly: Health and Society* 57 (1979): 234–264; A. B. Flood and W. R. Scott, "Professional Power and Professional Effectiveness: The Power of the Surgical Staff and the Quality of Surgical Care in Hospitals," *Journal of Health and Social Behavior* 19 (1978): 240–254; A. B. Flood, W. Ewy, W. R. Scott, W. H. Forrest, Jr., and B. W. Brown, "The Relationship Between Intensity and Duration of Medical Services and Outcomes for Hospitalized Patients," *Medical Care* 17 (1979): 1088–1102; A. B. Flood, W. R. Scott, and E. Wayne, "Does Practice Make Perfect? 1: The Relation Between Hospital Volume and Outcomes for Selected Diagnostic Categories," *Medical Care* 22 (1984): 98–114; A. B. Flood, W. R. Scott, and E. Wayne, "Does Practice Make Perfect? 2: The Relation Between Volume and Outcomes and Other Hospital Characteristics," *Medical Care* 22 (1984): 115–125.

18. New York Academy of Medicine, Committee on Public Health Relations, *Maternal Mortality in New York City: A Study of All Puerperal Deaths 1930–1932* (New York: Oxford University Press, for the Commonwealth Fund, 1933).

19. M. A. Morehead et al., *A Study of the Quality of Hospital Care Secured by a Sample of Teamster Family Members in New York City* (New York: Columbia University, School of Public Health and Administrative Medicine, 1964); L. S. Rosenfeld, "Quality of Medical Care in Hospitals," *American Journal of Public Health* 47 (1957); 856–865; S.-O. Rhee, "Relative Influence of Specialty Status, Organization of Office Care and Organization of Hospital Care on the Quality of Medical Care: A Multivariate Analysis" (doctoral dissertation, University of Michigan, 1975); S.-O. Rhee, "Factors Determining the Quality of Physician Performance in Patient Care," *Medical Care* 14 (1976): 733–750.

20. B. C. Payne, T. F. Lyons, E. Neuhaus, M. Kolton, and L. Dwarshius, *Method for Evaluating and Improving Ambulatory Care* (Ann Arbor, MI: Health Services Research Center, 1978); M. A. Morehead, R. S. Donaldson, and M. R. Seravelli, "Comparisons Between OEO Neighborhood Health Centers and Other Health Care Providers of Ratings of the Quality of Health Care," *American Journal of Public Health* 61 (1971): 1294–1306.

21. W. A. Ray, C. E. Federspiel, and W. Schaffner, "Prescribing of Chloramphenicol in Ambulatory Practice: An Epidemiologic Study Among Tennessee Medicaid Recipients," *Annals of Internal Medicine* 84 (1976): 266–270.

22. R. H. Brook and K. N. Williams, "Evaluation of the New Mexico Peer Review System, 1971 to 1973," *Medical Care* 14, suppl. (December 1976): 1–122.

23. Gittelsohn and Wennberg (note 4).

24. R. J. Nickerson, T. Colton, O. L. Peterson, B. S. Bloom, and W. W. Hauck, Jr., "Doctors Who Perform Operations: A Study on In-Hospital Surgery in Four Diverse Geographic Areas," *New England Journal of Medicine* 295 (1976): 921–926, 982–989.

25. Peterson et al. (note 7); Morehead (note 9).

26. Morehead (note 9).

27. Ibid.; Peterson et al. (note 7).

28. Ibid.

29. A. W. Childs and E. D. Hunter, "Non-Medical Factors Influencing use of Diagnostic X-Ray by Physicians," *Medical Care* 10 (1972): 323–325.

30. Brook and Williams (note 22).

31. B. C. Payne, T. F. Lyons, L. Dwarshius, M. Kolton, and W. Morris, *The Quality of Medical Care: Evaluation and Improvement* (Chicago: Hospital Research and Educational Trust, 1976); Morehead et al. (note 9).

32. Ibid.

33. R. L. Riedel and D. C. Riedel, *Practice and Performance: An Assessment of Ambulatory Care* (Ann Arbor, MI: Health Administration Press, 1979): Payne et al. (note 20).

34. S. G. Kohl, *Perinatal Mortality in New York City: Responsible Factors* (Cambridge, MA: Harvard University Press, for the Commonwealth Fund, 1955).

35. S.-O. Rhee, R. D. Luke, T. F. Lyons, and B. C. Payne, "Domain of Practice and the Quality of Physician Performance," *Medical Care* 19 (1981): 14–23; Rhee, "Relative Influence of Specialty Status" (note 19); Payne et al. (note 20); Payne et al. (note 31).

36. New York Academy of Medicine (note 18); Morehead et al. (note 20).

37. Rhee, "Relative Influence of Specialty Status" (note 19); Rhee, "Factors Determining the Quality of Physician Performance" (note 19).

38. G. V. Fleming, "Hospital Structure and Consumer Satisfaction," *Health Services Research* 16 (1981): 43–63.

39. H. S. Luft, J. P. Bunker, and A. C. Enthoven, "Should Operations Be Regionalized? The Empirical Relation Between Surgical Volume and Mortality," *New England Journal of Medicine* 301 (1979): 1364–1369; Flood et al. (note 17), parts 1 and 2.

40. New York Academy of Medicine (note 18).

41. American College of Obstetricians and Gynecologists, Committee on Maternal Health, *National Study of Maternity Care: Survey of Obstetric Practice and Associated Services in Hospitals in the United States* (Chicago: American College of Obstetricians and Gynecologists, 1970).

42. Eisenberg and Nicklin (note 12).

43. Childs and Hunter (note 29).

44. Brook and Williams (note 22).

45. Peterson et al. (note 7); Clute (note 7).

46. Morehead (note 9).

47. Payne et al. (note 20); Payne et al. (note 31).

48. Rhee, "Factors Determining the Quality of Physician Performance" (note 19).

49. Riedel and Riedel (note 33).

50. Peterson et al. (note 7).

51. Ibid.

52. Clute (note 7).

53. Morehead (note 9).

54. Ibid.

55. Payne et al. (note 20).

56. Hulka et al. (note 8).

57. Childs and Hunter (note 29).

58. United Steelworkers of America, Public Relations Department, *Special Study on the Medical Care Program for Steelworkers and Their Families* (Pittsburgh: USA, 1969).

59. Sparling (note 15).

60. R. B. Fitzpatrick, D. C. Riedel, and B. C. Payne, "Appropriateness of Admissions and Length of Stay," in *Hospital and Medical Economics: A Study of Population, Services, Costs, Methods of Payment, and Controls,* vol. 1, by W. J. McNerney et al. (Chicago: Hospital Research and Educational Trust, 1962).

61. A. Donabedian, "An Evaluation of Prepaid Group Practice," *Inquiry* 6 (1969): 3–27; M. I. Roemer and W. Shonick, "HMO Performance: The Recent Evidence," *Milbank Memorial Fund Quarterly: Health and Society* 51 (1973): 271–317; H. S. Luft, "Assessing the Evidence on HMO Performance," *Milbank Memorial Fund Quarterly: Health and Society* 58 (1980): 501–536.

62. Riedel and Riedel (note 33).

63. Peterson et al. (note 7).

64. Clute (note 7).

65. Payne et al. (note 31).

66. Ibid.

67. Rhee, "Relative Influence of Specialty Status" (note 19); Rhee, "Factors Determining the Quality of Physician Performance" (note 19).

68. Morehead (note 9).

69. Ibid.

70. Peterson et al. (note 7).

71. L. Gordis, "Effectiveness of Comprehensive-Care Programs in Preventing Rheumatic Fever," *New England Journal of Medicine* 289 (1973): 331–335.

72. S. Shapiro, L. Weiner, and P. M. Densen, "Comparison of Prematurity and Perinatal Mortality in a General Population and in the Population of a Prepaid Group Practice Medical Care Plan," *American Journal of Public Health* 48 (1958): 170–187.

73. J. D. Quick, M. R. Greenlick, and K. J. Roghmann, "Prenatal Care and Pregnancy Outcome in an HMO and General Population: A Multivariate Cohort Analysis," *American Journal of Public Health* 71 (1981): 381–390.

74. Morehead et al. (note 19).

75. Sparling (note 15).

76. J. Find and M. A. Morehead, "Study of Peer Review of Inhospital Patient Care," *New York State Journal of Medicine* 71 (1971): 1963–1973; Morehead et al. (note 19); Rhee, "Relative Influence of Specialty Status" (note 19); Rhee, "Factors Determining the Quality of Physician Performance" (note 19).

77. L. Lipworth, J. A. H. Lee, and J. N. Morris, "Case-Fatality in Teaching and Non-Teaching Hospitals 1956–59," *Medical Care* 1 (1963): 71–76.

78. Kohl (note 34).

79. American College of Obstetricians and Gynecologists (note 41).

80. Stanford Center for Health Care Research, *Study of Institutional Differences in Postoperative Mortality* (Springfield, VA: U.S. Department of Commerce, National Technical Information Service, 1974); Scott et al., "Hospital Structure" (note 17).

81. Luft et al. (note 39).

82. M. I. Roemer, A. T. Moustafa, and C. E. Hopkins, "A Proposed Hospital Quality Index: Hospital Death Rates Adjusted for Case Severity," *Health Services Research* 3 (1968): 96–118.

83. M. E. W. Goss and J. I. Reed, "Evaluating the Quality of Hospital Care Through Severity-Adjusted Death Rates: Some Pitfalls," *Medical Care* 12 (1974): 202–213.

84. Kohl (note 34).

85. Morehead et al. (note 19).

86. Stanford Center for Health Care Research (note 80).

87. Roemer et al. (note 82).

88. Morehead et al. (note 19).

89. D. Neuhauser, *The Relationship Between Administrative Activities and Hospital Performance,* Research Series 28 (Chicago: University of Chicago, Center for Health Administrative Studies, 1971).

90. Morehead et al. (note 19).

91. Rhee, "Relative Influence of Specialty Status" (note 19).

92. B. S. Georgopoulos and F. C. Mann, *The Community General Hospital* (New York: Macmillan Co., 1962); S. M. Shortell, S. W. Becker, and D. Neuhauser, "The Effects of Managerial Practices on Hospital Efficiency and Quality of Care," in *Organizational Research in Hospitals,* ed. S. M. Shortell and M. Brown (Chicago: Blue Cross Association, 1976). Scott et al., "Hospital Structure" (note 17); Scott et al., "Organizational Determinants" (note 17); Flood and Scott (note 17); Neuhauser (note 89).

93. Scott et al., "Hospital Structure" (note 17); Scott et al., "Organizational Determinants" (note 17); Shortell et al. (note 92).

94. Scott et al., "Hospital Structure" (note 17); Flood and Scott (note 17).

95. Flood and Scott (note 17).

96. Scott et al., "Organizational Determinants" (note 17).

97. L. Wyzewianski and A. Donabedian, "Equity in the Distribution of Quality of Care," *Medical Care* 19, suppl. (December 1981): 28–56.

98. R. H. Brook, *Quality of Care Assessment: A Comparison of Five Methods of Peer Review* (Washington, DC: Department of Health, Education and Welfare, Public Health Service, Health Resources Administration, Bureau of Health Services Research and Evaluation, 1973).

99. Ray et al. (note 21).

100. C. Bombardier, V. R. Fuchs, L. A. Lillard, and K. E. Warner, "Socioeconomic Factors Affecting the Utilization of Surgical Operations," *New England Journal of Medicine* 297 (1977): 699–705.

101. Lembcke (note 4).

102. T. F. Lyons and B. C. Payne, "The Quality of Physicians' Health Care Performance: A Comparison Against Optimal Criteria for Treatment of the Elderly and Younger Adults in Community Hospitals," *Journal of the American Medical Association* 227 (1974): 925–928; T. F. Lyons and B. C. Payne, "Quality of Physicians' Office-Care Performance: Different for Elderly Than for Younger Adults?" *Journal of the American Medical Association* 229 (1974): 1621–1622.

103. E. Janzen, "Quality Nursing Care Assurance: Initial Survey" (paper presented at the American Public Health Association annual meeting, New Orleans, Oct. 23, 1974).

104. S. Lichtner and M. Pflanz, "Appendectomy in the Federal Republic of Germany: Epidemiology and Medical Care Patterns," *Medical Care* 9 (1971): 311–330.

105. S.-O. Rhee, T. F. Lyons, and B. C. Payne, "Patient Race and Physician Performances: Quality of Medical Care, Hospital Admissions and Hospital Stays," *Medical Care* 17 (1979): 737–747.

106. Bombardier et al. (note 100).

107. Janzen (note 103).

108. L. D. Egbert and I. L. Rothman, "Relation Between the Race and Economic Status of Patients and Who Performs Their Surgery," *New England Journal of Medicine* 297 (1977): 90–91.

109. Morehead et al. (note 19).

110. Kohl (note 34).

111. J. P. Bunker and B. W. Brown, Jr., "The Physician-Patient as an Informed Consumer of Surgical Services," *New England Journal of Medicine* 290 (1974): 1051–1055.

112. Ibid.

113. P. A. Lembcke, "Medical Auditing by Scientific Methods: Illustrated by Major Female Pelvic Surgery," *Journal of the American Medical Association* 162 (1956): 646–655; E. G. McCarthy, M. L. Finkel, and H. S. Ruchlin, *Second Opinion Elective Surgery* (Boston: Auburn House, 1981); Doyle (note 16).

114. Lichtner and Pflanz (note 104).

115. J. G. R. Howie, "The Place of Appendectomy in the Treatment of Young Adult Patients With Possible Appendicitis," *Lancet*, 1968, pp. 1365–1367.

116. Fitzpatrick et al. (note 60).

117. Sparling (note 15).

118. Flood and Scott (note 17).

119. New York Academy of Medicine (note 18).

120. Kohn (note 34).

121. Shapiro et al. (note 72).

# Chapter 25

# The Outcomes Movement—Will It Get Us Where We Want to Go?

Arnold M. Epstein, M.D., M.A.

Arnold Relman, editor-in-chief of the *Journal,* has dubbed it "the third revolution in medical care."[1] That description of what I call the outcomes movement may be hyperbole, but clearly we have entered an era of unprecedented growth in activity directed at the assessment of outcomes, the analysis of effectiveness, and quality assurance.

There are many conspicuous manifestations of this type of activity. For example, the Joint Commission on Accreditation of Hospitals, moving away from its traditional reliance on structural measures, has formally embraced quality assessment based on severity-adjusted outcomes as the cornerstone of its future strategy for monitoring hospitals.[2,3] Paul Ellwood, who popularized the concept of health maintenance organizations, has now called for a major initiative in what he terms "outcomes management"[4]—a national program in which clinical standards and guidelines are based systematically on patient outcomes.

In line with this vision, the federal government, through the Health Care Financing Administration[5] and the newly established Agency for Health Care Policy and Research,[6] has launched a program directed at gauging the effectiveness of medical interventions and developing guidelines for medical practice through the assessment of patient outcomes. These activities will be pursued with the help of substantial increases in research funding. Two years ago federal funding devoted to this kind of activity, through the National Center for Health Services Research, was limited to $1.9 million; last year it rose to $5.5 million. More than $30 million is allotted for such research in this year's budget.

Proponents of the new emphasis on measuring the outcomes of medical practice[1,4,5] predict myriad social benefits, including better information for both physicians and patients, improved guidelines for medical practice, and wiser decisions by purchasers of health care. But will these efforts really pay off? Will the era of outcomes assessment and accountability actually provide what Ellwood says we need—"a central nervous system that can help us cope with the complexities of modern medicine."[4]

I believe that research on outcomes can tell us more about the effectiveness of different interventions and may help increase the efficiency of existing systems for monitoring the quality of care. At the same time, I question whether this information is all we need to formulate guidelines that will serve as a rational basis for decision making and make medical care for a broad range of conditions more efficient. In this article I shall first consider the forces that have brought about the outcomes

Reprinted with permission from Arnold M. Epstein, M.D., M.A., The Outcomes Movement—Will It Get Us Where We Want to Go?, *The New England Journal of Medicine,* Vol. 323 No. 4, pp. 266–270, 1990.

movement and the directions it has taken thus far. I shall then examine the goals of the movement and the likely impediments to its progress. I hope that the recognition of these impediments will lead us to modify our expectations appropriately and will help us funnel our efforts into the activities that will be most productive.

## THE ORIGINS OF THE OUTCOMES MOVEMENT

At least three important factors have led to the current emphasis on the assessment of effectiveness and outcomes. The first is the need for cost containment. Growth of managed care and the initiation of state and federal prospective-payment systems have engendered substantial fear that administrative and payment policies designed to control the increase in medical services will have deleterious effects on the quality of care. In the context of cost containment, the emphasis on outcomes is seen in two ways: as an index of the relative effectiveness of different interventions that allows the elimination of unnecessary expenditure and as part of a vital monitoring system directed not so much to improving the quality of care as to detecting its deterioration.[7]

The second factor is a renewed sense of competition. Since 1970, the number of health maintenance organizations has grown nearly 20-fold.[8,9] Using a variety of structures, these insurers now compete vigorously for the industrial buyer's dollar. Without question this competition has taken place on the battlefield of price, but there is concern that price alone is an inadequate basis for competition. Buyers need, in Walter McClure's words, to "buy right," to compare outcomes and quality, and to incorporate their findings into their ultimate buying decisions.[10]

The third, and perhaps the most important, factor leading to the outcomes movement has been the work of researchers such as John Wennberg, who have documented substantial geographic differences in the use of various medical procedures.[11–13] These differences, which appear to persist even after control for the severity of illness, raise questions about whether they reflect unnecessary costs in high-use areas or less-than-optimal care in low-use areas; the focus on outcomes is the obvious first step in answering these questions.

## NEW DIRECTIONS IN ASSESSING OUTCOMES

The surge of interest in outcomes has not meant simply an increase in the amount of attention paid to outcomes. Rather, the movement has taken some very specific directions that affect the types of data that are collected and used, the types of studies that are performed, and the types of outcomes that are assessed.

First, there has been a much greater emphasis on the use of large computerized data bases—for several reasons. One is the continuing accumulation of data by state rate-setting commissions and third-party payers, including the Health Care Financing Administration, that use computerized clinical and billing data in determining reimbursement. At the same time, the availability of portable computers and work-stations now facilitates the analysis of these data. There are currently 40–pound computers that can easily be used to analyze treatment patterns for literally hundreds of thousands of patients. Finally, vested interests have become involved. Government research initiatives have clearly been directed toward making use of the Health Care Financing Administration's files on Medicare beneficiaries, among other data.[4]

The existence of large computerized data bases also offers the potential for natural experiments of tremendous size. We have seen the resurgence of the quasi-experimental design or the nonrandomized study over the randomized, controlled trial. The latter is excellent for assessing efficacy—that is, for determining whether an intervention will reliably produce the desired effect under well-controlled, essentially ideal circumstances. On the other hand, randomized, controlled trials may not tell us much about how effective treatments are when they are used in everyday practice by ordinary clinicians and patients. The Lipid Research Clinics Coronary Primary Prevention Trial, for example, showed that cholestyramine is extremely efficacious in lowering cholesterol levels and diminishing the risk of coronary heart disease under controlled circumstances.[14,15] Yet many clinicians have questioned whether its adverse side effects will limit its effectiveness in everyday practice.

There are, of course, obvious trade-offs when one uses a nonrandomized design. Randomization allows one to compare different interventions while controlling for both known and unknown confounders. In nonrandomized trials, we can use statistical techniques such as matching, stratification, and structural modeling for this purpose. However, these techniques are most effective when the data available include detailed measures of the severity of illness. Thus, there has been a growing interest in expanding the data on coexisting diseases and severity that are routinely incorporated into large data bases.

Perhaps the most important effect of the outcomes movement has been a broadening of our focus to include a wider range of outcomes. For many years we have studied differences in the use of medical services; it was only a short step to the consideration of differences in the rates of mortality, readmission, and complications and in other traditional measures of clinical outcome. During the past few years, however, we have seen a dramatic expansion in the range of outcomes that physicians and policy makers are willing to consider valid indicators of health. These go far beyond traditional clinical indexes and include a series of variables assessed through interviews: functional status, emotional health, social interaction, cognitive function, degree of disability, and so forth. There is growing appreciation in the medical community that, although they are still imperfect, instruments based on subjective data from patients can provide important information that may not be evident from physiologic measurements and may be as reliable as—or more reliable than—many of the clinical, biochemical, or physiologic indexes on which doctors have traditionally relied.[16]

## THE GOALS AND LIMITATIONS OF THE OUTCOMES MOVEMENT

Proponents of the increased emphasis on outcomes believe this approach may help us achieve several related goals. These include increased understanding of the effectiveness of different interventions, the use of this information to make possible better decision making by physicians and patients, and the development of standards to guide physicians and aid third-party payers in optimizing the use of resources.

The effort to determine the outcomes and effectiveness of different medical interventions and to use that information as an aid to clinical decision making is, I believe, a useful extension of basic clinical research. We are seeing efforts not only to expand our medical knowledge but also to develop more effective ways to communicate new findings to physicians and make them accessible to patients. In recent years, for example, we have learned a substantial amount about the efficacy of prostatectomy to relieve the symptoms of benign prostatic hypertrophy, in terms of both the probability of success and the risk of mortality and adverse consequences such as impotence. A group of researchers, including Michael Barry, Floyd Fowler, Al Mulley, John Wennberg, and colleagues, have recently developed innovative videotapes to convey more accurately to patients who are considering prostatectomy the broad range of possible outcomes and the impact they may expect on their quality of life if they undergo the procedure (personal communication). Efforts to educate patients are, of course, not new. Yet the emphasis on outcomes that may be more meaningful to patients (i.e., the presence or absence of dribbling rather than urine-flow measurements) and the use of sophisticated audio-visual aids appear to be improvements on previous efforts. Additional work is now under way to refine this approach and apply it in other clinical situations—for example, for patients with breast cancer who are considering mastectomy and for patients with chronic low back pain who are considering orthopedic surgery.

A much more controversial aspect of the outcomes movement is the effort to develop guidelines that can be used by physicians in providing care and by third-party payers attempting to ensure the appropriate use of services.[1,4,5,17] In a review of more than 4500 hospital records of Medicare patients, Chassin et al. found that one sixth of those undergoing coronary angiography and upper-gastrointestinal endoscopy and one third of those undergoing carotid endarterectomy had procedures that a consensus panel considered inappropriate.[18] Because this study, carried out at the Rand Corporation, was based on a retrospective review of charts, some proportion of the identified instances probably represented inadequate documentation of appropriate care rather than truly inappropriate care. Nevertheless, the reported results suggest the potential magnitude of the problem.

Conceptually, the steps in the process of moving from outcomes to guidelines are straightforward.[4] We first use large data bases to establish monitoring systems; we identify variations in outcome in different areas and differences in procedures or interventions that are associated with the differences in outcome; we use nonrandomized trials or, if necessary, meta-analyses, decision analyses, or randomized, controlled trials to assess the results of the different interventions; we incorporate the results of data analysis into appropriate guidelines; and we use education and feedback to modify the behavior of physicians in the appropriate direction. Throughout the process we continue to monitor care, with the goal of modifying the initial guidelines over time as practice changes and as new technologies are developed.

Although the path to progress appears clear, numerous difficulties are likely to limit our ability to apply this approach to a broad range of conditions. The production of guidelines will be expensive and time-consuming and therefore will be justifiable only for common procedures or those that have a substantial impact on cost or outcome. It will also be most appropriate to develop guidelines for interventions in cases in which therapeutic options are stable.

The development of guidelines may be especially difficult when patients' preferences are an important factor in clinical decision making. In the case of prostatectomy, a 70–year-old man may have nocturia and urinary hesitancy and dribbling because of benign prostatic hypertrophy. Data show that prostatectomy is likely to relieve his symptoms but that the procedure entails a low risk of surgery-related death and a 5 to 25 percent risk of impotence.[19] Patients clearly differ in how they evaluate these potential benefits and risks. Better information on effectiveness may help determine the best decision for individual patients, but formal guidelines will be difficult to establish when appropriate care for persons with identical clinical characteristics differs because of their different priorities.

Progress in assessing the relative effectiveness of interventions may also be slow. Variations often arise in situations in which different groups of physicians believe different approaches are preferable. This is not a random occurrence. Controversies in medicine occur when, for one reason or another, effectiveness is difficult to gauge and the available data conflict. Should one perform a transurethral prostatectomy or an open prostatectomy for patients who need prostate surgery? Several studies have shown that the transurethral approach (used in approximately 95 percent of proctectomies[20]) can be effective.[21-23] Other studies show however, that open prostatectomy is more effective.[20] Will additional studies give a definitive answer?

Moreover, generally accepted standards for an appropriate level of cost effectiveness are still lacking. Today the results of hundreds of studies tell us that the cost effectiveness of various interventions ranges from a few thousand dollars to may hundreds of thousands of dollars per year of life saved. At the extremes, the decision is relatively simple. What do we do, however, for most interventions, which fall in the middle? We know, for example, that the use of cholestyramine to lower the serum cholesterol level of a 35–to–64–year–old male smoker with a serum total cholesterol level of 7.50 mmol per liter (290 mg per deciliter) and a low-density lipoprotein cholesterol level of 4.65 mmol per liter (180 mg per deciliter) will cost somewhere between $65,000 and $200,000 per year of life saved, depending on the patient's exact age.[24] Consensus guidelines developed by the National Cholesterol Educational Program tell us to treat that patient with cholestyramine,[25] but the consensus guidelines disagree.[26] Which set of guidelines is correct? Unfortunately, at present we have no universally accepted standards to help us develop appropriate clinical guidelines.

The consensus process will certainly be a focal point in the development of standards. To the extent that consensus merely provides an algorithm for clinical behavior that is supported by strong and consistent evidence, the task will be straightforward and worthwhile. When the data conflict or when cost effectiveness is not extreme, however, the process will be more problematic. In these situations, a panel of experts may be able to reach consensus on a guideline, but this agreement will not necessarily define the most appropriate course of care. Clearly, different panels of experts often disagree. We still have a surprisingly limited understanding of important aspects of the consensus process, including the impact of specialty training and geographic region in the composition of panels and the effects of structuring existing data in different ways.

Finally, there are potential difficulties with implemen-

tation and monitoring. Ideally, the promulgation and enforcement of guidelines should be designed strictly to make the use of health care services more appropriate. But virtually all studies on appropriateness so far and much of the attendant dialogue have focused on patients who undergo unnecessary procedures rather than on patients who do not receive appropriate care. I suspect that a reduction in the cost of care is high on the silent agenda of many who promote the use of guidelines. As a result, administrative efforts are more likely to be focused on decreasing inappropriate care than on increasing access to beneficial procedures.

Even if efforts at implementation are balanced, physicians are likely to resist unless the guidelines can be made sufficiently comprehensive to incorporate all the data that bear on the clinical decision. The establishment of such all-encompassing guidelines will, in some instances, be difficult. Previous study has shown that even when physicians view particular guidelines favorably, they are slow to change their patterns of practice.[27] This reluctance will be especially evident in controversial areas, in which guidelines may be arbitrary and open to challenge on the basis of contradictory data. In addition, our understanding of how to induce physicians to change their patterns of practice is incomplete.[28] Education, monitoring, and feedback may be helpful strategies but are costly in terms of administrative effort and expense.

Although none of these problems are insurmountable, collectively they represent a substantial impediment. Numerous studies have documented the prevalence of inappropriate use.[29,30] Although I am sympathetic to those who would move now to curtail practice patterns that fall outside the usual range,[31] I worry that extending this approach to a broad range of conditions will be difficult.

## IMPLICATIONS FOR THE FUTURE

The outcomes movement is well under way. The increased allotment of funds for research is real. Already greater attention is being devoted to determining the outcomes of different interventions, and this research is likely to yield insights into efficacy and rational behavior. I believe that expanding our research focus to a broader set of outcomes will reap rewards, since traditional physiologic and clinical indexes have important limitations. Understanding how different interventions affect such factors as physical and emotional function, social activity, and return to work will provide a more sensitive gauge. Developing new and more effective methods to convey such information to doctors and patients can only lead to wiser decisions. At the same time, however, we must realize that clinical research is not a new endeavor. Will the expansion of our research effort and the development and increased accessibility of larger computerized data bases lead to a revolutionary increase in our understanding? Will these changes truly be instrumental in creating a "central nervous system" for health care? Certainly they will help, but I believe our expectations should be modest.

What about guidelines? The political tide here is strong. Images of the "rogue surgeon" practicing beyond the acceptable bounds argue strongly for an aggressive approach. The proponents of guidelines would have us develop, implement, and enforce standards for a broad set of therapies now. Is that feasible? Clearly, the consensus process can provide an answer, and when the education of physicians is ineffective in changing practice, stronger administrative and financial levers can be used. But will such efforts make the provision of care more rational and lead to a more efficient system?

I believe the call for increased assessment and accountability is healthy, but in many instances guidelines are not likely to produce more rational or more efficient care. Our efforts should continue, but our energy should be focused and metered; progress will be made, but slowly. Our expectations must be moderate if we are to avoid disappointment. The danger we face is that we will undermine a health evolution and allow revolutionary zeal to lead us to carry a good thing too fast and too far.

## References

1. Relman AS, Assessment and accountability: the third revolution in medical care. *N Engl J Med* 1988; 319:1220–2.
2. O'Leary DS. The Joint Commission looks to the future. *JAMA* 1987; 258:951–2.
3. Roberts JS, Coale JG, Redman RR. A history of the Joint Commission on Accreditation of Hospitals. *JAMA* 1987; 258:936–40.
4. Ellwood PM. Outcomes management: a technology of patient experience. *N Engl J Med* 1988; 318:1549–56.
5. Roper WL, Winkenwerder W, Hackbarth GM, Krakauer H. Effectiveness in health care: an initiative to evaluate and improve medical practice. *N Engl J Med* 1988; 319:1197–202.
6. Public Law 101–239. The Omnibus Budget Reconciliation Act of 1989.
7. Wyszewianski L. Quality of care: past achievements and future challenges. *Inquiry* 1988; 25:13–22.
8. Mayer TR, Mayer GG, HMOs: origins and development. *N Engl J Med* 1985; 312:590–4.
9. HMO industry profile. Vol. 1. Benefits, premiums and market structure in 1988. Washington, D.C.: Research and Analysis Department. Group Health Association of America, 1989.
10. Inglehart JK. Competition and the pursuit of quality: a conversation with Walter McClure. *Health Aff* (Millwood) 1988; 7(1):79–90.
11. Wennberg J, Gittelsohn A. Small area variations in health care delivery. *Science* 1973; 182:1102–8.
12. Wennberg JE, Freeman JL, Shelton RM, Bubolz TA. Hospital use and mortality among Medicare beneficiaries in Boston and New Haven. *N Engl J Med* 1989; 321:1168–73.
13. Wennberg JE, Freeman JL, Culp WJ. Are hospital services rationed in New Haven or over-utilised in Boston? *Lancet* 1987; 1:1185–9.
14. Lipid Research Clinics Program. The Lipid Research Clinics Coronary Primary Prevention Trial results. I. Reduction in incidence of coronary heart disease. *JAMA* 1984; 251:351–64.
15. *Idem.* The Lipid Research Clinics Coronary Primary Prevention Trial results. II. The relationship of reduction in incidence of coronary heart disease to cholesterol lowering. *JAMA* 1984; 251:365–74.
16. Lohr KN. Advances in health status assessment: overview of the conference. *Med Care* 1989; 27:Suppl 3:S1–S11.
17. Lee PR, Ginsburg PB, LeRoy LB, Hammons GT. The Physician Payment Review Commission report to Congress. *JAMA* 1989; 261:2382–5.
18. Chassin MR, Kosecoff J, Park RE, et al. The appropriateness of use of selected medical and surgical procedures and its relationship to geographic variations in their use. Ann Arbor, Mich.: Health Administration Press, 1989.
19. Fowler FJ Jr, Wennberg JE, Timothy RP, Barry MJ, Mulley AG Jr, Hanley D. Symptom status and quality of life following prostatectomy. *JAMA* 1988; 259:3018–22.
20. Roos NP, Wennberg JE, Malenka DJ, et al. Mortality and reoperation after open and transurethral resection of the prostate for benign prostatic hyperplasia. *N Engl J Med* 1989; 320:1120–4.
21. Kolmert T, Norlen H. Transurethral resection of the prostate: a review of 1111 cases. *Int Urol Nephrol* 1989; 21:47–55.
22. Mebust WK. Surgical management of benign prostatic obstruction. *Urology* 1988; 32:Suppl 6:12–5.
23. Abddalla M, Davin JL, Granier B, Levallois M. Complications de la résection transurétrale dans la cure de l'hypertrophie prostatique bénigne: à propos d'une serie de 1 180 adénomes—1976–1986. *J Urol* (Paris) 1989; 95:15–21.
24. Oster G, Epstein AM. Cost-effectiveness of antihyperlipemic therapy in the prevention of coronary heart disease: the case of cholestyramine, *JAMA* 1987; 258:2381–7.
25. The Expert Panel. Report of the National Cholesterol Education Program Expert Panel on Detection, Evaluation, and Treatment of High Blood Cholesterol in Adults. *Arch Intern Med* 1988; 148:36–69.
26. Task Force on the Use and Provision of Medical Services. Report on the detection and management of asymptomatic hypercholesterolemia. Ontario Ministry of Health and the Ontario Medical Association, 1989.
27. Lomas J, Anderson GM, Dominick-Pierre K, Vayda E, Enkin MW, Hannah WJ. Do practice guidelines guide practice? The effect of a consensus statement on the practice of physicians. *N Engl J Med* 1989; 321:1306–11.

28. Eisenberg JM, Williams SV. Cost containment and changing physicians' practice behavior: can the fox learn to guard the chicken coop? *JAMA* 1981; 246:2195–201.
29. Chassin MR, Kosecoff J, Park RE, et al. Does inappropriate use explain geographic variations in the use of health care services? A study of three procedures. *JAMA* 1987; 258:2533–7.
30. Leape LL, Park RE, Solomon DH, Chassin MR, Kosecoff J, Brook RH. Does inappropriate use explain small-area variations in the use of health care services? *JAMA* 1990; 263:669–72.
31. Brook RH. Practice guidelines and practicing medicine: are they compatible? *JAMA* 1989; 262:3027–30.

# Chapter 26
# Total Quality Management in Health: Making It Work

Curtis P. McLaughlin, D.B.A., and
Arnold D. Kaluzny, Ph.D.

*Many health organizations are trying total quality management (TQM). This approach represents a total paradigm shift in health care management and presents a series of potential conflict areas in the way health organizations are managed. These areas include TQM's participatory approach versus professional and managerial authority, collective versus individual responsibility, quality assurance and standards versus continuous improvement, and flexible versus rigid objectives and plans. This article reviews the areas of conflict and suggests a number of action guidelines for the successful implementation of TQM.*

Interest in total quality management (TQM), a major managerial innovation, is running high. The Joint Commission on Accreditation of Healthcare Organizations (Joint Commission) has placed its "agenda for change" squarely within the philosophical context of TQM.[1] The Hospital Research and Educational Trust of the American Hospital Association has recently published a report to help hospitals "organize for, communicate about, monitor and continuously improve all aspects of health care delivery."[2(p.2)] This report is part of a three-year quality improvement initiative sponsored by fifteen hospital systems and alliances.

TQM, first developed in the United States and successfully implemented in Japan, is obviously receiving serious attention by U.S. health service organizations as they try to improve quality with fewer resources.[3–5] A growing number of hospitals and health maintenance organizations (HMOs) are implementing TQM. Some will succeed; many will fail. This article argues that TQM represents a fundamental paradigm shift in health care management and explores a series of potential conflicts between TQM and the way that health care institutions normally are managed. A number of action guidelines are suggested to better ensure that TQM fulfills its potential and functions effectively within health service organizations.

## TQM AS A PARADIGM SHIFT

Total quality management is a conceptual approach different from quality assurance (QA) and quality inspection and runs counter to many underlying assumptions of professional bureaucracies. It calls for continuous and relentless improvement in the total process that provides care, not simply in the improved actions of individual professionals. Improvement is thus based on both outcome and process.

Batalden et al.[6] outline what the health leadership must learn to implement TQM successfully.

Reprinted from *Health Care Management Review,* Vol. 15 No. 3, pp. 7–14, with permission of Aspen Publishers, Inc., copyright 1990.

- Management must learn the meaning of quality, including an understanding of the importance of the customer, and that there are multiple customers in the production process.
- Top management must sponsor and encourage the continuous improvement of quality, including the wise use of teams that can work together effectively to improve systems and of other processes, including group processes and organization and system change skills.
- Management must learn the meaning of statistical thinking: how to speak with data and manage with facts; how to take the guesswork out of decision making; how to reduce variation and unnecessary complexity through the use of the seven standard tools of data analysis and display (cause-and-effect diagram, Pareto chart, histogram, scatter diagram, flow chart, run or trend chart, and control chart); and how to link the results of the use of these tools with appropriate management action.[6]

TQM demands that change be based on the needs of the customer, not the values of the providers. It requires the meaningful participation of all personnel and a rapid and thoughtful response from top management to suggestions made by participating personnel. Management is no longer able to stifle the suggestions of personnel by requiring additional study or by requiring that all decisions be reviewed by a higher level of management.

TQM is more than a change in values and responsiveness by top management. It requires rigorous process flow and statistical analysis, evaluation of all ongoing activities, and the recognition and application of underlying psychosocial principles affecting individuals and groups within an organization. It requires accepting the fundamental assumption that most problems encountered in a health care organization are the result of not errors by administrative or clinical professionals, but the inability of the structure—within which all personnel function—to perform adequately.

An obvious conflict is between the relentless inquiry of TQM and the established norms of professional autonomy. This is not merely a conflict between administrators and clinical professionals: It is a fundamental challenge to the way all professionals think about quality, evaluate and regulate themselves, and gain and protect their professional domains and autonomy. TQM does not respect existing professional standards; it is continually demanding new ones.

TQM places primary emphasis for problem characterization on the system rather than the individual. Deming[7] estimates that 85% of errors introduced into a process are the result of problems with the system rather than the type of random errors and mistakes introduced by individuals. This runs counter to the prevailing assumption in health services that a problem is a result of one individual's error rather than of the larger structure or system within which the individual functions. For example, one of the authors was hospitalized briefly last summer and experienced a number of scheduling and coordination difficulties that unnecessarily complicated the stay. In an effort to provide constructive feedback to management, the author described his experience and displeasure to a staff member, suggesting that these problems could be improved, if not eliminated. A few weeks later at a social occasion, the supervisor of one of the departments involved approached him and started asking questions such as, "What did the person look like? Was the employee short or tall? I checked the records the day you were in, and the person who was on duty was the one least likely to do that." Unfortunately, the normal response to complaints is to "take names and kick butts."

Similarly, at a recent executive training program, a group of midlevel managers was asked to consider programmatic issues such as "Why does it take one to two hours to get a discharged patient from the floor to the front door?" Obviously, the solution to this problem lies in coordinating several departments, and the group members agreed that they could resolve the problem. However, they argued that upper management had not asked them to solve the problem. They knew it was a systems problem, but they felt responsible for managing only their own functions, not a system; therefore, the problem continued.

Finally, TQM challenges the prevailing model of who the customer is. The customer in TQM is not only the patient, but also the many users of a department's output. Here again, the criterion is not whether or not the work meets professional standards, but whether the user, often a member of a different profession, is satisfied with its timeliness and utility.

The reality is that both models—TQM and the professional bureaucracy—must be accommodated if TQM is to make a difference in health care organizations. For example, Galbraith[8] outlines the importance of the professional model in handling the flood of technical information that medical research has developed. He suggests that specialization is a way of handling information overload, especially in the absence of other information-processing alternatives such as a common management information system or lateral linkages for information coordination. In fact, one can see TQM as a methodology for developing lateral linkages in the health care organization that transfer information between disciplines as needed. It is a powerful method of lateral technology transfer in the traditionally highly compartmentalized organization.

## CONFLICTS BETWEEN THE TWO MODELS

The nature of the organizational change required to implement TQM can be outlined by contrasting the two models and evaluating points of conflict (see Figure 1). While they are not mutually exclusive and while the

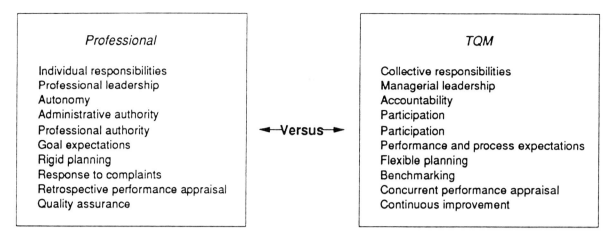

**Figure 1.** Areas of conflict between two organizational models: Professional and TQM

observed points of conflict will vary between organizations, each of the models requires explicit recognition.

### Individual versus Collective Responsibility

The professional model places the responsibility for performance squarely on the individual professional. As described by Mintzberg, "the Professional Bureaucracy . . . hires duly trained and indoctrinated specialists—professionals—and then gives them control over their own work."[9(p.349)] He goes on to state that such control means that the professional works independently of colleagues but closely with clients. If the professional makes a mistake, then that professional is primarily liable for damages. If the error is blatant, a QA committee, and the professional society in the very worst cases, sanctions the individual. Only in the most grievous cases is the organization itself at risk for damages.

The TQM model focuses on the system. If errors or problems occur (e.g., if individuals were not properly trained, key information was not transferred, or procedures were not adequate to the variety of possible situations), the TQM model focuses on the process, not the individual provider. To correct problems and errors, a group—usually interdisciplinary—of individuals in the organization is asked to assume ownership of each process and joint responsibility for its improvement.

### Clinical versus Managerial Leadership

In the health service organization, a continuing source of conflict is the relationship between the various levels of administrative management and the clinical professional leadership. At a time when the management is trying to gain more control over the clinical professional in the face of pressures for cost-containment purposes, TQM comes along and demands that management take a more participative approach. Managers are required to involve clinical professionals in the decision-making pro-

cess, leaving it up to them to solve quality problems as they arise. Yet, while this is a participative program, it is clearly a managerial initiative. Paradoxically, participation may be perceived as a threat to professional autonomy while at the same time contributing to individual and group autonomy.

### Autonomy versus Accountability

Autonomy is central to the clinical professional model. Under this model, clinical professionals have the special privilege of freedom from the control of outsiders. This privilege is justified by three claims:

1. Unusual degrees of skill and knowledge are involved in clinical professional work, and administrative professionals are not equipped to evaluate or regulate it.
2. Clinicians are responsible, and they may be trusted to work conscientiously without supervision.
3. Clinical professionals themselves may be trusted to undertake the proper regulatory action on those rare occasions where an individual does not perform work competently or ethically.[10]

Clinical professionals are thus suspicious of managerial actions in the areas of cost control and QA, and TQM may look like another in a progression of management steps designed to reduce their professional autonomy. TQM is a technique that is likely to increase personal autonomy in undertaking task-oriented change. It does not, however, respect professional autonomy as much as it respects personal autonomy. At the same time, it demands that clinical professionals hold themselves accountable for both outcome and process performance on a continuous basis.

### Administrative Authority versus Participation

TQM, through the use of quality circles, puts responsibility for quality control in the province of the frontline managers and employees. Quality circles are small groups of employees from the same areas who work on a range of problems to increase productivity and efficiency. Maintaining quality no longer means taking names and booting bottoms; it means monitoring and teaching employees to monitor their own performance and taking corrective action.

## Professional Authority versus Participation

The TQM approach diffuses responsibility for quality among the members of the team responsible for the delivery of care. The criteria are not necessarily those selected by physicians and other professional groups. TQM emphasizes that criteria are selected by the users of the output. It was best described by the director of a major teaching hospital, who defined his objective in starting a TQM program as wanting to "make this a customer-driven instead of a doctor-dominated hospital." Teams are likely to be multidisciplinary, and the creativity and worth of every team member must be respected equally. This has been reported frequently as a perceived threat to the status of middle managers. The same is quite likely to be the case with high-status professionals.

## Goal versus Process and Performance Expectations

The usual expectation in health care is that one has an objective goal for every act; that there is a "gold standard" for care. This means that each activity has a protocol for behavior and an expected outcome, and that the protocol remains in effect until a technological change makes it obsolete. That is not the case with TQM. The objective for TQM is one of continuous improvement. While this is not totally foreign to health care (e.g., the history of organ transplants has been one of continuous improvement), the hospital does not measure the success ratios of many of its basic procedures, such as getting the discharged patient out the door more quickly.

## Rigid versus Flexible Planning

A major teaching hospital tried forming quality circles and, like many other hospitals, developed a series of major cost-saving actions. As might be expected, these proposals often had associated capital requirements, and the hospital had already planned its capital investments for three or more years. The proposals were not implemented quickly, and the quality circles lost interest.

TQM requires that management be responsive to quality improvement suggestions. New priorities are necessary, and they must be addressed aggressively through flexible, ongoing planning rather than through rigid, preprogrammed activities.

TQM includes a concept called *benchmarking* of products and processes. This involves comparing current activities and performance against the best of the competition, the idea being to develop a product and process that significantly betters the competition. This implies several changes to existing approaches in health care, where the primary stimulus for change is the recognition of a problem vis-à-vis the established norm. First, TQM explicitly acknowledges that there is a competition to be studied and surpassed. Second, it recognizes the customer's experience as the basis of comparison. Third, it expects that the organization and its processes should be improving all the time, regardless of whether or not a complaint is registered or a problem identified. It means that the accepted way of doing things does not last long. It requires continuous growth and learning on the part of everyone, no matter how old or how educated.

## Retrospective versus Concurrent Performance Appraisal Systems

Most performance appraisal systems are based on setting goals and then meeting them. TQM appraisals focus on gaining skills to contribute to the process of quality improvement. Therefore, the reward system is based on contribution to a team effort to improve outcomes rather than on whether specific set objectives have been met. If TQM is in effect, the objectives will be changing almost daily: as some are achieved, new ones are immediately set. This case illustrates the concept of TQM.

> A European company won a contract to deliver headlamps to a Japanese car manufacturer. The initial contract allowed 50 defective lamps per 100,000. The lamp manufacturer modified its process to meet that standard painlessly. The next contract called for 20 defective lamps per 100,000. The lamp manufacturer managed to meet that too, so the next contract called for 5 per 100,000. Once again, the supplier struggled and met the new requirement. The next contract called for 10 per 1,000,000. This time the lamp manufacturer complained, "Why didn't you ask for that standard the first time?" "We didn't know what you could do, when we started," the Japanese replied.

The concept of Kaizen,[11] or "continuous improvement," is what drives a TQM program. No matter how well one does, one should be preparing and attempting to do better.

## Quality Assurance versus Continuous Improvement

The underlying premise of QA has been to identify human errors in the process, to follow established protocols, and to search for failures to meet the gold standard. This is the traditional Joint Commission approach: Either the standard is met or it is not. TQM emphasizes system errors and the continuous nature of improvement. Moreover, it requires that improvement be the responsibility of all personnel, not just those designated as "QA" personnel. Fortunately, the new Joint Commission standards are planned to reflect the TQM approach, emphasizing a process for continuous improvement rather than a go versus no-go measure.

## PREPARING FOR CHANGE

The implementation of TQM requires that administrative and medical managers mediate areas of conflict. How well management functions during the transition will depend on its ability to follow the action guidelines presented below.

### Action 1: Redefine the Role of the Professional

Most health care organizations have hired professionals on the basis of their possession of technical skills and standards certified by the training programs from which they were hired. Management has had relatively little control over professionals once they are hired, so they must have the right work habits, standards, and methods when hired. It has been assumed that the possession of this training and these work habits would lead to decision making that would meet the gold standard for an extended period of time.

The new set of decision-making skills required by TQM will have to include not only technical skills, but also the ability and flexibility to be guided by a quest for continuous improvement. This requires fundamental skills for statistical analysis of procedures and the ability to work with and in multidisciplinary teams. In essence, the routine tasks of the physician, nurse, and other providers will have to include basic epidemiology, statistics, and a variety of group process skills.

### Action 2: Redefine the Corporate Culture

Americans tend to look for the quick fix, the home run, and the Nobel Prize. While TQM may yield a home run early on, the basic philosophy is one of incessant change, the hitting of lots of singles, and the tortoise over the hare. Imai observes that Westerners are concerned with performance, while Easterners are concerned with both performance and process.[11] The Eastern philosophy calls for continuous employee training to assist with continuous improvement. This means that there must be a change in what Kilmann[12] refers to as culture, management skills, team-building strategy, structure, and reward system. Failure to address each in a systematic effort will greatly limit the implementation of TQM.

### Action 3: Redefine the Role of Management

In TQM, the manager becomes a symphony conductor, orchestrating the independent actions of a variety of professionals and project-oriented teams. This change really modifies current leadership roles at the top, middle, and bottom of the management hierarchy.[13] The top managers will do less of the decision making, leaving it to lower and middle levels of management to make the majority of the decisions involved. The role of top management, then, is to manage the culture and to allocate resources to support the change process. Top management will have to establish a planning process that is flexible enough to adapt to the propositions that the TQM process develops. Top management will have to be the spokespersons for the clients who are not represented in the system, especially the patients. Middle management has responsibility for monitoring the process of TQM and authorizing the implementation of the process changes that are identified for improvement of both quality and cost. Front-line management acquires the key role in TQM. The first-line manager has to lead the process and at the same time give people enough room to make it work. All levels of management must be evaluated as role models for TQM, and top managers have especially key roles in modeling, teaching, and providing feedback as part of the TQM process.

### Action 4: Empower the Staff to Analyze and Solve Problems

The most important challenge for management is to empower the staff to gather data, analyze it, and make recommendations. This involves convincing the staff that it is safe to collect data and do something with the results. This means that management must overcome status barriers; must be diligent in convincing people to try out statistical quality control techniques, making sure that people get rapid feedback to their proposals; and must be diplomatic. Supervisors also have to act as liaisons if problems turn out to have multiple causation (as they so often do). They have to be able to see the system in a systems way, focusing not first on their own units but on a component in a complex system. Most of all, they must all be supporters of the massive social changes that TQM can require.

### Action 5: Change Organizational Objectives

The organization's objectives need to be expressed in terms of both performance objectives and process objectives. This means that programs will have to set their own quality objectives period by period as they develop the capacity to measure, follow, and modify their own processes.

## Action 6: Develop Mentoring Capacity

The professionals and the managers will both perceive the changes as risky to implement and threatening to their professional identity. They will need models of behavior to follow and mentors with whom they can discuss their plans and feelings about the risks involved. Senior executives who are convinced of the importance of TQM are going to provide advice and support. In fact, in one industrial organization, a criterion for promotion among mid- and upper-level managers is how subordinates judge their abilities to function as role models.

## Action 7: Drive the Benchmarking Process from the Top

The hardest process step will be the benchmarking process, a process that must be led from the top of the organization. Top management is the group responsible for assessing the outside environment. They have the capacity to identify the best performance of competitive organizations and compare internal operations with these high-performance organizations. This will not happen effectively without strong leadership from the top down.

The unit of analysis for benchmarking is critical. It is not just "Do we have the best radiology department in the country?" It is also "Do we give our patients the best experience? Do we serve the attending physicians better than anyone else? Are we making fewer processing errors and fewer delayed reports than last month, and are we working to make this the best in the world?"

## Action 8: Modify the Reward System

The reward system of health care is constrained to a high degree by professional status and prerogatives. The health care institution, however, must reserve some rewards for those who cooperate most wholeheartedly and effectively. The rewards are most likely to be psychic rather than financial payments. They can effectively include travel, entertainment, employee recognition (best used for teams), and vacation time. For example, one major U.S. company that is very successful at TQM has eliminated all financial awards in its suggestion system. It now gives books on how to improve job performance and trips to continuing education programs instead. The ideal reward system should reward both performance and process development.

## Action 9: Go Outside the Health Industry for Models

Xerox Corporation of Stamford, Connecticut, has been one of the most successful adherents of TQM. TQM has helped the company to thrive in the highly competitive copier market and to compete well enough to recover some of its market from the Japanese. David T. Kearns, Chairman and Chief Executive Officer of Xerox, has suggested that the next benchmark for Xerox copiers after Japanese copiers is the telephone, with its attributes of both high reliability and low cost. Health managers should not hesitate to go outside of the health industry for its models of consumer-driven quality. The obvious future targets are highly successful consumer service organizations such as Walt Disney, American Airlines, Marriott, and American Express.

## Action 10: Set Realistic Time Expectations

The process of adopting and institutionalizing TQM, like all organizational change processes, takes time under the best of circumstances, most likely three to five years. It is likely to take longer in a large, complex organization like a teaching hospital. People will have to start with a realistic estimate of the time required. Two types of time are required—hours of input by already busy managers and professionals and calendar time required to implement the program. The latter is illustrated even in the case of a very tightly controlled organization such as Xerox, where new issues concerning TQM institutionalization continue to surface five years after implementation. For example, employee evaluation systems were not changed to include management commitment and role modeling for TQM, and college employment recruiters were not using TQM-related selection criteria until shortly before the firm received the Malcolm Baldrige Prize in 1989 in recognition of its successful implementation of TQM.

## Action 11: Make the TQM Program a Model for Continuous Improvement

The cases cited above highlight possibilities for using the TQM program to model a continuous improvement orientation for the total organization. Those who are responsible for program oversight must consciously challenge the TQM staff to suggest improvements in the program and respond rapidly and effectively. The professionals will be especially sensitive to any gaps between what is preached and what is practiced by those associated with this program. They have already seen many programs come and go in recent years, and they must be convinced that management is serious about TQM. Here actions will truly speak louder than words.

Health service organizations are facing new challenges, challenges that require a new look at how and why resources are organized and managed. The expectations are high for TQM. A recent survey by Peat, Marwick, Main & Co. of Chicago reports that 69% of institutional providers and 78% of physicians, purchasers, and third party payers believe that the cost of poor quality is so great that quality improvement should pay for itself.[14] Industrial organizations have reduced their operating expenses by 20% to 40%. If health care organizations can do half as well, quality improvement programs will have a major impact on the field.

TQM represents an approach with a great deal of potential, yet it presents some basic conflicts with underlying norms and expectations that guide professional bureaucracies. While the conflict exists, the problems are not intractable and, if recognized, represent opportunities not only to improve quality of care but also improve the system designed to provide quality care.

## References

1. Ente, B.H. *Brief Overview of the Joint Commission's "Agenda for Change."* Chicago, Ill.: Joint Commission, 1989.
2. James, B.C. *Quality Management for Health Care Delivery.* Chicago, Ill.: The Hospital Research and Educational Trust of the American Hospital Association, 1989.
3. Berwick, D. "Continuous Improvement as an Ideal in Health Care." *New England Journal of Medicine* 320, no. 1 (1989): 53–56.
4. Berwick, D. "Health Services Research and Quality of Care." *Medical Care* 27, no. 8 (1989): 763–71.
5. Goldfield, N., and Nash, D.B. *Providing Quality Care: The Challenge to Clinicians.* Philadelphia, Pa.: American College of Physicians, 1989.
6. Batalden, P., et al. "Quality Improvement: The Role and Application of Research Methods." *The Journal of Health Administration Education 7,* no. 3 (1989): 577–83.
7. Deming, W.E. *Out of Crisis.* Cambridge, Mass.: MIT Press, 1986.
8. Galbraith, J. *Designing Complex Organizations.* Reading, Mass.: Addison-Wesley, 1973.
9. Mintzberg, H. *The Structuring of Organizations.* Englewood Cliffs, N.J.: Prentice Hall, 1979.
10. Freidson, E. *Profession of Medicine.* New York, N.Y.: Dodd, Mead, 1975.
11. Imai, M. Kaizen. *The Key to Japan's Competitive Success.* New York, N.Y.: Random House, 1986.
12. Kilmann, R. *Beyond the Quick Fix.* San Francisco, Calif.: Jossey-Bass, 1989.
13. Kaluzny, A.D. "Revitalizing Decision-making at the Middle Management Level." *Hospital and Health Services Administration* 34, No. 1 (1989): 39–51.
14. Peat, Marwick, Main & Co. *Setting Quality Standards in Health Care: Balancing Purchaser, Provider and Patient Expectations.* Chicago, Ill.: KMPG Peat Marwick, 1988.

# PART SEVEN
## Health Policy

This final section of the book addresses national health policy. While all of the articles in this book related to health policy, the selection of articles presented in this section is designed to focus specifically on national decision making and on some of the complex trade-offs that must be addressed relatively soon.

The first two articles in this section deal with past failures and suggest some prospects for future difficulties in addressing and resolving national health care policy. The first article, by William B. Schwartz, looks at the failure of past cost containment strategies, while the second article, by Uwe E. Rheinhardt, looks at the failure to establish comprehensive national policies in health services and the limited prospects for doing so in the future.

The next two articles address alternative approaches to providing more comprehensive health services for all Americans. Numerous proposals have been presented over the past fifteen years, and others even earlier than that, suggesting ways in which health care systems and services can be better structured and organized to facilitate access for all of our citizens. These two articles present provocative and particularly interesting approaches that can be considered in the current debate over national health policy. The first, by Karen Davis, suggests avenues for expanding existing Medicare and employer plans to achieve universal health insurance, while the second, by Alain C. Enthoven and Richard Kronick, presents another approach to universal health insurance through managed competition.

The realities and implications of limited resource availability for health care are addressed by the last two articles in this section. The first, by David C. Hadorn, describes the efforts of the State of Oregon in setting health care priorities, particularly for medically indigent individuals under the state Medicaid program. Much attention has been paid to Oregon's attempt to determine where to draw the line in the provision of services when financial resources are constrained, and this article nicely sets out the issues and current thinking as addressed by the State of Oregon.

The final article in this section, by Robert G. Evans and associates, takes an international perspective by examining the Canadian experience in providing health services through provincial universal health care programs. The reality of the Canadian approach and its applicability to United States health policy decision making is addressed in a challenging discussion.

# Chapter 27

# The Inevitable Failure of Current Cost-Containment Strategies

## Why They Can Provide Only Temporary Relief

### William B. Schwartz, M.D.

**Abstract:** Current strategies for controlling hospital costs have focused primarily on eliminating care that is presumed to be of no medical value. These efforts have neglected the central fact that eliminating such care reduces current expenditures, but has little or no influence on three key factors responsible for the upward trend in real costs—population growth, rising input prices ("the hospital market basket"), and technologic innovation and diffusion. Aging of the population and the rising costs of malpractice insurance have received undue attention; together they can account for only three tenths of a percentage point in the upward trend. Gradual elimination of presumably useless care, perhaps as much as 30% of inpatient-days, can save many billions of dollars, but can only offset for a few years the forces causing costs to rise in US community hospitals. Indeed, in 1984, the reduction in patient days and resultant slowing in the real rate of rise to 2.1% appear simply to have concealed an underlying real rate of increase that was close to 7%. After all unnecessary days have been eliminated, the underlying rate of increase will reemerge unless limitations are placed on technologic innovation or beneficial services are rationed. (*JAMA* 1987;257:220–224)

The problem of hospital costs is not simply that they are high, but that they have been rising rapidly and consuming an even larger fraction of gross national product (GNP). If the fraction of GNP spent on hospital care were reactively constant, the current level might still be criticized but with little sense that a crisis is impending. This distinction between the level of current expenditures and the upward trend in expenditures is critical, but it has not figured in the discussion of policy options such as encouragement to the growth of health maintenance organizations (HMOs) and preferred provider organizations. In principle, the attempt to control rising costs can have either of two quite distinct effects. One of these is to lower current baseline expenditures. The other is to restrict the rate at which expenditures are growing, without cutting current outlays. It is possible, of course, that a particular intervention will have both effects, but the more interesting and important possibility is that one of these outcomes will be mistaken for the other. In the long run, only measures that reduce the growth in costs can solve the fundamental problem of a cost spiral.

Reprinted with permission from *Journal of the American Medical Association*, Jan 9, 1987, Vol. 257 No. 2, pp. 220–224. Copyright 1987, American Medical Association.

The opinions and conclusions expressed herein are solely those of the author and should not be construed as representing the opinions or policies of the Commonwealth Fund, New York, and the Robert Wood Johnson Foundation, Princeton, N.J.

# WHY ELIMINATING "UNNECESSARY" CARE CANNOT PROVIDE LONG-TERM COST CONTAINMENT

With this vital distinction in mind, let us consider the HMO as an example of a widely promoted approach to limiting expenditures. At any given time, enrollees in HMOs spend less than patients receiving fee-for-service care, chiefly because they avoid "unnecessary" admissions and thus use an average of 30% fewer hospital days per year than individuals in the fee-for-service sector.[1] Proponents of the HMO as a mode of providing care argue that little or nothing is lost as a result of this pattern of practice, although this point remains unresolved.

Even if we accept the premise that HMOs eliminate hospital days that have no medical justification, we may not infer that eliminating such care would achieve long-term control of rising costs. Although the average expenditures of HMO enrollees are below those in the fee-for-service sector at any given time, costs in both sectors must rise if they are to provide the full benefits of new technology to their patients. Indeed, a study covering the period 1961 to 1974 showed that fee-for-service and HMO costs rose at approximately the same rate, even though at each point in time the overall costs of HMOs were substantially lower.[2] A comparison between the Kaiser-Oregon hospital (HMO-run) and the Oregon community hospitals reveals that over a 20-year period ending in the early 1970s, the increase in expense per patient-day was almost identical in the two types of hospitals.[2] A more recent study covering the five-year period from 1976 to 1981 also demonstrates that the rate of rise in the two sectors has not been significantly different.[3]

This experience illustrates an important principle: even if all useless care were gradually eliminated, we could anticipate only a temporary respite from rising costs unless the forces sustaining the real rate of change—chiefly technologic innovation and rising input prices—were simultaneously brought under control.

## HOW LONG A RESPITE?

If all presumably useless days of hospital care were eliminated, there would be a period in which the rate of rise in hospital costs would slow. But how long would this period of respite last?

Calculations based on the Rand health insurance study indicate that, when adjusted for current fee-for-service copayments, HMO enrollees used 31% fewer days than did matched individuals in the fee-for-service section.[4,5] They also incurred 17% fewer expenditures. Extrapolating these findings to the United States as a whole yields an estimate that reducing inpatient-days by some 30%

would save about $20 billion, expressed in 1983 dollars. We can infer that if the whole country were instantaneously converted to the HMO style of practice, the national health care budget would fall $20 to $25 billion and then proceed to grow in following years at about the same rate as before. The saving would be instantly recognizable for what it was—a measure that lowered costs without reducing growth. But a more realistic scenario is that the elimination of useless hospitalization would take place gradually. Each year would yield a saving that would not be perceived as an outright reduction in expenditures, but as an attenuation in the rate of increase. We can estimate the effect as follows.

In 1984, inpatient-days in US community hospitals were reduced by 6.1% (4.7% after adjustment for an increase in hospital ambulatory visits).[6,7] If reductions in subsequent years were to continue at about the same rate, say 6% of inpatient-days during each of four years beginning in 1985, the realizable saving of about $4 to $5 billion per year would probably be exhausted by the end of 1988 or 1989. Assuming that the 6.8% average annual rise in expenditures prevailing from 1977 through 1983 (Table 1) becomes the underlying rate of rise throughout the middle and late 1980s, the net effect of the cutback in days would be an observed real rate of increase of less than 4% per year. Because this increase is slightly larger than the average annual increase in GNP over the last two decades[8] (US Department of Commerce Bureau of Economic Analysis, unpublished data, 1985), it seems likely that the percentage of GNP devoted to hospital care would rise, albeit less than in the past. But once the full reduction in baseline expenditures is achieved, costs (and the fraction of GNP devoted to health care) could be expected to increase once again unless regulatory measures or changes in reimbursement mechanisms were implemented.

Other scenarios are certainly possible. It is unlikely, for example, that the full theoretical saving will be achieved because many real-world impediments are likely to prevent the complete elimination of unnecessary care. Furthermore, any cutback in useless care might take place

Table 1.—Increase in Community Hospital Costs*

|  | % Increase | |
| --- | --- | --- |
|  | 1977-1983 (Average Annual) | 1984 |
| Nominal increase in costs | 14.5 (±2.2) | 5.9 |
| Real increase in costs | 6.8 (±1.6) | 2.1 |
| Real increase in costs per capita | 5.7 (±1.6) | 1.2 |

*Data are derived from the American Hospital Association[6] (hospital costs); current population reports from the US Department of Commerce, Bureau of the Census, data to April 1985, Series P-25, No. 969, June 1985 (population); and US Bureau of the Census[6] (gross national product implicit price deflator).

over a period longer than the envisioned five years, in which case the impact on the annual rate of increase would be smaller. However, data recently released show a reduction in inpatient-days in 1985 similar to that observed in 1984; inpatient-days fell by 7.8% (adjusted patient days by 5.5%) while real costs rose by 2.6%. In contrast to 1984, more days were saved by reducing admissions than by shortening length of stay.[6,9]

## THE UNDERLYING REAL RATE OF INCREASE AND ITS CAUSES

The forces driving hospital costs upward must obviously be the major target of any long-term cost-containment program. Three variables appear to account for most of the current increase in hospital costs: population growth, rising real input prices ("hospital market basket"), and increased intensity of services, caused almost entirely by technologic innovation and diffusion. A fourth factor that is commonly invoked—the anticipated growth in the proportion of older people between now and the year 2000—will not be an important contributor; it can be calculated that they will increase costs by only about 0.2 percentage points a year.[10,11]

Of the three important factors, two are out of reach. Population growth, projected at about 0.9% per year,[12] cannot be directly or rapidly influenced by any policy action. Input prices likewise cannot be much affected by hospital management because hospitals must compete for their labor and supplies (note that in the case of inputs that are specialized to hospitals, such as nurses, this statement holds only for the long run). Moreover, labor-intensive industries such as hospitals are particularly vulnerable to rising costs because wages tend to increase faster than the costs of capital.[13] So it is not surprising that for the past decade, real hospital input prices have increased at a rate which averaged 2.2 percentage points higher than the GNP implicit price deflator.[10] . . .

Only one element remains readily susceptible to control: the introduction and diffusion of new technology. How much this factor contributes to the growth of hospital costs must be determined by subtracting the contribution of other factors: population growth, rising input prices, and changes in the number of adjusted patient days per capita. The difference—an average of 3.5 percentage points annually from 1977 through 1983—reflects increased intensity of services, resulting mainly from technologic change. Because there was no appreciable annual change in the number of adjusted patient-days per capita (an average of -0.1% annually),[7,14-20] the influence of technologic change is captured by the change in intensity of care per adjusted patient-day. If anything, the value for intensity may be low because an additional component of technologic change, increased

skill levels of hospital personnel, is almost certainly hidden in the Hospital Input Price Index.

## 1984 AS A TEST CASE

In 1984, the cost of care in community hospitals rose only 5.9%, as reflected in a survey conducted by the American Hospital Association.[6] This figure was dramatically reduced from the 14.5% average annual rate of increase for all community hospitals between 1977 and 1983 (Table 1), a period unaffected by the hospital cost-containment program of President Richard M. Nixon. Even when corrected to real terms by applying the GNP implicit price deflator, this improvement appears striking; the real rate of increase was only 2.1%, as compared with an average figure of 6.8% during the previous seven years (Table 1). This finding was greeted by many key observers as evidence that the problem of hospital costs had been solved (New York Times, July 10, 1984, p. 1).[21,22] But the theoretical considerations already discussed herein suggest that the optimism may not have been warranted.

In the following two sections, the data for the year 1984 are analyzed to provide a conceptual framework for evaluating year-to-year changes in expenditures and their policy significance. The results of this analysis are consistent with the view that current cost-containment efforts have, in effect, largely masked an underlying real rate of increase of nearly 7%.

### The Expected Rise Without Cost Containment

As noted earlier, we have calculated that the average real rate of increase in community hospital costs for the period 1977 to 1983 was 6.8%. This suggests that the underlying real rate of increase in 1984 was probably also close to 7%. Given that the observed rate of rise in 1984 was 2.1%, it would appear that a little less than 5% of costs was saved as a result of cost-containment efforts. In a separate calculation, the saving induced by cost containment during 1984 was estimated by determining the degree to which expenditures on labor and on supplies and equipment fell below their historical trend lines; this calculation also indicated a saving of approximately 5%. . . .

### What Kinds of Services Were Eliminated?

The evidence that costs would have risen by close to 7% in the absence of containment efforts raises the question of how the reduction of 2.1% was achieved. There are three possibilities: (1) days of care that were unnecessary, in the sense that nobody benefited medically, could have been eliminated; (2) beneficial services that would have been rendered in the past (conventional care) could have been withheld; (3) introduction of new technology might have been constrained.

The first and second of these options—cutting back either unnecessary days or those providing only conventional benefits—share the characteristic that they simply produce a once-and-for-all reduction in costs without affecting the upward trend. The point is obvious with regard to unnecessary admissions: there can be only so many of them; after a certain point, one must begin to reduce useful hospitalizations. Likewise, a given reduction in the number of worthwhile cholecystectomies will not slow the rate of growth in total expenditures unless the cutbacks are made more severe in the following year. Because only a modest reduction in the amount of conventional care is likely to be tolerated, the aggregate saving would soon be exhausted.

Analysis of the data for 1984, carried out within the framework just described, strongly suggests that rationing of any kind made little contribution to cost containment in 1984 and that the saving was achieved almost entirely as the consequence of cutbacks in baseline (current) expenditures. Unnecessary admissions were a large target for cost-conscious physicians—so large that there is little reason to believe that more than a few admissions perceived to be beneficial would have been included in the cutbacks. Much the same kind of reasoning applies to length of stay. One would expect unnecessary days (which mainly occur at the end of a stay) to be the first target. I have nevertheless made the implausible assumption that, of the 10.5 million days eliminated from length of stay (Table 2), as many as 10% to 20% entailed denial of beneficial care; this level of rationing would have reduced the rate of growth in costs by no more than 0.3 to 0.6 percentage points, even assuming that the last days of care are as expensive

as an average day. I have also assumed, again implausibly, that of the 6.0 million days saved by admitting fewer patients (Table 2), 10% to 20% reflected rationing of beneficial care, and that this reduced the rate of growth by 0.2 to 0.4 percentage points. Together, these two forms of rationing could have lowered the rate of growth by 0.5 to 1.0 percentage points.

In any case, most—indeed, nearly all—of the rationing in 1984 was likely to have affected conventional rather than innovative care. Reduced lengths of stay, in particular, would not be expected to involve the appreciable denial of new services (if only because it is highly unlikely that such care is applied at the end rather than the beginning of a hospitalization). Even if as much as a quarter of the saving that might be attributed to withheld benefits resulted from the denial of new services, the effect on the upward trend in costs would be only several tenths of a percentage point. Moreover, that minimal amount would in reality be an overstatement because the costs incurred in caring for sick patients outside the hospital would to some degree offset the reduction in hospital costs.

So it seems highly unlikely that the 5.7% rise in per capita cost (which would have been expected without cost-containment efforts) was much attenuated because novel medical technologies were withheld from people who might have benefited from them. In sum, the underlying real rate of increase was probably at least 5.5% per capita in 1984, as compared with the 1.2% increase per capita that was observed. (If the effect of population growth is included, these figures become 6.5% and 2.1%, respectively.)

## THE TECHNOLOGIC AND FISCAL FUTURE

There is good reason to believe that the future rate of technologic change will be at least as great as in the past ten or 15 years. We can thus anticipate serious problems in controlling costs unless we are willing to forgo, at least in part, introduction and diffusion of innovative diagnostic and therapeutic measures. A host of expensive new technologies is now being deployed and an equally promising group is currently being developed. Consider, for example, expensive diagnostic methods such as magnetic resonance imaging (MRI) and spectroscopic examinations of tissues by MRI, positron emission tomography, and laser holography. Therapeutic advances promise to have an even larger impact. Transplantation of organs, the artificial heart, monoclonal antibodies, interventional cardiology, implantable defibrillators, genetic engineering, cochlear implants, and treatments for metastatic tumors (such as interleukin 2) are simply examples of technologies that are likely to add billions to costs if all the benefits they offer are to be exploited.

Table 2.—How 17 Million Inpatient-Days Were Saved in 1984*

| | Thousands of Days (%) Saved by Reduced Length of Stay† | Thousands of Days (%) Saved by Reduced Admissions† |
|---|---|---|
| Medicare patients | 9297 (56) | 1776 (11) |
| Non-Medicare patients | 1250 (8) | 4271 (26) |
| Total | 10 547 (64) | 6047 (36)‡ |

*Calculations based on unpublished data from the Bureau of Data Management and Strategy, Health Care Financing Administration; Health Care Spending Bulletin, No. 85-02, April 1985; and the American Hospital Association.[6]
†Days saved by the reduction in average length of stay were calculated by multiplying the number of 1984 admissions by the reduction in average length of stay between 1983 and 1984. Days saved by reduced admissions in 1984 were calculated by subtracting the days saved by the reduction in average length of stay from the total days saved.
‡The 1% discrepancy between individual values and the sum is due to rounding.

Although there is hope that future research will lead to the development of technologies that will check the rise in costs, the near or midrange prospects for such an outcome appear to be small. One major reason is the ongoing development of noninvasive diagnostic technologies. Such new devices may provide a unit of service more cheaply than their predecessors, but they can be used on many more patients because the level of risk and pain is negligible. They can thus be employed even when the likelihood of obtaining useful information is small. Moreover, many new technologies cannot be fully substituted for their predecessors even when both are noninvasive. For example, MRI will not eliminate certain applications of computed tomographic scanning, so both instruments must be available with appropriate personnel. Furthermore, its use is contraindicated in some patients, such as those with pacemakers or who are claustrophobic. The same applies to cardiac catheterization where there has been a steady accretion of technologies, including thallium imaging, digital subtraction angiography, gated blood-pool scans, and ever more sophisticated Doppler probes.

Even the occasional therapeutic advance that seems at first to promise an overall reduction in costs may fall short of expectations. Angioplasty is cheaper than open heart surgery, but given the number of immediate complications and the frequency of restenosis, the net saving one year after the initial procedure has been performed is only 15%.[23] Moreover, because angioplasty is less traumatic than bypass surgery, it has opened the door to treatment of patients who are not candidates for surgery. As a result, the net saving from lowering the cost per procedure is likely to be offset by wider and more frequent application. The same may prove to be true with lithotripsy if many patients with renal stones in the absence of acute renal colic are eventually viewed as candidates for therapy.

It is reasonable to anticipate, of course, that cost consciousness will encourage manufacturers to focus new attention on designing equipment that will produce the same unit of service more efficiently. But it seems highly improbable that such efficiencies will do more than slightly slow the rapid rise in costs generated by the tide of new technology. On the other hand, it is likely that in the long run, fundamental scientific advances will do much to contain the costs of care—even the high costs associated with terminal illnesses and diseases of aging. But in the foreseeable future, there appears to be little prospect of such a happy outcome. Policy decisions between now and the year 2000 cannot be predicated on optimism that technologic innovation will sharply limit the rise in expenditures.

Another factor that will add to the upward trend in costs, at least in the near future, is a growth in the number of cases of AIDS. Recent estimates suggest that by 1991 we will spend $8 to $16 billion on the treatment of AIDS,[24] $2 to $4 billion of which will represent an increase over the previous year. To the extent that new treatments prolong the illness but do not lead to a cure, the rise in costs will be still greater.

## LONG-TERM STRATEGIES

If, as I have argued, the essence of cost containment hinges on limiting the introduction and diffusion of beneficial new technology, there must eventually be some kind of society-wide decision that this is a necessary step. What then?

One possibility is to limit the amount of money invested by the federal government in research on new technology that promises to increase health care costs. But it is highly unlikely that we will opt to freeze the health care system at its present level of quality and sophistication. A recent recommendation that the National Institutes of Health proceed with funding for artificial heart research is a striking example of our reluctance to limit costs in this way (*Washington Post,* May 24, 1984, p A4).[25]

Price competition, budget limits, and changes in reimbursement are economic measures that are far more likely to restrict technologic innovation and diffusion. If the size of the market for expensive new technology shrinks sharply, industry will invest much less in the development of new products. Finally, regulatory measures and reimbursement mechanisms—either tailored for the purpose or inadvertently—may have the effect of rationing care that requires high technology.

Some observers have suggested that eliminating unnecessary laboratory tests and x-ray examinations could make a major contribution to cost-containment efforts. Indeed, within the last year, it has been stated that such ancillary activities "are the most rapidly swelling component of health-care costs."[26] This statement appears to be without foundation. From 1950 to the early 1970s, the use of "little ticket" tests (x-ray examinations, chemical laboratory tests, immunologic studies, etc) did rise dramatically,[27-30] but since then standard laboratory tests and diagnostic procedures have not been used with increased frequency and have therefore not contributed to rising costs for a given episode of illness.[31-33] Rather, new procedures and high-technology care have been the major culprits.[32,33]

A one-time saving can, of course, be achieved by eliminating the wasteful use of diagnostic x-ray examinations, electrocardiograms and electroencephalograms, pulmonary function tests, respiratory therapy, and laboratory tests, but the potential saving is relatively small. "Little ticket" items in 1983 accounted for only about 10% of hospital expenditures.[34] If we were to eliminate 30% of inpatient-days (24% of adjusted patient-days) assumed to be useless, costs would be reduced by about one fourth simply as a result of this action—but this saving is already reflected in the calculation of the saving attributable to reduced patient-days. If one third of the remaining tests were eliminated on the ground that they have no value, the saving would be only about 1% to 2% of hospital expenditures; the saving is no larger because costs of the omitted tests are substantially lower than the average cost of performing a test or procedure.

## COMMENT

A substantial saving, probably on the order of $20 to $25 billion (of total expenditures in 1983 of $116 billion), could be achieved if some 30% of days (presumably useless) were to be eliminated. If the 6.1% reduction in hospital-days that occurred in 1984 were followed by similar reductions over the next four or five years, the underlying rapid growth in costs would be partially offset. Consequently, the share of GNP devoted to hospital care would remain the same or even fall slightly. But by the end of the decade, all of the saving from this policy would be exhausted and the underlying rate of increase in expenditures would become the observed real rate of increase. Even if there were then a slowing in the absolute increase in expenditures (eg, due to elimination of the useless application of new technology), the rate of increase on the lower base of expenditures would probably remain at about 7%; if both useless baseline care and useless novel care were reduced by the same amount, say 20%, the rate of change would be about the same as in the past. Long-term control of the rate of increase in expenditures thus requires that we curb the development and diffusion of clinically useful technology. Moreover, for the attenuation achieved in year 1 to be maintained in subsequent years, additional rationing of equal magnitude must be imposed in each successive year.

Contrary to widespread belief, aging of the population and the rising costs of hospital malpractice insurance are only small contributors to the rise in costs; aging will add only 0.2 percentage points annually to costs between now and the year 2000, and an annual increase in malpractice insurance costs of about $250 million ($90 million in real terms), such as occurred in 1984, would add less than another 0.1 of a percentage point.[35]

Analysis of the data for 1984 suggests that the observed slowing in the real rate of increase in hospital costs to 2.1% concealed an underlying real rate of increase of nearly 7.0%. Moreover, the relatively low 2.1% rate exaggerates the saving in heath care that was accomplished from reducing hospital days; to the extent that home health care and out-of-hospital surgical and medical care replaced inpatient care, the net societal saving has been overstated.

If rationing is to be used as a method for controlling costs, it seems clear that the first target should be cutting back on kinds of care that have the lowest expected value (expected value is defined as the probability of improving the clinical outcome multiplied by the value placed on that outcome). A good example of a low-value procedure would be a computed tomographic scan in someone with recurrent headaches unaccompanied by neurologic signs. A scan carried out in a patient with a severe head injury will have a much higher expected value and would not be a likely target for rationing. Because an investment in any given type of care produces different expected benefits under various clinical circumstances, the systematic use of so-called benefits curves will be essential to the appropriate allocation of limited resources.[36]

The mechanisms used for rationing might range from diagnosis related groups and budget caps to the evolution of powerful competitive forces. Whatever the cost-containment strategy, it appears that painful choices lie ahead once we have exhausted the easy savings that can be achieved by eliminating unnecessary hospital care.

This research was supported in part by grants from the Commonwealth Fund, New York, and the Robert Wood Johnson Foundation, Princeton, NJ.

I am grateful to Joseph Newhouse, PhD, The Rand Corporation, Santa Monica, Calif; Frank Sloan, PhD, Vanderbilt University, Nashville, Tenn; and William Bennett, MD, Harvard Medical School, Boston, for their insightful criticisms and comments.

## References

1. Luft HS: How do health-maintenance organizations achieve their 'savings'? Rhetoric and evidence. N Engl J Med 1978;298:1336–1343.
2. Luft HS: Trends in medical care costs: Do HMOs lower the rate of growth? Med Care 1980;18:1–16.
3. Newhouse JP, Schwartz WB, Williams AP, et al: Are fee-for-service costs increasing faster than HMO costs? Med Care 1985;23:960–966.
4. Manning WG, Leibowitz A, Goldberg GA, et al: A controlled trial of the effect of a prepaid group practice on use of services. N Engl J Med 1984;310:1505–1510.
5. Newhouse JP, Manning WG, Morris CN, et al: Some interim results from a controlled trial of cost sharing in health insurance. N Engl J Med 1981;305:1501–1507.
6. Hospital Statistics, 1985. Chicago, American Hospital Association, 1985.
7. Hospital Statistics, 1984. Chicago, American Hospital Association, 1984.
8. Statistical Abstract of the United States: 1986, ed 106. US Bureau of the Census, 1985.

9. *Hospital Statistics, 1986.* Chicago, American Hospital Association, 1986.

10. Freeland MS, Schendler CE: Health spending in the 1980's: Integration of clinical practice patterns with management. *Health Care Financ Rev* 1984;5:1–68.

11. Fisher CR: Differences by age groups in health care spending. *Health Care Financ Rev* 1980;1:65–90.

12. Arnett RH III, McKusick DR, Sonnefeld ST, et al: Projections of health care spending to 1990. *Health Care Financ Rev* 1986;7:1–36.

13. Baumol WJ, Bowen WG: *Performing Arts—The Economic Dilemma.* New York, Twentieth Century Fund, 1966.

14. *Hospital Statistics, 1983.* Chicago, American Hospital Association, 1983.

15. *Hospital Statistics, 1982.* Chicago, American Hospital Association, 1982.

16. *Hospital Statistics, 1981.* Chicago, American Hospital Association, 1981.

17. *Hospital Statistics, 1980.* Chicago, American Hospital Association, 1980.

18. *Hospital Statistics, 1979.* Chicago, American Hospital Association, 1979.

19. *Hospital Statistics, 1978.* Chicago, American Hospital Association, 1978.

20. *Hospital Statistics, 1977.* Chicago, American Hospital Association, 1977.

21. Richmond JB: *Annual Report: Overview of the First Five Years.* Boston, Division of Health Policy Research and Education, Harvard University, 1985.

22. Heckler MM: Remarks. Read before the National Association of Counties, Seattle, July 9, 1984.

23. Reeder GS, Krishan I, Nobrega FT, et al: Is percutaneous coronary angioplasty less expensive than bypass surgery? *N Engl J Med* 184;311:1157–1162.

24. Barnes DM: Grim projections for AIDS epidemic. *Science* 1986;232:1589–1590.

25. The Working Group on Mechanical Circulatory Support of the National Heart, Lung, and Blood Institute: *Artificial Heart and Assist Devices: Directions, Needs, Costs, So-cietal and Ethical Issues,* publication 85–2723. National Institutes of Health, 1985.

26. Angell M: Cost containment and the physician. *JAMA* 1985;254:1203–1207.

27. Scitovsky AA: Changes in the costs of treatment of selected illnesses, 1951–65. *Am Econ Rev* 1967;57:1182–1195.

28. Scitovsky AA, McCall N: *Changes in the Costs of Treatment of Selected Illnesses 1951–1964–1971,* US Dept of Health, Education and Welfare publication (HRA) 77–3161. Rockville, Md, National Center for Health Services Research, 1976.

29. Sheeley DR, Sherman H: Conservation in hospital resource use: Treatment of pneumonias: An investigation of care in four hospitals over the past decade. *Ann Intern Med* 1976;85:648–652.

30. Martin SP, Donaldson MC, London CD, et al: Inputs into coronary care during 30 years: A cost effectiveness study. *Ann Intern Med* 1974;81:289–293.

31. Showstack JA, Schroeder SA, Matsumoto MF: Changes in the use of medical technologies, 1972–1977: A study of ten inpatient diagnoses. *N Engl J Med* 1982;306:706–712.

32. Showstack JA, Stone MH, Schroeder SA: The role of changing clinical practices in the rising costs of hospital care. *N Engl J Med* 1985;313:1201–1207.

33. Scitovsky AA: Changes in the costs of treatment of selected illnesses, 1971–1981. *Med Care* 1985;23:1345–1357.

34. *HAS/Monitrend: Discharge Based Data Book: For the Period Ending December 31, 1983.* Chicago, American Hospital Association, 1984.

35. *Medical Malpractice: Insurance Costs Increased But Varied Among Physicians and Hospitals,* publication GAO/HRD-86–112. US General Accounting Office, 1986.

36. Aaron HA, Schwartz WB: *The Painful Prescription: Rationing Hospital Care.* Washington, DC, Brookings Institution, 1984.

# Chapter 28

## Breaking American Health Policy Gridlock

### Uwe E. Reinhardt

In summer 1990, *Health Affairs* published the remarkable findings of a ten-nation survey of the public's view of their health care system.[1] In that survey, the United States ranked lowest in the percentage of respondents who agreed with the statement: "On the whole, our health system works pretty well, and only minor changes are necessary to make it work better." About 60 percent of the American respondents concurred with the statement: "There are some good things in our health care system, but fundamental changes are needed to make it work better." Close to 30 percent went so far as to agree that "our health care system has so much wrong with it that we need to completely rebuild it." Only the Italian health system came even close to earning so dismal a rating.

If Americans seek fundamental reform or complete rebuilding of their health system, there is no dearth of proposals to accomplish these goals. Most proposals seek to achieve two objectives at once. First, they seek to extend health insurance coverage to the thirty-four to thirty-seven million or so Americans who now lack that coverage. Second, they seek to offer those who pay for health care—patients, business, and government—instruments to control both the cost of benefits and total expenditures.

In a recent publication by the Pharmaceutical Manufacturers Association (PMA), there is a giant matrix spanning several pages, which lists the numerous proposals and positions taken by the many stakeholders in the health sector.[2] Not included in the matrix is any inkling of what the Bush administration might eventually propose, what might eventually emerge from the ongoing deliberations of the Advisory Council on Social Security, or what might eventually be proposed by the hardworking National Coalition on Health Care, an outgrowth of the erstwhile National Leadership Commission on Health Care.[3]

Entered into each cell of the PMA matrix is a symbol signifying whether the stakeholder or proponent represented by the corresponding column of the matrix either supports or opposes the particular design feature shown in the corresponding row of the matrix, or whether no attitude has been explicitly registered so far. Although many of the cells remain yet to be filled with "favor" or "oppose," those that are completed follow a predictable pattern.

Totally unsurprising, for example, is the Health Insurance Association of America's (HIAA's) opposition to the oft-proposed taxation of employer-paid health insurance benefits. We should not expect that industry to give up easily the public tax subsidy it has enjoyed for so long.

Reinhardt, UE, *Breaking American Health Policy Gridlock,* Princeton University. By permission of *Health Affairs,* Summer 1991; 10(2): 96–103.

Such subsidies expand one's market. Just as unsurprising is the opposition to the idea by the National Association of Manufacturers and the U.S. Chamber of Commerce. These organizations, too, appreciate that the current tax treatment of fringe benefits strengthens their members' hands in the labor market, for it enables them to do for employees what employees cannot do for themselves: buy things with pretax dollars. Remarkably, what the AFL-CIO thinks on the matter is not shown in the matrix. If an economist had to place a bet on the matter, however, he or she would bet that labor would be loath to give up that public tax subsidy to private spending as well.

Similarly, the opposition of the American Medical Association (AMA) and the American Society of Internal Medicine (ASIM) to negotiate and/or control prices in health care is not unexpected. Although, in principle, all American providers of health care support the idea that health care should be cost-effective and that those who pay for health care must have some sense of budgetary control at the onset of their fiscal year, we must not forget that every health dollar debited by some payer to an expense account is credited by some provider of health care to a revenue account. Each side of the ledger tends to color rather differently one's perception of proper cost control. For example, as part of the budget compact passed in late 1990, Congress confidently determined that U.S. physicians can treat the nation's aged adequately in 1991 if total Medicare outlays on physician services in fiscal year 1991 were raised by 7.3 percent above such outlays in fiscal year 1990. By contrast, the AMA has determined just as confidently that the job can be done properly only if these expenditures were raised by no less than 13.7 percent, and possibly by as much as 14.9 percent.[4]

If one were to summarize broadly the positions taken by major stakeholders in the issues of access and costs, the following would be a reasonable synopsis.

Government, business, and the American taxpayer would dearly love to see health insurance and access to needed health care extended to every American, but they believe that there is so much waste and overpayment within the present health system that added millions of people could easily be brought into the fold in a budget-neutral way.

The providers of health care would dearly love to see health insurance and access to needed health care extended to every American, but they argue that America spends only the barest minimum needed to finance the care being delivered now, and that added numbers of Americans can be properly cared for only if society is willing to spend an extra $30 to $60 billion or so on top of the $700 billion this nation already spends on health care.

The private health insurance industry would dearly love to see health insurance and access to needed care extended to every American, as long as policies aimed at that goal do not eat into the industry's market.

Each position, taken by itself, makes perfect sense from the stakeholder's own narrow perspective. Alas, jointly they spell gridlock for American health policy. No single interest group now seems strong enough to shepherd a coherent health care reform package into legislation, because every such group seems powerful enough to sabotage whatever someone else proposes. One must wonder whether even President Bush, master builder of the Mideast Coalition, would be capable of forging a directed American health care coalition under our Byzantine system of governance.

This raises a fundamental question: In the probable absence of any coherent, politically viable strategy for health care reform, whither the American health sector in the 1990s? Will it simply lumber on with the status quo? Or will it look drastically different by the end of the decade?

## HEALTH CARE IN THE 1990S

The following seems a plausible scenario: A generally sluggish economy, the public's unwillingness to suffer tax increases, coupled with its clamoring for ever more government services and assistance—including sundry bailouts—will beget government deficits of unprecedented size. It may be possible to finance these deficits with a combination of home-grown and foreign savings, as long as the demand for financing by the private sector of the U.S. economy remains sluggish and as long as Eastern Europe and mainland China remain too risky for Western capital. Eventually, however, the world's suppliers of funds are apt to tire of holding ever larger mountains of American paper and will seek greener pastures for their funds. They will accept additional American IOUs only at commensurately higher real interest rates.

Long before that upward pressure on real interest rates actually will be felt, the U.S. government is likely to begin a series of increasingly strident assaults upon domestic spending. The Medicare budget remains an inviting target for such assaults. Apparently unbeknownst to the providers of health care, who have bemoaned that program's "brutal budget cuts" throughout the 1980s, the Medicare budget actually tripled during that period, from $34 billion in 1980 to over $100 billion in 1990. One must wonder whether Congress will let it triple again during the 1990s. There is apt to be much more concerted pressure to curb the annual growth in that program's outlay.

In seeking these curbs, the Medicare program can rely upon a powerful arsenal that the market devotees in the Reagan administration, wittingly or unwittingly—and, surely, quite ironically—took right out of the pages of Soviet economic textbooks: a system of administered prices set by the central government.[5] For better or for worse, this system of centrally administered prices has endowed the federal government with the lever of a clever hydraulic tax system.

It is now generally agreed that Medicaid pays the typical American hospital less than fully allocated costs for services rendered to Medicaid patients. During the past few years, Medicare, too, appears to have paid the typical hospital something short of fully allocated costs. For the most part, uninsured patients who are treated by hospitals pay them less even than truly incremental costs, let alone fully allocated costs. Jointly, these three groups of patients therefore leave the hospital with substantial uncovered fixed costs. The shortfall is made up by charging privately insured patients commensurately more than fully allocated costs. Large private payers with some market clout may be able to escape a part of this so-called cost shift by way of discounts garnered through preferred provider organizations (PPOs) or contracts with health maintenance organizations (HMOs).[6] Private payers who lack that market power, however, bear the full brunt of the shift. They pay full charges. Big business has, so far, played along with this system with amazing passivity.

As noted, small business firms now appear to be the main target of the cost shift. But they are victims of yet another major cost driver, namely, the extraordinarily high loading factor for administrative costs typically incorporated into the premiums for group health insurance policies sold to small business firms. [Table] 1 illustrates this phenomenon. Clearly, through their health insurance premiums, many small American firms now support almost as much paper pushing as they do health care proper.

During the past two decades or so, the annual growth in total national health spending has exceeded the annual growth in nonhealth gross national product (GNP) by close to three percentage points.[7] That trend is likely to persist through much of the 1990s, particularly if nonhealth GNP remains in recession for some time. IF federal and state governments continue to operate the hydraulic tax system as they have in recent years, if big business finally bestirs itself and resists the cost shift from government (leaving it to be absorbed mainly by small business), and if small American business continues to be the victim of the heavy loading factors shown in [Table] 1, then we can expect more and more small firms simply to drop health insurance as a fringe benefit or not to put it on their books at all. Thus, there is likely to be growth in the number of uninsured low-income and middle-class working Americans—a group not as easily overlooked by politicians as are members of the so-called underclass.

## GOVERNMENT OPTIONS

Government has three major options to respond to this development. First, it can simply look the other way, assuming that the problem will be taken care of by America's fabled thousand points of light. In practice, of course, these points of light will be the emergency rooms of the nation's hospitals. When 20 to 30 percent of the residents in a hospital's market area go without health insurance—as is already the case in many parts of the nation—the thousand-points-of-light approach will mean severe fiscal pressure upon the hospitals and doctors who feel morally obligated to treat critically ill uninsured patients. These providers, naturally, will do their part in the aforementioned hydraulic tax system. They will pass on the cost of their charity care to those private payers least able to resist higher charges, small business firms

Table 1
Administrative Expense Breakdown For Conventionally Insured Plans, As A Percentage Of Incurred Claims

| Number of employees | Claims administration | General administration | Interest credit | Risk and profit | Commissions | Premium taxes | Total |
|---|---|---|---|---|---|---|---|
| 1 to 4 | 9.3% | 12.5% | −1.5% | 8.5% | 8.4% | 2.8% | 40.0% |
| 5 to 9 | 8.6 | 11.2 | −1.5 | 8.0 | 6.0 | 2.7 | 35.0 |
| 10 to 19 | 7.2 | 9.2 | −1.5 | 7.5 | 5.0 | 2.6 | 30.0 |
| 20 to 49 | 6.3 | 7.6 | −1.5 | 6.8 | 3.3 | 2.5 | 25.0 |
| 50 to 99 | 4.3 | 4.8 | −1.5 | 6.0 | 2.0 | 2.4 | 18.0 |
| 100 to 499 | 4.1 | 4.0 | −1.5 | 5.5 | 1.6 | 2.3 | 16.0 |
| 500 to 2,499 | 3.9 | 3.2 | −1.5 | 3.5 | 0.7 | 2.2 | 12.0 |
| 2,500 to 9,999 | 3.8 | 1.4 | −1.5 | 1.8 | 0.3 | 2.2 | 8.0 |
| 10,000 or more | 3.0 | 0.7 | −1.5 | 1.1 | 0.1 | 2.1 | 5.5 |

Source: U.S. Library of Congress, Congressional Research Service, *Costs and Effects of Extending Health Insurance Coverage*, Report prepared for the House Committees on Education and Labor and Energy and Commerce and the Senate Special Committee on Aging, Washington, D.C., October 1988. Estimates by Hay/Huggins Company based on underwriting practices of major insurers.

prominent among them. As a result, those small firms that still offer their employees health insurance coverage are likely to see their premiums shoot up ever more rapidly. The erosion of insurance coverage among small business firms is likely to accelerate. This first option is a short-run remedy likely to set off a vicious cycle that feeds upon itself.

Government's second option would be to face the problem squarely and cover anyone not privately insured by a public fail-safe insurance system.[8] That option, of course, would require politicians openly to utter the dreaded *t*-word (taxes), for the approach would saddle the government with added outlays anywhere up from $60 billion or so. Furthermore, if the government sought to control the cost of such a program by activating ever more vigorously its lever of the hydraulic health tax system—simply by lowering fees to doctors and hospitals unilaterally—the second option also would likely drive up the health insurance premiums of small business firms, thereby triggering part of the same vicious cycle described under the first option above. The second option, then, is not an attractive remedy either.

This leaves us with government's third option, namely, mandated employer-provided health insurance. With one stroke of the legislative pen, that option would seep roughly two-thirds of the currently uninsured into mainstream American health insurance and, thus, health care. The remainder of the uninsured presumably could be absorbed into an expanded Medicaid program or, more probably, left as a more manageable problem for the thousand points of light in the nation's emergency rooms.

To be sure, a mandate upon employers to provide their employees with health insurance is a tax, pure and simple. If the mandate is to provide an insurance policy, it becomes a head tax on employment, that is, a tax whose magnitude is not linked to the wages of the employee. If the mandate is a so-called pay-or-play plan, under which employers must either offer their employees health insurance or pay *x* percent of payroll into a government health insurance trust fund, the mandate becomes a form of payroll tax. From the politician's perspective, however, this form of taxation is relatively attractive, because it can be artfully referred to in words that spare one's lips from having to trace out even the semblance of the dreaded letter *t*. Furthermore, if business is mandated to provide insurance outright, government can redirect added funds toward health care within the private sector without having these funds flow through its own budget.

The third option strikes me as the option most likely to be adopted first by various state governments and eventually by the federal government. Quite aside from its appeal among politicians, it now appears also to have the widest support among the providers of health care whose powerful hands have always guided the pen of

those who write health policy. The option has already found explicit endorsement by the AMA. It is likely to be supported also by the American Hospital Association, should that organization ever be able to reach an internal consensus on a preferred health care reform strategy. Although President Bush had tarred the idea as outright socialism during his election campaign, it should be possible to relabel the package more felicitously for eventual approval all around.[9] After all, the idea is really former President Richard Nixon's, who was wise enough to label it "Community Health Insurance Partnership" (CHIP).[10] Besides, what the president may not sign, many governors will.

## REPERCUSSIONS IN THE SYSTEM

One would expect large business firms, which currently underwrite so much of the cost of the uninsured through the hydraulic tax system, tacitly to endorse an employer mandate as well, although no self-respecting American chief executive officer is likely to campaign openly for the idea as long as it remains stigmatized as "socialism." Organizations representing small businesses, on the other hand, would be likely to offer genuine opposition. Indeed, it is improbable that the small-business sector would ever accept a mandate to provide employees health insurance so long as its insurance premiums remain experience rated over even small, single firms; so long as 30 to 40 percent of these premiums go up in administrative smoke; and so long as small business firms remain the ultimate, most heavily taxed repository of health care costs in our health tax system. It can be doubted that small business firms will forever be willing to pay their neighborhood hospitals much more for standard medical procedures than do large business firms with greater market muscle. That form of pricing will be labeled "unfair," market be damned.[11]

If mandated employer-provided health insurance passes into legislation at all, it is likely to be accompanied, at the behest of small business and possibly even the U.S. Chamber of Commerce, by severe regulation of the private health insurance industry. In the end, the policies sold by that industry are likely to be subject to (1) mandatory open enrollment; (2) mandatory community-rated premiums; and (3) a mandated all-payer reimbursement system, under which every payer within a given region will pay the same provider the same fee for the same service.

Such fees, of course, would have to be negotiated, at both the national and regional levels, between associations of payers and the corresponding associations of providers.[12] Bodies to perform that task would have to be established by legislation and endowed with the power to negotiate binding schedules of fees or capitation payments. Both government and the providers of health care would be wise to begin exploring the nature of this novel, semiprivate, semipublic institutional framework. Fortunately, Western Europe—particularly the Statutory Health Insurance System of Germany—offers a rich set of working models. Europe more so than Canada will provide insights for U.S. health policy during the 1990s.

The development I forecast is not likely to be the product of a bold, visionary, preemptive strategy and of sweeping legislation at any one time. Instead, it is likely to emerge gradually, as the product of a tortuous lurching by the health sector along the only logical path left open, absent a more coherent strategy. Very elegant the approach is not. One may aptly describe it as "health policy keister-backwards," as our health sector is inexorably backed into this particular corner, not by anyone in particular, but simply by the march of events and government's piecemeal reactions to them. It is a plausible default option for a health policy that has for so long now been stuck in gridlock.

## Notes

1. R.J. Blendon et al., "Satisfaction with Health Systems in Ten Nations," *Health Affairs* (Summer 1990): 185–192.

2. Pharmaceutical Manufacturers' Association, *Approaches to Improving Access to Health Care for the Uninsured: Proposals and Positions* (Washington, D.C.: PMA, August 1990).

3. The Department of Health and Human Services (HHS) is said to be working on a proposed reform package, although little about that effort has leaked to the outside, possibly because there is little to leak.

4. S. McIlrath, "Hold Medicare Spending Growth for Doctors to 7.3 Percent in 1991—HHS," *American Medical News* (21 January 1991):1, 23.

5. Diagnosis-related groups (DRGs) are nothing other than an accounting-cost relative value scale for hospitals. They become a fee schedule only when a monetary value is assigned to the basic DRG unit. That value could have been set through competitive bidding, or by negotiation. Instead, the Reagan administration chose to let it be set more or less unilaterally by Congress. Furthermore, throughout most of the Reagan and Bush administrations, there have been government-imposed controls on physician fees under Medicare. All told, these resemble more the pricing policies of centrally planned economies than the "procompetitive" strategy heralded by the Reagan administration.

6. Actually, the term *cost shift* is not a felicitous one in this context. The phenomenon is nothing other than straightforward price discrimination of the sort routinely practiced by the hotel and airline industries. It is found where the fixed unit costs of a good or service are high relative to incremental costs and where customers cannot resell the good or service among themselves.

7. V.R. Fuchs, "The Health Sector's Share of the Gross National Product," *Science* (2 February 1990):534–538.

8. For a proposal along this line, see U.E. Reinhardt, "Health Insurance for the Nation's Poor," *Health Affairs* (Spring 1987):101–112.

9. My favorite is "The All-American, Private-Public Sector, Judeo-Christian Health-Care Partnership Act."

10. See President Nixon's *Health Message to the U.S. Congress,* 18 February 1971.

11. The allocation of fixed costs among the customers of firms with high fixed costs and low incremental costs is rarely "fair."

12. Relative value scales would probably be set nationally. The monetary points of the base units would be set regionally.

# Chapter 29

# Expanding Medicare and Employer Plans to Achieve Universal Health Insurance

Karen Davis, Ph.D.

**Abstract:** This article presents a proposal for expanding Medicare and employer-based health insurance plans to achieve universal health insurance. Under this proposed health care financing system, employers would provide basic health insurance coverage to workers and dependents, or pay a payroll tax contribution toward the cost of their coverage under Medicare. States would have the option of buying all Medicaid beneficiaries and other poor individuals into Medicare by paying the Medicare premiums and cost sharing. Other uninsured individuals would be automatically covered by Medicare. Employer plans would incorporate Medicare's provider payment methods. This proposal would result in incremental federal governmental outlays on the order of $25 billion annually. These new federal budgetary costs would be met through a combination of premiums, employer payroll tax, income tax, and general tax revenues. The principal advantage of this plan is that it draws on the strengths of the current system while simplifying the benefit and provider payment structure and instituting innovations to promote efficiency.
(*JAMA.* 1991;265:2525–2528)

The United States has a mixed public-private system of financing health care. In 1988, of 244 million Americans, 13% were covered by Medicare, 6% by Medicaid, 57% by employer health plans, 9% by individual insurance or other sources, and 15% were uninsured.[1] This patchwork approach to health insurance coverage, while it serves some Americans well, contributes to a complex, costly health care system. The United States spends 12% of its gross national product on health care—far more than any other industrialized nation. Of greatest concern, an estimated 37 million uninsured people are vulnerable to receiving inadequate health care in the event of illness or injury and are exposed to the risk of severe financial hardship from health care bills.[2-4]

This article presents a plan to cover the entire US population by building on the two strongest elements of the current system—employer-provided health insurance and the Medicare program, which currently covers elderly and disabled persons—while instituting a new universal provider payment system to control rising costs. This plan would achieve greater efficiency and simplicity by establishing a common basic benefit package under both Medicare and employer plans, and establishing common provider payment methods applicable to both Medicare and employer plans. It would be financed through a combination of employer and individual premium contributions, payroll taxes, personal income taxes, and other general tax revenues.

Reprinted with permission from *Journal of the American Medical Association,* May 15, 1991, Vol. 265 No. 19, pp. 2525–2528. Copyright 1991, American Medical Association.

## RATIONALE

The strongest elements of the current US health financing system are the Medicare program and health insurance provided through large employer-based plans. Both are popular with beneficiaries and have a proven record of administrative efficiency with a low ratio of administrative expenses to benefits. Medicare has adopted new methods of paying hospitals and physicians that provide incentives for provider efficiency, simplify administration for both the program and providers, improve the equity of payment among providers, and give the federal government an enhanced ability to moderate the historical rates of spending growth.[5,6] Many large employer plans have been innovative in the establishment of incentives for employees to join lower-cost health maintenance organizations and other managed care plans.[6]

The Medicaid program is an important source of health financing for the poor and has been instrumental in improving access to health care for many of the nation's poor.[7–9] It is the only significant source of financing for long-term care—with over 40% of Medicaid expenditures devoted to nursing home care. However, the program has a number of limitations. Medicaid provider payment rates are clearly substandard. The program is administratively complex, causing many eligible people to fail to participate.

The most unsatisfactory sources of insurance coverage are individual insurance plans and small group insurance. Such plans have high administrative costs, charge high premiums, exclude individuals who are major health risks, and exclude coverage for preexisting conditions.[9,10]

Building on the strongest parts of the current US health financing system would have several advantages. With an existing administrative structure, expanded coverage could be implemented relatively quickly with minimal disruption of current coverage. Further, by building on current programs rather than replacing them, current revenue sources would be maintained. Any new taxes or other revenues could be targeted for care of the uninsured, rather than, for example, requiring major tax increases to replace existing private coverage.

## BASIC STRUCTURE

All employers would be required to provide basic health insurance coverage to full-time and part-time workers and dependents, or pay a payroll tax contribution toward the cost of their coverage under Medicare. Required employer financial obligations under either private insurance or Medicare would be limited to 6% of workers' wages. This would expand coverage to two thirds of the uninsured who are members of working families. States would be given the option of buying all current Medicaid beneficiaries and others below the poverty income level into Medicare, shifting most of the cost of basic hospital and physician benefits to the federal government. The remaining uninsured would be covered under Medicare, and would be assessed an income-related premium through the income tax system.

### Benefits

The current Medicare benefit package would be expanded to include preventive care for pregnant women and children, in addition to the current benefit package of hospital services, physician services, limited home care and nursing home care, limited mental health services, and limited adult preventive services. The cost-sharing structure of Medicare would be revised to include a maximum $250 per person, or $500 per family deductible—rather than separate deductibles for hospital and physician services. A coinsurance of 20% would apply to all services other than hospital care. Cost sharing would be limited to $1500 for an individual, or $3000 for a family annually.

### Employer Responsibilities

Employers would be required to contribute toward the health insurance coverage of full-time and part-time (defined as at least 10 hours per week) workers and dependents. Since all employers would be subject to this requirement, working spouses would be covered under their own employer's plan.

Employer coverage under private plans would be required to cover benefits at least as comprehensive as the Medicare benefit package. Employers could choose to provide benefits beyond this benefit package, without penalty to employers or workers.

Employers would be required to contribute at least 6% of employee earnings on average toward private plan coverage, not to exceed the cost of the basic benefit plan. Employees would be responsible for the remainder of the premium, but could negotiate with employers to cover a higher percentage. Alternatively, employers could meet this obligation by paying a 6% payroll tax to Medicare, resulting in coverage of workers and dependents under Medicare. Families bought into coverage under Medicare by employers would also contribute 2% of their family income toward coverage. Contributions to health coverage under either private plans or Medicare for low-income families would be offset by an increase in the earned income tax credit to ensure that such coverage would be affordable for low-wage workers.

## State Medicaid Plans

States would be given the option of buying all Medicaid beneficiaries and other individuals below the federal poverty income level into Medicare. Currently, states are required to buy Medicare coverage for all elderly and disabled Medicare beneficiaries with incomes below the federal poverty level, and recent legislation will require Medicaid programs to pay the Medicare premiums for those with incomes up to 120% of the federal poverty level. In addition, under recent legislation states will be required to provide Medicaid coverage to all children up to age 18 years in families with incomes below the federal poverty level.

Under the proposal, states would be given the option of enrolling all Medicaid beneficiaries in Medicare. However, states electing this option would be required to extend this option to all uninsured poor adults as well as children. States would be responsible for sharing with the federal government the cost of the Medicare Part B premium (currently $32 monthly), deductibles, and coinsurance on covered services. The effect of this provision is to shift most of the cost of hospital and physician services for Medicaid beneficiaries to the federal government, and nearly all states could be expected to do so. In addition, states could elect to supplement the Medicare benefit package, covering prescription drugs, dental care, and other optional services with full state funding.

The federal government would continue to share in the cost of long-term care services for Medicaid beneficiaries according to the current federal-state matching rate. Reform of long-term care financing is also an important issue for the national health policy agenda, but is not addressed herein. It adds significantly to the cost of any health insurance reform proposal, and is, in my view, best addressed separately on its own merits.

The Medicare provider payment rates for hospitals, physicians, and other providers would apply to services provided to low-income beneficiaries bought into Medicare coverage by the states. Physicians would not be permitted to charge low-income beneficiaries fees in excess of the Medicare allowable fees.

## Remaining Uninsured

An estimated 5 to 8 million nonpoor individuals would remain uninsured after expansion of employer coverage to all working families and Medicaid buy-in to Medicare of all poor individuals. Some of these individuals are early retirees who do not have retiree health benefits; some are disabled individuals who have not met the 2-year waiting period for Medicare coverage.[11]

All remaining uninsured individuals would be automatically covered under Medicare. They would be assessed a tax equal to 2% of their income, prorated over the year for any portion of the year during which the individual was not covered by private insurance. This would guarantee that all individuals who fail to be covered under an employer plan, an individual health insurance plan, or a state Medicare buy-in plan would be protected from the risk of financial catastrophe in the event of a serious illness or injury.

## Medicare Beneficiaries

Medicare beneficiaries would experience some changes under the plan. The cost-sharing structure would be modified to include a single deductible of $250 per person for all services, rather than separate hospital and physician deductibles. A ceiling on out-of-pocket expenses of $1500 per person would be established. On average, beneficiary cost-sharing burdens could be expected to decline, especially for those who have catastrophic illnesses or injuries.

## Financing

The current Medicare Trust Funds would be replaced with two new trust funds: the Medicare Elderly and Disabled Beneficiaries Trust Fund and the Medicare Employed Families and Individuals Trust Fund. Current Medicare beneficiaries services would be financed by revenue flows into the Medicare Elderly and Disabled Beneficiaries Trust Fund. Newly covered Medicare beneficiaries, including those bought in by employer contributions and by state Medicaid plans, would be covered under the Medicare Employed Families and Individuals Trust Fund.

The current financing of care for the elderly and disabled would be modified somewhat. Payroll tax contributions of 1.45% of earnings up to $125,000 for employers and employees would continue to be assessed and would flow into the Medicare Elderly and Disabled Beneficiaries Trust Fund. The current Medicare Part B flat premium would be replaced by a premium set at 2% of family income, not to exceed the full actuarial value of Medicare. Revenues from this income-related premium would be approximately equal to current part B premium receipts, although the distribution of the financial burden of the premium would clearly be shifted to higher-income Medicare beneficiaries. The premium would be collected through the income tax system, and forgiven for anyone with no net tax liability.[12] The premium would no longer be voluntary, but required of all Medicare beneficiaries. General tax revenues would continue to subsidize care for elderly and disabled beneficiaries, at a rate equivalent to the current general tax revenue contribution to Part B of Medicare.

Financing of the Medicare Employed Families and Individuals Trust Fund would be based on the 6% of payroll contributions by employers and 2% of income contributions of families and individuals newly covered under Medicare. States would contribute the state share of Medicare Part B premiums and cost sharing for Medicaid and other poor beneficiaries based on the current state matching rate under Medicaid. Federal general tax revenues would be used to provide any additional subsidies required to cover the remaining cost of employed families and nonworking individuals.

Provider Payment and System Reform

Employer plans would incorporate Medicare's provider payment methods. Specifically, physicians would be paid according to the Medicare Fee Schedule for all services, and a maximum limit on balance billing would be set on all services similar to that in the Medicare program. Employers electing to pay the balance bills for workers and dependents would be permitted to do so.

The Medicare Fee Schedule would result in lower physician payments than is currently the case in some private employer plans. Physicians would receive higher payments for Medicaid and uninsured patients. This would provide greater equity to physicians who currently provide a disproportionate share of care to low-income patients, and expand availability of care to such patients.

The Medicare Volume Performance Standard that now establishes a target for growth in expenditures for physician services under Medicare would be modified to include employer plans. This economic incentive to control unnecessary growth in the volume of services would be supplemented by the development of appropriateness guidelines and expanded research on effectiveness of medical procedures and treatment.

Hospitals would be paid a flat rate for the care of inpatients covered under employer plans based on the diagnosis related group prospective payment system. Hospitals would not be permitted to charge patients over and above the allowed rate. Again, while Medicare rates are lower than in some employer plans, bad debts for care of the uninsured and low payments by Medicaid would be eliminated under the plan.

Beneficiaries enrolled in both Medicare and employer plans would be given the option of enrolling in health maintenance organizations or other managed care plans. Employers would be permitted to pay a higher percentage of the premium, reduce cost sharing, or otherwise provide financial incentives to workers and dependents to enroll in more cost-effective managed care plans. However, the current practice by which larger employers obtain favorable price discounts through preferred provider organizations would no longer be permitted. Instead preferred provider organizations would be required to compete on the basis of the effectiveness of their utilization review and other managed care techniques.

## COST

While careful cost analysis would be required to estimate the fiscal impact of the proposal, a rough estimate can be obtained by drawing on the work of the Pepper Commission.[13] The benefits and coverage of the proposal are quite similar to the Pepper proposal, although the sources of financing, cost-containment methods including universal provider payment, role of private insurance, and administrative mechanisms differ. Like the Pepper plan, it can be expected that the incremental federal governmental outlays will be on the order of $25 billion annually (my estimate). These costs would be somewhat lower given the expansions of Medicaid that have occurred since the cost of the Pepper proposal was estimated. The cost-containment mechanisms set forth may also result in lower costs over time.

The new federal budgetary costs would be met through a combination of employer payroll tax contributions set at 6% of earnings for those newly covered under Medicare and individual contributions set at 2% of earnings for those covered under Medicare. Any remaining revenues could be met either through a 2% income tax surcharge on all tax-paying households or the establishment of a new upper income tax bracket of 38%.

## COMMENT

The principal advantage of the plan is that it is a feasible approach that draws on the strengths of the current system while simplifying the benefit and provider payment structure and instituting innovations to promote efficiency. It minimizes the need for additional federal outlays, spreads the financial burden of health spending more equitably among employers and states, and makes health insurance more affordable to small businesses, self-employed, and nonworking individuals.

The plan achieves greater equity within the health care system by reducing the fiscal burden of hospitals, physicians, and primary care centers providing charity care to the uninsured and contributes to their financial survival. It protects all Americans from the financial hardship of health care bills, and it helps get all children off to a healthy start in life through comprehensive coverage of material and infant health care.

It builds on the existing administrative system for employer-provided health insurance and Medicare and, most important, realizes savings from lower administrative costs of these plans.

The combination of a universal provider payment system, coupled with expenditure constraints and incentives for managed care, should greatly improve the ability of government and employers to constrain rising health care costs. It preserves pluralism in the health system, while permitting effective cost containment through a unified payer approach to setting physician and hospital payment rates similar to those of other industrialized nations.

This approach has a minimal disruptive economic impact and is likely to have a negligible impact on employment in small firms, with some expansion of jobs in the health sector. Its design minimizes any inflationary impact on the health sector, while making American products more competitive in international markets through effective cost controls and more equitable sharing of costs among employers.

The plan differs from the plan advanced by the Pepper Commission [13] and other mixed public-private plans in that it does not stress reform of the private health insurance market—such as requiring community-rating, prohibiting the exclusion of preexisting conditions, or establishing risk-sharing pools. While these measures are commendable and perhaps worthy of trial, they are working against the economic incentives insurers have to avoid bad risks and are likely to be circumvented through imaginative marketing practices.

Rather, the proposal gives all employers and non-working individuals the option of coverage under Medicare, with its administrative efficiency and strong cost-containment provisions. This should provide an incentive to private insurers to offer plans with good benefits at competitive premiums to avoid loss of enrollees to Medicare. However, it can be expected that the Medicare alternative will be relatively more attractive to low-wage employers, groups with greater than average health risk, and small firms that do not wish to search for a less costly private plan.

The tendency of low-wage employers to seek Medicare coverage, however, can be viewed as an advantage. It should help increase the stability of coverage of low-income individuals as they gain employment and leave welfare. Their coverage under state purchase of Medicare will continue as employer purchase of Medicare.

The option of purchasing Medicare should also reduce the extent of variation in experience-rated premiums among employer private insurance plans, by permitting high-risk groups to choose Medicare coverage. Dumping individuals identified as poor risks on Medicare should be mitigated by the requirement that an employer make an all-or-nothing decision to cover employees under Medicare. Persons deemed bad risks could not be singled out for public plan coverage. Medicare coverage, however, could be expected to be attractive to early retirees with health problems who do not have employer retiree health benefits or who cannot purchase private insurance individually at an attractive premium. Medicare becomes, in effect, the mechanism for pooling the cost of many high-risk persons, with necessary subsidies provided by general tax revenues.

The United States cannot afford to continue on its present course with a costly health system that subjects many of its most vulnerable citizens to inadequate health care. It is hoped that this article will contribute to shaping a consensus for change.

## References

1. *Overview of Entitlement Programs: 1990 Green Book.* Washington, DC: US House of Representatives, Committee on Ways and Means; 1990.
2. Davis K. Availability of medical care and its financing. In: Rogers DE, ed. *Doctoring America.* Baltimore, Md: The Johns Hopkins School of Medicine; 1990.
3. Freeman HE, Blendon RJ, Aiken L, Sudman S, Mullimix C, Corey C. Americans report on their access to health care. *Health Aff.* 1987;6:6–18.
4. Blendon RJ. What should be done about the uninsured poor? *JAMA.* 1988;260:3176–3177.
5. Ginsburg PB, LeRoy LB, Hammons GT. Medicare physician payment reform. *Health Aff.* 1990;9:178–188.
6. Davis K, Anderson GF, Rowland D, Steinberg EP. *Health Care Cost Containment.* Baltimore, Md: The Johns Hopkins Press; 1990.
7. Davis K, Rowland R. Financing health care for the poor: contribution of health services research. In: Eli Ginzberg, ed. *Health Services Research: Key to Health Policy.* Cambridge, Mass: Harvard University Press; 1991:93–125.
8. Rogers DE, Blendon RJ, Moloney TW. Who needs Medicaid? *N Engl J Med.* 1982;307:13–18.
9. Davis K. *National Health Insurance: Benefits, Costs, and Consequences.* Washington, DC: The Brookings Institution; 1975.
10. Davis K. National health insurance: a proposal. *Am Econ Rev.* 1989;79:349–352.
11. Davis K. Uninsured older adults: the need for a Medicare buy-in option. In: *Health Insurance Options: Expanding Coverage Under Medicare and Other Public Health Insurance Programs.* Washington, DC: US House of Representatives, Committee on Ways and Means; 1990.
12. Davis K, Rowland D. *Medicare Policy: New Directions for Health and Long-term Care.* Baltimore, Md: The Johns Hopkins Press; 1986.
13. US Bipartisan Commission on Comprehensive Health Care. *A Call for Action.* Washington, DC: The Pepper Commission on Comprehensive Health Care; 1990.

# Chapter 30

# Universal Health Insurance through Incentives Reform

Alain C. Enthoven, Ph.D., Richard Kronick, Ph.D.

**Abstract:** Roughly 35 million Americans have no health care coverage. Health care expenditures are out of control. The problems of access and cost are inextricably related. Important correctable causes include cost-unconscious demand, a system not organized for quality and economy, market failure, and public funds not distributed equitably or effectively to motivate widespread coverage. We propose Public Sponsor agencies to offer subsidized coverage to those otherwise uninsured, mandated employer-provided health insurance, premium contributions from all employers and employees, a limit on tax-free employer contributions to employee health insurance, and "managed competition." Our proposed new government revenues equal proposed new outlays. We believe our proposal will work because efficient managed care does exist and can provide satisfactory care for a cost far below that of the traditional fee-for-service third-party payment system. Presented with an opportunity to make an economically responsible choice, people choose value for money; the dynamic created by these individual choices will give providers strong incentives to render high-quality, economical care. We believe that providers will respond to these incentives. (*JAMA.* 1991;265:2532–2536)

## THE PARADOX OF EXCESS AND DEPRIVATION

American national health expenditures are now about 13% of the gross national product, up from 9.1% in 1980, and they are projected to reach 15% by 2000, far more than in any other country.[1-3] These expenditures are straining public finances at all levels of government. At the same time, roughly 35 million Americans have no health care coverage at all, public or private, and the number appears to be rising.[4-7] Millions more have inadequate insurance that leaves them vulnerable to large expenses, that excludes care of preexisting conditions, or that may be lost if they become seriously ill. The American health care financing and delivery system is becoming increasingly unsatisfactory and cannot be sustained. Comprehensive reform is urgently needed.

## DIAGNOSIS

The etiology of this worsening paradox is extremely complex; many factors enter in. Some factors we would not change if we could (eg, advancing medical technology, people living longer). We emphasize factors that are important and correctable.

First, our health care financing and delivery system contains more incentives to spend than to not spend. It is based on *cost-unconscious demand*. Key decision makers have little or no incentive to seek value for money

Reprinted with permission from *Journal of the American Medical Association,* May 15, 1991, Vol. 265 No. 19, pp. 2532–2536. Copyright 1991, American Medical Association.

in health care purchases. The dominant open-ended fee-for-service (FFS) system pays providers more for doing more, whether or not more is appropriate. ("Open ended" means that no budget is set in advance within which the job must be done.) Once insured, consumers are not cost conscious. Deductibles and coinsurance at the point of service have little or no effect on most spending, which is on sick people who have exceeded their out-of-pocket spending limits. "Free choice of provider insurance" blocks cost consciousness on the demand side by depriving the insurer of bargaining power. This approach is rapidly yielding in the marketplace to preferred provider insurance. In its present forms, preferred provider insurance helps to regulate price but is not yet very effective in controlling the volume of services. Medicare, Medicaid, and the subsidies to employer-provided health care coverage built into the income and payroll tax laws are all open ended and encourage decisions in favor of more costly care. These incentives are reinforced by a medical culture that esteems use of the most advanced technology, high patient expectations, and the threat of malpractice litigation if these expectations are not met.

Contrary to a widespread impression, America has not yet tried *competition* of alternative health care financing and delivery plans, using the term in the normal economic sense, ie, *price* competition to serve cost-conscious purchasers. When there is price competition, the purchaser who chooses the more expensive product pays the full difference in price and is thus motivated to seek value for money. However, in offering health care coverage to employees, most employers provide a larger subsidy to the FFS system than to health maintenance organizations (HMOs), thereby destroying the incentive for consumers and providers to choose the economical alternative. Many employers offer no choice but FFS coverage.[8,9] Others offer choices but pay the whole premium, whichever choice the employee makes. In such a case, the HMO has no incentive to hold down its premium; it is better off to charge more and use the money to improve service. In many other cases, employers offer a choice of plan, but the employer pays 80% or 90% of the premium or all but some fixed amount, whichever plan the employee chooses. In all these cases, the effect is that the employer pays more on behalf of the more costly system and deprives the efficient alternatives of the opportunity to attract more customers by cutting cost and price.

The rational policy from an economic point of view would be for employers to structure health plan offerings to employees so that those who choose the less costly plans get to keep the full savings. Several factors discourage them from doing this. Employers became committed to paying the price of the FFS plan in the 1960s and 1970s, when costs were much lower and HMOs were few. Now this commitment is hard to break. When an employment group considers more costly and less costly health plans, it knows that government will pay about one third of the extra cost of the more costly plan through tax remission. Labor unions see management commitment to full payment of costs of the open-ended system as a precious bargaining prize. There is a need for collective action. If one employer attempts to convert to cost-conscious employee choice while other employers remain with the employer-pay-all system, the employer will get disgruntled employees in the short run but no reformed, cost-effective health care system in the long run. For the latter to happen, most employers in a geographic area must convert to cost-conscious choice.

The second major problem is that our present health care financing and delivery system is not organized for quality and economy. One of the main drives in the present system is for each specialist to exercise his or her specialty, not to produce desired outcomes at reasonable cost. In a system designed for quality and economy, managed care organizations would attract the responsible participation of physicians who would understand that, ultimately, their patients bear the costs of care, and they would accept the need for an economical practice style. Data would be gathered on outcomes, treatments, and resource use, and providers would base clinical decisions on such data. We have few outcome data today. The FSS system often pays more to poor performers who have high rates of complications than to good performers who solve patients' medical problems quickly and economically. High-quality performers are not rewarded, because of the payment system and because employers and consumers do not have the data to identify them.

There are too many beds and too many specialists in relation to the number of primary care physicians. A high-quality cost-effective system would carefully match the numbers and types of physicians retained and other resources to the needs of the population served so that each specialist and subspecialist would be busy seeing just the type of patient she or he was trained to treat. We have a proliferation of costly specialized services that are underutilized. For example, in 1986, more than one third of the hospitals in California doing open-heart surgery performed fewer than 150 operations, the minimum annual volume recommended by the American College of Surgeons (*Los Angeles Times.* December 27, 1988:3).

The third major problem area is "market failure." The market for health insurance does not naturally produce results that are fair or efficient. It is plagued by problems of biased risk selection, market segmentation, inadequate information, "free riders," and the like.[10] Insurers profit most by avoiding coverage of those who need it most. The insurance market for small employment groups is breaking down as small employers find insurance unavailable or unaffordable, especially if a group member has a costly medical condition. Most employment groups are too small for risk spreading or economical purchase of health insurance. Systematic action by large collective purchasers is needed to manage competition to reward providers of high-quality economical care and to make affordable coverage available to individuals and small groups.

Fourth, public funds are not distributed equitably or effectively to motivate widespread coverage. The unlimited exclusion of employer health benefit contributions from the taxable incomes of employees is the second-largest federal government health care "expenditure," trailing only expenditures for the Medicare program. While providing incentives for the well-covered well-to-do to choose even more generous coverage, this provision does little or nothing for those (mainly lower-income) people without employer-provided coverage. Most of the $46 billion the federal budget lost to this tax break in 1990 went to households with above-average incomes, many of whom would have brought at least catastrophic expense protection without the tax subsidy, while little went to households with below-average incomes, people whose decisions to insure could be substantially affected by such subsidies. The system works backwards: the most powerful incentives to insure go to those in the highest income tax brackets. From a tax effectiveness point of view, it should be the reverse. Government-provided subsidies should give everyone strong incentives to purchase coverage and to choose economically.

In brief, powerful *incentives* that shape behavior in the health care system and that influence the distribution of services point the system in the wrong direction: services too costly for those who are covered, and the exclusion of millions from any coverage at all.

## OUR PROPOSAL

We propose a set of public policies and institutions designed to give everyone access to a subsidized but responsible choice of efficient, managed care (HMO, preferred provider insurance plans, etc).[11,12] We propose *comprehensive reform of the economic incentives* that drive the system. We propose cost-conscious informed consumer and employer (or other sponsor) choice of managed care so that plans competing to serve such purchasers will have strong incentives to give value for money. We also propose a strategy of *managed competition* to be executed by large employers and public sponsors (explained below), designed to reward with more subscribers those health care financing and delivery plans that offer high-quality care at relatively low cost. The goal of these policies would be the gradual

transformation of the health care financing and delivery system, through voluntary private action, into an array of managed care plans, each competing to attract providers and subscribers by finding ways to improve the quality of care and service while cutting costs. We propose restructuring the tax subsidies to create incentives to cover the uninsured and to encourage the insured to be cost conscious in their choice of plan. We propose the creation of public institutions to broker and market subsidized coverage for all who do not obtain it through large employers. We favor substantial public investments in outcomes and effectiveness research to improve the information base for medical practice and consumer/employer choice.

### Public Sponsor Agencies

The Public Sponsor, a quasi-public agency (like the Federal Reserve) in each state, would contract with a number of private-sector health care financing and delivery plans typical of those offered to the employed population and would offer subsidized enrollment to all those who do not have employment-based coverage. Except in the case of the poor, the Public Sponsor would contribute a fixed amount equal to 80% of the cost of the average plan that just meets federal standards. The enrollee would pay the rest. (The 80% level was chosen to balance two incentives. First, we wanted the subsidy level to be low enough so that there would be room for efficient plans to compete by lowering prices and taking subscribers away from inefficient plans. Second, we wanted the subsidy to be high enough so that the purchase of health insurance would appear very attractive even to those who expect to have no medical expenses.) To the enrollee, the Public Sponsor would look like the employee benefits office.

In the case of the poor, we propose additional subsidies. People at or below the poverty line would be able to choose any health plan with a premium at or below the average and have it fully paid. For people with incomes between 100% and 150% of the poverty line, we propose public sharing of the premium contribution on a sliding scale related to income.

Public Sponsors would also act as collective purchasing agents for small employers who wished to take advantage of economies of scale and of the ability of Public Sponsors to spread and manage risk. Small employers could obtain coverage for their groups by payment of a maximum of 8% of their payroll.

Today, a substantial part of the money required to pay for care of the uninsured comes from more or less broadly based state and local sources, including employers' payments to private hospitals for bad debt or free care and direct appropriations from state and local governments to acute-care hospitals. In our proposal, federal funds (the sources of which are described below) would be the main source of support for the Public Sponsors. These funds would be supplemented by funds from state and local sources.

## Mandated Employer-Provided Health Insurance

For better or worse, we have an employment-based system of health insurance for most people under age 65 years. It can be modified gradually but not replaced overnight. Most employers and employees agree that health care will be included in the compensation package. This is responsible behavior; if one of the group gets sick, the group pays the cost. Some employers and employees do not include health care in the package. The effect is irresponsible behavior; if an employee becomes seriously ill, these employers and employees count on someone else to pay. They are taking a "free ride." It is hard to justify raising taxes on the insured to pay for coverage for the employed uninsured unless those uninsured are required to contribute their fair share.

The existence of Public Sponsors would give all employers access to large-scale efficient health care coverage arrangements. However, in the absence of corrective action, the availability of subsidized coverage for uninsured individuals would create an incentive for employers to drop coverage of their employees. This would create additional expense for the Public Sponsor without compensating revenue. To prevent this, our proposal requires employers to cover their full-time employees (employers would make a defined contribution equal to 80% of the cost of an average plan meeting federal standards and would offer a choice of health plans meeting federal standards).

## Premium Contributions from All Employers and Employees

Many people who are self-employed, who have part-time or seasonal work, or who are retired and under age 65 years do not have enough attachment to one employer to justify requiring the employer to provide coverage. Thus, an employer mandate for full-time employees would leave out millions of people. Moreover, in the absence of corrective action, a requirement that employers cover full-time employees creates a powerful incentive to use part-time employees.

We propose that employers be required to pay an 8% payroll tax on the first $22,500 of the wages and salaries of part-time and seasonal employees, unless the employer covered the employee with a health insurance plan meeting federal standards. Self-employed persons, early retirees, and everyone else not covered through employment would be required to contribute through the income tax system. An 8% tax would apply to adjusted gross income up to an income ceiling related to the size of the household. The ceiling would be calculated to ensure that households with sufficient income paid for approximately the total subsidy that would be made available to them through the Public Sponsor.

The proceeds of these taxes would be paid by the federal government to the states, on a per-person-covered basis, for use by Public Sponsors in offering subsidized coverage to persons without employment-based coverage.

This tax would be at the federal level because individual states might be deterred from levying such a tax by employer threats to move to a state without the tax.

## Limit on Tax-Free Employer Contributions

We propose that Congress change the income and payroll tax laws to limit the tax-free employer contribution to 80% of the average price of a comprehensive plan meeting federal standards. The average price of a qualified health plan in 1991 might be roughly $290 per family per month. As a condition of tax exemption, employer health plans would be required to use fixed-dollar defined contributions, independent of employee choice of plan, not to exceed the limit, so that people who choose more costly health care plans must do so with their *own* money, not with that of the taxpayer or employer.

The purposes of this measure are two-fold. First, it would save the federal budget some $11.2 billion in 1988 dollars. This money could be used to help finance subsidies for the uninsured comparable to those received by the employed insured. Second, making people cost conscious would help enlist all employed Americans in a search for value for money in health care, would stimulate the development of cost-effective care, and would create a market for cost-effective managed care. Thus, this tax reform is defensible on grounds of both equity and efficiency.

## Budget Neutrality

The Congressional Budget Office has estimated the effects of our proposal on coverage, costs, and the federal budget and has found that our proposed new revenues would equal the added outlays.[13] We have not done a state-by-state analysis, but, in the aggregate, required state and local contributions appear to approximately equal outlays for care of the uninsured.

## Managed Competition

The market for health insurance does not naturally produce results that are fair or efficient. It is plagued by problems of biased risk selection, market segmentation, inadequate information, etc. In fact, the market for health insurance cannot work at the individual level. To counteract these problems, large employers and Public Sponsors must structure and manage the demand side of this market.[10] They must act as intelligent, active, collective purchasing agents and manage a process of informed cost-conscious consumer choice of "managed care" plans to reward providers of high-quality economical care. Tools of effectively managed competition include the annual open-enrollment process; full employee consciousness of premium differences; a standardized benefit package within each sponsored group; risk-adjusted sponsor contributions, so that a plan that attracts predictably sicker people is compensated; monitoring disenrollments; surveillance; ongoing quality measurement; and improved consumer information.

### Outcomes Management and Effectiveness Research

As Ellwood[14] and Roper et al[15] have pointed out, there is a poverty of relevant data linking outcomes, treatments, and resource use. Although such data are costly to gather, they constitute a public good, and their production ought to be publicly mandated and supported. Combined with the incentives built into our proposal, such data could be of great value to providers and patients seeking more effective and less costly treatments. Without incentives for efficiency, such data are likely to have little impact on health care costs.

### Mutually Supportive Components

Some components of our proposal have been proposed individually. However, they would be much more effective as parts of an integrated, comprehensive reform program than they would be alone. Consider, for example, a law that employers must cover their full-time employees. Alone, this law would leave out people who are not employed on a full-time basis and their dependents—12 million people. Without a payroll tax on uninsured employees, employers would have a strong incentive to escape the mandate by using part-time employees. Without Public Sponsors, the law would not address the problem of availability of affordable coverage for small employers. Without the limit on tax-free employer contributions, the law would not address the need for a cost-containment strategy.

We recognize the propensity of the American political system to seek minimal, incremental change. Some components of our proposal would be viable and helpful on their own. However, we believe that effective solution of the problems of access and cost requires a comprehensive strategy, and the merits of the combined package exceed the merits of the individual components.

## WILL IT WORK?

Our confidence that a reasonably well-managed comprehensive reform plan along these lines can be made to work rests on two propositions.

First, efficiently managed care does exist. It is possible to improve economic performance substantially over the nonselective FFS, solo practice, third-party intermediary model. The best documented example was a randomized comparison of per capita resource use between Group Health Cooperative of Puget Sound and traditional third-party insurance and FFS providers in Seattle, Wash, in the Health Insurance Experiment of the RAND Corp.[16] Group Health Cooperative of Puget Sound cared for its assigned patients at a cost about 28% lower than that in the FFS sector, resulting in essentially equal health outcomes and overall patient satisfaction about 95% as high. Satisfaction with interpersonal aspects of care and technical quality was 98% as high as in the FFS sector.[17,18] Group Health Cooperative of Puget Sound accomplished this without much cost-conscious demand and without any significant competing organized system. One wonders how much better they might have done if there had been several such organizations competing to serve cost-conscious consumers. Other nonrandomized studies have produced similar results.[19]

Many physicians and patients may prefer practice styles other than prepaid group practice. We do not have similar experimental evidence on the economic performance of independent practice associations and preferred provider insurance plans. However, we have observed wide variation in the performance of providers. For example, in Los Angeles, Calif, in 1986, one hospital performed 44 coronary artery bypass grafts with an 11.4% death rate and median charges of $59,000, while another hospital performed 770 coronary artery bypass grafts with a 3.8% death rate and median charges of $16,000 (*Los Angeles Times.* July 24, 1988:3). Some managed care plans would find ways of selecting economical providers of high quality and would channel business to them, improving quality and cutting costs substantially.

Second, people do choose value for money. Our limited experience with even attenuated price competition in employment groups such as federal employees, California state employees, and Stanford University suggests that, over time, people do migrate to cost-effective systems. A recent study of health plan choice in the Twin Cities, Minnesota, area found that employees' decisions are quite sensitive to health plan prices.[20,21] This accords with generally accepted principles of economic behavior.

We have been asked, "Why, if non-profit HMOs are so much more efficient and desirable, have they failed to grow except very modestly?" In times past, legal and professional barriers were important, including illegal restraints of trade.[22] In recent years, the main inhibitor of the growth of HMOs has been the employer contribution policies we have discussed; that is, most employers do not structure their health plan offerings in such a way that the employee who chooses the most economical plan gets to keep the savings. Nevertheless, some nonprofit HMOs have been growing rapidly; through the 1980s, Harvard Community Health Plan averaged membership growth of more than 11% per year, and the Kaiser-Permanente Medical Care Program averaged 5.2% growth on a much larger base. However, the success of our proposal does not depend only on nonprofit HMOs. Other forms of cost-effective managed care may do the job. What we propose is a restructured market system in which the efficient prosper and the inefficient must improve or fail.

## COMPREHENSIVE REFORM THAT RELIES ON INCENTIVES IS PREFERABLE TO DIRECT GOVERNMENT CONTROLS

One alternative to the system we have proposed is a system like Canada's, in which the government is the sole payer for physician and hospital services. While Canada's system has evident strengths, there would be major difficulties in successfully adopting or implementing it in the United States. First, it would require a political sea change to adopt such a system here. A tax increase of approximately $250 billion per year would be required, the intense opposition of insurers and many provider groups would need to be overcome, and the concerns of many employers and citizens about the effects of such a system on access and quality would need to be allayed. In the era in which the Berlin wall has been torn down, one must be cautious about branding any proposal as politically infeasible, but it is difficult to imagine a politician winning election on a platform including an extremely large tax increase. Second, government regulatory processes tend to freeze industries and often penalize efficiency. The Canadian system is not as frozen as it might be because proximity to the United States exposes Canadians to our innovations. If American medical care were also entirely financed and regulated by the government, the negative effects of regulation would likely loom larger.

A second alternative would be to leave the financing of health insurance for the employed population in the private sector but to have the government regulate physician and hospital prices for all payers. It is possible to imagine a political compromise in which such a system could be adopted—in the midst of a recession, providers might agree to accept all payer price controls in exchange for an employer mandate, and employers might acquiesce to a mandate in exchange for price controls—

but it is hard to imagine that such a regulatory structure could be effective over time in promoting quality or economy. Such price controls would be met by continuing provider efforts to circumvent and modify them. Providers would lobby for adjustments and exceptions deemed to enhance equity, increasing the complexity of the regulations and the incentives for those who were not favored to seek favor. Congress would have created a rich new barrel of pork to reward electoral supporters and contributors—an especially attractive source, because price increases for private sector rates could be granted without requiring a tax increase.

Furthermore, such a system does not contain incentives to shift medical care resources from less productive to more productive uses. The current mantra in cost containment is the development of practice guidelines and the application of these guidelines to eliminate the ineffective practices that exist in our medical care system today. While we strongly support the development of better outcomes data and practice guidelines, in the absence of change in the financial incentives created by the FFS system, such guidelines will do little either to control costs or to lead to improvements in efficiency. For guideline development to succeed, medical care would have to be much more of a science and much less of an art than it is likely to be at any time in the foreseeable future.

Finally, administrative costs in the present system are high and increasing.[23] These costs arise from many causes: the multiplicity of payers, each with its own forms, processes, and data requirements; the high marketing costs associated with the coverage of individuals and small groups; the costs of determining eligibility for coverage in a system in which millions have no coverage; the costs of billing patients for covered services; the costs of payers attempting to determine whether services were actually provided and were appropriate; and others. We believe administrative costs would be greatly reduced under our proposal. After a competitive shakedown, there would be relatively few managed care organizations in each geographic area. Everyone would get coverage through large group arrangements. Eligibility determination would be simple in a system of universal coverage. Today, the best managed care organizations do not bill patients for services. Providers are paid by health plans in simplified ways using prospective payments for global units of care. In a system with relatively few managed care organizations competing to serve competent sponsors and cost-conscious consumers, payers would not have to attempt to micromanage the delivery of care because providers would be at risk. Administrative costs and the "hassle factor" would be much lower than they are today. However, the most important economies would be in the effective organization of the process of care itself.

Over time, we would expect slowed growth in the price of the average health plan and continuing improvements in efficiency comparable to those in other competitive industries.

The authors gratefully acknowledge support from the Robert Wood Johnson Foundation, Princeton, NJ, and the Henry J. Kaiser Family Foundation, Menlo Park, Calif.

# References

1. Office of the Actuary, Health Care Financing Administration. National health expenditures, 1986–2000. *Health Care Financ Rev.* Summer 1987;8:1–36.
2. Schieber GJ, Poullier JP. Recent trends in international health care spending. *Health Aff.* Fall 1987;6:105–112.
3. *1991 US Industrial Outlook.* Washington, DC: US Dept of Commerce; 1991.
4. Kronick R. *The Slippery Slope of Health Care Finance: Business, Hospitals and Health Care for the Poor in Massachusetts.* Rochester, NY: University of Rochester; 1990. Thesis.
5. Wilensky GR. Filling the gaps in health insurance: impact on competition. *Health Aff.* Summer 1988;7:133–149.
6. Ries P. Health care coverage by age, sex, race, and family income: United States, 1986. In: *Advance Data From Vital and Health Statistics of the National Center for Health Statistics: No. 139.* Hyattsville, Md: Public Health Service; 1987. US Dept of Health and Human Services publication PHS 87–1250.
7. *Health Insurance and the Uninsured: Background Data and Analysis.* Washington, DC: Congressinal Research Service, Library of Congress; 1988.
8. Jensen GA, Morrisey MA, Marcus JW. Cost sharing and the changing pattern of employer-sponsored health benefits. *Milbank Q.* 1987;65:521–542.
9. Foster Higgins Health Care Benefits Survey. *Managed Care Plans.* New York, NY: Foster Higgins; 1989.
10. Enthoven A. *Theory and Practice of Managed Competition in Health Care Finance.* Amsterdam, the Netherlands: Elsevier Science Publishers; 1988.
11. Enthoven A, Kronick R. A consumer choice health plan for the 1990s: universal health insurance in a system designed to promote quality and economy, I. *N Engl J Med.* 1989;320:29–37.
12. Enthoven A, Kronick R. A consumer choice health plan for the 1990s: universal health insurance in a system designed to promote quality and economy, II. *N Engl J Med.* 1989;320:94–101.
13. Long S, Rodgers J. *Enthoven-Kronick Plan for Universal Health Insurance.* Washington, DC: Congressional Budget Office; 1988.
14. Ellwood PM. Outcomes management: a technology of patient experience. *N Engl J Med.* 1988;318:1549–1556.
15. Roper WL, Winkenwerder W, Hackbarth GM, Krakauer H. Effectiveness in health care. *N Engl J Med.* 1988;319:1197–1202.
16. Manning WG, Leibowitz A, Goldberg GA, Rogers WH, Newhouse JP. A controlled trial of the effect of a prepaid group practice on use of services. *N Engl J Med.* 1984;310:1505–1510.
17. Davies AR, Ware JE, Brook RH, Peterson JR, Newhouse JP. Consumer acceptance of prepaid and fee-for-service medical care: results from a randomized controlled trial. *Health Serv Res.* 1986;23:429–452.
18. Sloss, EM, Keeler EB, Brook RH, Operskalski BH, Goldberg GA, Newhouse JP. Effect of a health maintenance organization on physiologic health. *Ann Intern Med.* 1987;106:130–138.
19. Luft HS. How do health-maintenance organizations achieve their 'savings?' rhetoric and evidence. *N Engl J Med.* 1978;298:1336–1343.
20. Feldman R, Dowd B, Finch M, Cassou S. *Employee-Based Health Insurance.* Rockville, Md: National Center for Health Services Research; 1989. US Dept of Health and Human Services publication PHS 89–3434.
21. Feldman R, Finch M, Dowd B, Cassou S. The demand for employment-based health insurance plans. *J Hum Res.* 1989;24:115–142.
22. Weller CD. 'Free choice' as a restraint of trade in American health care delivery and insurance. *Iowa Law Rev.* 1984;69:1351–1392.
23. Himmelstein DU, Woolhandler S. Cost without benefit: administrative waste in US health care. *N Engl J Med.* 1986;314:441–445.

# Chapter 31

## Setting Health Care Priorities in Oregon

### Cost-Effectiveness Meets the Rule of Rescue

**David C. Hadorn, M.D., M.A.**

**Abstract:** The Oregon Health Services Commission recently completed work on its principal charge: creation of a prioritized list of health care services, ranging from the most important to the least important. Oregon's draft priority list was criticized because it seemed to favor minor treatments over lifesaving ones. This reaction reflects a fundamental and irreconcilable conflict between cost-effectiveness analysis and the powerful human proclivity to rescue endangered life: the "Rule of Rescue." Oregon's *final* priority list was generated without reference to costs and is, therefore, more intuitively sensible than the initial list. However, the utility of the final list is limited by its lack of specificity with regard to conditions and treatments. An alternative approach for setting health care priorities would circumvent the Rule of Rescue by carefully defining necessary indications for treatment. Such an approach might be applied to Oregon's final list in order to achieve better specificity. (*JAMA* 1991;265:2218–2225)

On May 2, 1990, the Oregon Health Services Commission (OHSC) released a draft priority list of health care services. This list was prepared in response to Oregon Senate Bill 27, which, contingent on receipt of a federal waiver, would expand Medicaid coverage to 100% of poor Oregonians while providing coverage only for those services deemed to be of relatively high priority.

As reported by Egan (*New York Times,* July 30, 1990; sect A:6), "Some doctors and consumer groups were highly critical of the draft list, asking why some procedures they deemed beneficial or lifesaving were placed below routine procedures like headache treatment." In response to these criticisms, OHSC blamed "incomplete or inaccurate information" and further postponed completion of the final priority list,[1] which had originally been scheduled for March 1990.

Although faulty data no doubt contributed to the perceived problems with Oregon's initial priority list, an even more systematic factor was also at work. Specifically, the cost-effectiveness analysis approach used to create the initial list conflicted directly with the powerful "Rule of Rescue"—people's perceived duty to save endangered life whenever possible.

## COST-EFFECTIVENESS ANALYSIS

Traditional cost-effectiveness theory dictates that in developing a priority list of services the cost of each service should be divided by some measure of the health benefit that is expected from treatment. Benefit is often defined in terms of "quality-adjusted life years" in order to integrate the expected longevity benefit or harm of a treatment with its overall impact on quality of life.[2]

Reprinted with permission from *Journal of the American Medical Association,* May 1, 1991, Vol. 265 No. 17, pp. 2218–2225. Copyright 1991, American Medical Association.

An excellent example of traditional cost-effectiveness teaching comes from the classic treatise by Weinstein and Stason[3] presented as follows:

> The ratio of costs to benefits, expressed as cost per year of life saved or cost per quality-adjusted year of life saved, becomes the cost-effectiveness measure. Alternative programs or services are then ranked, from the lowest value of this cost-per-effectiveness ratio to the highest, and selected from the top until available resources are exhausted. The point on the priority list at which the available resources are examined, or at which society is no longer willing to pay the price for the benefits achieved, becomes society's cutoff level of permissible cost-per-unit effectiveness.

As described below, OHSC followed this prescription exactly in generating its draft priority list.

Weinstein and Stason continue by observing that "[a]pplication of this procedure ensures that the maximum possible expected health benefit is realized, subject to whatever resource constraint is in effect." This statement assumes a utilitarian framework, in which the overall goal is to maximize health benefits within society—without regard to any effects on given individuals. Weinstein and Stason acknowledge that disregarding individual welfare is a limitation of the approach, at least when "the equitable distribution of benefits and costs across individuals or groups [is] of concern." Nevertheless, they assert, ". . . as economists are wont to argue, over large numbers of programs and practices the inequities are likely to even themselves out and, with some exceptions, may reasonably be ignored."[3]

This critical claim is effectively refuted by the Oregon draft priority list—and by public reaction to it. Specific examples taken from a single page of the 161-page list illustrate the problem. Surgical treatment for ectopic pregnancy and for appendicitis are rated just below, or as less important than, dental caps for "pulp or near pulp exposure" and splints for temporomandibular joint disorder, respectively. This priority order occurred despite the fact that the former surgical procedures are virtually 100% effective in treating otherwise generally fatal conditions, while the latter conditions are minor

and may resolve even without treatment. This counterintuitive preference order did not occur as a result of faulty data, as was suggested by OHSC, or by chance, but as an inevitable consequence of the application of cost-effectiveness analysis.

Table 1 depicts the factors that were combined to produce the priority ratings for the four treatments just specified; similar line items were generated for each of the more than 1600 condition and treatment pairs (eg, appendectomy for appendicitis) contained in the list. Three factors were estimated for each line item: (1) the expected net benefit from treatment, (2) the expected duration of this benefit, and (3) the direct costs of providing the treatment. Priority ratings were then obtained using the following formula: Priority Rating = Cost of treatment/(Net Expected Benefit x Duration of Benefit). This formula is a faithful reflection of classic cost-effectiveness theory, including the calculation of quality-adjusted life years in the denominator.

While a description of the procedures used to arrive at the various estimates of cost and outcomes is beyond the scope of this article,[4] the estimates in Table 1 appear reasonable. Dental caps, for example, were estimated to produce an average quality-of-life improvement of about 8% vs nontreatment, whereas an appendectomy was expected to produce a 97% improvement (virtually the difference between being alive and being dead).

These reasonable estimates did not translate into reasonable (relative) priority ratings, however. Although both surgical procedures for appendectomy and ectopic pregnancy were correctly estimated to entail a far higher level and duration of benefit than either of the two minor treatments, the relatively high costs of surgery effectively neutralized these outcome considerations, producing nearly identical priority ratings for all four treatments.

## THE RULE OF RESCUE

What's wrong with the priority order of Oregon's initial list? After all, in an economic or utilitarian sense it may be true, as implied by the relative location of services on the draft list, that the overall value to society of treating

Table 1.—Factors Producing the Priority Scores of Four Treatments in Oregon's Draft List

| Treatment | Expected Net Benefit From Treatment* | Expected Duration of Benefit, y | Cost, $ | Priority Rating† | Priority Ranking |
|---|---|---|---|---|---|
| Tooth capping | .08 | 4 | 38.10 | 117.6 | 371 |
| Surgery for ectopic pregnancy | .71‡ | 48 | 40¹5 | 117.8 | 372 |
| Splints for temporomandibular joint disorder | .16 | 5 | 98.51 | 122.2 | 376 |
| Appendectomy | .97 | 48 | 5744 | 122.5 | 377 |

*Maximum achievable benefit = 1.0.
 †Priority ratings were obtained using the following formula: Priority Rating = Cost of Treatment/(Net Expected Benefit × Duration of Benefit). Ratings ranged from 1.45 (highest priority) to 999 998 (lowest priority).
 ‡The net benefit is relatively low because Oregon's consultant physicians estimated that (only) 70% of patients with ectopic pregnancy would die if not operated on. Increasing the estimated net benefit from surgery to 1.0 would move this treatment to 326 on the draft priority list.

50 to 100 patients who have temporomandibular joint disorders or dental pulp exposures is comparable to the value of a single life. Treating many patients for a painful condition could, in theory, be considered equivalent to saving one life.

However, any plan to distribute health care services must take human nature into account if the plan is to be acceptable to society. In this regard, there is a fact about the human psyche that will inevitably trump the utilitarian rationality that is implicit in cost-effectiveness analysis: people cannot stand idly by when an identified person's life is visibly threatened if effective rescue measures are available. This strong proclivity has been dubbed the "Rule of Rescue" by Jonsen,[5] who recognized the difficulties posed by the Rule for resource allocation planning:

> Many of the technologies under assessment relieve illness or pain or disability, but do not directly save life, do not rescue people from imminent death. Those technologies that do stave off death pose a particularly daunting problem [for resource allocation planners] . . . a barrier difficult to climb, a chasm difficult to leap: namely, the imperative to rescue endangered life.[5]

This duty-based imperative, Jonsen believes, cannot be "expunged from our collective moral conscience," even by the "most evangelical utilitarian." Moreover, although the Rule of Rescue clearly is most compelling in the context of lifesaving interventions, it is also a factor whenever an identified patient is in need of treatment (eg, for a fractured arm).

Ironically, it was a graphic example of the Rule of Rescue that stimulated current events in Oregon. In June 1987, the Oregon legislature decided to stop funding pancreas, liver, heart, and bone marrow transplants under its Medicaid system.[6] Some 6 months later, a 7-year-old boy, named Coby Howard, died of acute lymphocytic leukemia after trying but failing to receive a bone marrow transplant under Medicaid. His mother raised $80,000 of the necessary $100,000 hospital deposit before Coby died. Amid the glare of cameras, the state and nation watched the little boy die, apparently for want of a medical procedure that would have been available just a few months earlier. The *New York Times* (May 1, 1988;sect A:12) ran a story entitled "Oregon Cut in Transplant Aid Spurs Victim to Turn Actor to Avert Death," referring to the child's "performances" at fundraising events.

The "Coby Howard factor," as it might be called, would likely resurface every time an identified patient was denied access to a treatment that was acknowledged to be substantially beneficial, or "lifesaving." The extent of media exposure would vary with the patient's age and attractiveness,[7] but would represent a source of continual societal discomfort and shame.

Is the Rule of Rescue justified or simply an emotional reaction of some kind? Very likely, it is both. Depending on one's conception of distributive justice (ie, what we owe each other), the Rule might be seen as facilitating a sense of fairness in providing for the needs of others—a sense that might be poorly developed otherwise. Clearly, however, as noted above, there is also an emotional component to the Rule of Rescue that can interfere with the development and implementation of fair allocation systems. Society cannot afford to provide every possible beneficial service to every patient—identified or not—as Oregon's planners realized when they embarked on their priority-setting mission. Yielding to the Rule of Rescue in every case of apparent need would lead to an impossibly expensive system.

How then should we cope with the Rule of Rescue when setting health care priorities, as we surely must do if equitable and rational systems of resource allocation are to be developed?[8] To answer this question, let's look at how OHSC proceeded following the release of its draft priority list.

## DEVELOPMENT OF THE FINAL PRIORITY LIST

Strung by public criticism of its initial list, and themselves dismayed by the intuitive unacceptability of the draft list's priority order, OHSC moved swiftly to adopt a different method for purposes of developing its final priority list. Thus, while attributing the problems in their draft list to flaws in the data, OHCS immediately established an Alternative Methodology Subcommittee to investigate other methods for complying with the mandates of Oregon Senate Bill 27. The Alternative Methodology Subcommittee promptly focused on a distinctly different, cost-free method for setting health care priorities—one that OHSC had considered previously but rejected in favor of the cost-effectiveness formula described above. This alternate method, which was based on a suggestion I originally put forth in an unpublished grant proposal (D. Hadorn, *Health Care Effectiveness Research and Public Policy*, November 23, 1988), consisted of two steps: (1) developing a set of categories that depict varying types or degrees of expected health benefit from treatments, and (2) assigning each condition and treatment pair to a single category.

At the recommendation of the Alternative Methodology Subcommittee, OHSC again explored this categorization approach. After trimming the Alternative Methodology Subcommittee's draft set of 26 categories to 17, OHSC ranked the final set of categories (Table 2) in order of importance, based on three criteria: (1) the category's perceived value to the individual, (2) its value to society, and (3) the "necessity" of the category. Next, OHSC assigned each line item (eg, appendectomy for appendicitis) to one specific category. Several runs were

Table 2.—Oregon Health Services Commission's Service Category Definitions (in Rank Order of Deemed Importance)*

1. Treatment of acute life-threatening conditions† where treatment prevents imminent death‡ with a full recovery§ and return to previous health state§
    *Examples:* Appendectomy for appendicitis
    Repair of deep, open wound of neck
2. Maternity care, including disorders of newborn
    *Examples:* Obstetrical care for pregnancy
    Medical therapy for low birth-weight babies
3. Treatment of acute life-threatening conditions† where treatment prevents imminent death‡ without a full recovery§ or return to previous health state§
    *Examples:* Surgical treatment for head injury with prolonged loss of consciousness
    Medical therapy for acute bacterial meningitis
4. Prevention care for children (includes well-child care)∥
    *Examples:* Immunizations
    Screening for vision or hearing problems
5. Treatment of a fatal, chronic condition where, with treatment, one would have improvement in life span‡ and QWB¶
    *Examples:* Medical therapy for type I diabetes mellitus
    Medical therapy for asthma
6. Reproductive services (excluding maternity and infertility)#
    *Examples:* Contraceptive management, vasectomy, tubal ligation
7. Comfort care**
8. Preventive dental care
    *Example:* Cleaning and fluoride
9. Preventive (A, B, C), adults∥
    *Examples:* Mammograms, blood pressure screening
10. Treatment of acute,§ nonfatal†† non–self-limited§ conditions with return to previous health state§
    *Examples:* Medical therapy for acute thyroiditis
    Medical therapy for vaginitis
11. One-time treatment of nonfatal,†† chronic§ conditions with improvement in QWB¶
    *Examples:* Hip replacement
    Laser surgery for diabetic retinopathy
12. Treatment of acute,§ nonfatal†† conditions where treatment will improve QWB¶ without return to prior health state§
    *Examples:* Relocation of dislocated elbow
    Arthroscopic repair of internal derangement of knee
13. Repetitive treatment§ of nonfatal,†† chronic§ (with recurrent or continuous symptoms) conditions with improvement in QWB¶ with short-term benefit§
    *Examples:* Medical therapy for chronic sinusitis
    Medical therapy for migraine headache
14. Treatment of acute,§ nonfatal,†† self-limited§ condition where treatment will expedite return to prior health state§
    *Examples:* Medical therapy for diaper rash
    Medical therapy for acute conjunctivitis
15. Infertility services
    *Examples:* Medical therapy for anovulation
    Microsurgery for tubal disease
16. Preventive (D, E), adults∥
    *Examples:* Dipstick urinalysis for hematuria in adults who are younger than 60 years
    Sigmoidoscopy for persons who are younger than 40 years
17. Treatment of fatal† or nonfatal†† conditions with minimal or no improvement in QWB¶ or life span§
    *Examples:* Medical therapy for gallstones without cholecystitis
    Medical therapy for viral warts

*OHSC refers to Oregon Health Services Commission. Category descriptions are verbatim from working documents used by the OHSC. Examples are taken from material released by OHSC for its press conference on February 20, 1991, at which the final list was announced.
†Five-year mortality rate estimated at 1% or greater.
‡Reduces expected 5-year mortality rate by 25% or more.
§Not defined, left to the judgment of commissioners.
∥Defined by reference to the US Preventive Services Task Force Report, except that well-child care is defined using American Academy of Pediatrics guidelines.
¶QWB refers to quality of well-being, the Commission's term for quality of life; derived from the QWB Index of Robert Kaplan and colleagues.*
#Also includes abortion for "unwanted pregnancy." OHSC will issue a separate disclaimer stating that it advises no change in current Oregon Medicaid policy with respect to abortion.
**Patients with estimated remaining life span of 1 year or less.
††Five-year mortality rate <1%.

made through the categories by different commissioners in an attempt to achieve consensus and relative consistency in category assignments.

Encouraged by the results of these exercises, OHSC voted on September 5, 1990, to adopt the categorization approach as an alternative to cost-effectiveness analysis for preparing its final list. The next 5 months were spent adjusting category descriptions and definitions, assigning and reassigning line items to the various categories, and continuing to make line item data corrections. Final adjustments in category ranking and line item assignments were made by OHSC on February 2, 1991.

The final priority list was prepared by "stacking" categories on top of each other in rank order so that all the line items in the top-ranked category were deemed to be of higher priority than all the items in the second-ranked category, and so on. Services were ordered within each category according to the net benefit component of the cost-effectiveness ratio. This criterion was selected because in earlier test runs it had seemed to generate the most sensible priority order. Thus, cost was eliminated as a systematic factor in the ordering of services on the final priority list.

To a very minor extent, cost was reintroduced in the concluding step of the process, during which OHSC rearranged line items "by hand." Between February 13 and February 20 (the date of OHSC's meeting, at which time the final priority list was released), the commissioners of OHSC moved individual line items higher or lower on the priority list based on their collective judgment concerning the overall importance of each item in relation to the others. These judgments were guided informally by several factors (as articulated by the commissioners during their discussion and debate), including the number of people who were expected to benefit from a treatment, the value placed on the treatment by society (eg, higher weights on prevention and maternal and child care), and on the item's cost-effectiveness ratio (ie, priority rating [Table 1]). Thus, service costs were factored into Oregon's final priority list to a minor extent; the influence of cost on the final ordering of services was negligible, however, in comparison with the effect of the categories and the initial within-category ranking of services by net benefit.

Approximately 33% to 50% of the line items contained in the final list were rearranged, although only about 5% to 10% were moved more than 50 positions from the locations arrived at by the prioritization method just described. This rearrangement rate seems reasonable in view of the tremendous complexity of the prioritization task. Surely far more "list jockeying" (as the commissioners sometimes called the process) would have been necessary had the original cost-effectiveness formula been retained, since the Rule of Rescue would still have been a factor. Because service costs were essentially eliminated from Oregon's final priority list, however, the Rule of Rescue was quiescent; as a result, the priority order of the final list generally appears to be far more sensible than the initial list. For example, surgery for appendicitis and for ectopic pregnancy are now both ranked in the top 10 services, while splints for temporomandibular joint disorder dropped near the bottom of the list and dental caps were eliminated entirely as a separate line item.

Events in Oregon continue to evolve. An actuarial analysis of the final priority list will be completed by May 1, which will furnish estimates of the costs required for the state to provide the various services on the priority list—based on historical conjunctions of the various diagnosis and treatment codes used by OHSC to define each line item. These codes were taken from the *International Classification of Diseases, Ninth Revision (ICD-9)* and *Current Procedural Terminology, Fourth Edition (CPT-4)* manuals. Multiple copies of these man-

uals were always present (and heavily used) during OHSC's meetings.

After estimating the costs of line items, actuaries will calculate the total cost of providing services down to each of several possible "cut points" in the final list. The Oregon Legislative Assembly will then review the final list and decide, by late spring 1991, whether to accept it as the basis for changing the Oregon Medicaid program. If the list is accepted, legislators will "draw a line" somewhere on the list to divide the services that will be covered under Oregon's Medicaid program (those "above the line") from services that will not to be covered (those "below the line"). Legislators are not authorized to change the order of the priority list.

In its final report, scheduled for release May 1, 1991, OHSC will issue a series of findings and recommendations, including the finding that "essential health care" consists of almost all of the services in categories 1 through 9 (Table 2) and most of the services in categories 10 through 13. Services in categories 14 through 17 are deemed nonessential. Based on the location of services on the final list (a total of 714 items), a line drawn somewhere between item 450 (removal of an ovary or fallopian tube for benign conditions) and item 500 (lobectomy for benign pulmonary neoplasm) would appear to fulfill OHSC's definition of essential care.

Finally, if Oregon's Legislative Assembly accepts the priority list and specifies a funding cutoff point, Oregon's leaders will petition both the US Congress and the Health Care Financing Administration for a Medicaid waiver—required for the restructuring of Oregon's Medical program to proceed. Prospects for a waiver will be dim if the Legislative Assembly fails to find services in accordance with OHSC's definition of essential care.

Waiver legislation, as currently drafted, would permit the federal government to "pull the waiver at any time if basic health needs of the poor are threatened" (*Healthweek*, March 11, 1991:12). In addition, and problematically, the bill would include "safeguards that prevent other states from following Oregon's lead" (*Healthweek*, March 11, 1991:12) for a period of 3 years. This latter provision was contained in the original waiver legislation, drafted by Rep Ron Wyden (D, Ore) in November 1988 (in anticipation of what later became Oregon Senate Bill 27), and is being carried forward in current versions of the bill.

Although Oregon was probably 3 years ahead of the field in 1988, many other states are today also interested in the concept of prioritization. For example, in March 1991, the Colorado legislature narrowly defeated (for the second year in a row) a bill that would have established health care priorities for all basic-level health plans, including (but not limited to) Medicaid. Similar legislation is likely to be reintroduced next year. Colorado and other states may, therefore, be expected to oppose Oregon's proposed exclusionary provision, especially in view of the desperate financial status of state Medicaid programs across the country—and because setting priorities will be an inevitable part of any long-term solution to the health care cost-access problem. In my opinion, states other than Oregon should be permitted to implement their own carefully considered prioritization programs, assuming that adequate oversight and evaluation is maintained.

## MODIFIED COST-EFFECTIVENESS ANALYSIS

Returning to our discussion of the Oregon process, we have seen how Oregon's final priority list was generated primarily by reference to category assignment, which in turn was based on the expected health benefit of treatment. Moreover, services were arranged within categories (prior to hand-rearranging) according to the net benefit component of the cost-effectiveness formula. Thus, service costs were effectively eliminated in generating the final priority list. It was also noted that the Oregon legislature will specify a cutoff point for funding under Medicaid (assuming the final priority list is deemed acceptable). The cutoff point would determine the balance between the range of services covered under Oregon's Medicaid program and the cost of that program.

This two-stage process represents a modification rather than an abandonment of traditional cost-effectiveness theory, since services are still ranked and "selected from the top until resources are exhausted."[3] The key difference, of course, is that Oregon's final list was not constructed using cost-effectiveness ratios as the initial criterion of priority, as posited by traditional theory.

In my view, this two-stage, modified approach represents a significant advance over traditional cost-effectiveness analysis for purposes of setting health care priorities. Setting priorities first on the basis of net expected health benefit, followed by a determination of the degree of benefit required before services are deemed necessary (eg, how close to the top of the list they must be for coverage), provides a reasonable compromise between a public-good, utilitarian framework and the need to accommodate the Rule of Rescue.

Using this two-stage process for setting priorities, a patient, such as Coby Howard, would not be denied access to a desired treatment (ie, the patient would not be denied coverage under his or her insurance plan) unless that treatment had been judged relatively non-beneficial from the perspective of health outcomes alone and without explicit consideration of cost (this point is pursued below). Thus, coverage would be denied only when the desired treatment had been duly deemed not to work (well enough) for patients with that particular problem. Therefore, in cases of coverage denial, there

would be fewer distressing implications to the effect that society had judged a patient's life to be of insufficient value (ie, the cost of the service) to warrant receiving a particular treatment, or had decided to "sacrifice" him or her for the greater good. Once it was clear that no reasonably effective rescue measure existed for a patient—that there is "nothing [effective] we can do"—obedience to the Rule of Rescue becomes futile and pointless, and in most cases can be expected to give way to resignation and acceptance.

## THE PROBLEM OF HIGH-COST AND HIGH-BENEFIT SERVICES

A major potential problem with this approach is that some highly beneficial treatments might cost so much that giving priority to them would distort the priority structure. Other treatments of moderate to high benefit might be "squeezed out" if no consideration was given to the costs of services within the highest levels of care.

Pending actuarial analysis of Oregon's final list, it is not possible to say whether and to what extent this problem occurred using Oregon's method. However, any reasonable method for integrating the expected longevity and quality-of-life benefits of treatment would likely place relatively few very expensive treatments within the top tiers of beneficial care. It is difficult to think of even a single instance of an expensive treatment that offers benefits on the order of, say, a simple appendectomy or, for that matter, comparable to prenatal care and immunizations. Most exotic and costly health services have not been demonstrated to provide a high degree of benefit with any degree of certainty.

Even when a very expensive treatment is considered highly beneficial, this level of benefit is usually expected for only a few indications. For example, liver transplants were recently evaluated by the Agency for Health Care Policy and Research and found to be of convincing benefit only for patients who suffer from primary biliary cirrhosis or primary sclerosing cholangitis.[10] Similarly, low osmolar contrast media, a relatively expensive alternative to standard roentgenographic contrast media, probably cannot reasonably be expected to be of significant net benefit for patients other than those who are at high risk for an adverse reaction.[11] (Unfortunately, as will be discussed below, Oregon's final priority list does not permit an adequate degree of resolution among different types of patients.)

The above considerations notwithstanding, what would happen if the number of expensive and important treatments did in fact overly distort the priority list (by virtue of cost's not being a factor in developing the list)? If this were to happen, the following three responses would be available under the two-stage process: (1) raise more money (eg, through taxes or premiums) in order to provide for all health care needs as currently defined, eg, above the line; (2) permit people who cannot pay for some care that is deemed necessary to go without; or (3) redefine necessary care by selecting a more stringent standard for judging when services are necessary (eg, moving the cutoff point on the prioritized list of services closer to the top).

The first approach to the problem of inadequate resources for necessary care is the most straightforward, and would be the most effective in keeping the Rule of Rescue under control. This option may not always be politically feasible, however. The second alternative, by contrast, conflicts directly with the Rule of Rescue—and with the tenets of distributive justice—and should, therefore, be resisted. It is this second alternative, the withholding of care that is acknowledged to be necessary, which can legitimately be labeled "rationing."[12]

The third alternative, redefining needs based on a more stringent standard of health benefit, would result in the systematic elimination of coverage for services of marginal expected benefit. Redefining health care needs in this way may seem arbitrary and disingenuous, since a treatment once considered "necessary" could suddenly become "unnecessary" after needs were redefined. However, from the perspective of distributive justice[13] and society's duty to respond to need-claims,[14] such a change is perfectly justified and simply reflects society's evolving preferences for health care vs other goods. All that is required to fulfill the dictates of distributive justice is that needs be defined by reference to objective criteria,[14] and that these objective criteria be systematically applied in defining the "adequate level of care."[15]

Despite these theoretical considerations, the Rule of Rescue would, to some extent, be reactivated if health care needs were redefined "downward," causing some once-covered services to no longer be covered and, therefore, often become unavailable. This process might be viewed as "bending" the Rule of Rescue, which, while potentially troubling, is clearly preferable to the overt breaking of the Rule (ie, withholding care that is acknowledged to be necessary [rationing]). As long as we can say in a justifiable and systematic manner that a desired health care service has been duly deemed unnecessary by virtue of relatively little net expected benefit, the Rule of Rescue should stay under relatively good control. Meanwhile, the democratic process can determine whether the collective malaise produced by bending the Rule warrants the allocation of more resources to health care.

## THE NEED TO SPECIFY TREATMENTS AND INDICATIONS

Summarizing the discussion so far, I have argued that the alternative method selected by OHSC is preferred to cost-effectiveness analysis for purposes of setting health care priorities. This process entails a two-stage approach: (1) initial assessment and prioritization of services based only on expected benefit, and (2) determination of how beneficial a treatment must be to warrant coverage as necessary care. I have also argued that it is acceptable for society to redefine necessary care according to evolving societal values and preference, as long as objective criteria are used.

Implicit in these arguments has been a key assumption: that the cost-free initial priority structure (eg, priority list) is constructed with enough detail to permit providers and payers to distinguish among relevantly different types of patients who stand to receive different degrees of benefit from a given treatment. Unfortunately, Oregon's priority list, as it stands now, comes up short on this critical point.

In developing a priority list based on net expected health benefit, everything depends on the specific indication for a particular treatment or procedure. In a recent article on the problem of defining essential services, David Eddy[16] noted that descriptions of services such as

"hospital care," "surgical care," "diagnostic tests," and even "prenatal care" are far too broad to enable any useful estimates of benefits, harms, and costs. Furthermore, for many interventions it will be necessary to narrow the target to specific indications. Carotid endarterectomy might well be considered essential for a 65-year-old man with transient ischemic attacks, 80% stenosis, and a history of stroke, but not for a 50-year-old asymptomatic man with 20% stenosis.

Thus, the same service might be ranked high with respect to one indication and much lower in relation to other indications. This degree of distinction among different treatments and indications is largely lacking in Oregon's list. The following items from the final priority list illustrate the problem:

- Medical therapy for cholera or ratbite fever, or toxic effects of mushrooms, fish, berries, etc.
- Medical therapy for accidents involving exposure to natural elements (eg, lightning strike or heatstroke)
- Medical and surgical therapy for ("treatable") breast cancer

Obviously, many types of patients and treatments are encompassed within each of these broad descriptions—in each case ranging from simple treatments for relatively minor problems to potentially life-threatening conditions and heroic therapy. With regard to breast cancer (and all other cancers), no distinction is made among different stages, cell types, or other factors that are likely to influence the choice of treatment and expected outcomes, nor are different treatments distinguished (eg, chemotherapy, radiation therapy, immunotherapy, or surgery).

This lack of specificity in large part reflects OHSC's reliance on *ICD-9* (diagnosis) and *CPT-4* (treatment) codes to define the line items. As indicated earlier, this method of specifying services and indications was adopted to facilitate actuarial analysis of the final priority list. OHSC was aware of the limitations imposed on indication and treatment specificity by the use of these codes; indeed, the commissioners sometimes referred to the "tyranny of the *ICD-9* codes" during development of the final list. Nevertheless, given the time constraints imposed on their efforts, the commissioners were unable to overcome this limitation. The result is that the final priority list will likely require additional specification before it can be fully implemented.

## NECESSARY-CARE GUIDELINES

How might the requisite degree of specification be accomplished? By way of answer, I will outline an alternative approach to setting health care priorities that relies on clinical guidelines to specify when treatments are necessary. This concept is described more fully elsewhere[17] and will only be briefly summarized for purposes of the present discussion. I will then relate this approach back to Oregon's final priority list.

The suggested alternative process revolves around the concept of health care needs and entails the creation of clinical practice guidelines that depict the indications (ie, types of patients) for which specified services are necessary. These necessary-care guidelines would be developed by duly constituted panels or bodies, using appropriate consensus processes to estimate outcomes, and would incorporate available public preference data.

Necessary-care guidelines would specify the clinical indications for which services have been "reasonably well-demonstrated to provide significant net health benefit versus no or alternative treatments." A determination

of "significant benefit" would be treated as the threshold that must be crossed before a service is deemed necessary. Services judged to offer only minimal (ie, nonsignificant) benefit would not be considered necessary. Table 3 illustrates model necessary-care guidelines.

The terms *significant* and *reasonably* cannot be defined operationally and indeed constitute the crux of judgment. As in the legal-judicial arena (eg, "beyond a reasonable doubt"), such qualitative descriptors permit the exercise of an adequate degree of discretion across the nearly limitless number of individual situations. The panel of decision makers would function much like a grand jury, hearing evidence concerning the expected outcomes of care (based in large part on literature reviews) and judging when indications meet the stipulated standard of demonstrated benefit. "Net benefit" would be defined simply as overall enhancements or improvements in longevity and/or quality of life, including the effects of treatment on pain, functional status, and other important health outcomes.

Using this method of priority setting, basic-level health plans would provide coverage for a given service or treatment only for patients whose condition corresponded to applicable necessary-care guidelines. (Appeals processes would be employed to accommodate atypical cases or extenuating circumstances). Patients with conditions other than those depicted in the guidelines could not (in most cases) legitimately claim to need that service—since significant health benefit had not been adequately demonstrated for patients with their particular problems or conditions. These latter patients would, therefore, either go without the service—perhaps the best approach since it has been deemed unnecessary—or purchase it with private funds.

The approach to setting health care priorities just outlined resembles the final Oregon method in two important respects. First, cost is not considered in de-

Table 3.—Model Necessary-Care Guidelines*

---

### Coronary Artery Bypass Surgery
High-grade (>70%) left main coronary artery obstruction
Triple-vessel disease (>70% each vessel) with impaired left ventricular function (ejection fraction <40%)
Unstable or persistent angina that is unresponsive to maximal medical therapy or in which side effects are incapacitating

### Cancer Chemotherapy
Nonseminomatous testicular carcinoma
Advanced stages of Hodgkin's disease and aggressive lymphomas
Acute lymphocytic leukemia in children and acute myelogenous leukemia in adults
Ovarian cancer, stages III and IV

### Computed Tomographic Scanning of the Head
History of recent head trauma and
  Patient unconscious or with rapidly decreasing mental status
  Clearly abnormal mental status, beyond drowsy
  Drowsy or initially alert with slow decrease in mental status with focal findings on neurological examination
Headache of sudden or recent onset, with abnormal neurological signs
Any significant, new-onset neurological abnormality, including recent abnormal neurological signs

---

*These model guidelines represent my interpretation of informal conversations with physician colleagues, each of whom was asked to specify the indications for which the procedures have been "clearly demonstrated to provide significant net health benefit vs nontreatment." "Benefit" was restricted to final outcomes (ie, longevity plus quality of life), rather than considering intermediate outcomes (eg, tumor shrinkage, improved blood flow). These model guidelines are presented for purposes of illustration only and do not necessarily resemble the necessary-care guidelines that would be developed after a formal consideration of evidence and appropriate consensus process.[17]

termining the importance of treatment. Thus, in both cases the Rule of Rescue would be attenuated, since treatments that are not covered for a given indication would have been officially deemed unnecessary, ie, of insignificant or inadequately demonstrated benefit. As mentioned earlier, if no effective rescue measure exists for an endangered person, our perceived duty to help is much diminished.

The second similarity between the two approaches is that in both cases the range of covered services can be expanded or contracted by varying the standard against which treatments are judged. Thus, in the case of Oregon's final method, a cutoff point can be moved commensurate with society's relative priority for health care. Similarly, using the necessary-care guideline approach the standard of proof required for demonstrating "significant net benefit" could be varied from "reasonably well demonstrated" (as suggested above) to "clearly demonstrated" (a stricter standard, resulting in fewer covered services) to "reasonably expected" (a looser standard, resulting in more covered services).[17]

The use of variously stringent standards of proof to define the balance between access to care and the cost of an insurance plan is modeled on the use of standards in the legal-judicial system. Here, more stringent standards (eg, beyond a reasonable doubt) are imposed in criminal trials when a defendant stands to lose life or liberty; looser standards (eg, preponderance of evidence) are used in most civil trials, since "only" property or money is at stake. This dichotomy exists because our society values life and liberty more highly than money and property; standards of proof reflect these values by making it more difficult for the state to deprive citizens of the former goods, compared with the latter.

Just as variously stringent standards of proof are used in the legal arena to reflect societal values, so too would society's values be reflected in the choice of the standard for defining health care needs. Different standards of proof of net expected benefit would result in the creation of necessary-care guidelines of varying stringency, just as the movable cutoff point in Oregon's final list would alter the degree of benefit demanded of services before they are covered (ie, deemed necessary). Such flexibility is essential if society is to balance its conflicting imperatives to allocate resources efficiently and to keep the Rule of Rescue under control.

Although similar to Oregon's final priority list in the respects just noted, the use of necessary-care guidelines offers two important advantages over the current version of Oregon's list. First, the problem of inadequate specification of indications for treatment is directly resolved, since the guidelines clearly define the particular indications for which a given treatment is necessary.

Second, OHSC never explicitly considered health care needs during the prioritization process. OHSC's post-

hoc definition of "essential care," by reference to service categories (see above), falls short of addressing medical need, only in part because of the lack of treatment and indication specificity described earlier. Oregon's planners are, therefore, vulnerable to charges (whether justified or not) that medically necessary services will be omitted from coverage (ie, fall below the line). A more explicit consideration of health care needs, as entailed by the necessary-care guideline approach, would ensure the provision of all deemed-necessary care.

In principle, it may be possible to dovetail Oregon's final priority list with the sort of guideline approach outlined above. Specific indication and treatment pairs could be dissected out of broad line items in the form of guidelines—and assigned individual expected benefit (ie, priority) ratings. Physicians could be asked to consider many of the existing, overly broad indications for treatment to identify clinical indications that entail benefit. Once specified, indications entailing high degrees of benefit would be moved higher on the priority list; indications for which not much benefit was expected would be moved lower. If a standard of proof approach were used, indications deemed necessary would automatically be moved (or remain) above the line; those deemed unnecessary would be moved (or remain) "below the line." Costs of providing treatment for these specific indications could be estimated using physicians' judgments concerning the prevalence of the various indications.

## CRITICISMS OF THE OREGON EFFORT

Even if I am correct in thinking that Oregon's priority list may require further work prior to implementation, this conclusion in no way minimizes the efforts and accomplishments of Oregon's leaders and of OHSC. The American health care system is in desperate, even shameful condition, and immediate action is clearly required. As Oregon's leaders have realized for several years, any good-faith effort to expand access to an adequate array of services is probably preferable to continued toleration of the status quo. Moreover, the Oregon exercise has provided a wealth of information for future efforts to set health care priorities. Indeed, the problems inherent in the literal application of cost-effectiveness theory were in part brought to light by these efforts.

Despite the obvious need for undertakings like the Oregon priority-setting exercise, leaders in that state and members of OHSC have endured sustained volleys of criticism (Am Med News, February 16, 1990:3, 45–47). Perhaps the most commonly heard objection is that "it is wrong to ration care to the poor." These "most vulnerable and defenseless patients," it has often been said, should not be singled out and subjected to benefit reduction.

What critics may not realize is that if and when Oregon succeeds in its ultimate goal, services above the line will collectively constitute the long sought-after adequate level of care,[15] providing for all legitimate health care needs. As such, the benefit package defined for Medicaid recipients may actually represent an improvement in quality over the excessively rich package of often inappropriate (even harmful) services currently available to well-insured patients. Moreover, if Oregon succeeds in its efforts, the designated benefit package would likely be widely embraced and adopted outside the Medicaid arena. Such a package could even become the basis for a fair and affordable system of national health insurance.

With regard to technical criticisms, it is sometimes claimed that Oregon's approach is fatally flawed because OHSC lacks valid outcome data. Indeed, much remains to be accomplished both in Oregon and elsewhere with regard to measuring and estimating outcomes and preferences. Nevertheless, millions of treatment decisions are made every day on real patients despite the same lack of outcome information that hampers Oregon's (and everyone else's) efforts to evaluate medical services. Nobody is suggesting, however, that physicians stop making treatment decisions because of a lack of information. Oregon's planners merely asked physicians to make explicit the outcome estimates on which they currently (and implicitly) base their decisions. The relative lack of formal outcome data does not mean that Oregon and other states should not do the best they can to develop reasonable outcome (and preference) estimates. The American health care cost and access problem is too critical to await the development of perfect methods for performing these difficult tasks.

In this regard, certain assumptions used in Oregon's method could be criticized, such as the lack of consideration of the costs associated with no or alternative treatment and the various arbitrary definitions of key terms in the service category labels, as shown in Table 2. Moreover, no reliability or validity studies of the methods used to estimate outcomes and preferences have been performed. While troubling, these limitations in method are, in my view, justifiable initial simplifications given the complexity of the task undertaken by OHSC. It has been acknowledged by Oregon's planners and OHSC's commissioners that their method will become more sophisticated in time. In fact, the commissioners noted at a February 20 press conference (at which time the release of the final list was announced) that their "final" priority list is actually just a "first-generation" product.

The criticisms that have plagued the Oregon project, coupled with inevitable misunderstandings concerning the project's rationale and complex methods, now threaten to undermine efforts in other states to set health care priorities. For example, during recent legislative debate on the Colorado prioritization bill (which, as stated earlier, was narrowly defeated) "opponents [of the bill] mentioned a similar 'rationing' attempt undertaken in Oregon, saying 2 years of efforts to start up that system have led to confusion and failure" (*Denver Post,* March 22, 1991;sect B:3). While this epitaph for the Oregon exercise is obviously premature, similar sentiments will likely be heard again and may continue to handicap future efforts to set health care priorities. It is my hope that the present article will clarify Oregon's purpose and methods so that this important exercise does not unwittingly and unreservedly become an albatross for subsequent prioritization projects.

## CONCLUSIONS

Perhaps that most fundamental lesson to be learned from the Oregon experience is that the use of cost-effectiveness analysis is unlikely to produce a socially or politically acceptable definition of necessary care. This is an important conclusion, especially since it is at odds with opinions expressed by most health economists and by certain health scholars, notably David Eddy. Eddy has recently advocated (in rather strong terms) that service costs be considered on an equal footing with net health benefits in defining "essential care":

> . . . to remove [costs] from the equation would render the concept of essential care meaningless. . . . An operational definition of essential care that is not based on its benefits, harms, and costs is like an automobile without a steering wheel.[16]

Eddy is willing, apparently, to relegate to "nonessential" status services that are highly beneficial but whose costs exceed some threshold. The Oregon experience tells us that the Rule of Rescue would make this approach highly problematic in modern American society.

Obviously, Eddy's "essential care" concept differs substantially from "necessary care," which, as used throughout this article (and in most other contexts), refers to services that are required to meet health care needs. By contrast, Eddy purposely eschews the concept of needs (oral communication, March 25, 1991), and instead defines "essential care" as the set of services deemed to be "worth paying for" by some representative sample of "patients."[16] Aside from the limitations inherent in such willingness-to-pay methods,[8] however, one must wonder whether attempting to "finesse" the notion of health care needs can lead to a satisfactory system of health care resource allocation.

One final point about costs deserves mention. Setting priorities based on net expected health benefit alone is likely to be financially feasible today because, as discussed earlier, few very expensive services have been demonstrated to provide significant benefit for many types of patients. Moreover, at least 30% to 50% of current health services would probably fail to meet the "reasonably well demonstrated to provide significant net health benefit" standard suggested herein,[18] resulting in sufficient cost savings to provide necessary care for all.

As Aron and Schwartz[19] have observed, however, eliminating services deemed to offer inadequate benefit will not protect society's purse from the highly beneficial (and often expensive) services that will be developed in the coming years. Relentless technological progress might some day swamp even a "clearly demonstrated" standard (although not in the foreseeable future). If so, it might eventually become necessary to "ration medical progress," as recommended recently by Callahan.[20]

With regard to Oregon's (and other) efforts to set health care priorities, in the end, what may matter most is that the "product" of priority-setting efforts—whether a prioritized list, a set of guidelines, or some combination thereof—appears intuitively sensible. Absent a gold standard of validity, there can be no "right" way to set health care priorities, nor any single "correct" list or set of guidelines. Like the laws by which our society is governed, priority lists and guidelines will be flawed, and will change over time. Inevitably, and despite our best efforts, mistakes will be made in allocating services to patients who don't need them, and in withholding care from those who do.

We must learn to tolerate these imperfections as we strive for equality and rationality in our health care system—just as we continue to live under the rule of law despite the fact that courtroom verdicts are sometimes in error. What Oregon's leaders realize, and others as of yet do not, is that laws of allocation are desperately needed in the US health care system—that the anarchy that reigns today is totally unacceptable.

By deleting cost as a factor in developing its final priority list, OHSC laid the groundwork for successfully attenuating the Rule of Rescue—a necessary first step if the fair allocation of resources is to be accomplished. What remains to be done is to better specify services and indications in order to distinguish among relevantly different treatments, types of patients, and degrees of expected benefit. When this final step is concluded, we will all have reason to be grateful for Oregon's efforts.

This work was supported by Research Service Award T32 HS 00007 from the Agency for Health Care Policy and Research, Rockville, Md, and by a grant from the Pew Charitable Trusts, Philadelphia, Pa.

I gratefully acknowledge the helpful comments made on earlier drafts of the report by Robert Brook, MD, ScD, Shan Cretin, MD, Allan Detsky, MD, PhD, Emmett Keeler, PhD, Don Hoagland, LLB, Forrest Adams, MD, and two anonymous reviewers.

## References

1. Morell V. Oregon puts bold health plan on ice. *Science*. 1990;249:468–471.
2. Loomes G, McKenzie L. The use of QALYs in health care decision making. *Soc Sci Med*. 1989;28:299–308.
3. Weinstein MC, Stason WB. Foundations of cost-effectiveness analysis for health and medical practices. *N Engl J Med*. 1976;296:716–721.
4. Hadorn DC. The Oregon priority-setting exercise: quality of life and public policy. *Hastings Cent Rep*. In press.
5. Jonsen A. Bentham in a box: technology assessment and health care allocation. *Law Med Health Care*. 1986;14:172–174.
6. Welch HG, Larson EB. Dealing with limited resources: the Oregon decision to curtail funding for organ transplantation. *N Engl J Med*. 1988;319:171–173.
7. Boisaubin EV. Charity, the media, and limited medical resources. *JAMA*. 1988;259:1375–1376.
8. Hadorn DC. The role of public values in setting health care priorities. *Soc Sci Med*. 1991;52:773–781.
9. Kaplan RM, Anderson JD. A general health policy model: update and applications. *Health Serv Res*. 1988;23:203–235.
10. Agency for Health Care Policy and Research. *Health Technology Assessment Reports: Assessment of Liver Transplantation*. Washington, DC: US Dept of Health and Human Services; 1990.
11. Goel V, Deber RB, Detsky AS. Nonionic contrast media: economic analysis and health policy development. *Can Med Assoc J*. 1989;140:389–395.
12. Hadorn DC, Brook RH. The health care resource allocation debate: defining our terms. Presented at "Designing a Fair and Reasonable Basic Benefit Package Using Clinical Guidelines: A California Proposal," a conference sponsored by the California Public Employees' Retirement System; April 24, 1991; Sacramento, Calif.
13. Rawls J. *A Theory of Justice*. Cambridge, Mass: Harvard University Press; 1971.
14. Scanlon W. Preference and urgency. *J Philosophy*. 1975:19:655–669.
15. President's Commission for the Study of Ethical Problems in Medicine and Biomedical and Behavioral Research. *Securing Access to Health Care*. Washington, DC: US Government Printing Office; 1983;1.
16. Eddy DM. What care is 'essential'? what services are 'basic'? *JAMA* 1991;265:782, 786–788.
17. Hadorn D. Necessary-care guidelines: using an explicit standard of proof to define health care needs. Presented at "Designing a Fair and Reasonable Basic Benefit Package Using Clinical Guidelines: A California Proposal," a conference sponsored by the California Public Employees' Retirement System; April 24, 1991; Sacramento, Calif.
18. Brook RH, Lohr KN. Will we need to ration effective health care? *Issues Sci Technol*. 1986;3:68–77.
19. Aaron H, Schwartz WB. Rationing health care: the choice before us. *Science*. 1990;247:418–422.
20. Callahan D. Rationing medical progress: the way to affordable health care. *N Engl J Med*. 1990;322:1810–1813.

# Chapter 32

# Controlling Health Expenditures—The Canadian Reality

Robert G. Evans, Ph.D., Jonathan Lomas, M.A., Morris L. Barer, M.B.A., Ph.D., Roberta J. Labelle, M.A., Catherine Fooks, M.A., Gregory L. Stoddart, Ph.D., Geoffrey M. Anderson, M.D., Ph.D., David Feeny, Ph.D., Amiram Gafni, Ph.D., George W. Torrance, Ph.D., and William G. Tholl

**Abstract:** Canada and the United States have conducted a large-scale social experiment on the effects of alternative ways of funding expenditures for health care. Two very similar societies, with (until recently) very similar systems of providing health care, have adopted radically different systems of reimbursement. The results of this experiment are of increasing interest to Americans, because the Canadian approach has avoided or solved several of the more intractable problems facing the United States. In particular, overall health expenditures have been constrained to a stable share of national income, and universality of coverage (without user charges) eliminates the problems of uncompensated care, individual burdens of catastrophic illness, and uninsured populations.

The combination of cost control with universal, comprehensive coverage has surprised some American observers, who have questioned its reality, its sustainability, or both. We present a comparison of the Canadian and American data on expenditures, identifying the sectors in which the experience of the two nations diverges most, and describing the processes of control. In any system, cost control involves conflict between providers and payers. Political processes focus this conflict, whereas market processes diffuse it. But the stylized political combat in Canada may result in less intrusion on the professional autonomy of the individual physician than is occurring in the United States. (*N Engl J Med* 1989;320:571–7.)

American interest in the Canadian health care system appears to be on the rise, as evidenced in a recent three-part article by Iglehart[1-3] in the *Journal.* Such interest has been intermittent in the past, depending in part on the position of national health insurance on the U.S. political agenda. In the early 1970s, the most recent period during which national health insurance seemed imminent, Americans paid considerable attention to the structure, logic, and history of the Canadian system.[4] At the time, that system had just been established in its entirety. Although its origins and organization were documented, there had been little experience with universal, public coverage, and data were not yet available on its performance. Universal hospital coverage was a decade or more old (in Saskatchewan, a quarter century), but the extension of insurance to cover physicians' services was very new. Then the moment passed, national health insurance moved off the American agenda, and after a variety of attempts to regulate the health care system at arm's length, competition and the marketplace became the dominant ideas of the 1980s. In this context the Canadian experience was of little relevance.

Reprinted with permission from Robert G. Evans, Ph.D.; Jonathan Lomas, M.A.; Morris L. Barer, M.B.A., Ph.D.; Roberta J. LaBelle, M.A.; Catherine Fooks, M.A.; Gregory L. Stoddart, Ph.D.; Geoffrey M. Anderson, M.D., Ph.D.; David Feeny, Ph.D.; Amiram Gafni, Ph.D.; George W. Torrance, Ph.D.; and William G. Tholl, Controlling Health Expenditures—The Canadian Reality, *The New England Journal of Medicine,* Vol. 320 No. 9, pp. 571–577, 1989.

So far, however, market forces, at least as applied in practice, have been even less successful in containing the growth of health care expenditures than were the regulatory efforts of the 1970s.[5,6] The one major success in this field, prospective payment and diagnosis-related groups, is virtually a pure type of regulatory intervention, despite its being occasionally clothed in market rhetoric. At the same time, the proportion of the American population with no insurance coverage or grossly inadequate coverage is believed to be both large and growing,[7,8] and there is increasing uneasiness about the effect of market forces in health care on the interests of both patients and providers.[9-11] In this context, the radically different Canadian approach to funding may deserve a second look—not as a panacea, but as evidence that perhaps things could be different. By now that system has generated nearly two decades of experience that can be compared with the American record.

To an American audience, the most striking feature of the Canadian experience may be the association of universal coverage with substantially lower expenditures for health services. Despite (or, as many Canadians would argue, because of) universal access on equal terms and conditions, overall costs in Canada have risen more or less in line with the growth of national income, rather than eating up a steadily increasing share of it, as in the United States.

Before 1971, when the Canadian funding system was more similar to the American one, health care costs consumed a share of national income that was virtually identical in both countries and was rising steadily. In 1971 it reached 74 percent in Canada, as compared with 7.6 percent in the United States. After 1971, however, the Canadian share remained stable, whereas in the United States it continued to rise.[5,12-14] By 1981 their spending shares were 7.7 and 9.2 percent, respectively. In the 1982 recession, the share of expenditures for health care rose sharply in both countries, to 8.6 and 10.2 percent.[12,14] In both systems, health care escaped the effects of the recession—an interesting and unstudied observation. But the Canadian share stabilized at its new level; preliminary estimates for 1987 show it still at 8.6 percent. In contrast, the United States share continued to rise. Estimates for 1987 are in excess of 11 percent.[5,15]

The large and growing gap between the United States and Canada drives home the point that, for good or ill, the form of funding adopted by Canada does permit a society to control its overall outlays on health care. Furthermore, it is unnecessary to impose financial barriers to access in the process. In this paper we sketch some of the basic institutional and statistical facts of that process, and their implications for physicians in particular.

Cost control, although successful in general, can be a bruising political process, producing much sound and fury. External observers who rely on newspaper reports may not always get a clear picture, either of the critical issues in dispute or of the distinction between facts and rhetoric. Further confusion arises from casual interpretations of the comparative data, such as that by Feder et al.[16] Looking at the period from 1970 to 1984, they noted that health spending in Canada rose faster than in the United States, but that the gross national product (GNP) rose faster still. They concluded that the apparent success of the Canadian system with cost control was illusory, and that the stability of the share of the GNP applied to health care was simply the result of rapid economic growth. A more detailed look at the data shows this conclusion to be incorrect.

## NATIONAL INCOME AND HEALTH EXPENDITURES IN CANADA AND THE UNITED STATES

Table 1 provides the relevant data for Canada and the United States over the period referred to by Feder et al. The Canadian GNP does in fact outpace the American by 2 percent per year. But after adjustment for the more rapid rate of inflation in Canada, our advantage shrinks to 0.7 percent. When adjusted further for the slightly faster growth of the Canadian population, the difference in real per capita growth rates is less than half a percent per year—respectable enough over the long term, but not enough to account for the divergence in the shares of the GNP spent on health. The oversight of confusing nominal with real rates of GNP growth leads Feder et al. to their erroneous conclusion.

The relevant base year for examining the effect of national health insurance on health spending is not 1970, however, but 1971. Quebec, the second-largest province, with about a quarter of the Canadian population, adopted its health plan in October 1970, and New Brunswick began its plan on January 1, 1971. Correspondingly there was a substantial jump, from 7.1 to 7.4

Table 1. Average Annual Percentage Increases in Gross National Product (GNP), 1970 to 1984.*

| MEASURES OF GNP | CANADA | UNITED STATES | DIFFERENCE† |
|---|---|---|---|
| | | percent | |
| Current dollars | 12.1 | 9.8 | 2.0 |
| Constant dollars | 3.4 | 2.7 | 0.7 |
| Constant dollars per capita | 2.2 | 1.7 | 0.4 |

*Data for the United States are from the Health Care Financing Administration[5] and the Bureau of Economic Analysis[17]; data for Canada are from the Department of Finance.[18,19]

†Differences in annual growth rates must be calculated geometrically, not by subtraction [d = (1 + r₁)/(1 + r₂) − 1]. Rates have been rounded after calculation.

percent, in the share of the GNP applied to health care for all of Canada.

Table 2 shows the annual rates of increase in total health spending in Canada and the United States since the completion of universal Medicare coverage in Canada. Spending in nominal dollars did rise somewhat faster in Canada, by 0.7 percent per year. But when account is taken of the more rapid rate of general inflation in Canada and the slightly faster rate of population growth, health spending in constant dollars per capita rose more slowly in Canada, by 1.6 percent per year.

To put this more concretely, in 1985 Americans spent an average of $1,710 each on health care.[5] If their rate of cost escalation since 1971, in real terms, had been the same as that in Canada, they would have spent only $1,362, or 20 percent less. Preliminary estimates for 1987 show Americans spending just under $2,000 each for health care. Detailed Canadian data are not yet available, but the spending gap is clearly continuing to widen. One may estimate conservatively that if the Canadian rates of escalation in real cost since 1971 had prevailed in the United States, health spending would by 1987 be about $450 less, on average, for every person in the country, or at least $100 billion less in all.

## THE PROCESS OF COST CONTROL IN CANADA

How much control has been achieved, and with what effects, continues to form a major part of the agenda for research on health services in Canada.[20] As Iglehart pointed out,[2] virtually the entire difference between Canada and the United States in the share of GNP that is spent on health is accounted for by three components: insurance overhead, or costs of prepayment and administration; payments to hospitals; and payments for physicians' services. In 1985, these three items took up

0.59, 4.18, and 2.07 percent, respectively, of the U.S. GNP, and 0.11, 3.48, and 1.35 percent of the Canadian GNP.

Relative to the expenditures that might have been generated by a system comparable to Canada's, in 1985 Americans spent about $20 billion more for insurance and prepayment costs, and just under $30 billion more for each of physicians' services and hospital costs.

### Administration and Prepayment Expenses

In relative terms, the most extraordinary difference between Canadian and American spending is in the area of administration and prepayment expenses. In 1985 the overhead component of health insurance—the share of premiums that goes not to the reimbursement of physicians, hospitals, and other providers, but to paying for the handling of the flow of paper and dollars—cost Americans $95 each, out of their overall $1,710. Canadians spent $21—and those were Canadian dollars. Indeed, Canadians spent less per capita to administer universal comprehensive coverage than Americans spent to administer Medicare and Medicaid alone (about $26 U.S. per capita[5]).

A universal, tax-financed system can simply be much less costly to administer, at all levels, and the Canadian system is. On the review side, once a tax system is in place, as it is in all modern societies—with income tax, sales tax, and everything else—the additional cost of raising more funds is minimal. (Some Canadian provinces continue to collect premiums, which are taxes in all but name. They are related to family size, but not to risk status; they cover only a portion of the total plan outlays; they are compulsory for most of the population; and most important, coverage is not conditional on payment.)

On the expense side, all the costs of determining coverage and eligibility are avoided—everyone is eligible, and for the same benefits. Patients drop out of the payment system entirely, and reimbursement takes place between the public insurer and the provider. There are no marketing expenses, no costs of estimating risk status in order to set differential premiums or decide whom to cover, and no allocations for shareholder profits; the process of claims payment, although not free of costs, is greatly simplified and much cheaper. In this area it is obvious that the public sector is more efficient and less costly than the private sector,[21] a fact that was recognized early on in Canada. The 1964 Royal Commission on Health Services, which drew up the blueprint for Canada's universal system, described the private administration of insurance as "an uneconomic use of . . . limited resources."[22] This "uneconomic use" accounts for nearly one quarter of the difference in cost for health insurance between Canada and the United States.

Table 2. Average Annual Percentage Increases in Total Expenditures for Health Care, 1971 to 1985.*

| MEASURES OF HEALTH EXPENDITURES | CANADA | UNITED STATES | DIFFERENCE+ |
|---|---|---|---|
| | | *percent* | |
| Current dollars | 13.1 | 12.3 | 0.7 |
| Constant dollars‡ | 4.3 | 5.8 | -1.4 |
| Constant dollars per capita‡ | 3.1 | 4.8 | -1.6 |

*Data for the United States are from the Health Care Financing Administration.[5] Gibson et al.,[14] and the Department of Commerce[17], data for Canada are from Health and Welfare Canada[12,13] and the Department of Finance.[18,19]

†Differences in annual growth rates must be calculated geometrically, not by subtraction [d = (1 + r₁)/(1 + r₂) − 1]. Rates have been rounded after calculation.

‡These constant-dollar measures are not real output measures for the health sector, they have not been adjusted by price indexes specific to the health sector. Rather, they are adjusted for changes in the general level of prices, economy-wide, as reflected in price indexes based on gross national expenditures, and they therefore reflect the increase in generalized purchasing power that is absorbed by the health care sector, in the form of either increased resource inputs or health sector–specific inflation.

Nor is that the end of the story. Himmelstein and Woolhandler[23] calculate that in the United States, the provider-borne overheads for hospitals, nursing homes, and doctors' offices (the accounting costs of complying with the requirements for documentation by a multiplicity of insurers, as well as coping with the determination of eligibility, direct billing of patients, and collections) amounted to $62.1 billion in 1983. They estimate that shifting to a national health insurance system could save $21.4 billion in the administrative costs of hospitals and physicians' offices. This would be 6 percent of total health care costs, or 0.63 percent of the GNP in 1983— leading to the startling conclusion that the costs of running the American payment system itself, independent of the costs of patient care, may account for more than half the difference in cost between the Canadian and the U.S. systems.

For the Canadian physician, differences in the costs of insurance administration show up as a lower overhead for practice. The problems of determining insurance status and managing the collections process disappear, along with the problem of uncollectible accounts. The costs of compliance with the requirements of the health care reimbursement system also show up outside the area of health expenditures as it is normally defined, particularly in the budgets of the social welfare services, and to no inconsiderable degree in the monetary and nonmonetary costs borne by individual patients and their families. Furthermore, the considerable research, legal, and regulatory efforts required to put the complex and varied reporting and compliance requirements in place are not without cost, but will be counted as outside the health care system.

There is private insurance for some forms of health care in Canada. But for hospital and medical care, such coverage is prohibited for services that are included in the public plans. The original intent was quite explicit— to prevent private firms from skimming off the good risks, supporting the development of multiclass service, or both. But the restriction also has the very important effect of making provincial governments to all intents and purposes the sole funders of hospital and medical care, and of creating a bilateral bargaining situation as the foundation for cost control in these sectors.

## The Effect on Hospitals

In Canada, controlling hospital costs is a two-part process. Operating budgets are approved, and funded almost entirely, by the Ministry of Health in each province, but they include no allowance for capital expenditures. New facilities, equipment, major renovations, and the like are funded from a variety of sources, but they require the approval of the same provincial agency, which generally also contributes the major share of financing. This process of centralized approval prohibits hospitals from accessing private capital markets, and has historically limited their efforts to support expansions of capacity from community sources. So far, it has been relatively successful in limiting such expansion,[24] but somewhat less successful in managing the diffusion of major equipment.[25,26]

Centralized control over operating costs is more complete. Annual global budgets are negotiated between ministries and individual hospitals. Although political pressures have often forced governments to pick up the deficits of hospitals that are unable or unwilling to stay within these budgets, this process has resulted in a significantly less rapid rise in hospital expenditures in Canada than in the United States.[27,28]

The more rapid rate of escalation of hospital costs in the United States since 1971 has been shown to result from major differences in the growth in hospital costs per patient day at constant hospital input prices, or intensity of servicing.[27–30] This measure increases in response to increases in the number of nursing hours or drugs, or in the use of operating rooms, magnetic resonance imaging, and other such complex technology, per day of inpatient care. In the case of particular technologies that are embodied in specifically countable items like machines, capacities available per capita have tended to increase less rapidly in Canada. On the other hand, changes in the intensity of servicing in hospitals also include relative increases in internal administrative costs. Therefore, some portion of the apparent relative increase in servicing intensity simply reflects the increasing administrative intensity of the American hospital system.

But the different trends in servicing intensity also reflect quite different patterns in the use of beds in acute care hospitals. In Canada, a growing share of such beds has been occupied by patients over 54 years of age, whose stays exceed 60 days and whose daily care requirements are well below average. These patients prevent physicians from using the beds in question to treat short-term patients.[31]

Thus, Canada can have higher rates of hospitalization and greater average lengths of stay than the United States, yet also have lower per capita hospital expenditures.[32] Even if such expenditures, in terms of the cost of hospital care, are less different than is usually believed (because so much of the U.S. expenditure is for administrative activity), it does appear that the resulting mix of hospital activities favors intensive, high-technology services in the United States and long-term, chronic care in Canada. Nor should this come as a surprise, given the history of cost and procedural reimbursement in the United States, and of global budget-constrained funding in Canada. Which is preferable, in terms of value for money or benefits to patients, is harder to say. Possibly, each system generates its own forms of overuse and underuse.

One product that is clearly generated by the Canadian system, structured as it is to place the sole responsibility for control of hospital resources on the provincial governments, is intense, continuing public debate. The rhetoric of underfunding, shortages, excessive waiting lists, and so on is an important part of the process by which providers negotiate their share of public resources—including their own incomes.[33] Furthermore, there are reasons for the noticeable recent increase in such rhetoric. Increases in the supply of physicians per capita, in the face of a relatively constant supply of beds, have resulted in steady reductions in the number of short-term hospital beds available to each physician since 1971.[27] As bed availability and operating budgets have undergone increasing scrutiny, hospital administrators responded first (in the mid-1970s) by rationalizing administrative operations, and more recently by joining physicians in stepped-up rhetoric and pressure about underfunding.[34]

The difficulty for health policy and funding is that, since the boy always cries wolf (and must do so, given the political system of funding), one does not know if the wolf is really there. The political dramatics should not mislead external observers into believing that the wolf is always at hand. What varies most between the two nations in the method of establishing total hospital expenditures is the centralized, overtly political process in Canada, in contrast to the largely decentralized, institution-centered, and only implicitly political process in the United States. The Canadian controls on hospital expenditures impinge on individual physicians by limiting the complementary resources that are available to them. In this way, the environment of medical practice is changed, and practice patterns change in response. But individual physicians are not subject to any substantial direct intervention by hospital management or third parties. In this sense, Canadian physicians are actually much more autonomous than their American counterparts.

The Effect on Physicians

From 1971 to 1985, the share of the American GNP going to physicians has risen by over 40 percent. By contrast, Canadian physicians had an increase of only 10 percent. The stories that U.S. physicians hear about disaffected Canadian physicians, outmigration, underfunding, and occasional strikes correspond to an underlying reality of less generous funding. Despite the rhetoric, however, there has been no mass bailout of physicians from Canada. The supply of physicians per capita has risen throughout the period, is currently growing at between 1.5 and 2 percent per year, and is

projected to continue its growth for the foreseeable future.[35] At the end of 1985 there were about 490 people per physician in Canada—very similar to the U.S. ratio. As in the United States, the policy concern is with surpluses, not shortages.[36] There may be some loss of superstars to the United States, but this is hard to document—individual anecdotes do not make a trend. In any case there is always some leakage of stars in any field from countries with small populations to populous neighbors (the Gretzky effect).

The main explanation for the difference in outlays to physicians is that real fees have increased much faster in the United States than in Canada.[27,37] This difference, in turn, has resulted from the effect of universal public coverage on the process of fee determination. Increases in the general levels of fees and rules of payment are negotiated periodically between provincial medical associations and Ministries of Health. Over the long term, this complex negotiation process has had a major impact on the overall rate of escalation of fees.[37] Ironically, for a society that believes in the influence of competitive markets, the increasing supply of physicians in the United States seems to be associated with an acceleration in fee increases. In 1986, the rise in fees relative to the overall Consumer Price Index was one of the largest on record.[5]

Two other related issues have been particularly contentious for Canadian physicians—billing at rates above those reimbursed by the provincial plans ("extra billing") and the growth in the use of services per physician. Since 1971 these factors have become increasingly prominent in the political negotiating process, although the first one may at last have been pushed off center stage.

With the passage of the Canada Health Act in 1984,[38] the right to "extra bill" was removed in all provinces in which such billing had previously occurred. This act, passed unanimously by the House of Commons, was a response to public perceptions that extra billing was undermining the fundamental principle of universal access on uniform terms and conditions. The termination of extra billing was met with intense opposition from physicians in some provinces, however, culminating in a lengthy strike in Ontario.[2,39] Physicians argued that the threat of widespread extra billing was a safety valve, protecting them against overly aggressive bargaining by the Ministries of Health and helping to push up public reimbursement rates. Although relatively few physicians engaged in extra billing, the majority strongly supported the option. They were unable to mobilize any sizable public support, however.

The extreme distress among physicians in Ontario appears to have been based largely on symbolic considerations. The right of ultimate access to the patient's economic resources seems to have had a meaning difficult for nonphysicians to understand. In fact, no change has occurred in the prevailing pattern of private, fee-for-service practice with reimbursement at uniform, negotiated rates. But Canadian physicians do have real concerns about the future, which have been linked to the extra-billing issue.

Once governments have achieved control over fee levels by ensuring that the public reimbursement rates represent payment in full, it is feared that the next step in cost control will be to restrict the amount or type of care provided, or at least the number and mix of services for which reimbursement will be made. This is particularly likely if physicians increase their delivery of services to compensate for the loss of extra billing, for a stagnant fee structure, or both.

The latter possibility has been an important consideration in recent American discussions of physicians' reimbursement under Medicare.[40,41] Analyses of the U.S. experience with fee freezes in the early 1970s clearly demonstrated that increased billing occurred as a response.[42,43] Billing activity per physician has risen faster in Canada than in the United States since 1971, in a manner consistent with this concern, although in Canada fee controls have clearly moderated the rate of escalation of expenditures for physicians' services, not just that of fees. Until recently, the provincial governments have been willing to accept an additional rise in expenditures (increases in physicians' productivity or more creative billing, depending on one's point of view) over and above increases in fees and numbers of physicians. Nationally, this has averaged 1 to 2 percent per year since 1971.[37]

The exception was Quebec, where over a four-year period of unchanged fees (1971 to 1975) the increase became so large as to create a fiscal problem.[37,44] Starting in 1976, Quebec introduced modifications to the reimbursement process that limited its liability for increases in services, billings, or both (per practitioner and in the aggregate) that exceeded preset target levels. From a billing standpoint, 26 office-based diagnostic and therapeutic procedures were bundled into the office visit. These procedures had been billable separately, in addition to the basic visit fee, and during the early 1970s their number and cost per office visit had risen rapidly. Their consolidation into the office-visit fee removed one of the principal mechanisms by which Quebec physicians had been able to stem some of the erosion in their real incomes during the period of unchanged fees.[37]

In addition, there are ceilings on the quarterly gross billings of individual practitioners, above which physicians are reimbursed at only 25 percent of the allowable fee. For the profession as a whole, negotiated fee increases are implemented in steps, conditional on the rate of increase in use. If the rate of use per physician (i.e., average gross receipts) rises faster than a predetermined percentage, subsequent fee increases are scaled down or eliminated.

None of these measures impinge directly on the autonomy of individual physicians in their practices, however. Specific clinical decisions are not reviewed by the reimbursement agency, nor are therapeutic protocols established. If the aggregated bill for all clinical decisions exceeds the limits, then fees to either the individual or the group as a whole will be scaled down, but physicians remain free to determine their own practice patterns.

Committees to review patterns of practice have existed for years in each province, under various names. But they were established to monitor a very small number of practitioners whose patterns deviated radically from those of their peers, and to look for fraud or incompetence. Such committees have neither the mandate nor the resources to go beyond statistical outliers in their investigations; even in this role, a recent commentary suggests that they are not very aggressive or effective.[45]

Since 1985, British Columbia, Alberta, Saskatchewan, Manitoba, and Ontario have all negotiated contracts setting limits on aggregate billings. British Columbia attempted to go further, by restricting the numbers of new physicians entitled to reimbursement by the provincial plan and controlling their locations of practice.[46] This policy, however, was successfully challenged on constitutional grounds. It was sustained at the provincial court, but overturned on appeal, and leave to appeal further was denied by the Supreme Court of Canada.

The absence of intrusion by any of these measures into the autonomy of individual practice contrasts markedly with the situation in the United States, where managed care systems and prospective payment, designed to alter individual physicians' care of individual patients, have become the principal tools for the control of expenditures for physicians' services. In the absence of a centralized bargaining mechanism between physicians and payers—a single-source payer—there is no way to limit the overall levels of billings. Hence the leap from constraints on capacity (as by a certificate of need) straight to the level of minute scrutiny of the behavior of individual physicians or the treatment of specific diseases.

Thus, many Americans already feel the threats to clinical freedom that Canadian physicians fear for the future. Whether such fears actually materialize will probably depend in large part on whether the provincial governments can continue to contain overall expenditures. What is disturbing, however, is that the current aggregate approaches to control of the use of services leave unexplored the cost-effectiveness, and even the efficacy, of the actual services provided. Such concerns, if left unaddressed by the profession itself, may become the catalysts for more detailed scrutiny of the use of services within the fee-negotiation process in Canada.

To date, we see little evidence of this, but a decade ago there was little sign of the now widespread practice of bargaining over aggregate use along with fees. The context of policy decisions changes more slowly in Canada than in the United States, but it does move forward.

### Orchestrated Outrage versus Diffuse Distress

Thus, the major difference between the two countries with respect to health expenditures lies in the degree of centralization of the cost-control process. In the United States the battles are fought in a myriad of private struggles between physicians and their employers, or their hospitals (or their competitors). When the struggle becomes public, as in the call by Minnesota physicians for unionization,[47] it takes the form of a series of isolated and localized incidents. The general pattern is obscured. In Canada, by contrast, the struggle over shares of income between physicians and the rest of the society is played out as large-scale public theater, with all the rhetorical threats and flourishes that political clashes require.[48] Physicians in Canada, and perhaps also in the United States, may perceive the Canadian conflicts as more severe and as arising from the presence of a universal public-payment system. That system serves to focus and channel such conflicts and to bring them into the headlines, but it has also afforded Canadian physicians a greater degree of professional autonomy.

Whatever the liabilities of such an overt and at times rancorous process, the Canadian approach has controlled health care costs more effectively. In the end, this may be the root of the sense of unease among Canadian physicians, who face a problem common to physicians in every country with a rapidly rising supply, including the United States. In such circumstances, every community of physicians must struggle for an ever-increasing share of national income or accept falling personal incomes. In the process, they must urge on the rest of society the benefits of buying the additional services that the additional numbers of physicians make possible (some would say inevitable)—and of doing so at fees that will sustain their own incomes. Whether such benefits are real or illusory is important from the standpoint of health policy, but irrelevant to the needs of the medical community.

The rest of society, or at least a sector of it, attempts to resist this expansion under the banner of cost control. When such resistance is organized collectively through public insurance, it is relatively successful. When it is disorganized and fragmented, an inconsistent and contradictory mix of strategies, as in the United States, it has so far been unsuccessful. Again, that observation is logically independent of whether the lack of success in the United States reflects waste, or whether the Canadian success leads to "underfunding."

In such an environment the pressure on physicians can only grow. To the extent that they resist such pressures successfully and continue to expand their share of the national income, as in the United States, the public and private responses to cost escalation will become increasingly radical. Major institutional changes are already transforming thee American health care system to an extent much greater than has been the case in the more conservative Canadian environment. Fears and anecdotes about the erosion of professional autonomy, and even of incomes, are becoming increasingly widespread. In the United States, corporate competitors or employers may turn out to be more ruthless than public regulators.

Such are the costs of economic success. The Canadian environment is more stable and predictable precisely because its cost-control processes work relatively well. But in Canada, whatever has happened or may happen can be blamed on government and on the evils of "socialized medicine." Anxiety and dissatisfaction are easily, if not always accurately, focused and channeled collectively through the process of public negotiation. In the United States, it is harder for individual practitioners to find the villains, and still harder to identify an effective response. At the same time, it is easier to misinterpret the experience of other countries with more visible bargaining processes.

We are indebted to Sidney Lee, Theodore R. Marmor, and Uwe E. Reinhardt for helpful discussions.

## References

1. Iglehart JK. Canada's health care system. N Engl J Med 1986; 315:202–8.
2. Idem. Canada's health care system. N Engl J Med 1986; 315:778–84.
3. Idem. Canada's health care system: addressing the problem of physician supply. N Engl J Med 1986; 315:1623–8.
4. Adreopoulos S, ed. National health insurance: can we learn from Canada? New York: John Wiley, 1975.
5. Division of National Cost Estimates, Health Care Financing Administration. National health expenditures, 1986–2000. Health Care Financ Rev 1987; 8(4):1–35.
6. Fein R. Medical care, medical costs: the search for a health insurance policy. Cambridge, Mass: Harvard University Press, 1986.
7. Wilensky GR. Variable strategies for dealing with the uninsured. Health Aff (Millwood) 1987; 6(1):33–46.
8. Library of Congress, Congressional Research Service. Health insurance and the uninsured: background data and analysis. Washington, D.C.: Government Printing Office, 1988.
9. Fuchs VR. The "competition revolution" in health care. Health Aff (Millwood) 1988; 7(3):5–24.
10. Brook RH. Kosecoff JB. Competition and quality. Health Aff (Millwood) 1988; 7(3):150–61.

11. Gray BH, ed. for the Institute of Medicine. For-profit enterprise in health care. Washington, D.C.: National Academy Press, 1986.

12. Canada, Health and Welfare Canada. National health expenditures in Canada 1975–1987. Ottawa: Health and Welfare Canada, 1985.

13. Idem. National health expenditures in Canada 1970–1982. Ottawa: Health and Welfare Canada, 1985.

14. Gibson R, Levit K, Lazenby H, Waldo D. National health expenditures, 1983. Health Care Financ Rev 1984; 6(2):1–29.

15. Ginzberg E. A hard look at cost containment. N Engl J Med 1987; 316:1151–4.

16. Feder J, Scanlon W, Clark J. Canada's health care system. N Engl J Med 1987; 317:320.

17. Department of Commerce, Bureau of Economic Analysis. Survey of Current Business, September 1987; 67(9).

18. Canada, Department of Finance. Quarterly economic review: annual reference tables, June 1987. Ottawa: Department of Finance, 1987.

19. Idem. Economic review April, 1985. Ottawa: Department of Finance, 1985.

20. Evans RG. Finding the levers, finding the courage: lessons from cost containment in North America. J Health Polit Policy Law 1986; 11:585–615.

21. Reinhadt UE. On the B-factor in American health care. Washington Post. August 9, 1988:20.

22. Canada, Royal Commission on Health Services (Hall Commission). Report Vol. 1. Ottawa: Queen's Printer, 1964:745.

23. Himmelstein DU, Woolhandler S. Cost without benefit: administrative waste in U.S. health care. N Engl J Med 1986; 314:441–5.

24. Bellerose P-P, Tholl W. Capital spending in the health sector. Presented at the Annual Meeting of the Canadian Health Economics Research Association, Halifax, Canada, June 8, 1987.

25. Feeny D, Guyatt G, Tugwell P. Health care technology: effectiveness, efficiency and public policy. Montreal: Institute for Research in Public Policy, 1986.

26. Deber RB, Leatt P. Technology acquisition in Ontario hospitals: you can lead a hospital to policy, but can you make it stick? In: Horne JM, ed. Proceedings of the Third Canadian Conference on Health Economics. Winnipeg: University of Manitoba, 1987:259–77.

27. Barer ML, Evans RG. Riding north on a south-bound horse? Expenditures, prices, utilization and incomes in the Canadian health care system. In: Evans RG, Stoddart GL, eds. Medicare at maturity: achievements, lessons and challenges. Calgary: University of Calgary Press, 1986:53–163.

28. Detsky AS, Stacey SR, Bombardier C. The effectiveness of a regulatory strategy in containing hospital costs: the Ontario experience, 1967–1981. N Engl J Med 1983; 309:151–9.

29. Barer M, Evans RG. Prices, proxies and productivity: an historical analysis of hospital and medical care in Canada. In: Diewert E, Montmarquette C, eds. Price level measurement. Ottawa: Statistics Canada, 1983:705–77.

30. Detsky AS, Abrams HB, Ladha L, Stacey SR. Global budgeting and the teaching hospital in Ontario. Med Care 1986; 24:89–94.

31. Evans RG, Barer ML, Hertzman C, Anderson GM, Pulcins IR, Lomas J. The long goodbye: the great transformation of the British Columbia hospital system. Health Serv Res (in press).

32. Newhouse JP, Anderson GM, Roos LL. What accounts for differences in hospital spending between the United States and Canada: a first look. Health Aff (Millwood) 1988; 7(5):6–16.

33. Reinhardt UE. Resource allocation in health care: the allocation of lifestyles to providers. Milbank Q 1987; 65:153–76.

34. Murray VV, Jick TD, Bradshaw P. Hospital funding constraints: strategic and tactical decision responses to sustained moderate levels of crisis in six Canadian hospitals. Soc Sci Med 1984; 18:211–9.

35. Barer ML, Gafni A, Lomas J. Accommodating rapid growth in physician supply: lessons from Israel, warnings for Canada. Int J Health Serv 1989; 19:95–115.

36. Lomas J, Barer ML, Stoddart GL. Physician manpower planning: lessons from the MacDonald Report. Toronto: Ontario Economic Council, 1985.

37. Barer ML, Evans RG, Labelle RJ. Fee controls as cost control: tales from the frozen north. Milbank Q 1988; 66:1–64.

38. Heiber S, Deber R. Banning extra-billing in Canada: just what the doctor didn't order. Can Public Policy 1987; 13:62–74.

39. Barer ML, Antioch K. Bill 94 and the Ontario physicians' strike: lobbying as professional emasculation. Vancouver: University of British Columbia, 1987.

40. United States Congress, Office of Technology Assessment. Payment for physician services: strategies for Medicare. Washington, D.C.: Government Printing Office, 1986:146–50.

41. United States Congress, Congressional Budget Office, Physician reimbursement under Medicare: options for change. Washington, D.C.: Government Printing Office, 1986:10–2.

42. Holahan J, Scanlon W. Price controls, physician fees and physician incomes from Medicare and Medicaid. Working paper no. 998–5. Washington, D.C.: Urban Institute, 1978.

43. Gabel JR, Rice TH. Reducing public expenditures for physician services: the price of paying less. J Health Polit Policy Law 1985; 9:595–609.

44. Contandriopoulos A-P. Cost containment through payment mechanisms: the Quebec experience. J Public Health Policy 1986; 7:224–38.

45. Wilson PR, Chappell D, Lincoln R. Policing physician abuse in British Columbia: an analysis of current policies. Can Public Policy 1986; 12:236–44.

46. Barer ML. Regulating physician supply: the evolution of British Columbia's Bill 41. J Health Polit Policy Law 1988; 13:1–25.

47. Doctors' dilemma: unionizing. New York Times, July 11, 1987:13, 21.

48. Tuohy CJ. Conflict and accommodation in the Canadian health care system. In: Evans RG, Stoddart GL, eds. Medicare at maturity: achievements, lessons and challenges. Calgary: University of Calgary Press, 1986:393–434.